THE JOHNS HOPKINS
MANUAL OF GYNECOLOGY
AND OBSTETRICS

Fourth Edition

D1241985

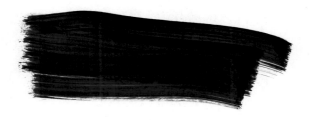

THE JOHNS HOPKINS MANUAL OF GYNECOLOGY AND OBSTETRICS

Fourth Edition

Department of Gynecology and Obstetrics
The Johns Hopkins University School of Medicine
Baltimore, Maryland

Editors

K. Joseph Hurt, MD, PhD

Matthew W. Guile, MD, MS

Jessica L. Bienstock, MD, MPH

Harold E. Fox, MD, MSc

Edward E. Wallach, MD

Wolters Kluwer | Lippincott Williams & Wilkins
Health

Philadelphia · Baltimore · New York · London
Buenos Aires · Hong Kong · Sydney · Tokyo

Acquisitions Editor: Sonya Seigafuse
Product Manager: Nicole Walz
Vendor Manager: Alicia Jackson
Senior Manufacturing Manager: Benjamin Rivera
Marketing Manager: Kim Schonberger
Design Coordinator: Terry Mallon
Production Service: SPi Technologies

Library of Congress Cataloging-in-Publication Data
   The Johns Hopkins manual of gynecology and obstetrics. — 4th ed. / Department of Gynecology and Obstet-
rics, The Johns Hopkins University School of Medicine, Baltimore, Maryland ; editors, K. Joseph Hurt ... [et al.].
      p. ; cm.
   Other title: Manual of gynecology and obstetrics
   Includes bibliographical references and index.
   ISBN 978-1-60547-433-5
   1. Gynecology—Handbooks, manuals, etc. I. Hurt, K. Joseph. II. Johns Hopkins University. Dept. of
Gynecology and Obstetrics. III. Title: Manual of gynecology and obstetrics.
   [DNLM: 1. Genital Diseases, Female—Handbooks. 2. Obstetrics—Handbooks. 3. Pregnancy
Complications—Handbooks. 4. Women's Health—Handbooks. WQ 39]
   RG110.J64   2011
   618—dc22
                                                                                            2010029167

RRS1010

*This book is dedicated to our many excellent teachers in gynecology, obstetrics, surgery, and medicine—to those true mentors who have inspired and motivated us in our training and careers.
Their dedication, support, and encouragement inform our development and shape our work for a lifetime.*

Contents

Introduction

When I was a resident at Kings County Hospital, standard text books in obstetrics and gynecology all seemed to originate from Johns Hopkins. To begin with, there were Emil Novak's *Gynecological and Obstetrical Pathology* and *Novak's Textbook of Gynecology*. The obstetrical text in vogue at that time was the Eleventh edition of *Williams Obstetrics* by Nicholson Eastman. It did not stop there because Richard TeLinde's *Operative Gynecology* was the surgical bible. If this were not enough, the *Obstetrical and Gynecological Survey* was edited by Drs. TeLinde and Eastman and then by Drs. Howard and Georgeanna Jones. For nearly a century, it was almost as if obstetrics and gynecology revolved around Johns Hopkins.

Although times have changed dramatically, 11 years ago the First edition of *The Johns Hopkins Manual of Gynecology and Obstetrics* was published. The popularity of this text prompted a Second edition in 2002 and then the Third in 2007. The Johns Hopkins Manual has ultimately become a fixture. The content, format, and size have had great appeal for practicing physicians, house officers, medical students, and medical teachers. Each edition of the manual has been serially updated in content and in format. The book's new format makes for easy reading and for portability. It contains many new attractive and helpful figures and tables. What can be more convenient than a concise but complete text that virtually fits in your pocket?

Where the manual has not changed is in the unique manner in which it is developed. Each chapter has been caringly created by the collaborative efforts of a resident, a faculty preceptor, and a senior faculty editor at Hopkins. It has thus been prepared and overseen by a triad of physicians who have combined their expertise to provide a book with practical appeal at many levels. The widespread popularity of previous editions has prompted translation into Portuguese, Spanish, and Chinese. The manual is used regularly in a number of Japanese medical centers. This global popularity attests to the manual's readability and usefulness.

Collaboration tends to bring out the best in any group endeavor. The esprit de corps established among the residents who are responsible for the first draft, preceptors, and editors, is a by-product of this educational endeavor. In utilizing our manual, we hope you too will appreciate the degree of input for each chapter and recognize the camaraderie with which the manual was created. The spirit of scholastic and collaborative dedication has obviously been perpetuated in publications originating at Johns Hopkins.

Edward E. Wallach, MD
Harold E. Fox, MD, MSc
Jessica L. Bienstock, MD, MPH

Acknowledgments

We gratefully acknowledge the support and effort of crucial behind-the-scenes personnel. Our assistant editor, Brigitte Pocta, had the necessary persistence and patience to format all of the pieces and document the permissions for the final manuscript. Nicole Walz, our editor at Lippincott Williams & Wilkins, assisted us in assembling and copyediting a sometimes unwieldy multiauthor work. We want to thank, especially, the loved ones who energize and inspire us—they allow us to pursue this project and others while balancing the duties of home, work, and scholarship. Only with their assistance and understanding is such a publication possible.

Contributors

Frank Aguirre, MD
*Resident, Department of Gynecology and
  Obstetrics*
Johns Hopkins University School of Medicine
Baltimore, Maryland

Janyne E. Althaus, MD
*Assistant Professor of Gynecology and
  Obstetrics*
Division of Maternal Fetal Medicine
Johns Hopkins University School of Medicine
Baltimore, Maryland

Kristiina Altman, MD, PhD
*Assistant Professor of Gynecology and
  Obstetrics*
*Director, Johns Hopkins Women's Services at
  White Marsh*
Johns Hopkins Bayview Medical Center
Baltimore, Maryland

Alejandra Alvarez, MD
*Resident, Department of Gynecology and
  Obstetrics*
Johns Hopkins University School of Medicine
Baltimore, Maryland

Jean Anderson, MD
Professor of Gynecology and Obstetrics
*Director of the Division of Gynecologic
  Specialties*
Johns Hopkins University School of Medicine
Baltimore, Maryland

Cynthia Holcroft Argani, MD
*Assistant Professor of Gynecology and
  Obstetrics*
Division of Maternal Fetal Medicine
Director of Labor and Delivery
Johns Hopkins Bayview Medical Center
Johns Hopkins University School of Medicine
Baltimore, Maryland

Anya J. Bailis, MD
*Fellow, Division of Maternal Fetal
  Medicine*
Department of Gynecology and Obstetrics
Johns Hopkins University School of Medicine
Baltimore, Maryland

Joyce N. Barlin, MD
*Resident, Department of Gynecology and
  Obstetrics*
Johns Hopkins University School of Medicine
Baltimore, Maryland

Jacqueline Baselice, MD
*Resident, Department of Gynecology and
  Obstetrics*
Johns Hopkins University School of Medicine
Baltimore, Maryland

Jessica L. Bienstock, MD, MPH
*Associate Professor of Gynecology and
  Obstetrics*
Division of Maternal Fetal Medicine
Residency Program Director
Johns Hopkins University School of Medicine
Baltimore, Maryland

Meredith Birsner, MD
*Resident, Department of Gynecology and
  Obstetrics*
Johns Hopkins University School of Medicine
Baltimore, Maryland

Robert E. Bristow, MD, MBA
Professor of Gynecology and Obstetrics
Professor of Oncology
Director, Kelly Gynecologic Oncology Service
*Director, F.J. Montz Fellowship in
  Gynecologic Oncology*
Division of Gynecologic Oncology
Johns Hopkins University School of Medicine
Baltimore, Maryland

Anne E. Burke, MD, MPH
*Assistant Professor of Gynecology and
  Obstetrics*
Director of Family Planning
Johns Hopkins Bayview Medical Center
Baltimore, Maryland

Chi Chiung Grace Chen, MD
*Assistant Professor of Gynecology and
  Obstetrics*
*Division of Female Pelvic Medicine and
  Reconstructive Surgery*
Johns Hopkins Bayview Medical Center
Baltimore, Maryland

Betty Chou, MD
Assistant Professor of Gynecology and Obstetrics
Director, Johns Hopkins Women's Services at Odenton
Johns Hopkins Bayview Medical Center
Baltimore, Maryland

Mindy S. Christianson, MD
Resident, Department of Gynecology and Obstetrics
Johns Hopkins University School of Medicine
Baltimore, Maryland

Sarah Cohen, MD
Resident, Department of Gynecology and Obstetrics
Johns Hopkins University School of Medicine
Baltimore, Maryland

Kathleen A. Costigan, RN, MPH
Coordinator, Fetal Assessment Center
Department of Gynecology and Obstetrics
Johns Hopkins University School of Medicine
Baltimore, Maryland

Alexandre Buckley de Meritens, MD
Resident, Department of Gynecology and Obstetrics
Johns Hopkins University School of Medicine
Baltimore, Maryland

Elizabeth Wood Denne, MS, CGC
Assistant Professor
Division of Maternal Fetal Medicine
Department of Gynecology and Obstetrics
Johns Hopkins University School of Medicine
Baltimore, Maryland

Abigail E. Dennis, MD
Resident, Department of Gynecology and Obstetrics
Johns Hopkins University School of Medicine
Baltimore, Maryland

Teresa P. Díaz-Montes, MD, MPH
Assistant Professor of Gynecology and Obstetrics
Division of Gynecologic Oncology
Johns Hopkins University School of Medicine
Baltimore, Maryland

Jennifer Ducie, MD
Resident, Department of Gynecology and Obstetrics
Johns Hopkins University School of Medicine
Baltimore, Maryland

Sydney Dy, MD, MSc
Associate Professor of Medicine and Oncology
Physician Leader, Duffey Pain and Palliative Care Program
Johns Hopkins University School of Medicine
Baltimore, Maryland

Jill Edwardson, MD
Resident, Department of Gynecology and Obstetrics
Johns Hopkins University School of Medicine
Baltimore, Maryland

Catherine Eppes, MD
Resident, Department of Gynecology and Obstetrics
Johns Hopkins University School of Medicine
Baltimore, Maryland

Dayna Finkenzeller, MD
Assistant Professor of Gynecology and Obstetrics
Johns Hopkins Bayview Medical Center
Baltimore, Maryland

Harold E. Fox, MD, MSc
Professor and Director
Obstetrician/Gynecologist-in-Chief
Dorothy Edwards Professor of Gynecology and Obstetrics
Johns Hopkins University School of Medicine
Baltimore, Maryland

Robert L. Giuntoli, II, MD
Assistant Professor of Gynecology and Obstetrics
Assistant Professor of Oncology
Division of Gynecologic Oncology
Johns Hopkins University School of Medicine
Baltimore, Maryland

Ernest M. Graham, MD
Associate Professor of Gynecology and Obstetrics
Division of Maternal Fetal Medicine
Johns Hopkins University School of Medicine
Baltimore, Maryland

Isabel C. Green, MD
*Assistant Professor of Gynecology and
  Obstetrics*
*Medical Director, Resident Outpatient
  Services in Gynecology and Obstetrics*
Johns Hopkins University School of Medicine
Baltimore, Maryland

Cara L. Grimes, MD
*Resident, Department of Gynecology and
  Obstetrics*
Johns Hopkins University School of Medicine
Baltimore, Maryland

Maureen Grundy, MD
*Resident, Department of Gynecology and
  Obstetrics*
Johns Hopkins University School of Medicine
Baltimore, Maryland

Matthew W. Guile, MD, MS
*Resident, Department of Gynecology and
  Obstetrics*
Johns Hopkins University School of Medicine
Baltimore, Maryland

Camille Gunderson, MD
*Resident, Department of Gynecology and
  Obstetrics*
Johns Hopkins University School of Medicine
Baltimore, Maryland

Natalia A. Colón Guzmán, MD
*Resident, Department of Gynecology and
  Obstetrics*
Johns Hopkins University School of Medicine
Baltimore, Maryland

S.J. Hanson, MD
*Resident, Department of Gynecology and
  Obstetrics*
Johns Hopkins University School of Medicine
Baltimore, Maryland

Janice Henderson, MD
*Assistant Professor of Gynecology and
  Obstetrics*
Division of Maternal Fetal Medicine
Johns Hopkins University School of Medicine
Baltimore, Maryland

Nancy A. Hueppchen, MD
*Assistant Professor of Gynecology and
  Obstetrics*
Division of Maternal Fetal Medicine
Director of Medical Student Education
Johns Hopkins University School of Medicine
Baltimore, Maryland

K. Joseph Hurt, MD, PhD
*Resident, Department of Gynecology and
  Obstetrics*
Johns Hopkins University School of Medicine
Baltimore, Maryland

Sherrine A. Ibrahim, MD, MS
*Resident, Department of Gynecology and
  Obstetrics*
Johns Hopkins University School of Medicine
Baltimore, Maryland

Lisa K. Jacobs, MD
Assistant Professor of Surgery
Director of Clinical Breast Cancer Research
Division of Surgical Oncology
Johns Hopkins University School of Medicine
Baltimore, Maryland

Alaina Johnson, MD
*Resident, Department of Gynecology and
  Obstetrics*
Johns Hopkins University School of Medicine
Baltimore, Maryland

Valerie A. Jones, MD
*Resident, Department of Gynecology and
  Obstetrics*
Johns Hopkins University School of Medicine
Baltimore, Maryland

Jean Keller, PA
Assistant Professor
Division of Gynecologic Specialties
*Manager, Johns Hopkins HIV Women's
  Health Program*
Department of Gynecology and Obstetrics
Johns Hopkins University School of Medicine
Baltimore, Maryland

Michelle Khan, MD, MPH
*Resident, Department of Gynecology and
Obstetrics*
Johns Hopkins University School of Medicine
Baltimore, Maryland

Mary Kimmel, MD
*Resident, Department of Gynecology and
Obstetrics*
Johns Hopkins University School of Medicine
Baltimore, Maryland

Lisa Kolp, MD
*Assistant Professor of Gynecology and
Obstetrics*
*Division of Reproductive Endocrinology and
Infertility*
Johns Hopkins University School of Medicine
Baltimore, Maryland

Lauren Krill, MD
*Resident, Department of Gynecology and
Obstetrics*
Johns Hopkins University School of Medicine
Baltimore, Maryland

Shari Lawson, MD
*Assistant Professor of Gynecology and
Obstetrics*
*Medical Director, Johns Hopkins Women's
Services at Bayview Medical Center*
Johns Hopkins Bayview Medical Center
Baltimore, Maryland

Amy S.D. Lee, MS, WHCRNP
Nurse Practitioner, Gynecology
Department of Gynecology and Obstetrics
Johns Hopkins Hospital
Baltimore, Maryland

Judy M. Lee, MD, MPH, MBA
*Assistant Professor of Gynecology and
Obstetrics*
Johns Hopkins University School of Medicine
Baltimore, Maryland

Kimberly Levinson, MD, MPH
*Resident, Department of Gynecology and
Obstetrics*
Johns Hopkins University School of Medicine
Baltimore, Maryland

Pamela A. Lipsett, MD
*Professor of Surgery, Anesthesia and Critical
Care Medicine, and Nursing*
*Program Director, General Surgery and
Surgical Critical Care*
*Department of Surgery and Surgical
Sciences*
Johns Hopkins University School of Medicine
Baltimore, Maryland

Meredith Buonanno Loveless, MD
*Assistant Professor of Gynecology and
Obstetrics*
Director of Pediatric Gynecology
Johns Hopkins Bayview Medical Center
Baltimore, Maryland

Amr Madkour, MD
*Resident, Department of Gynecology and
Obstetrics*
Johns Hopkins University School of Medicine
Baltimore, Maryland

Teresa Martino, DO
Fellow, Division of Maternal Fetal Medicine
Department of Gynecology and Obstetrics
Johns Hopkins University School of Medicine
Baltimore, Maryland

Richard P. Marvel, MD
Director of the Center for Pelvic Pain
Greater Baltimore Medical Center
*Adjunct Assistant Professor of Gynecology
and Obstetrics*
Johns Hopkins University School of Medicine
Baltimore, Maryland

Colleen McCormick, MD, MPH
Fellow, Division of Gynecologic Oncology
Department of Gynecology and Obstetrics
Johns Hopkins University School of Medicine
Baltimore, Maryland

Tiffany McNair, MD
*Resident, Department of Gynecology and
Obstetrics*
Johns Hopkins University School of Medicine
Baltimore, Maryland

Lorraine A. Milio, MD
*Assistant Professor of Gynecology and
    Obstetrics*
Division of Maternal Fetal Medicine
Johns Hopkins University School of Medicine
Baltimore, Maryland

Jamie Murphy, MD
Assistant Professor of Anesthesia
Director of Obstetric Anesthesia
Johns Hopkins University School of Medicine
Baltimore, Maryland

Maria Palmquist, MD
*Fellow, Division of Maternal Fetal
    Medicine*
Department of Gynecology and Obstetrics
Johns Hopkins University School of Medicine
Baltimore, Maryland

Alok C. Pant, MD
*Resident, Department of Gynecology and
    Obstetrics*
Johns Hopkins University School of Medicine
Baltimore, Maryland

Elizabeth Purcell, MD
*Resident, Department of Gynecology and
    Obstetrics*
Johns Hopkins University School of Medicine
Baltimore, Maryland

Linda Rogers, CRNP
*Nurse Practitioner, Gynecology and
    Obstetrics*
Johns Hopkins Bayview Medical Center
Baltimore, Maryland

Jessica B. Russell, MD
*Resident, Department of Gynecology and
    Obstetrics*
Johns Hopkins University School of Medicine
Baltimore, Maryland

Melissa L. Russo, MD
*Resident, Department of Gynecology and
    Obstetrics*
Johns Hopkins University School of Medicine
Baltimore, Maryland

Andrew J. Satin, MD
*Professor and Vice Chair of Gynecology and
    Obstetrics*
*Chair, Johns Hopkins Bayview Medical
    Center*
Johns Hopkins University School of Medicine
Baltimore, Maryland

David Schwartz, MD
*Chief, Department of Obstetrics and
    Gynecology*
Sinai Hospital of Baltimore
Professor, Obstetrics & Gynecology
Wayne State University Medical School
Detroit, Michigan
*Associate Professor, Gynecology and
    Obstetrics*
Johns Hopkins University School of Medicine
Baltimore, Maryland

Catherine Sewell, MD
*Assistant Professor of Gynecology and
    Obstetrics*
Director, Johns Hopkins Fibroid Center
Johns Hopkins University School of Medicine
Baltimore, Maryland

Stuart Shippey, MD
*Assistant Professor, Gynecology and
    Obstetrics*
*Division of Female Pelvic Medicine and
    Reconstructive Surgery*
Johns Hopkins Bayview Medical Center
Baltimore, Maryland

Samuel Smith, MD
*Chair, Department of Obstetrics and
    Gynecology*
Franklin Square Hospital
*Associate Professor, Division of Reproductive
    Endocrinology and Infertility*
Johns Hopkins University School of Medicine
Baltimore, Maryland

Hindi Stohl, MD
*Resident, Department of Gynecology and
    Obstetrics*
Johns Hopkins University School of Medicine
Baltimore, Maryland

Linda M. Szymanski, MD, PhD
Fellow, Division of Maternal Fetal Medicine
Department of Gynecology and Obstetrics
Johns Hopkins University School of Medicine
Baltimore, Maryland

Cornelia Liu Trimble, MD
Associate Professor
Division of Gynecologic Specialties
Department of Gynecology and Obstetrics
Johns Hopkins University School of Medicine
Baltimore, Maryland

Edward Trimble, MD, PhD
Head of the Surgery Section — Cancer
  Therapy Evaluation Program
National Cancer Institute
Associate Professor of Gynecology and
  Obstetrics
Associate Professor of Oncology
Division of Gynecologic Oncology
Johns Hopkins University School of Medicine
Baltimore, Maryland

Sayeedha Uddin, MD
Assistant Professor
Department of Gynecology and Obstetrics
Johns Hopkins University School of Medicine
Baltimore, Maryland

Stefanie Ueda, MD
Fellow, Division of Gynecologic Oncology
Department of Gynecology and Obstetrics
Johns Hopkins University School of Medicine
Baltimore, Maryland

Edward E. Wallach, MD
J. Donald Woodruff Professor of Gynecology
Division of Reproductive Endocrinology
Department of Gynecology and Obstetrics
Johns Hopkins University School of Medicine
Baltimore, Maryland

Frank R. Witter, MD
Professor of Gynecology and Obstetrics
Director, Labor and Delivery
Division of Maternal Fetal Medicine
Department of Gynecology and Obstetrics
Johns Hopkins University School of Medicine
Baltimore, Maryland

Melissa Yates, MD
Fellow, Division of Reproductive
  Endocrinology
Department of Gynecology and Obstetrics
Johns Hopkins University School of Medicine
Baltimore, Maryland

Howard Zacur, MD, PhD
Professor of Gynecology and Obstetrics
Director, Division of Reproductive
  Endocrinology and Infertility
Johns Hopkins University School of Medicine
Baltimore, Maryland

Women's Health Care

Primary and Preventive Care

Sarah Cohen and Sayeedha Uddin

Obstetrician-gynecologists are in a unique position to interact with women across the reproductive and age spectrum, and are seen by many patients as the sole provider of **primary and preventive health care**. The responsibilities of a primary care physician include screening and treatment of selected diseases, counseling, and providing immunizations. Additionally, common nongynecologic conditions that the ObGyn should be familiar with include asthma, allergic rhinitis, respiratory tract infections, gastrointestinal disorders, urinary tract disorders, headache, low back pain, and skin disorders.

SCREENING AND TREATMENT

- The majority of deaths among women under the age of 65 are preventable (see Table 1-1)
- *Primary prevention*: identification and control of risk factors before disease occurs
- *Secondary prevention*: early diagnosis of disease to reduce morbidity/mortality
- A condition which is a good target for screening should have the following:
  - A significant effect on the quality and quantity of life
  - An acceptable and available treatment
  - An asymptomatic period during which detection and treatment significantly reduce the risk for morbidity and mortality
  - An incidence sufficient to justify the cost of the screening
  - An asymptomatic phase during which treatment yields therapeutic results superior to those obtained by delaying treatment until symptoms develop
- The screening test should be:
  - Acceptable to patients and available at a reasonable cost
  - Reasonably accurate with acceptable sensitivity and specificity
    - Test sensitivity: percentage of patients with the disease who test positive
    - Test specificity: percentage of patients without disease who test negative

1

TABLE 1-1 Leading Causes of Death Among Females of All Races in the United States (2002–2007)

Rank	Age 15–24	Age 25–34	Age 35–44	Age 45–54	Age 55–64	Age 65+	All ages
1	Unintentional injury	Unintentional injury	Malignant neoplasm	Malignant neoplasm	Malignant neoplasm	Heart disease	Heart disease
2	Homicide	Malignant neoplasm	Unintentional injury	Heart disease	Heart disease	Malignant neoplasm	Malignant neoplasm
3	Malignant neoplasm	Heart disease	Heart disease	Unintentional injury	Chronic respiratory disease	Cerebrovascular disease	Cerebrovascular disease
4	Suicide	Suicide	Suicide	Cerebrovascular disease	Diabetes mellitus	Chronic respiratory disease	Chronic respiratory disease
5	Heart disease	Homicide	HIV	Diabetes mellitus	Cerebrovascular disease	Alzheimer's disease	Alzheimer's disease

Adapted from Office of Statistics and Programming, National Center for Injury Prevention and Control, Centers for Disease Control and Prevention—Web-based Injury Statistics Query and Reporting System (WISQARS). Data from National Center for Health Statistics, National Vital Statistics System. Available at http://webappa.cdc.gov/saweb/ncipc/leadcause/0.html. Accessed August 6, 2010.

CANCER

Screening for Breast Cancer

- See Chapter 2.
- Breast cancer is the most common cancer in women, with a lifetime incidence of 12%. For those at average risk, the American College of Obstetricians and Gynecologists (ACOG) and the U.S. Preventive Services Task Force (USPSTF) recommend routine mammography every 1 to 2 years for women in their 40s and annually thereafter. In addition, ACOG recommends annual clinical breast examination.
- Women should be referred for genetic counseling and BRCA testing if they have the following family history:
  - Two first-degree relatives with breast cancer, at least one diagnosed before age 50
  - Three or more first- or second-degree relatives with breast cancer, any age at diagnosis
  - A combination of first- and second-degree relatives with breast and ovarian cancer
  - A first-degree relative with bilateral breast cancer
  - Two or more first- or second-degree relatives with ovarian cancer
  - A first- or second-degree relative with both breast and ovarian cancer
  - A male relative with breast cancer
- Ashkenazi Jewish women should be referred for genetic counseling and evaluation for BRCA testing if they have one first- or two second-degree relatives with breast or ovarian cancer.

Screening for Lung Cancer

- Lung cancer, the second most common cancer in women, is the leading cause of cancer-related death. There were over 1 million deaths due to lung cancer worldwide in the year 2000.
- Risk factors include cigarette smoking (associated with 90% of lung cancers), radiation therapy, environmental toxins such as asbestos, and pulmonary fibrosis.
- None of the screening methods for lung cancer (chest x-ray, sputum cytology, CT scan) has been consistently shown to have mortality benefit. Screening is not currently recommended for asymptomatic people, and prevention via smoking cessation campaigns remains crucial.
- Smoking may confer a greater relative risk for women than men; however, many of the early studies on lung cancer screening did not include women. It is theorized that screening in women may have different outcomes due to higher rates of peripherally located adenocarcinoma.

Screening for Colorectal Cancer

- Colorectal cancer is the third most commonly diagnosed cancer and the third leading cause of cancer-related death in women; lifetime incidence is 5%.
- Risk factors include a family history of colorectal cancer, a personal history of colon polyps or cancer, a personal history of inflammatory bowel disease, and the genetic syndromes familial adenomatous polyposis and hereditary nonpolyposis colon cancer. High-risk individuals should be screened with colonoscopy beginning at earlier ages depending on risk.
  - Women should initiate screening at age 40 if they have a relative diagnosed with colon cancer before the age of 60 or two first-degree relatives diagnosed with colon cancer at any age.

- Women with a diagnosis of hereditary nonpolyposis colon cancer (HNPCC) should initiate screening at age 20 to 25 or 10 years before the youngest age of colon cancer diagnosis in the family.
- The USPSTF recommends screening for colorectal cancer for all persons aged 50 and older. The American College of Gastroenterology recommends beginning screening at age 45 in African Americans due to higher incidence and earlier age of onset.
- Many screening protocols exist, including flexible sigmoidoscopy every 5 years, colonoscopy every 10 years, double-contrast barium enema every 5 years, computed tomographic colonography every 5 years, guaiac-based fecal occult blood test annually (two samples from each of three consecutive stools), fecal immunochemical test annually, and stool DNA test. The 2007 multi-society guidelines support any of the above regimens; however, ACOG encourages colonoscopy.

Screening for Endometrial Cancer

- See Chapter 44.
- No routine screening is recommended for asymptomatic women. Certain high-risk groups may undergo screening such as endometrial biopsy, pelvic ultrasound, or both. All episodes of postmenopausal bleeding should be investigated.

Screening for Skin Cancer

- Melanoma is the sixth leading cancer in women; risk factors include light skin tone and ultraviolet ray exposure, particularly childhood sunburns. People with between 50 and 100 typical nevi or large congenital nevi are also at increased risk (relative risk of 5 to 17 and >100, respectively).
- Although there are no consensus guidelines for total skin examination, ACOG recommends evaluation in those patients at high risk. All patients should be educated regarding sunscreen use and UV ray avoidance.
- Guidelines regarding suspicious lesions are as follows:
  - **A**symmetry
  - **B**order irregularities
  - **C**olor variegation
  - **D**iameter >6 mm
  - **E**nlargement/**E**volution of color change, shape, or symptoms

Screening for Ovarian Cancer

- See Chapter 45.
- No North American expert groups recommend routine screening for ovarian cancer. Instead, a careful family history and an annual pelvic exam are recommended for all women.

Screening for Cervical Cancer

- See Chapter 42.
- Routine screening for cervical cancer with Papanicolaou (pap) testing is recommended to begin 3 years after a patient becomes sexually active, no later than age 21, and should be repeated yearly. The American Cancer Society and ACOG have suggested that Pap smears may be obtained every 3 years once results are normal on three consecutive tests, and provided the patient does not have a history of CIN2 or worse, is not HIV positive or immunocompromised, and has no history of diethylstilbestrol exposure. Insufficient evidence exists to recommend for or against an upper age limit for pap testing.

- ACOG and the USPSTF both agree that cervical cancer screening may be discontinued for women who have had a total hysterectomy for benign indications and no history of CIN2 or worse.
- In women 30 years and older, a combination of HPV testing for high-risk types and cytology may be performed. If both are negative, rescreening should be done no earlier than 3 years.

HEART AND VASCULAR CONDITIONS

Screening for Coronary Heart Disease (CHD)

- Rates of CHD in women increase with age, ranging between 5% and 15%. Risk factors include hypertension, dyslipidemia, diabetes, smoking, and family history of premature CHD (age <55 years in male first-degree relative or age <65 years in first-degree female relative).
- Validated risk stratification models include the Framingham risk score that predicts 10-year risk of a CHD event. The Framingham model was updated by the National Cholesterol Education Program (NCEP) Adult Treatment Panel III (ATP III), and adjusts for the following variables: age, gender, LDL-cholesterol, HDL-cholesterol, blood pressure, diabetes, and smoking. The USPSTF recommends against routine screening of asymptomatic low-risk patients for CHD using resting electrocardiogram (ECG), ambulatory ECG, or exercise ECG.

Aspirin for Primary Prevention of Cardiovascular Events

- The USPSTF *strongly* recommends that physicians consider aspirin prophylaxis in patients at high risk for CHD, including postmenopausal women, premenopausal women with high cholesterol, high blood pressure, or diabetes, or those who smoke. Benefits of prevention of CHD should be weighed against the risks of gastrointestinal and intracranial bleeding.
- A dose of 75 mg/day appears as effective as higher doses.

Screening for Dyslipidemia

- Dyslipidemia is a direct and modifiable risk factor for CHD, and the USPSTF *strongly* recommends screening with fasting lipid profile for women aged >45 if they are at increased risk of CHD. Screening of high-risk women aged 20 to 45 is recommended, and screening of low-risk women is neither recommended nor discouraged.
- Table 1-2 summarizes NCEP/ATPIII treatment recommendations.
  - Lifestyle changes include limiting fat intake (particularly *trans* and saturated fat), increasing dietary fiber and plant sterol intake, weight loss, and increasing physical activity.
  - The most commonly used options for pharmacologic treatment of dyslipidemia include bile acid–binding resins, statins, nicotinic acid, fibric acid derivatives, and cholesterol absorption inhibitors. Choice of drug depends on the particular lipid profile, however, statins are the drug of choice for cardioprotection.

Screening for Hypertension

- Hypertension (defined as blood pressure ≥140/90 mm Hg or requirement for antihypertensive medication) is a leading risk factor for CHD, congestive heart failure, stroke, ruptured aortic aneurysm, renal disease, and retinopathy. Suboptimal blood pressure has been reported as the number one risk factor for death worldwide.

TABLE 1-2	NCEP/ATPIII Cholesterol Treatment Recommendations (2002)		
Risk Group	**LDL Goal (mg/dL)**	**LDL Level to Start Lifestyle Changes**	**LDL Level to Start Drug Therapy**
CHD or risk-equivalent[a]	<100	≥100	100–130
2+ risk factors[b]	≤130	≥130	130–160
0–1 risk factor[b]	≤160	≥160	≥190

[a]CHD risk equivalent = diabetes mellitus, abdominal aortic aneurysm, peripheral artery disease, symptomatic carotid artery disease. [b]Risk factors = smoking, hypertension, HDL cholesterol <40 mg/dL, family history of premature CHD, age (men 45 y; women 55 y). HDL cholesterol >60 mg/dL is a negative risk factor. Adapted from ATPIII Guidelines and Grundy SM, Cleeman JI, Bairey Merz CN, et al. Implications of recent clinical trials for national cholesterol education program adult treatment panel III guidelines. *Circulation* 2004;110:227–239.

- Essential or primary hypertension may result from excess salt intake, obesity, low fruit/vegetable intake, low potassium, or excessive alcohol use. Secondary causes of hypertension may include chronic renal disease, aortic coarctation, pheochromocytoma, Cushing disease, primary aldosteronism, renovascular disease, sleep apnea, or thyroid disease.
- The USPSTF recommends screening for hypertension in adults age ≥18 every 1 to 2 years (more frequently if prehypertension).

TABLE 1-3	JNC-7 Treatment Guidelines for Hypertension (2003)	
Blood Pressure (mm Hg)	**Lifestyle Modification**	**Drug Therapy**
Normal (<120/<80)	Encouraged	No
Prehypertension (120–139/80–89)	Yes	Only for compelling indication[a]
Stage I hypertension (140–159/90–99)	Yes	Thiazide (may consider ACE, ARB, BB, CCB)
Stage II hypertension (≥160/≥100)	Yes	Two drug combination: usually thiazide and ACE or ARB or BB or CCB

Goal blood pressure is <140/90. [a]Compelling indications include diabetes or chronic kidney disease where goal is <130/80 mm Hg. From Chobanian AV, Bakris GL, Black HR, et al., and the National High Blood Pressure Education Program Coordinating Committee. The Seventh Report of the Joint National Committee on Prevention, Detection, Evaluation, and Treatment of High Blood Pressure: the JNC 7 report. *JAMA* 2003;289:2560–2572.

- The 2003 Joint National Committee on Prevention, Detection, Evaluation, and Treatment of High Blood Pressure (JNC-7) guidelines for treatment are summarized in Table 1-3.
- Lifestyle modifications include weight reduction, reduction in dietary sodium intake, moderate alcohol consumption, increased physical activity, and eating a balanced DASH (Dietary Approaches to Stop Hypertension) diet.
- Drug choice is determined by comorbid conditions and contraindications, and as noted in Table 1-3 may include thiazide diuretics, angiotensin converting enzyme inhibitors (ACE), angiotensin II receptor blockers (ARB), beta-blockers (BB), calcium channel blockers (CCB), or a combination.

INFECTIOUS DISEASES

People at highest risk for sexually transmitted disease include those with a history of multiple sexual partners, sexually transmitted diseases, inconsistent condom use, commercial sex work, and drug use. Preventive strategies such as abstinence, reduction in number of sexual partners, and barrier contraceptive methods should be discussed with all patients.

Screening for HIV

- The 2006 CDC guidelines recommend that all individuals between 13 and 64 years of age be screened for HIV regardless of recognized risk factors using opt-out screening protocols.

Screening for Chlamydia

- The 2006 CDC Sexually Transmitted Diseases Treatment Guidelines support chlamydia screening annually in all sexually active women under age 25 and in older women with new/multiple sex partners or high-risk behavior. See Chapter 25.
- The USPSTF and CDC recommend against routine screening for hepatitis B, hepatitis C, gonorrhea, or syphilis in low-risk nonpregnant patients.

METABOLIC, ENDOCRINE, AND NUTRITIONAL CONDITIONS

Screening for Diabetes

- See Chapter 13.
- The USPSTF recommends screening for type II diabetes in asymptomatic adults with sustained blood pressure >135/80 mm Hg.
- Proposed risk factors for screening normotensive adults include: age >45 years, obesity, family history of diabetes in first-degree relative, non-Caucasian ethnicity, history of gestational diabetes or delivering a baby >9 pounds, inactivity, dyslipidemia, polycystic ovarian syndrome, and vascular disease.
- Screening tests: fasting plasma glucose (FPG) or the 2-hr 75 g glucose challenge test (GCT).
  - Diabetes = FPG ≥126 mL/dL *OR*
    GCT ≥200 mg/dL *OR*
    random plasma glucose ≥200 mg/dL with symptoms
    classic symptoms include polyuria, polydipsia, and weight loss

- Impaired glucose regulation = FPG 100–125 mg/dL *OR*
  GCT 140–199 mg/dL
- Patients with impaired glucose regulation should be referred for counseling on weight loss and exercise; medical therapy may be initiated in high-risk obese patients.
- Upon diagnosis of diabetes, screening should be performed to evaluate for retinopathy, nephropathy, neuropathy, CHD, cerebrovascular disease, peripheral artery disease, and dental disease.

Screening for Thyroid Disorders

- See Chapter 13.
- The USPSTF does not recommend screening asymptomatic people for hypothyroidism. ACOG recommends testing with thyroid-stimulating hormone serum levels in patients with autoimmune disease or strong family history of thyroid disease.

Counseling on Nutrition

- The 2005 USDA Dietary Guidelines recommend consumption of a variety of nutrient-dense foods and beverages within and among the basic food groups while choosing foods that limit the intake of saturated and *trans* fats, cholesterol, added sugars, salt, and alcohol. Specific recommendations include:
  - Adults over age 50 should consume supplemental vitamin B_{12}.
  - Women of childbearing age should consume foods high in iron and folic acid. Preferably, iron-rich foods should be taken with vitamin C to enhance absorption.
  - Older adults, people with darker skin tones, and those with minimal exposure to sunlight should consume at least 400 IU/day of supplemental vitamin D.
- Estimated caloric requirement for adult women varies between 1,800 and 2,400 kcal based on level of activity.

Counseling on Obesity

- The National Health and Nutrition Examination Survey results from 2005 to 2006 report that up to 35% of adult women are obese. It is estimated that up to 60% of Americans are either overweight or obese.
- Obesity is associated with an increased risk of morbidity including type II diabetes, hypertension, infertility, heart disease, gallbladder disease, uterine cancer, and colon cancer.
- Screening for obesity should include calculation of Body Mass Index (BMI), measurement of waist circumference, and evaluation of overall risk due to comorbid conditions.
- BMI is a measure of obesity which correlates with body fat content.
  Underweight = BMI <18.5 kg/m^2
  Overweight = BMI 25–29.9 kg/m^2
  Obese = BMI >30 kg/m^2
  Class I obesity = BMI 30–34.9 kg/m^2
  Class II obesity = BMI 35–39.9 kg/m^2
  Class III (morbid) obesity = BMI ≥40 kg/m^2
- The USPSTF recommends that all patients identified as obese are offered intensive counseling and behavioral interventions to improve diet and physical activity.

Medications, such as orlistat and sibutramine, or surgery may be necessary for some women.

SCREENING FOR OTHER MEDICAL CONDITIONS

Screening for Osteoporosis

- See Chapter 40.
- Bone mineral density examinations should be performed routinely at age 65 (or age 60 for women with risk factors), or in any postmenopausal woman with a fracture.
  - Risk factors for low bone mineral density include low body weight (<70 kg), smoking, family history of osteoporosis, chronic corticosteroid use, sedentary lifestyle, alcohol or caffeine use, or low calcium or vitamin D intake.
  - A T-score of –1.5 to –2.5 indicates osteopenia.
  - A T-score of less than –2.5 indicates osteoporosis.
- Intervals between successive bone mineral density examinations should not be <2 years.
- Treat osteopenia with risk factors with 35 mg/week of alendronate or 35 mg/week of risedronate.
- Treat osteoporosis with 70 mg/week of alendronate or 35 mg/week of risedronate.
- Total daily calcium intake should be 1,200 mg and total daily vitamin D intake should be 800 IU.

Screening for Depression

- Depression affects over 30 million American adults yearly. The lifetime risk for women of developing a major depressive disorder is 10% to 25%, two to three times higher than for men.
- Factors that may predispose women to depression include perinatal loss, infertility, or miscarriage; physical or sexual abuse; socioeconomic deprivation; lack of support, isolation, and feelings of helplessness; family history of mood disorders; loss of a parent during childhood (before age 10); history of substance abuse; and menopause.
- The symptoms of depression are summarized by the mnemonic SIG EM CAPS (five out of nine symptoms must be present for over 2 weeks to fulfill the definition of major depression, including either depressed mood or loss of interest)
  - **S**leep—insomnia or hypersomnia
  - **I**nterest—markedly decreased interest or pleasure in activities
  - **G**uilt—feelings of worthlessness or inappropriate guilt nearly every day
  - **E**nergy—fatigue or loss of energy
  - **M**ood—depressed mood most of the day
  - **C**oncentration—diminished ability to think, concentrate, or make decisions
  - **A**ppetite—significant appetite or weight change
  - **P**sychomotor—observable psychomotor retardation or agitation
  - **S**uicide—recurrent thoughts of death or suicide
- Dysthymic disorder is characterized by chronically depressed mood on most days for 2 or more years, plus at least two of the symptoms from the list defining a major depressive episode.
- The USPSTF recommends screening adults for depression. Many patient questionnaires for self-reporting exist.

- *Psychosocial treatment* may be used alone or in conjunction with antidepressant medication. For patients with mild to moderate depression, psychosocial therapies have been found to be as effective as pharmacologic treatment. Commonly used methods include behavioral therapy, cognitive-behavioral therapy, and interpersonal therapy.
- *Pharmacologic treatment* for depression includes selective serotonin reuptake inhibitors, selective norepinephrine reuptake inhibitors, and tricyclic antidepressants. Patients with severe or chronic depression, or failure to respond after 12 weeks of psychotherapy should be started on medication. A large percentage of women experience significant improvement or even complete remission with medical treatment.

Screening for Domestic Violence

- See Chapter 30.
- Health maintenance visits should include assessment for domestic violence, utilizing direct interview, patient questionnaires, or both.

Screening and Counseling for Substance Abuse

- The 2007 National Survey on Drug Use and Health found that approximately 20 million Americans (8%) use illicit drugs, 58 million (23%) engage in binge drinking, and 71 million (29%) use tobacco products.
- All patients should be questioned on substance abuse; a number of screening tools exist (e.g., the CAGE questions—Have you ever tried to **C**ut down? Do you get **A**nnoyed when others comment on your use? Do you feel **G**uilty about your drinking? Do you ever need an **E**ye-opener?)
  - The USPSTF recommends counseling for reducing alcohol abuse; brief 15-minute counseling interventions have been shown to reduce hazardous drinking.
- The USPSTF *strongly* recommends screening for tobacco use and counseling for cessation as it has been shown that 1 to 3 minutes of counseling significantly increases abstinence rates.
  - Medical interventions include nicotine replacement therapy, bupropion, and varenicline.

COUNSELING

- The routine health maintenance visit is an ideal time to counsel patients regarding many health-related behaviors.
- Several techniques for brief physician counseling have been developed, including the five A's model:
  - *Assess* for problem
  - *Advise* making a change
  - *Agree* on action to be taken
  - *Assist* with self-care support to make the change
  - *Arrange* follow-up to support the change

- It is important to recognize a patient's state of readiness, as an estimated 80% of people are unprepared to commit to a lifestyle change at initial encounter. The Stages of Change Model includes the following:
  - Precontemplation: no intention of changing behavior. Goal of counseling = introduce ambivalence.
  - Contemplation: considering making a change. Goal of counseling = explore both sides of the patient's attitude and help resolve behavior.
  - Preparation: resolved to make a change. Goal of counseling = identify successful strategies for change.
  - Action: making a change in behavior. Goal of counseling = provide solutions to deal with specific relapse triggers.
  - Maintenance: committed to change. Goal of counseling = solidify the patient's commitment to a continued change.

IMMUNIZATIONS

- Immunizations are an integral component of primary and preventive health care. A patient's vaccination history should be reviewed at regular intervals and updated as appropriate (see Figs. 1-1 and 1-2).

OTHER PRIMARY CARE PROBLEMS

- **Urinary Tract Infections:** for uncomplicated cystitis, a 3-day course of trimethoprim-sulfamethoxazole is generally the first-line recommendation. Alternatives include floroquinolones or nitrofurantoin. Empiric antibiotic treatment without urine culture is appropriate in the nongravid patient if the patient displays dysuria and has urine leukocytes and nitrites present on urinalysis. The presence of fever or costovertebral angle tenderness is suggestive of an upper tract infection which requires more aggressive treatment. See Chapter 16.
- **Upper Respiratory Infections:** typically viral in origin, mild upper respiratory infections should be treated symptomatically with a combination of cough suppressants and decongestants. The presence of secondary bacterial infection is suggested by persistence of rhinosinusitis symptoms for >7 days and purulent nasal discharge, unilateral tooth, facial, or maxillary sinus pain, or worsening symptoms after initial improvement. Patients with severe pain, fever, and failure of improvement after a period of observation should be treated with narrow-spectrum antibiotics such as amoxicillin, trimethoprim-sulfamethoxazole, or a macrolide for 10 to 14 days. See Chapter 15.
- **Asthma:** in addition to monitoring lung function and reducing exposure to triggers, pharmacologic treatment is conducted in a step-wise fashion. Mild intermittent asthma may be treated with quick-acting inhaled beta-agonists such as albuterol. For mild persistent asthma, add a low-dose inhaled glucocorticoid or leukotriene blocker. Patients with moderate persistent asthma may be treated with medium-dose inhaled glucocorticoid plus long-acting inhaled beta-agonist or a high-dose inhaled glucocorticoid. Patients with severe asthma should be referred to a pulmonologist or allergist for management. See Chapter 15.

Vaccine	Age group (yrs)		
	19–49	50–64	≥65
Tetanus, diphtheria, pertussis (Td/Tdap)*	1-dose Td booster every 10 yrs / Substitute 1 dose of Tdap for Td		
Human papillomavirus (HPV)*	3 doses (females) (0, 2, 6 mos)		
Measles, mumps, rubella (MMR)*	1 or 2 doses	1 dose	
Varicella*	2 doses (0, 4–8 wks)		
Influenza*	1 dose annually	1 dose annually	
Pneumococcal (polysaccharide)	1–2 doses		1 dose
Hepatitis A*	2 doses (0, 6–12 mos, or 0, 6–18 mos)		
Hepatitis B*	3 doses (0, 1–2, 4–6 mos)		
Meningococcal*	1 or more doses		
Zoster		1 dose	

*Covered by the Vaccine Injury Compensation Program.

☐ For all persons in this category who meet the age requirements and who lack evidence of immunity (e.g., lack documentation of vaccination or have no evidence of prior infection)

☐ Recommended if some other risk factor is present (e.g., on the basis of medical, occupational, lifestyle, or other indications)

Figure 1-1. Adapted from Recommended United States Adult Immunization Schedule, 2010. (Advisory Committee on Immunization Practices, Department of Health and Human Services, Centers for Disease Control and Prevention. More information available on the CDC website at: http://www.cdc.gov/vaccines/recs/schedules/adult-schedule.htm. Accessed September 28, 2008.)

	Indication								
Vaccine	Pregnancy	Immuno-compromising conditions (excluding human immunodeficiency virus [HIV]), medications, radiation	HIV infection — CD4+ T lymphocyte count <200 cells/µL	HIV infection — CD4+ T lymphocyte count ≥200 cells/µL	Diabetes, heart disease, chronic pulmonary disease, chronic alcoholism	Asplenia (including elective splenectomy and terminal complement component deficiencies)	Chronic liver disease	Kidney failure, end-stage renal disease, receipt of hemodialysis	Health-care personnel
Tetanus, diphtheria, pertussis (Td/Tdap)*	1 dose Td booster every 10 yrs / Substitute 1 dose of Tdap for Td								
Human papillomavirus (HPV)*	3 doses for females through age 26 yrs (0, 2, 6 mos)								
Measles, mumps, rubella (MMR)*	Contraindicated	Contraindicated	Contraindicated	1 or 2 doses					
Varicella*	Contraindicated	Contraindicated	Contraindicated	2 doses (0, 4–8 wks)					
Influenza*	1 dose TIV annually								1 dose TIV or LAIV annually
Pneumococcal (polysaccharide)	1–2 doses								
Hepatitis A*	2 doses (0, 6–12 mos, or 0, 6–18 mos)								
Hepatitis B*	3 doses (0, 1–2, 4–6 mos)								
Meningococcal*	1 or more doses								
Zoster	Contraindicated						1 dose		

*Covered by the Vaccine Injury Compensation Program.
TIV, trivalent inactivated vaccine;
LAIV, live attenuated influenza vaccine.

For all persons in this category who meet the age requirements and who lack evidence of immunity (e.g., lack documentation of vaccination or have no evidence of prior infection)

Recommended if some other risk factor is present (e.g., on the basis of medical, occupational, lifestyle, or other indications)

Figure 1-2. From: Vaccines that might be indicated for adults based on medical and other indications, United States, 2010. (From Advisory Committee on Immunization Practices, Department of Health and Human Services, Centers for Disease Control and Prevention. More information available on the CDC website at: http://www.cdc.gov/vaccines/recs/schedules/adult-schedule.htm. Accessed September 28, 2008.)

SUGGESTED READINGS

American Diabetes Association. Standards of medical care in diabetes—2008. *Diabetes Care* 2008;31(Suppl 1):S12–S54.

American Gastroenterological Association. American Gastroenterological Association medical position statement on Obesity. *Gastroenterology* 2002;123:879.

Centers for Disease Control and Prevention web site: http://www.cdc.gov/

Chobanian AV, Bakris GL, Black HR, et al. The seventh report of the Joint National Committee on prevention, detection, evaluation, and treatment of high blood pressure. *JAMA* 2003;289:2560–2572.

Levin B, Lieberman DA, McFarland B, et al. Screening and surveillance for the early detection of colorectal cancer and adenomatous polyps, 2008: a joint guideline from the American Cancer Society, the US Multi-Society Task Force on colorectal cancer, and the American College of Radiology. *Gastroenterology* 2008;134(5):1570–1595.

Primary and preventive care: periodic assessments. ACOG Committee Opinion Number 452. American College of Obstetricians and Gynecologists. *Obstet Gynecol* 2009;114:1444–1451.

Routine cancer screening. ACOG Committee Opinion Number 356. American College of Obstetricians and Gynecologists. *Obstet Gynecol* 2006;108:1611–1613.

Smith RA, Cokkinides V, Brawley OW. Cancer screening in the United States, 2008: a review of current American Cancer Society guidelines and cancer screening issues. *CA Cancer J Clin* 2008;58(3):161–179.

Third Report of the National Cholesterol Education Program (NCEP) expert panel on detection, evaluation, and treatment of high blood cholesterol in adults (Adult Treatment Panel III) final report. *Circulation* 2002;106(25):3143–3421.

U.S. Department of Health and Human Services, U.S. Department of Agriculture. *Dietary Guidelines for Americans, 2005*, 6th Ed. Washington, DC: U.S. Government Printing Office, 2005:vii,12,31.

U.S. Preventive Services Task Force web site: http://www.ahrq.gov/clinic/uspstfix.htm

Breast Diseases

Alejandra Alvarez and Lisa K. Jacobs

Breast cancer is a common and devastating health issue for many women. One in eight women will develop breast cancer in her lifetime. Benign breast disease can be difficult to differentiate from malignant breast disease, and it is crucial that the gynecologist be able to evaluate and treat breast disease.

ANATOMY (see Fig. 2-1)

- The borders of the adult breast are the second and sixth ribs in the vertical axis and the sternal edge and midaxillary line in the horizontal axis. A small portion of breast tissue also projects into the axilla, forming the *axillary tail of Spence.*
- The breast is composed of three major tissues: skin, subcutaneous tissue, and breast tissue. The breast tissue, in turn, consists of parenchyma and stroma. The parenchyma is divided into 15 to 20 segments that converge at the nipple in a radial arrangement. There are between 5 and 10 collecting ducts that open into the nipple. Each duct gives rise to buds that form 15 to 20 lobules, and each lobule consists of 10 to 100 alveoli, which constitute the gland.
- The breast is enveloped by fascial tissue. The superficial pectoral fascia envelops the breast and is continuous with the superficial abdominal fascia of Camper. The undersurface of the breast lies on the deep pectoral fascia, covering the pectoralis major and serratus anterior muscles. Connecting the two fascial layers are fibrous bands (Cooper suspensory ligaments) that are the natural support of the breast.
- The principal blood supply to the breast is the *internal mammary artery*, constituting two thirds of the total blood supply. The additional third, which supplies primarily the upper outer quadrant, is provided by the *lateral thoracic artery*. Nearly all of the lymphatic drainage of the breast is to the axillary nodes. The internal mammary nodes also receive drainage from all quadrants of the breast and are an unusual, but potential, site of metastasis.
- The majority of abnormalities in the breast that result in biopsy are due to benign breast disease. Benign abnormalities can result in pain, a mass, calcifications, and nipple discharge. Similar findings are present in malignant disease.
- For the purposes of delineating metastatic progression, the axillary lymph nodes are categorized into levels (Fig. 2-1). Level I lymph nodes lie lateral to the outer border of the pectoralis minor muscle, level II nodes lie behind the pectoralis minor muscle, and level III nodes are located medial to the medial border of the pectoralis minor muscle.

SCREENING AND DIAGNOSIS

The main screening modalities include clinical breast exam, breast self-exam, and screening mammography (see Table 2-1). Diagnostic modalities include diagnostic mammography and breast biopsy (including fine needle, core, and excisional). Additional diagnostic modalities include ultrasound and magnetic resonance imaging (MRI).

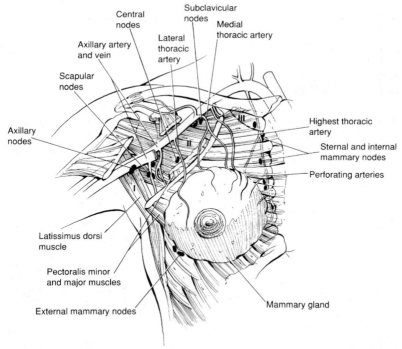

Figure 2-1. Anatomy of the breast. Roman numerals (I, II, III) indicate axillary lymph node levels. (From Green VL. Breast Diseases: Benign and Malignant. In Rock JA, Jones HW, eds. *TeLinde's Operative Gynecology.* 10th Ed. Philadelphia, PA: Lippincott Williams & Wilkins, 2008, with permission.)

Breast Exam

- The clinical breast examination (CBE) should be a routine part of the gynecologic examination (Fig. 2-2). The National Breast and Cervical Cancer Early Detection Program found that CBE detects approximately 5% of cancers that are not visible on mammography. Also, it offers an opportunity to demonstrate the technique of breast self-examination and to encourage women to perform this examination on a regular basis. The examination consists of:
  - Inspection and palpation of the breasts in the supine and sitting positions, with hands above the head and then on the hips. The supine position flattens the breast tissue against the chest, allowing for a more thorough exam.
  - Observation of the contour, symmetry, and vascular pattern of the breasts for signs of skin retraction, edema, or erythema in each of the previously mentioned positions.
  - Systematic palpation of each breast, the axilla, and supraclavicular areas in a circular motion using light, medium, and deep pressures. Use the pads of the three middle fingers to palpate for masses. A vertical strip pattern appears more thorough than concentric circles. To ensure that all breast tissue is examined, cover

TABLE 2-1   Breast Cancer Screening Techniques and Guidelines

	Application	Sensitivity/Efficacy	Limitations	Guidelines[a]
Mammography	Detects microcalcifications, abnormal shadowing, or soft tissue distortion	Sensitivity 74%–95% Specificity 89%–99% Sensitivity is decreased in women under age 50 and in women with dense breasts Reduces risk of cancer-related mortality by 16%–35%	Less sensitive for faster growing tumors (young women) Breast density Hormone therapy Breast implants	USPSTF: ≥40, every 1–2 years ACOG: 40–49, every 1–2 years ≥50 years, annually ACS: 40–69, annually NCI: ≥40, every 1–2 years
Clinical breast exam	Inspection and palpation in the supine and sitting positions, including axillary and supraclavicular lymph nodes as well as nipple and areola Recommended 6–10 min	Sensitivity 54% Specificity 94% Detects approximately 5% of cancers missed by mammography Most studies show efficiency in conjunction with mammography—likely that each contributes	Examiner dependent Less specificity than mammography—higher rate of biopsy for benign disease Limited in obese women	USPSTF: no recommendations for or against ACOG: annually ACS: 20–30, at least every 3 years ≥40, annually
Breast self-examination	Monthly exams, during approximately 10th day of cycle	Sensitivity 20%–30% Very few randomized trials Failed to show benefit in rate of diagnosis, cancer death, or tumor size	Examiner dependent Higher rate of biopsy for benign disease Studies limited	USPSTF: insufficient evidence to make recommendation ACS: inform women regarding benefits and limitations ACOG: routine teaching

Screening recommendations differ for patients with a family or personal history of breast cancer. [a]A summary of guidelines can be found at The National Guideline Clearing House. Available at: http://www.guidelines.gov. USPSTF, United States Preventive Services Task Force; ACOG, American College of Obstetricians and Gynecologists; ACS, American Cancer Society; NCI, National Cancer Institute.

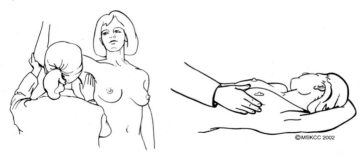

Figure 2-2. Breast examination. (From Scott JR, et al. *Danforth's Obstetrics and Gynecology*, 9th Ed. Philadelphia, PA: Lippincott Williams & Wilkins, 2003:892–893, with permission.)

a rectangular area bordered superiorly by the clavicle, laterally by the midaxillary line, and inferiorly by the bra line.
• Evaluation for nipple discharge, crusting, or ulceration.
• For the anatomic location and description of tumors or disease, the surface of the breast is divided into four quadrants and the numbers of the face of a clock are used as reference points (Fig. 2-3). A finding may be described as "a hard mass palpated in the upper inner quadrant of the right breast at the 2 o'clock position, approximately 2 cm from the nipple."

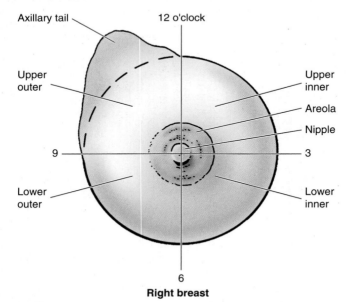

Figure 2-3. Breast quadrants. For the anatomical location and description of tumors, the surface of the breast is divided into four quadrants. (From Moore KL, Dalley AF. *Clinically Oriented Anatomy*, 4th Ed. Baltimore, MD: Lippincott Williams & Wilkins, 1999:74, with permission.)

Mammography

- Although mammography remains the primary screening modality, <40% of women actually undergo annual mammography. Breast cancers detected by mammography tend to be smaller and have more favorable histologic and biologic features. Limitations to mammography include patient age, rate of tumor growth, density of breast tissue, use of hormone replacement therapy (HRT), and breast implants.
  - **Screening mammography** is for women with no signs or symptoms of breast disease and consists of bilateral two-view images.
  - **Diagnostic mammography** presents various views (e.g., spot compression, magnification) and localization techniques and is usually used after the discovery of an abnormal finding on clinical exam, self-exam, or screening mammography. Mammography is an essential part of the evaluation of a patient with obvious breast cancer. In this situation, mammography is useful for evaluating other areas of the breast as well as the contralateral breast. Approximately 5% to 15% of cancers are not apparent on mammography, and all palpable lesions require biopsy.

Alternate Screening Modalities

- **Ultrasound.** Although ultrasound is not a substitute for mammography, it has become a common tool in the evaluation of breast lesions. Ultrasound is particularly useful in differentiating cystic from solid lesions and is most commonly used in evaluating lesions in young women, especially those younger than age 40. It can also be used as an additional screening tool in women with dense or cystic breasts or those with breast implants. Suspicious features include solid masses with ill-defined borders, acoustic shadowing, or complex cystic lesions. In women with dense breasts, ultrasound may increase detection of small, early-stage cancers not detected by other methods. Ultrasound guidance also assists in diagnostic procedures, including biopsy or fine-needle aspiration.
- **MRI.** Studies have shown MRI to be more sensitive but less specific and more expensive than mammography in the detection of breast cancers.
  - BRCA1-associated breast cancers are more likely to have round, pushing margins and rare calcifications and exhibit benign mammographic appearance, which makes MRI a better choice for their detection. It is likewise helpful in detecting infiltrating lobular carcinoma and ductal carcinoma in situ (DCIS) as they are difficult to see on mammography.
  - Childhood cancer survivors who were treated with radiation therapy are at increased risk for developing solid tumors, including breast cancer. Because their screening begins at a younger age, MRI is better than mammography in screening the dense breast tissue in this group.

COMMON BREAST DISORDERS AND COMPLAINTS

Approximately 16% of women ages 40 to 69 seek a physician's advice over breast-related complaints in any 10-year period, with the most common complaint being a breast lump (40%). Other common complaints include nipple discharge and breast pain. Breast cancer will account for only 10% of these complaints and the failure to diagnose breast cancer is high on the list of malpractice claims in the United States. The most common reasons for lawsuits against obstetrician-gynecologists are "physical findings failed to impress" and "failure to refer to the specialist for biopsy." Physicians must be prepared to fully evaluate, address, and educate patients regarding their concerns.

Mastalgia

- Breast pain may be cyclic or noncyclic. Cyclic breast pain is maximal premenstrually and is relieved with the onset of menses. It can be either unilateral or bilateral. Women with fibrocystic changes typically have breast pain and tenderness during the luteal phase; however, other women may also have this cyclic breast pain. Fibrocystic pain is also characterized by localization primarily to the subareolar or upper outer regions of the breast. This pain is likely due to stromal edema, ductal dilation, and some degree of inflammation. Microcysts in fibrocystic disease can progress to form palpable macrocysts.

- Noncyclic pain can have various causes, including hormonal fluctuations, firm adenomas, duct ectasia, and macrocysts. It may also arise from musculoskeletal structures, such as soreness in the pectoral muscles from exertion or trauma, stretching of the Cooper's ligaments, or costochondritis. Mastitis and hidradenitis suppurativa may present with breast pain. With most noncyclic breast pain, no definite cause is determined. Carcinoma can present with breast pain (<10%) but this is uncommon. The evaluation of breast pain includes a careful history and physical, as well as mammography for women over age 35. The primary value of mammography is to provide reassurance. Patients with no dominant mass can be reassured.

- In most cases, mastalgia resolves spontaneously, although sometimes only after months or years. Restriction of methylxanthine-containing substances (e.g., coffee, tea) has not been shown to be superior to placebo, but some patients may note relief. Pain from a macrocyst may be relieved with aspiration. Symptomatic relief may be achieved with a supportive brassiere, acetaminophen, or a nonsteroidal anti-inflammatory drug (NSAID). Finally, cyclic pain may be partially relieved with oral contraceptives, thiazide diuretic, danazol, or tamoxifen.

Breast Mass

- Evaluation of a palpable breast mass requires a careful personal history, family history, physical examination, and radiographic examination. A breast mass reported by the patient should undergo the same evaluation, even if it fails to be appreciated on physical exam.

- In general, breast tissue can be lumpy and irregular. The following are characteristics of cancerous lesions: single, hard, immobile, irregular margins, and >2 cm. In the majority of cases, the masses are painless. Ten percent of patients with cancer present with some symptoms of breast discomfort. Associated symptoms may include nipple discharge, nipple rash or ulceration, diffuse erythema of the breast, adenopathy, or symptoms associated with metastatic disease.

- Diagnostic mammography is recommended in the evaluation of any woman over age 35 with a palpable breast mass. Findings suspicious for cancer on mammography include increased density, irregular margins, spiculation, or an accompanying cluster of microcalcifications (see Fig. 2-4).

- In women under age 35, ultrasonography may be used to distinguish a simple cyst from a more worrisome complex cyst, solid mass, or tumor. Fine-needle aspiration, core-needle biopsy, or excisional biopsy can be used for ultimate tissue diagnosis of the palpable mass. Bloody fluid yielded on aspiration or persistence of a mass after aspiration should prompt excisional biopsy or surgical consultation. Finally, the combination of physical examination, mammography, and fine-needle aspiration biopsy is referred to as *triple diagnosis*. Fewer than 1% of breast cancers are missed using this diagnostic approach.

- **Benign breast masses** include fibroadenomas, breast cysts, or fat necrosis.

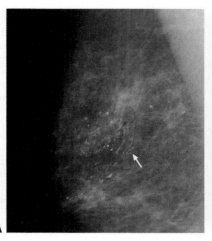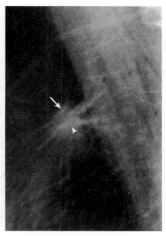

A **B**

Figure 2-4. (**A**) A 53-year-old woman with bloody discharge from the nipple. Mediolateral view of the right breast demonstrates casting calcifications involving a large part of the breast extending to the nipple. The calcifications are nonuniform, irregular, and branched (*arrow*), and they form a dot-dash linear pattern. They are aligned with the ductal system. (**B**) A 60-year-old woman with a palpable mass and no other pertinent history. Mediolateral view of the right breast reveals a spiculated mass (*arrow*) with architectural distortion. Within the center of the mass, irregular (pleomorphic) microcalcifications are present (*arrowhead*). The diagnosis is carcinoma, largely DCIS, of comedo type (**A**) and invasive ductal carcinoma, not otherwise specified (**B**). (From Pope TL Jr. *Aunt Minnie's Atlas and Imaging Specific Diagnosis*, 2nd Ed. Philadelphia, PA: Lippincott Williams & Wilkins, 2003:329, with permission.)

- **Fibroadenoma** is the most common mass lesion found in women younger than 25 years of age. Growth is gradual, and occasional cystic tenderness may be present. If the lesion is palpable, increasing in size, or psychologically disturbing, core or excisional biopsy should be considered. Conservative treatment may be appropriate for small lesions that are not palpable and have been identified as fibroadenomas. Carcinoma within a fibroadenoma is a rare occurrence. A rare malignant tumor that can be confused with fibroadenoma is *cystosarcoma phyllodes,* which is treated by wide resection with negative margins. Local recurrence is uncommon, and distant metastasis is very rare.
- **Breast cysts** can be found in premenopausal or postmenopausal women. Physical examination cannot distinguish cysts from solid masses. Ultrasonography and cyst aspiration are diagnostic. Simple cysts have a thin wall with no internal echoes and are benign. In these cases, no further therapy is required. Complex cysts have a thickened wall or internal septation and are considered suspicious. Complex cysts generally undergo some form of biopsy. If a cyst does not resolve with aspiration, yields a bloody aspirate, recurs within 6 weeks, or is complex on ultrasound evaluation, surgical consultation should be obtained.
- **Fat necrosis** is frequently associated with breast trauma resulting in a breast mass. It can occur after breast biopsy, infection, duct ectasia, reduction mammoplasty, lumpectomy, and radiotherapy for breast carcinoma. Fat necrosis is most common in the subareolar region. This process can be difficult to distinguish from breast cancer on both physical examination and mammography. The lesion needs

to be evaluated like any other palpable breast lesion. Only a benign histologic appearance affords reassurance.

Abnormal Mammogram

- Suspicious radiologic findings require surgical consultation and consideration of breast biopsy, even with an unremarkable physical examination.
- **Radiologic findings of concern on mammography:**
  - Soft tissue density, especially if borders are not well defined
  - Clustered microcalcifications in one area
  - Calcification within or closely associated with a soft tissue density
  - Asymmetric density or parenchymal distortion
  - New abnormality compared with previous mammogram
- When a woman's screening mammography is ambiguous, diagnostic mammography should be performed with possible radiographically directed biopsy. Biopsy techniques for radiographically identified nonpalpable lesions include needle localization, excisional biopsy, and stereotactic core biopsy. If the mammographic studies are inconclusive, a short-term follow-up study at 3 to 6 months can be considered. Table 2-2 describes the standardized reporting system used in mammography.

Breast Infections

- **Puerperal mastitis** is an acute cellulitis of the breast in a lactating woman. Prompt initiation of treatment reduces risk of abscess. Mastitis usually occurs in the early weeks of breast-feeding. On inspection, cellulitis is often present in a wedge-shaped pattern over a portion of the breast skin. Tissue is warm, red, and tender. The infection is around rather than within the duct system, leading to the absence of purulent discharge from the nipple. Patients may present with high fevers, chills, flulike malaise, and body aches. The most common causal organism is *Staphylococcus aureus*. The antibiotic usually recommended is dicloxacillin (500 mg by mouth four times a day for 10 days). Aggressive emptying of the affected breast is an important treatment. The patient should be encouraged to continue breast-feeding or pumping to promote drainage. Warm compresses and manual pressure are also beneficial. Microbiologic culture is indicated if the mastitis does not resolve or if an abscess develops. The latter case also warrants incision and drainage.
- **Nonpuerperal mastitis** is an uncommon, subareolar infection. In contrast to puerperal mastitis, nonpuerperal mastitis is usually a polymicrobial infection and the woman is generally not systemically ill. Antibiotic coverage typically includes clindamycin or metronidazole, in addition to a beta-lactam antibiotic. All breast inflammation must raise concern for inflammatory breast cancer, and the threshold for performing a skin biopsy should be low, particularly in the elderly population. Failure to respond to antibiotic treatment should prompt biopsy in any patient. Finally, the patient should be up-to-date with mammography screening.

Nipple Discharge

- **Nipple discharge** is a common complaint and finding on examination of the breast. Nipple discharge is usually benign (95% of cases). The causes of discharge range from physiologic to endocrine-related to pathologic. See Figure 2-5 for an algorithm for evaluation of nipple discharge.
- **Physiologic.** Secretion from the nipple during examination or nipple stimulation is a common occurrence. As many as 50% to 80% of women in their reproductive years can express one or more drops of fluid. This benign discharge is usually

TABLE 2-2	American College of Radiology Breast Imaging Reporting and Data System (BI-RADS) Mammography Assessment Categories		
Category	Assessment	Definition	Likelihood Ratio for Breast Cancer Diagnosis[a]
1	Negative	Breasts appear normal	0.1
2	Benign finding(s)	A negative mammogram result, but the interpreter wishes to describe a finding	0.1
3	Probably benign finding—short interval follow-up suggested	Lesion with a high probability of being benign	1.2
0	Need additional imaging evaluation and/ or previous mammograms for comparison	Lesion noted— additional imaging is needed; used almost always in a screening situation	7.0
4	Suspicious abnormality— biopsy should be considered	A lesion is noted for which the radi- ologist has suffi- cient concern to recommend biopsy	125
5	Highly suggestive of malignancy— appropriate action should be taken	A lesion is noted that has a high probability of being cancer	2,200

[a]Likelihood ratio at first screening mammography: ratio of diseased to nondiseased persons for a given test result. From Kerlikowske K, Smith-Bindman R, Ljung BM, et al. Evaluation of abnormal mammography results and palpable breast abnormalities. *Ann Intern Med* 2003;139:274–284, with permission.

nonspontaneous, bilateral, and serous in character. If the remainder of the breast exam is normal, reassurance is sufficient, and no further workup is necessary.

- **Galactorrhea.** Galactorrhea is milk production unrelated to nursing or preg- nancy and is typically a bilateral, multiduct discharge with a milky character. Several endocrine abnormalities give rise to galactorrhea and are frequently associ- ated with amenorrhea (e.g., dopamine inhibitors, hypothalamic/pituitary disease, hypothyroidism, postthoracotomy syndrome, chronic renal failure). Chronic breast

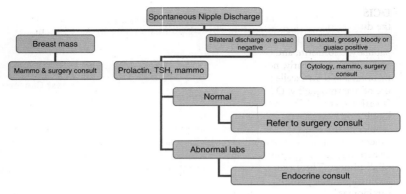

Figure 2-5. Algorithm for evaluation of nipple discharge.

stimulation or exogenous estrogen via oral contraceptive pills may cause galactorrhea. A third of cases are idiopathic. Evaluation includes a careful history reviewing medications and recent trauma/stimulation of the breast and physical exam. Questioning includes symptoms of amenorrhea, hypothyroid disease, visual field changes, or new-onset headaches. Further evaluation includes a prolactin level, thyroid function tests, and computed tomography (CT) brain scan if the prolactin level is elevated. Prolactin levels may be falsely elevated after meals, after breast examination, or based on diurnal variation.

- **Pathologic Discharge.** This discharge is typically unilateral and spontaneous. It may be greenish gray, serous, or bloody. Causes of pathologic discharge are carcinoma, intraductal papilloma (straw colored), duct ectasia, and fibrocystic changes. Only 5% of pathologic discharge is caused by carcinoma. A physical exam should attempt to identify the area of the breast and the specific duct from which the discharge is expressed. Skin lesions or an associated mass may be identified. If the fluid is not grossly bloody, guaiac testing may be performed to identify subtle bloody fluid. If grossly bloody or guaiac positive, cytology is performed; otherwise, the sensitivity is very low for malignancy. In addition, imaging with bilateral mammography is required. If the patient is younger than 35 years, ultrasound may also be used.

BREAST CANCER

Breast cancer is the most common cancer affecting women in the United States and second only to lung cancer in cancer mortality for women. Median age of diagnosis and that of death are 61 and 69 years, respectively. Primarily due to improved screening, the prevalence of breast cancer has doubled in the past 50 years. Based upon the National Cancer Institute's (NCI) Surveillance, Epidemiology, and End Results (SEER) Program, the lifetime risk of breast cancer for women is 12.7% (about 1 in 8).

Pathology

- Breast cancer most commonly arises in the upper outer quadrant of the breast, taking an average of 5 years to become palpable. It arises in the terminal duct-lobular unit of the breast and can be invasive or noninvasive (in situ). The growth pattern is described as comedo or noncomedo (solid, cribriform, micropapillary, and papillary).

- **DCIS**, also called **intraductal cancer**, refers to a proliferation of cancer cells within the ducts without invasion through the basement membrane into the surrounding stroma. Histologically, DCIS can be divided into multiple subtypes: solid, micropapillary, cribriform, and comedo. DCIS can also be graded as low, intermediate, or high. DCIS is an early, noninfiltrating form of breast cancer with minimal risk of metastasis and an excellent prognosis with local therapy alone. With the increased use of mammography, DCIS is being diagnosed more often.
- **Invasive Cancer.** The two most common types of invasive cancers are ductal and lobular. **Infiltrating lobular** carcinoma is a variant associated with microscopic lobular architecture. These carcinomas account for 10% to 15% of invasive breast cancers, are often multifocal, have a higher incidence of bilaterality, and are less evident on mammography. **Infiltrating ductal** carcinoma accounts for 60% to 75% of all tumors. These cancers account for a group of tumors classified by cell type, architecture, and pattern of spread. These include mucinous, tubular, and medullary carcinomas.

Premalignant Conditions

- **Atypical hyperplasia** is a proliferative lesion of the breast that possesses some of the features of carcinoma in situ. Atypical hyperplasia can be categorized as ductal or lobular. It should be considered premalignant and carries a four- to fivefold increased risk of breast cancer, usually in the ipsilateral breast. Complete excision is recommended. Proliferative lesions, such as sclerosing adenosis, ductal epithelium hyperplasia, and intraductal papillomas, also carry an increased risk of cancer.
- **Lobular carcinoma in situ (LCIS)**, sometimes called *lobular neoplasia*, is a nonpalpable, noninvasive lesion arising from the lobules. LCIS is more common in premenopausal women and is considered an indicator lesion or marker that identifies women at increased risk of subsequent invasive cancer. Absolute risk of developing invasive cancer is approximately 1% per year. It is often an incidental finding on biopsy, is usually multicentric, and is often bilateral. Management is controversial and includes observation, tamoxifen administration, or prophylactic mastectomy. Tamoxifen has been shown to decrease the risk of developing breast cancer in women with LCIS. Some women, particularly those at high risk for developing breast cancer, may choose prophylactic bilateral mastectomy.

Risk Factors

- The most commonly used model to determine breast cancer risk is the Gail model. The number of first-degree relatives with breast cancer, age at menarche, age at first live birth, number of breast biopsies, and presence of atypical hyperplasia on a breast biopsy are its components. Its accuracy is limited as it omits a detailed family history of breast and ovarian cancers and underestimates the risk in African American women and overestimates the risk in Asian American women. This model should not be used in women who have a history of breast cancer or women who are known gene mutation carriers.
- **Age** is the primary risk factor for breast cancer (Table 2-3). Approximately 95% of breast cancers occur in women over 40 years of age.
- **Family History and Genetic Predisposition.** Family history confers an increased risk for breast cancer, specifically with a history of premenopausal breast cancer in a first-degree relative, male breast cancer, bilateral breast cancer, or a combination of breast and ovarian cancers within a family. Inheriting BRCA1 or BRCA2 confers

TABLE 2-3	Age-Specific Probabilities of Developing Breast Cancer
Age	**Probability of Developing Breast Cancer in the Next 10 Years**
20	1:1,985
30	1:229
40	1:68
50	1:37
60	1:26
70	1:24
Lifetime	1:8

American Cancer Society. *Breast Cancer Facts and Figures 2005–2006*. Atlanta, GA: American Cancer Society, Inc., 2005.

a 40% to 85% lifetime risk of breast cancer, yet these cases account for <10% of all diagnoses. In addition, BRCA1 confers a 40% risk and BRCA2 a 20% risk for ovarian cancer; BRCA1 and BRCA2 are tumor suppressor genes with autosomal dominant inheritance, of either maternal or paternal lineage. Both are more common in the Ashkenazi Jewish population (1 in 40).
- A woman has 35% to 43% chance of developing a second primary breast cancer and a 7% to 13% chance of developing ovarian cancer within the first 10 years of her first breast cancer diagnosis if she carries these genes. In addition, she is at increased risk for pancreatic cancer. (See Chapter 45 for indications for referral for BRCA testing.)
- **Hormone Exposure.** Early menarche (<12 years), late natural menopause (>55 years), older age at first full-term pregnancy, and fewer pregnancies increase a woman's risk of developing breast cancer. Breast-feeding is associated with a lower risk of breast cancer. In addition, moderate alcohol use, which is related to an increase in estrogen, carries a higher risk. Finally, the role of exogenous estrogen use in the development of breast cancer remains controversial. Long-term oral contraceptive use (>10 years) and current hormone therapy use are associated with a nonsignificant increased risk of breast cancer.
- **Diet and Lifestyle.** Impressive differences in the incidence of breast cancer in different geographic and cultural areas have long raised the suspicion of dietary risk factors. High-fat diets have been implicated. Data are insufficient to support firm dietary advice for reduction in breast cancer risk. Lifestyle activities with protective effects include physical activity and weight control.
- **Personal History.** Women with a history of breast cancer are at a 0.5% to 1% risk per year of developing cancer in the contralateral breast, in addition to the risk of recurrence in the treated breast. The majority of recurrences occur within the first 5 years after diagnosis. A personal history of a benign breast biopsy or atypical hyperplasia also yields an increased risk.
- **Exposure to Radiation Therapy.** Previous exposure to ionizing radiation is associated with an increased risk for breast cancer, usually identified a decade after exposure (e.g., lymphoma mantle radiation). The lifetime risk is 35% for these women.

Staging and Prognostic Factors

- The American Joint Committee on Cancer's Tumor-Node-Metastasis (TNM) staging system for breast cancer uses tumor size, axillary node status (incorporating sentinel nodes), and metastasis status (see Tables 2-4 and 2-5). Prognosis is strongly correlated with tumor size and node status. Expression of estrogen and progesterone receptors in tumor tissue is associated with a better prognosis and can assist in systemic treatment. Other prognostic factors include tumor grade, S phase, DNA ploidy, and expression of the *human epidermal growth factor receptor 2 (HER2/neu)* oncogene.
- **HER2/neu** is a gene encoding transmembrane receptors for growth factors, thus regulating cellular growth and differentiation. Overexpression of this oncogene leads to a more aggressive subtype of breast cancer. These cancers tend to be poorly

TABLE 2-4	TNM Classification of Breast Cancer
Notation	**Description**
Tumor Size	
TX	Primary tumor cannot be assessed
T0	No evidence of primary tumor
Tis	Carcinoma in situ: intraductal carcinoma, LCIS, or Paget's disease of the nipple with no tumor
T1	Tumor 2 cm in greatest dimension
T1a	Tumor 0.5 cm in greatest dimension
T1b	Tumor >0.5 cm but 1 cm in greatest dimension
T1c	Tumor >1 cm but 2 cm in greatest dimension
T2	Tumor >2 cm but 5 cm in greatest dimension
T3	Tumor >5 cm in greatest dimension
T4	Tumor of any size with direct extension to the chest wall or skin
T4a	Extension to the chest wall
T4b	Edema (including *peau d'orange*) or ulceration of the skin of the breast or satellite skin
T4c	Both T4a and T4b
T4d	Inflammatory carcinoma
Lymph Node Metastases	
NX	Regional lymph nodes cannot be assessed (e.g., previously removed)
N0	No regional lymph node metastasis
N1	Metastasis to movable ipsilateral axillary lymph node(s)
N2	Metastasis to ipsilateral axillary lymph node(s), fixed to one another or other structures
N3	Metastasis to ipsilateral internal mammary lymph node(s)
Distant Metastases	
M	Presence of distant metastasis cannot be assessed
M0	No distant metastasis
M1	Distant metastasis (including metastasis to ipsilateral supra-clavicular lymph node[s])

TNM, Tumor-Node-Metastasis. From www.cancer.org/Cancer/BreastCancer/DetailedGuide/breast-cancer-staging

TABLE 2-5	TNM Staging System for Breast Cancer		
Stage	**Tumor Size**	**Lymph Node Metastases**	**Distant Metastases**
0	Tis	N0	M0
I	T1	N0	M0
IIa	T0	N1	M0
	T1	N1	M0
	T2	N0	M0
IIb	T2	N1	M0
	T3	N0	M0
IIIa	T0	N2	M0
	T1	N2	M0
	T2	N2	M0
	T3	N1, N2	M0
IIIb	T4	Any N	M0
	Any T	N3	M0
IV	Any T	Any N	M1

TNM, Tumor-Node-Metastasis. From www.cancer.org/Cancer/BreastCancer/DetailedGuide/breast-cancer-staging

differentiated and high grade. They have high rates of cellular proliferation and lymph node involvement and are resistant to chemotherapy. The decreased expression of progesterone and estrogen receptors is associated with resistance to the typical adjuvant hormonal therapies. This gene is overexpressed in 20% to 25% of breast cancers. The American Society of Clinical Oncology and the National Comprehensive Cancer Network strongly suggest that all newly diagnosed invasive breast cancer patients have the HER2 status checked.

TABLE 2-6	Prognosis by Stage: 10-Year Breast Cancer Survival Based on the National Cancer Database[a]
Stage	**10-Year Survival Rates**
Stage 0	95%
Stage I	88%
Stage II	66%
Stage III	36%
Stage IV	7%

[a]The National Cancer Database is a joint project of the Commission on Cancer of the American College of Surgeons and the American Cancer Society. It collects and analyzes data from a wide variety of sources throughout the United States, including small community hospitals. From Fremgen AM, Bland KI, McGinnis LS Jr, et al. Clinical highlights from the National Cancer Database, 1999. *CA Cancer J Clin* 1999;49:145–158.

TABLE 2-7	Therapy by Breast Cancer Stage	
Stage	**Surgery**	**Adjuvant Treatment**
Stage 0	Total mastectomy vs BCT (includes lumpectomy and breast irradiation)	
Stage I	Total mastectomy vs BCT (includes lumpectomy and breast irradiation) ± sentinel node biopsy/axillary lymph node dissection	Chemotherapy >1 cm ±tamoxifen
Stage II	Modified radical mastectomy vs BCT (includes lumpectomy and breast irradiation/axillary lymph node dissection)	Chemotherapy ± tamoxifen Radiation therapy of the supra-clavicular nodes ± chest wall if mastectomy performed or if ≥4 positive nodes
Stage III	Modified radical mastectomy vs BCT/axillary lymph node dissection	Chemotherapy ± neoadjuvant chemotherapy ± tamoxifen Radiation therapy of the supraclavicular nodes ± chest wall, if mastectomy performed Radiation therapy of the breast (inflammatory breast cancer)
Stage IV	Surgery for local control	±Chemotherapy ±Hormonal agents

From Gemignani ML. Breast cancer. In: Barakat RR, Beavers MW, Gershenson DM, et al., eds. *The Memorial Sloan-Kettering & MD Anderson Cancer Center Handbook of Gynecologic Oncology*, 2nd Ed. London: Martin Dunitz Publishers, 2002:297–319.

Treatment

Early detection is the key to improved survival (see Table 2-6). Treatment for invasive breast cancer includes lumpectomy with radiation (breast conservation therapy [BCT]) or modified radical mastectomy (Table 2-7).

Surgical or Local Treatment

• **Mastectomy** involves the complete removal of breast tissue with preservation of the pectoralis muscles. A total or **simple mastectomy** removes the breast with the nipple areolar complex but without lymph nodes. The **modified radical mastectomy** includes removal of the entire breast and levels I and II of the axillary lymph nodes. Mastectomy is recommended if the disease is multicentric, invades skin and chest wall, or has inflammatory features or if negative margins cannot be achieved with breast preservation. Any type of mastectomy can be performed with or without immediate reconstruction. The benefit of simultaneous reconstruction includes combining two surgeries; however, it is not optimal if the reconstruction would result in a delay in adjuvant irradiation or chemotherapy. Various types of reconstruction can be used, including autologous tissue reconstruction (e.g., deep inferior epigastric perforator [DIEP], free transverse rectus abdominis muscle [TRAM], or latissimus dorsi flaps) or using a tissue expander and subsequent prosthetic implant.

- In **BCT**, a wide local excision or lumpectomy is performed to achieve a 1- to 2-mm negative margin. Adjuvant radiation therapy is required. Radiation is delivered to the entire breast with a possible boost dose to the lumpectomy bed. Trials comparing BCT and mastectomy show comparable survival rates. In select patients with very low risk DCIS or patients >70 years of age, the radiation therapy can be eliminated.
- **Axillary lymph node staging** is important in prognosis, staging, and treatment planning. Axillary dissection is not free from complications. Patients may experience lymphedema (10% to 15%), pain, numbness, or weakness of the affected arm.
- **Sentinel lymph node biopsy** has evolved into the method of choice for axillary node staging in the clinically negative axilla. The sentinel lymph node is identified using radioactive tracer or dye injected into the periareolar region of the breast. When the isotope and dye are used in combination, the positive predictive value approaches 100%, the negative predictive value is close to 95%, and the false-negative rate is 5% to 10%.
- **Radiation therapy**, although most often administered as part of BCT, can also be used for other indications.

Systemic Therapy
- Systemic therapy (e.g., biologic, chemotherapy, and hormonal) given before surgery is termed **neoadjuvant therapy**. When given after surgery, the term used is **adjuvant therapy**, which is typically recommended to patients with positive lymph node findings or when the tumor size is >1 cm.
- **Hormonal therapy** is the most frequently recommended adjuvant systemic therapy and is aimed at targeting estrogen receptor– or progesterone receptor–positive breast cancer. Tamoxifen, a **selective estrogen receptor modulator**, has been used most commonly. Hormone therapy results in a 26% annual reduction in the risk of recurrence and a 14% annual reduction in the risk of death from breast cancer. Tamoxifen is administered at 20 mg/day for 5 years, after which its maximal effect is reached.
  - Tamoxifen has effects of both strong antagonism and weak agonism on the estrogen receptor. It acts as an agonist on the endometrium and doubles the risk of endometrial cancer. Bleeding, most often in the postmenopausal setting, is a common problem. Patients should be monitored for symptoms of postmenopausal bleeding, but routine imaging or endometrial sampling is not recommended.
  - More recently, **aromatase inhibitors** (e.g., letrozole, anastrozole, and exemestane) have been added to the field of hormonal therapy. These potent inhibitors of estrogen synthesis have been shown to be more effective than tamoxifen in treating breast cancer with a different set of side effects including osteoporosis, myalgias, elevated cholesterol, and joint pain. They carry a reduced risk of thromboembolic events and virtually no risk of endometrial hyperplasia when compared to tamoxifen. These agents are effective as first-line agents or as second-line agents in patients whose cancer has progressed during or after tamoxifen therapy. Letrozole and anastrozole improve disease-free survival better than tamoxifen, suggesting that aromatase inhibitors are better than tamoxifen as adjuvant therapy. In addition, letrozole has been shown to be superior to anastrozole in reducing the risk of distant metastasis, suggesting that letrozole is more effective at preventing breast cancer–related deaths. Studies are ongoing to see if this is a beneficial drug for prophylaxis.

- **Biologic Therapy.** Trastuzumab (Herceptin) is a genetically engineered monoclonal antibody to the *HER2 protein*. Three recent trials demonstrated revolutionary reductions in the risk of recurrence in patients with HER2-positive tumors treated with trastuzumab. Women taking trastuzumab in addition to chemotherapy were half as likely to experience a cancer recurrence as women treated with chemotherapy alone. Patients with HER2-positive cancers taking trastuzumab, who were originally thought to have a worse prognosis, appear to do better in response to chemotherapy than do HER2-negative cancer patients. Long-term follow-up and further recommendations regarding the best form of testing for the HER2 oncogene, timing of treatment, and use of additional chemotherapy have not been clearly delineated.
- **Chemotherapy** has been shown to improve overall survival and reduce the odds of death by 25% in selected patients. Chemotherapy is typically administered postoperatively over 3 to 6 months.

Metastatic or Advanced Disease
- Although breast cancer is uncommonly found to be metastatic at the time of presentation, approximately one third of patients subsequently develop distant metastatic disease. Median survival for patients with metastatic disease is 2 years, but fewer than 5% live beyond 5 years. Breast cancer metastasizes to the bone, liver, and brain. The goal of therapy in metastatic disease is palliation of symptoms.

Treatment of DCIS
- Patients who have DCIS can be offered the options of mastectomy or BCT. However, unlike infiltrating or invasive cancer, the risk for nodal involvement is <1% and lymph node sampling is not routinely recommended. As with infiltrating cancer, lumpectomy and BCT must achieve complete negative margins. In cases of multicentric disease, BCT is contraindicated.

Prevention

- **Chemoprevention** includes treatment with tamoxifen and raloxifene. Evidence from four randomized controlled trials show that **prophylactic tamoxifen** reduces the risk for estrogen receptor–positive breast cancer in women without previous breast cancer. Further analysis of the largest of these trials showed a possible reduction in breast cancer incidence for women with *BRCA2* mutations but not for those with *BRCA1* mutations, possibly because women with *BRCA1* mutations had predominantly estrogen receptor–negative tumors.
  - **Raloxifene** is a selective estrogen receptor modulator that has been demonstrated to reduce the incidence of breast cancer. It was studied in the Multiple Outcomes of Raloxifene Evaluation (MORE) and Continuing Outcomes Relevant to Evista (CORE) studies. These studies measured the effects of raloxifene on bone mineral density and studied as a secondary outcome the risk for breast cancer. It decreased risk of all breast cancers by 62% and invasive breast cancer by 72%.
- **Surgical prevention** can be considered in two groups of women: (a) patients positive for BRCA1 or BRCA2 and (b) patients with a strong family history suggestive of hereditary breast cancer but negative for BRCA1 or BRCA2. Surgical prevention includes contralateral mastectomy, prophylactic bilateral mastectomy, and bilateral salpingo-oophorectomy. Prophylactic bilateral mastectomies have been shown to reduce the risk of breast cancer by 90%. This is increased to 95% if combined with a bilateral salpingo-oophorectomy.

Pregnancy and Breast Cancer

- Breast cancer is the most common cancer in pregnancy, with an incidence of 1 in 3,000 gestations. The average patient age is 32 to 38 years. Breast cancer can be especially difficult to diagnose during pregnancy and lactation (secondary to increased glandular breast tissue), which may lead to a delay in diagnosis. Thus, cancers are often found at a later stage in pregnant women or immediately postpartum. Mammograms may be performed safely during pregnancy. Pregnant patients do as well as their nonpregnant counterparts at a similar disease stage.
- Treatment during pregnancy is generally the same as that for nonpregnant patients. The tumor can usually be fully excised or mastectomy performed during pregnancy. The agents used to identify the sentinel lymph node are not approved in pregnancy and therefore axillary dissection is commonly performed. Initiation of chemotherapy is generally considered safe after the first trimester. Radiotherapy should be avoided until after delivery. No evidence has been reported that aborting the fetus or interrupting the pregnancy leads to improved outcome.

SUGGESTED READINGS

Breast cancer screening. ACOG Practice Bulletin Number 42. American College of Obstetricians and Gynecologists. *Obstet Gynecol* (2003 reaffirmed) 2006;101:821–832.

Hereditary Breast and Ovarian Cancer Syndrome. ACOG Practice Bulletin Number 103. American College of Obstetricians and Gynecologists. *Obstet Gynecol* 2009;113:957–966.

Leach MO. Breast cancer screening in women at high risk using MRI. *NMR Biomed* 2009;22:17–27.

Speroff L, Fritz MA, eds. The breast. In *Clinical Gynecologic Endocrinology and Infertility*. Philadelphia, PA: Lippincott Williams & Wilkins, 2005:573–620.

Tang S-C. Reducing the risk of distant metastases: a better end point in adjuvant aromatase inhibitor breast cancer trials? *Cancer Investig* 2008;26(5):481–490.

Critical Care

K. Joseph Hurt and Pamela A. Lipsett

ROUTINE POSTOPERATIVE CARE

Postoperative care after gynecologic or obstetric surgery requires vigilant monitoring of fluid and hemodynamic status, appropriate institution of prophylactic measures, and timely identification of and intervention for complications.

- **Patient evaluation** after surgical procedures is determined by the severity of illness, comorbidities, and the type and degree of the procedure.
  - A written **night of surgery evaluation** should document assessment of respiratory effort and adequacy, hemodynamic stability, pain control, and recovery from anesthesia. Pulse, blood pressure, and fluid intake and output (including intraoperative fluids) should be recorded in the evaluation of hemodynamic status.
  - Intraoperative insensible fluid loss can be approximated as 5 to 15 mL/kg/hr, in addition to maintenance fluid, for the time that the abdomen is open. On our gynecology service, we approximate insensible losses as 250 mL/hr per quadrant of the incision (i.e., dividing the abdomen into four regions; a large vertical midline incision would, therefore, yield 1,000 mL/hr insensible losses). Whatever the method, the important point is to account for increased insensible loss in your total fluid calculations.
  - **Urine output** >0.5 mL/kg/hr in the absence of hyperosmotic disorders (e.g., diabetes) is generally adequate. Low postoperative urine output deserves assessment for bleeding, inadequate intraoperative fluid resuscitation, inflammatory "third space" intravascular volume loss, and urinary tract injury. An isotonic fluid bolus of 10 mL/kg can be given to assess the volume status by monitoring changes in urine output. A larger fluid bolus up to 20 mL/kg may be preferred for a hypotensive patient. In addition to **intake and output** measures, **daily weight** should be recorded for patients at high risk of postoperative fluid imbalance (e.g., with cardiovascular, pulmonary, or renal disorders, or for prolonged or extensive procedures).
- **Deep vein thrombosis (DVT) prophylaxis** with sequential compression devices (SCD; e.g., lower limb SCDs or foot pump) should be instituted prior to incision for all patients undergoing major surgery and for obstetric surgical patients. Anticoagulation with heparin or low molecular weight heparin is indicated for high-risk patients with malignancy, prior DVT or pulmonary embolism (PE), obesity, hypercoagulable states, and prolonged abdominal or pelvic surgery (see Chapters 17 and 24).
- **Perioperative beta adrenergic blockade** has been shown in multiple large clinical trials to decrease cardiac events and overall mortality in high-risk noncardiac surgical patients. High-risk factors include the following: age >55 years, diabetes, hypertension, hypercholesterolemia, and current tobacco use. Ideally, beta blockade is instituted preoperatively and continued for several weeks after surgery to reduce the deleterious effects of the stress-activated sympathetic response. Beta-blockade should not be administered in low-risk individuals.

- **Incentive spirometry** should be encouraged, with teaching and assistance initially, as well as deep breathing and coughing to clear pulmonary secretions.
- **Prophylactic antibiotics** are indicated just before incision (<1 hr) and during surgery; their use postoperatively and especially beyond 24 hr after a procedure should be strongly discouraged. Antibiotics for proven or suspected infection (i.e., as therapy) may be prescribed with a prolonged regimen if indicated.
- **Infection control** measures reduce the occurrence of multidrug-resistant organisms and prevent hospital-based transmission. Effective hand hygiene protocols produce a significant reduction in nosocomial infection rates. **Standard precautions**, protecting both patients and healthcare workers, should also be strictly employed.
- **Common postoperative problems** such as fever, infection, PE/DVT, bowel and bladder injury or dysfunction, nausea/vomiting, and pain control are discussed in Chapter 24.

POSTOPERATIVE COMPLICATIONS

Postoperative complications such as **severe hypotension and shock** require systems-based critical care management. Chapter 14 describes management of critical care hypertensive disorders during and after pregnancy.

Hypotension and Shock

Shock is a clinical syndrome in which decreased perfusion leads to symptoms of vital organ dysfunction, including hypotension, oliguria, and altered mentation. In patients with gynecologic malignancy, common postoperative causes include hemorrhage, PE, myocardial infarction, and sepsis. Oliguria is defined as urine output <0.5 mL/kg/hr. No absolute criteria for hypotension define shock, but systolic blood pressure (SBP) <100 mm Hg or a decrease in SBP of 40 mm Hg from baseline deserves further evaluation. Management starts with determination of the etiology and correction of the underlying disease process. Ensuring sufficient perfusion and adequate oxygenation is the primary goal.

- **Hypovolemic shock** is due to intravascular fluid loss (e.g., bleeding, nasogastric suction, diarrhea).
  - **Hemorrhagic shock** is classified by the volume of blood loss and physiologic response (Table 3-1). Expedient volume resuscitation is required when blood loss exceeds 30% to 40%.
    - It is important to **replace both volume and erythrocytes**, and perhaps coagulation factors, during massive hemorrhage. Restoring intravascular volume with crystalloid improves blood pressure, cardiac filling pressure, and organ perfusion. Though young healthy patients can tolerate hematocrits below 20% if intravascular volume is adequate, older adults and patients with comorbidities may benefit from earlier packed red blood cell (PRBC) transfusion. Ongoing myocardial ischemia or impaired oxygenation deserves transfusion with packed red cells to hemoglobin of 10 g/dL.
    - **Crystalloid** is typically available on any unit, inexpensive, and carries less risk than colloid administration. Ringer's lactate is less acidic than normal saline and can ameliorate the hyperchloremic metabolic acidosis that results from large volume saline infusion, though there is no important physiologic difference in the degree of resuscitation provided by Ringer's versus normal saline (Table 3-2).

TABLE 3-1 Classification of Hemorrhage by Extent of Blood Loss

Parameter	Class I	Class II	Class III	Class IV
Blood loss (mL)	750	750–1,500	1,500–2,000	>2,000
Blood volume lost (%)	<15	15–30	30–40	>40
Pulse rate (beats/min)	<100	>100	>120	>140
Supine blood pressure	Normal	Normal	Decreased	Decreased
Urine output (mL/hr)	>30	20–30	5–15	<5
Mental status	Anxious	Agitated	Confused	Lethargic

See Gutierrez G, Reines HD, Wulf-Guterrez ME. Clinical review: hemorrhagic shock. *Crit Care* 2004;8:373–381.

TABLE 3-2 Composition of Intravenous Crystalloid Fluids

Preparation	Na (mEq/L)	Cl (mEq/L)	K (mEq/L)	Ca (mEq/L)	Mg (mEq/L)	pH	Osmolality (mOsm/L)	Buffer (mEq/L)
Plasma	140	103	4	5	2	7.4	290	Bicarbonate (25)
0.9% NaCl	154	154	0	0	0	5.7	308	None
7.5% NaCl	1,283	1,283	0	0	0	5.7	2,567	None
Lactated Ringer's	130	109	4	3	0	6.4	273	Lactate (28)
Normosol/plasmalyte	140	98	5	0	3	7.4	295	Acetate (27), gluconate (23)

Adapted from Marino PL. *The ICU Book*, 3rd Ed. Philadelphia, PA: Lippincott Williams & Wilkins, 2007:235.

○ **Colloid** therapy is more costly but may provide better short-term volume expansion. The benefit may not last more than 60 minutes, however.

○ **Vasoactive pharmacotherapy** may be required along with fluid resuscitation. Intensive care and possibly invasive monitoring (i.e., Swan Ganz pulmonary artery catheter, see below) are required. Norepinephrine is often employed in the treatment of severe hypotensive shock (Table 3-3).

- **Distributive shock** is a consequence of venous pooling (e.g., early sepsis, peritonitis, anaphylaxis, neurologic injury).
- **Cardiogenic shock** occurs with decreased myocardial contractility and function (e.g., myocardial infarction, severe congestive heart failure). It may also occur along with septic or hemorrhagic shock, especially in patients with baseline cardiovascular disease.
- **Obstructive shock** is secondary to mechanical obstruction of blood flow (e.g., cardiac tamponade, tension pneumothorax, massive PE, prosthetic valve thrombosis).
- **Septic shock** occurs secondary to the vasodilation, complement activation, and increased vascular permeability that is stimulated by vasoactive substances released during a massive inflammatory process. In early septic shock, the etiology may be distributive. In later stages, sepsis can produce cardiogenic shock when hypotension, acidosis, and ischemia suppress myocardial function. Additionally, infection, tissue trauma, or obstetric accidents can activate the intrinsic coagulation pathway with subsequent intravascular thrombosis and fibrinolysis, causing disseminated intravascular coagulation and massive bleeding. Management of septic shock is done with aggressive fluid replacement, broad-spectrum antibiotics, vasopressor support, and eradication of the infectious source.
- **Toxic shock syndrome (TSS)** occurs in <5 per 100,000 reproductive age women. It results from *Staphylococcus aureus* (staphylococcal TSS [STSS]) or Group A streptococcus (GAS; *S. pyogenes* causing toxic shock-like syndrome [TSLS]) production of specific exotoxins that can cause dramatic and rapid critical illness. There is an association with extended or superabsorbant tampon use, surgical wounds, skin infection, and abscesses. The bacterial toxin (e.g., TSS toxin 1 from *S. aureus*; pyrogenic exotoxin from GAS) is absorbed systemically, causing illness in individuals who lack protective antitoxin antibodies. STSS can occur in otherwise healthy individuals while TSLS typically presents with a prior infection. Blood cultures can be negative.
  - The **diagnostic criteria** for STSS are the following: fever >39.9; diffuse blanching erythroderma progressing to desquamation at 10 to 14 days, especially on the palms and soles; hypotension with systolic BP <90 mm Hg or orthostasis; and involvement of three or more organ systems such as GI (diarrhea, vomiting), musculoskeletal (severe myalgia, CK > twice upper limit of normal), mucous membrane hyperemia (oropharynx, conjunctiva, vagina), renal dysfunction (BUN or creatining > twice upper limit), liver dysfunction (bilirubin, AST, or ALT > twice the upper limit), hematologic abnormalities (platelets <100,000/μL), or mental status changes without focal findings. Diagnostic criteria for TSLS are similar but require isolation of GAS and dysfunction in at least two organ systems.
  - The **differential diagnosis** includes: Rocky Mountain spotted fever, Stevens-Johnson syndrome, scarlet fever, viral exanthems, drug reaction, meningococcemia, leptospirosis, and heat stroke.
  - **Treatment** includes early recognition, elimination/debridement of infectious source if identified, anti-Staphylococcal antibiotics (e.g., vancomycin, nafcillin, oxacillin, or a first-generation cephalosporin; add clindamycin for toxin

TABLE 3-3	Selected Vasoactive Agents in Critical Care				
Drug	Main Effects	Dose	Mechanism	Use	Warnings
Dobutamine	Increased inotropy, and systemic vasodilation	3–15 μg/kg/min	Potent β_1 agonist, weak β_2 agonist.	Primarily for decompensated heart failure.	Adverse effects include tachycardia, ventricular ectopy. Contraindicated with hypertrophic cardiomyopathy.
Dopamine	Low-dose: renal and splanchnic vasodilation and natriuresis; medium dose: increased inotropy and systemic vasodilation; high dose: systemic vasoconstriction	1–3 μg/kg/min; or 3–10 μg/kg/min; or >10 μg/kg/min	Dose-dependent agonist for dopamine receptors (low), β adrenergic receptors (medium), and peripheral α adrenergic receptors (high)	May be useful for cardiogenic or hypotensive shock where both cardiac stimulation and peripheral vasoconstriction are needed	Low-dose dopamine is not appropriate for acute renal failure. Adverse effects include tachyarrhythmia, ischemic limb necrosis, increased intraocular pressure, and delayed gastric emptying
Epinephrine	Dose-dependent increase in cardiac output, increased systemic vascular resistance, relaxation of bronchial smooth muscle.	0.3–0.5 mg IM; 2–8 μg/min infusion	β adrenergic receptor agonist (low dose) and α agonist (high dose).	Drug of choice for anaphylaxis. Used in ACLS protocols for cardiac arrest. Nebulized racemic epimer used for laryngospasm and severe asthma exacerbation.	Contraindicated with narrow angle glaucoma, ischemic cardiac disease. Local infiltration can cause tissue necrosis.

(Continued)

TABLE 3-3	Selected Vasoactive Agents in Critical Care *(Continued)*			
Norepinephrine	Dose-dependent increase in systemic vascular resistance	α adrenergic receptor agonist and cardiac β agonist	Preferred vasopressor for septic shock or refractory hypotension.	Extreme vasoconstriction can exacerbate end-organ damage. Extravasation can produce local tissue necrosis.
Nitroglycerin	Low dose: venodilation; high dose: arteriodilation	Metabolized in endothelial cells to produce nitric oxide (NO) that stimulates cGMP production causing smooth muscle relaxation. Dose-dependent vasodilator.	Used for unstable angina, and to augment cardiac output in decompensated heart failure.	Rapid onset and metabolism. Tolerance develops quickly. Contraindicated for patients taking phosphodiesterase inhibitors.
Nitroprusside	Systemic vasodilation	Releases NO in bloodstream; similar mechanism to nitroglycerin.	Used for rapid control of severe hypertension and for decompensated heart failure.	Risk for accumulation of cyanide metabolite.

Adapted from material in Marino PL. *The ICU Book*, 3rd Ed. Philadelphia, PA: Lippincott Williams & Wilkins, 2007.

suppression), and ICU supportive care with fluids, oxygen, and vasopressors if needed. Mortality ranges from 5% to 60% depending on the bacterial strain and severity of illness.

CARDIOVASCULAR CRITICAL CARE

Cardiovascular function in critical care can be assessed with **invasive hemodynamic monitoring** using a pulmonary artery catheter (Swan-Ganz PA catheter) that provides information on the cardiac performance, fluid status, and oxygen transport capacity of critically ill patients. Indications include the following: distinguishing cardiogenic from other causes of pulmonary edema; managing perioperative fluids in high-risk patients with severe cardiac, pulmonary, or renal disease; guiding fluid resuscitation in patients with shock, renal failure, or unexplained acidosis; and calculating oxygen consumption and intrapulmonary shunt fraction in patients with acute respiratory failure. Despite its potential utility, no clinical trials have demonstrated improved patient outcomes from invasive monitoring, and recently it has become less popular in most ICUs. Understanding the principles of invasive monitoring is nonetheless instructive and comprises a necessary knowledge base for many board-type exams.

- The basic **PA catheter** is 110 cm long and 2.3 mm in diameter (7 French). It is placed via the subclavian or internal jugular vein (preferred) and has two lumens. One lumen opens 30 cm from the catheter tip (proximal port) and is positioned in the superior vena cava or right atrium. The other lumen extends the entire length of the catheter with its opening at the tip (distal port). The catheter tip has a 1.5-mL capacity balloon that, when inflated, encompasses the tip and helps guide (or "sail") the catheter through the right atrium and ventricle into the pulmonary artery. When the balloon is "wedged" into a branch of the pulmonary artery, the pulmonary capillary wedge pressure (PCWP) can be obtained. The balloon is then deflated to prevent complications. Ventricular arrhythmias are common during insertion, so waveforms are monitored continuously, and the physician placing the catheter should be trained to recognize and treat them.

- **Hemodynamic parameters** that can be measured with a PA catheter and their normal values are listed in Table 3-4. A parameter that is expressed relative to body surface area (BSA) is called an *index*.

  - **Central venous pressure (CVP)** is recorded from the proximal port of the catheter and reflects **right atrial pressure (RAP)**. When there is no obstruction between the right atrium and ventricle, CVP = RAP = right ventricular end-diastolic pressure. CVP is measured in the supine position, with the transducer held at the level of the right atrium (i.e., in the fourth intercostal space along the midaxillary line).

  - **Pulmonary capillary wedge pressure (PCWP)** is recorded with the PA catheter balloon inflated and wedged in a branch of the pulmonary artery. When there is no obstruction between the left atrium and ventricle, PCWP = left atrial pressure = left ventricular end-diastolic pressure. Left ventricular end-diastolic pressure reflects left ventricular preload only with normal ventricular compliance.

  - **Cardiac index (CI)** is cardiac output (stroke volume × heart rate)/BSA. Cardiac output is measured with a PA catheter using a thermodilution technique. A thermistor located 4 cm from the end of the PA catheter tip detects the flow of a cold fluid injected via the proximal port to calculate blood flow rate (equivalent to cardiac output).

  - **Right ventricular end-diastolic volume (RVEDV)** is the fraction of right ventricular volume ejected during systole.

TABLE 3-4	Cardiovascular and Oxygen-Transport Parameters Obtained with Invasive Monitoring	

Parameter	Abbreviation	Normal Value
Central venous pressure (=right ventricular end-diastolic pressure)	CVP	1–6 mm Hg
Pulmonary capillary wedge pressure (=left ventricular end-diastolic pressure)	PCWP	6–12 mm Hg
Cardiac index	CI	2.4–4 L/min/m^2
Stroke volume index	SVI	40–70 mL/beat/m^2
Right ventricular ejection fraction	RVEF	46–50%
Right ventricular end-diastolic volume	RVEDV	80–150 mL/m^2
Right ventricular stroke work index	RVSWI	4–8 g·m/m^2
Left ventricular stroke work index	LVSWI	40–60 g·m/m^2
Systemic vascular resistance index	SVRI	1,600–2,400 dynes s/cm^5/m^2
Pulmonary vascular resistance index	PVRI	200–400 dynes s/cm^5/m^2
Arterial oxygen delivery	DO$_2$	520–570 mL/min/m^2
Mixed venous oxygen saturation	SvO$_2$	70%–75%
Oxygen uptake	VO$_2$	110–160 mL/min/m^2
Oxygen extraction	O$_2$ER	20%–30%

Adapted from Marino PL. *The ICU Book*, 3rd Ed. Philadelphia, PA: Lippincott Williams & Wilkins, 2007.

- **Right ventricular stroke work index (RVSWI)** is the work performed by the right ventricle to eject the stroke volume across the pulmonary vessels/BSA.
- **Stroke volume index (SVI)** is the volume ejected by the left ventricle during systole/BSA.
- **Left ventricular stroke work index (LVSWI)** is the work performed by the left ventricle to eject the stroke volume into the aorta/BSA.
- **Systemic vascular resistance index (SVRI)** is the peripheral vascular resistance/BSA and **pulmonary vascular resistance index (PVRI)** is the pulmonary vascular resistance/BSA.
- **Oxygen transport parameters** that can be measured using a PA catheter are also listed in Table 3-4.
- **Arterial oxygen delivery (DO$_2$)** is the rate of oxygen transport in arterial blood.
- **Mixed venous oxygen saturation (SvO$_2$)** is the oxygen saturation in pulmonary arterial blood, measured from a blood sample drawn from the distal port or as a continuous reading using a specialized PA catheter. **Oxygen extraction ratio (O$_2$ER)** is the proportion of arterial O$_2$ that is taken up upon delivery to the peripheral tissues.
- **Diagnostic hemodynamic profiles** obtained with a PA catheter are presented in Table 3-5. They are especially useful in diagnosing congestive heart failure

TABLE 3-5	Hemodynamic Profiles for Critical Care Diagnosis					
Condition	**CVP**	**PCWP**	**CI**	**PVRI**	**SVRI**	**RAP**
Right heart failure	↑	nl or ↑	↓	↑	↑	↑
Left heart failure	↔	↑	↓	↑	↑	↔
Hypovolemic hypotension	↓	↓	↓	↔	↑	↓
Cardiogenic hypotension	↑	↑	↓↑	↑	↑	↑
Vasogenic hypotension	↓	↓	↑	↔	↓	↓

↑, increased; ↓, decreased; ↔, no change; ↓↑, either decreased or increased; nl, normal; CVP, central venous pressure; PCWP, pulmonary capillary wedge pressure; CI, cardiac index; PVRI, pulmonary vascular resistance index; SVRI, systemic vascular resistance index; RAP, right atrial pressure. Adapted from Marino PL. *The ICU Book,* 3rd Ed. Philadelphia, PA: Lippincott Williams & Wilkins, 2007.

versus cardiogenic shock and acute respiratory distress syndrome (ARDS) versus cardiogenic pulmonary edema.

RESPIRATORY CRITICAL CARE

Respiratory support is frequently required for critical care patients.
- **Hypoxic respiratory failure** is characterized by decreased arterial partial pressure of oxygen (Pa_{O_2}) <60 mm Hg and/or arterial oxygen saturation (Sa_{O_2}) <90% and is typically associated with tachypnea and hypocapnia. Initially, the Sa_{O_2} may be normal or elevated from baseline.
  - The differential diagnosis includes drug-induced hypoventilation, acute neuromuscular dysfunction, PE, heart failure, congestive obstructive pulmonary disease (COPD), pulmonary edema, pneumonia, atelectasis, and ARDS.
- **Hypercapnic respiratory failure** is characterized by increased arterial partial pressure of carbon dioxide (Pa_{CO_2}) >46 mm Hg and pH <7.35 and is associated with hypoventilation. Sa_{O_2} may be normal.
  - The differential diagnosis includes infection, seizures, overfeeding, shock, chronic neuromuscular disorder, electrolyte abnormalities, cardiac surgery, obesity, and drug-induced respiratory depression. Consider hypercapnia as a cause of hypertension in somnolent, tachycardic postoperative patients who may be overmedicated, and avoid administering additional narcotics.
- A stepwise **evaluation of respiratory failure** (i.e., hypoxemia or hypercapnia) begins with an arterial blood gas and calculation of the alveolar-arteriolar (A-a) oxygen gradient.
  - The **A-a gradient** $= 148 - 1.2(Pa_{CO_2}) - Pa_{O_2}$. It is the difference in the partial pressure of oxygen between the alveolus and the arterial blood, assuming that the patient is breathing room air ($FIO_2 = 0.21\%$ or 21%) at sea level. The **expected A-a gradient** can be estimated using the formula: Age/4 + 4. Supplemental oxygen increases the normal gradient by 5 to 7 mm Hg for every 10% increase in FIO_2.

- ○ *If the A-a gradient is normal/unchanged*, evaluate the maximum inspiratory effort (PI_{max}) for hypoventilation from a central or neuromuscular disorder. PI_{max} is measured by having the patient inspire maximally against a closed valve. For most adults, PI_{max} should be >80 cm H_2O but varies with age and sex. When PI_{max} is <40 mm H_2O, carbon dioxide may be retained, displacing alveolar oxygen.
  - If the PI_{max} is normal, consider drug-induced central hypoventilation.
  - If the PI_{max} is low, consider a neuromuscular cause of hypoventilation.
- ○ *If the A-a gradient is increased with hypoxemia*, measure the mixed venous oxygen pressure (Pv_{O2}) to assess for ventilation-perfusion (V/Q) abnormalities. Pv_{O2} is ideally measured from pulmonary arterial blood using a PA catheter, but superior vena caval blood can be used. Normal values from the pulmonary artery are 35 to 45 mm Hg.
  - If the Pv_{O2} is normal, consider a V/Q abnormality.
    - *V/Q* >1 indicates increased dead space ventilation and occurs with PE, CHF, emphysema, and alveolar overdistension from positive pressure ventilation.
    - *V/Q* <1 indicates intrapulmonary shunt and occurs with asthma, bronchitis, pulmonary edema, pneumonia, and atelectasis.
    - The portion of cardiac output in an intrapulmonary shunt is called the shunt fraction and is normally <10%. Shunt fractions >50% will not improve with oxygen supplementation.
  - If the Pv_{O2} is low, consider an imbalance in oxygen delivery/uptake (D_{O2}/V_{O2}).
    - Evaluate the hemoglobin concentration and cardiac output and optimize to improve oxygen delivery.
- ○ *If the A-a gradient is increased with hypercapnia*, measure the rate of CO_2 production (V_{CO2}) to assess metabolic versus other disorders. V_{CO2} is evaluated by a metabolic cart using infrared light to measure CO_2 in expired gas. Normal V_{CO2} is 90 to 130 mL/min/m^2.
  - If the V_{CO2} is increased, consider overfeeding (especially with carbohydrate load), fever, sepsis, and seizures.
  - If the V_{CO2} is normal, consider increased dead space ventilation (see above) and hypoventilation from respiratory weakness (e.g., shock, multisystem organ failure, prolonged neuromuscular blockade, electrolyte imbalances, cardiac surgery) or central hypoventilation (e.g., opiate or benzodiazepine depression, obesity).

Acute Respiratory Distress Syndrome (ARDS)

- ARDS is a leading cause of acute respiratory failure, resulting from a myriad of inflammatory primary disease processes. The pathophysiology is activation of diffuse pulmonary inflammation and endothelial damage producing inflammatory alveolar exudates, microvascular thrombosis, pulmonary fibrosis, and high mortality rates exceeding 50% to 60%. Predisposing conditions include sepsis, blood product transfusion, aspiration or chemical pneumonitis, pneumonia, pancreatitis, multiple or long bone fractures, intracranial hypertension, cardiopulmonary bypass, and amniotic fluid embolism. Clinically, ARDS is characterized by severe early hypoxemia, normal pulmonary capillary hydrostatic pressures, and diffuse pulmonary inflammatory injury.
  - **Diagnosis** is by clinical criteria: acute onset, predisposing condition, bilateral pulmonary infiltrates on chest radiograph, Pa_{O2}/FIO_2 ratio <200, and PCWP <18 mm Hg. Only careful evaluation distinguishes ARDS from severe pneumonia, PE, and cardiogenic pulmonary edema. ARDS may be confirmed with bronchoalveolar

lavage demonstrating an increased lavage/serum protein ratio (>0.7) and florid neutrophil invasion.

- **Management** of ARDS is essentially supportive. The underlying disorder should be corrected while respiratory support (i.e., mechanical ventilation) is provided. Recent clinical trials have demonstrated the value of low tidal volume (TV) ventilation (<6 mL/kg ideal body weight) with low-level positive end expiratory pressure (PEEP), permissive hypercapnia, and limitation of plateau pressure (<30 mm Hg) to avoid the destructive proinflammatory effects of ventilator-induced barotrauma. Lower Sa_{O_2} (>88%) and Pa_{O_2} (>55 mm Hg) can be tolerated. Protocols for ARDS management can be accessed online at www.ardsnet.org. Steroid treatment (2 to 3 mg methylprednisolone per kg/day) in the later fibroproliferative phase (7 to 14 days after onset) may improve overall survival.

Oxygen Therapy and Ventilators

- **Oxygen therapy** can be used in many patients to improve oxygenation of peripheral tissues but should be applied judiciously. Oxygen can contribute directly to cellular injury and pathophysiology: it increases toxic-free radical metabolites, stimulates peripheral vasoconstriction which decreases systemic blood flow, directly injures pulmonary tissues at high concentrations, and has a negative cardiac inotropic effect which reduces cardiac output. In critically ill patients with depleted antioxidant stores, any FIO_2 >21% (room air) may be toxic. An FIO_2 of >60% for longer than 48 hr can lead to undesirable outcomes, including ARDS. Therefore, oxygen supplementation should only be used when there is evidence or risk of inadequate tissue oxygenation such as Pa_{O_2} <60 mm Hg, venous oxygen saturation <50%, serum lactate >4 mmol/L, or CI <2 L/min/m². Selenium and vitamin E supplementation may help to maintain antioxidant supplies and reduce oxygen toxicity.
- **Oxygen delivery systems** are classified as low flow (e.g., nasal cannula, face mask with and without bags) and high flow. Use the lowest appropriate FIO_2 with the least invasive but effective delivery system as dictated by an individual patient's acute illness and recovery; respiratory treatments should be assessed and optimized frequently.
- **Nasal cannulas** use the patient's oro-nasopharynx as an oxygen reservoir (about 50 mL capacity). A patient with normal ventilation (i.e., TV 500 mL; respiratory rate 20 breaths per minute; inspiratory/expiratory ratio 1:2) increases their FIO_2 by 3% to 4% for each additional volume (L/min) of oxygen flow. The increase in FIO_2 is significantly reduced with hyperventilation when minute ventilation exceeds the system flow rate, and as the oxygen reservoir is drained, the patient inspires only room air. Above the maximum flow rate of 6 L/min, there is no increase in FIO_2 (~45%).
- **Face masks without bags** have an oxygen reservoir of 100 to 200 mL. In order to clear exhaled gases, a minimum flow rate of 5 L/min is required. The maximum flow rate of 10 L/min provides an FIO_2 of 60%.
- **Face masks with bags** have an oxygen reservoir of 600 to 1,000 mL. There are two types of reservoir mask devices:
  ○ A **partial rebreather** has a maximum FIO_2 of 70% to 80%. It "captures" initial exhaled air containing a higher proportion of O_2 from the upper airway (anatomic dead space) in the reservoir bag and releases the terminal exhaled air containing more CO_2. The reservoir bag maintains a high O_2 content.
  ○ A **nonrebreather** has a maximum FIO_2 of 100%. It requires a tight seal during use and can be used to administer nebulizer treatments but does not allow easy oral feeding. The reservoir bag maintains 100% O_2 content.

- **High flow oxygen masks** deliver a constant FIO_2 at a flow rate that exceeds the peak inspiratory rate, preventing the variability seen with low flow systems. They may be useful in patients with chronic hypercapnia who require a constant FIO_2 to avoid increased CO_2 retention. The maximum FIO_2 is 50%.
- **Noninvasive positive pressure ventilation (NIV)** can be a useful alternative to invasive (i.e., endotracheal or tracheostomy) intubation. It has been used to successfully manage obstructive sleep apnea in general medical patients but is also appropriate for critical care patients with moderate respiratory compromise due to mild neuromuscular weakness, congestive heart failure/cardiogenic pulmonary edema, and decompensated COPD. A cooperative patient with no risk for emergent intubation and moderate dyspnea, tachypnea, increased work of breathing, hypercapnia, or hypoxemia can be considered for NIV. Contraindications include cardiac or respiratory arrest or severe cardiopulmonary compromise, coma, status epilepticus, potential airway obstruction, patient inability to protect her airway, and emergent conditions.
  - NIV can be supplied via mouthpiece, nasal pillows, face mask, or helmet; the device must fit properly to avoid air leaks. FIO_2 is titrated to the necessary minimum and the backup rate, pressure support, and PEEP are adjusted to maintain an appropriate TV (5 to 7 mL/kg/breath). Complications with NIV include facial or nasal pressure sores, gastric distension, aspiration, and inspissated uncleared secretions.
  - Randomized trials show a consistent benefit of NIV for moderate-to-severe COPD with hypercapnic respiratory failure; the risk of intubation, complications, mortality and length of hospital stay are reduced. Treatment of CHF with NIV also decreases the rate of intubation. Postextubation NIV is gaining some popularity for early extubation of select patients or as part of the overall approach to weaning from invasive ventilation.
- **Mechanical ventilation** should be instituted for patients who cannot be adequately managed with the systems above, are in respiratory distress, or are at risk for cardiopulmonary collapse. Specific indicators for endotracheal intubation include tachypnea >35 breaths/min; Pa_{O_2} <60 mm Hg; Pa_{CO_2} >46 mm Hg with pH <7.35; absent gag reflex. Standard positive pressure ventilation is delivered with a preset volume-cycled device; additional modes of ventilation such as high frequency and proportional assist ventilation are not discussed here. Selection of ventilation modes is somewhat tailored to the patient, but one mode is not superior to the another and is largely selected by provider preference.
  - In **assist-control ventilation (ACV)**, the patient initiates breaths and the ventilator delivers a set TV. If the patient fails to initiate, the ventilator "assists" at a preset "controlled" rate and TV. Tachypnea is not well tolerated in this mode and can lead to overventilation, respiratory alkalosis, and hyperinflation. Patients with respiratory muscle weakness are appropriately ventilated with ACV.
  - In **intermittent mandatory ventilation (IMV)**, a breath is delivered at a preset rate and volume, but the patient can breathe spontaneously between machine breaths without assistance. In **synchronized IMV**, machine breaths are coordinated with spontaneous respirations to avoid respiratory alkalosis and "stacking" breaths. Asynchronous IMV is not ideal since it can deliver a breath at any time during the patient's spontaneous breaths (i.e., during expiration).
  - In **pressure-controlled ventilation (PCV)**, breaths are delivered at a constant pressure by regulating the inspiratory flow rate throughout each breath. PCV is well suited to patients with neuromuscular disease with stable lung mechanics.

- In **inverse-ratio ventilation (IRV)**, PCV is delivered with a prolonged inspiratory phase. A normal inspiratory:expiratory ratio is 1:2 to 1:4. In IRV, the ratio is reversed to 2:1, which prevents alveolar collapse and provides auto-PEEP, but may lead to reduced cardiac output. The main use of IRV is for ARDS with hypoxemia or hypercapnia that is refractory to conventional ventilation modes.
  - In **pressure support ventilation** (PSV), the patient breathes spontaneously and the machine adds extra support to maintain inspiratory pressures. It is a common weaning mode of ventilation.
- **Ventilator management** is a continuous and dynamic process, ideally leading to weaning from mechanical ventilation and extubation. The following basic parameters can be adjusted: mode, FIO_2, TV, PEEP, and pressure support.
  - **FIO_2** is initially set to 100% and then titrated to the minimum needed to maintain Pa_{O_2} above 60 mm Hg or Sa_{O_2} above 90%. Although oxygen can be toxic, in acute respiratory distress, treatment of hypoxemia takes precedence.
  - Normal **minute ventilation** (respiratory rate × TV) is 6 to 8 L/min. Infection, inflammation, and acid-base disorders can effect large variation in the required ventilation.
  - PEEP is the positive airway pressure at the end of respiration (i.e., alveolar pressure higher than atmospheric pressure) that prevents alveolar collapse.
    - **Extrinsic PEEP** is created by a device that stops exhalation at a preselected pressure. PEEP reduces the risk of oxygen toxicity by improving gas exchange, increasing lung compliance, and increasing the Pa_{O_2} which allows reduced FIO_2.
    - **Intrinsic PEEP** (auto-PEEP) is created by increasing minute ventilation or shortening the expiratory phase. It is common in patients with prolonged expiration such as during an asthma exacerbation.
    - PEEP can progress to the point of sudden cardiovascular collapse; elevated auto-PEEP requires immediate disconnection from the ventilator to allow the patient to fully exhale. This may take 30 to 60 seconds, but it is life saving.
- **Weaning from mechanical ventilation** is the gradual process of reducing ventilation to minimum settings (i.e., FIO_2 <50%, IMV, with PEEP and pressure support <5 cm H_2O each) or T-piece ventilation, followed by extubation. Duration of mechanical ventilation is directly related to complications, so extubation should be performed as soon as feasible. A daily sedation break and spontaneous breathing trial should be performed on all eligible patients. Criteria for extubation include progressive clinical recovery from illness; intact neurologic status (i.e., alert, oriented) with ability to follow commands; patent airway without concern for occlusion (see cuff test, below); and normal arterial blood gas on minimal supplemental oxygen.
  - Assessment of airway patency and **respiration mechanics** helps assess whether a patient is ready for extubation. Patients who cannot meet minimum criteria or are neurologically impaired and unable to cooperate with the evaluation may not be ready for unassisted respiration.
    - The **"cuff test"** can be used to assess the airway. The endotracheal tube cuff is deflated and the patient is asked to breathe while the tube is occluded. A normal upper airway with an appropriately sized tube will permit breaths both in and out around the tube. Extubation may need to be deferred for patients with abnormal findings.
    - **Forced vital capacity** should be at least 10 mL/kg and is typically at least 1,000 mL. Measurement can vary widely depending on technique and on patient effort.

- **Negative inspiratory force (NIF)** should be −25 to −30 cm H_2O. When performed as an "occlusion NIF," the test is not effort dependent. A normal person can generate NIF of −80 cm H_2O.
- **Rapid shallow breathing index (RSBI or Tobin index)** should be <80 and predicts the patient's ability to remain extubated for 24 hr. It is measured by switching from any ventilator mode to continuous positive airway pressure and assessing the patient's respiratory rate (f) and TV over 1 minute. The RSBI = f/TV.
  • Patients with RSBI <80 are eight- to ninefold more likely to remain extubated.
  • Patients with RSBI >100 are eight- to ninefold more likely to require reintubation.
  • Patients with RSBI between 80 and 100 require clinical judgment regarding suitable timing for extubation.
- After extubation, **secretions** should be cleared and humidified oxygen should be supplied by face mask. The patient should be encouraged to cough and breathe deeply at regular intervals. If reintubation is necessary, perform a complete assessment of the reasons for failure and attempt extubation again within 24 to 72 hr.

FLUIDS AND ELECTROLYTES

Fluid and electrolyte disorders are common for critically ill patients and for women with obstetric morbidity or undergoing major gynecologic surgery. Some of the most common issues are addressed here.
• **Maintenance fluid** for patients with no oral intake (and without preexisting renal, water metabolism, or electrolyte dysfunction) can be calculated using the "4-2-1 rule."
  • For the first 10 kg of weight, 4 mL/kg/hr (40 mL/hr) of IV fluid is given.
  • For the next 10 kg of weight, 2 mL/kg/hr (20 mL/hr) of IV fluid is given.
  • For each kg of weight after 20 kg, an additional 1 mL/kg/hr is given.
  • Although 0.25% normal saline with 20 mEq KCl/L and 5% dextrose is a technically correct maintenance fluid, surgical stress causes near universal hyponatremia if hypotonic fluid is used, especially in gynecologic surgery patients. Therefore, one-half normal saline with 20 mEq KCl is usually selected and typically administered at 125 mL/hr.
  • Fluids removed by nasogastric suction should be replaced 1:1 with half normal saline.
• **Hyponatremia** is defined as serum sodium <136 mEq/L. It is the most common disorder occurring in critically ill patients. It can be classified on the basis of volume status and further diagnosed with urine sodium and osmolality (Fig. 3-1). Management includes treating the underlying condition and replacing the sodium deficit if present.
  • Rapid **correction of chronic or severe hyponatremia** can cause cerebral edema and increased intracranial pressure leading to a demyelinating encephalopathy or central pontine myelinolysis. Calculate the total body water (TBW), sodium deficit, and infusion rate to correct the plasma sodium (P_{Na}) to 130 mEq/L for symptomatic patients as follows:
    ○ TBW in L = 50% lean body weight (kg) in women.
    ○ Sodium deficit in mEq = TBW × [130 − (current P_{Na})].
    ○ Hypertonic saline (3% NaCl = 513 mEq Na/L) needed to correct the calculated sodium deficit = sodium deficit/513 mEq/L.

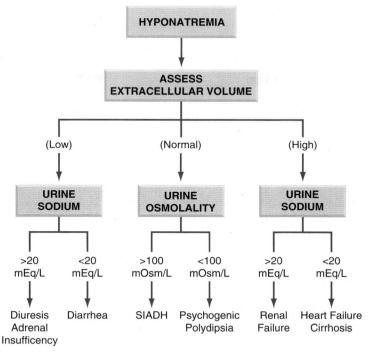

Figure 3-1. Classification and diagnosis of hyponatremia. SIADH, syndrome of inappropriate antidiuretic hormone secretion. (From Marino PL. *The ICU Book*, 3rd Ed. Philadelphia, PA: Lippincott Williams & Wilkins, 2007;606, with permission.)

- ○ Infusion rate should be adjusted to correct P_{Na} no more than 0.5 mEq/L/hr.
- ○ Hours to correct the hyponatremia = [130 mEq/L – (current P_{Na})]/0.5 hr.
- ○ Fluid infusion rate (mL/hr) = volume hypertonic saline needed/number hours needed.
    - For example, a 60-kg woman with a sodium level of 120 mEq/L has a calculated sodium deficit of 300 mEq that should be corrected by total infusion of 585 mL of 3% NaCl over 20 hr at a rate of 29 mL/hr.
- **Hypernatremia** is defined as serum sodium higher than 145 mEq/L. It reflects a relative deficiency of free water as occurs with vomiting, diarrhea, overdiuresis, diabetes mellitus with nonketotic hyperglycemia, and diabetes insipidus (see Chapter 13). Iatrogenic hypernatremia from hypertonic saline or sodium bicarbonate infusion is also possible. Clinical findings can vary from tachycardia and decreased urine output to encephalopathy, seizures, and coma.
    - **Management** is generally directed toward volume replacement with crystalloid or colloid and maintenance of cardiac output. It is based on accurate assessment of extracellular volume by invasive monitoring or clinical evaluation.
        - ○ **Hypovolemic hypernatremia** requires correction of plasma volume and total sodium deficit quickly, followed by gradual replacement of TBW over 48 to 72 hr.

- The free water deficit should be calculated and replaced at a rate that lowers serum sodium no more than 0.5 mEq/L/hr, in order to avoid cerebral edema.
  ○ **Euvolemic hypernatremia** is treated with isotonic saline to slowly replace the water deficit.
  ○ **Hypervolemic hypernatremia** will be corrected by the kidneys via renal sodium excretion. In some cases, diuresis may be helpful but care must be taken to avoid hypovolemia and exacerbating the problem.
- **Hypokalemia** is defined as serum potassium <3.5 mEq/L. It can be caused by artifactual dilution (i.e., drawn near an IV infusion site), decreased potassium intake, insufficient replacement of NG tube output, diuretic therapy, diarrhea, and laxative abuse.
  - **Clinical findings** of severe hypokalemia include muscle weakness and mental status changes. ECG changes can be seen, such as flattened T waves, prolonged QT intervals, and U waves. Chronic hypokalemia can result in renal tubular disorders with concentrating abnormalities, phosphaturia, and azotemia.
  - **Management** includes correcting the underlying cause (e.g., alkalosis) and replacing the potassium deficit. Typically, potassium repletion is not an emergency, except in the most severe cases with active arrhythmias or in patients who are on digoxin therapy. Bring the potassium level to 4 mEq/L.
    ○ For each 10 mEq oral or IV KCl, the serum potassium rises by about 1 mEq/L if there is no significant total body potassium deficit to restore.
    ○ Rapid increases in serum potassium can predispose to cardiac arrest, so the maximum rate of IV KCl infusion is 20 mEq/L via central catheter or 10 mEq/L via peripheral IV. The KCl solution is extremely hyperosmotic so should be diluted before infusion.
    ○ Hypomagnesemia can cause refractory hypokalemia and should be replaced along with potassium. Serum magnesium levels are not generally helpful unless the patient is receiving magnesium infusion (e.g., for preeclampsia) or the patient has impaired renal function.
    ○ Patients with significant kidney disease (i.e., GFR <25 mL/min) should have potassium therapy titrated using serial serum potassium levels. Patients taking potassium-sparing diuretics may also require close monitoring.
- **Hyperkalemia** is defined as serum potassium higher than 5.0 mEq/L. It is not as well tolerated as hypokalemia and can be life threatening. It can be caused by laboratory artifact (i.e., hemolyzed specimen), cellular redistribution associated with acidosis (e.g., diabetic ketoacidosis, sepsis), renal insufficiency, adrenal insufficiency, and tissue injury (e.g., hemolysis, rhabdomyolysis, crush injury, burns).
  - **Clinical findings** in the majority of patients are unimpressive. ECG changes are seen when serum potassium approaches 6 mEq/L; the earliest findings include peaked T waves, especially in precordial leads, flattened P waves, and prolonged PR intervals. This progresses to absent P waves, wide QRS complexes, and ultimately ventricular fibrillation and asystole.
  - **Management** in an asymptomatic patient with unexpected hyperkalemia starts with repeating the measurement and discontinuing any potassium supplementation. If the abnormal value is confirmed, acute management is guided by serum potassium and ECG findings, if any (Table 3-6).
- **Hypocalcemia** is defined as total serum calcium lower than 8.5 mg/dL or ionized serum calcium lower than 1.1 mmol/L. A "normal" plasma calcium is lower in patients with hypoalbuminemia, due to decreased protein binding. Causes of hypocalcemia include hypoparathyroidism, hypomagnesemia, alkalosis, blood

TABLE 3-6   Management of Hyperkalemia

Clinical Condition	Treatment	Warnings and Notes
K <6 mEq/L and no ECG changes	Treat underlying cause and monitor K levels and ECG changes.	
K 6–7 mEq/L and no ECG findings *Or* after acute treatment	30 g sodium polystyrene sulfonate (Kayexalate) orally in 50 mL 20% sorbitol.	Rectal administration can result in rare cases of colon necrosis; therefore, Kayexalate enema is *never* recommended.
K >7 mEq/L *Or* ECG findings with any hyperkalemia	10 mL calcium gluconate (10%) IV in 3 min. Repeat in 15–30 min. 10 U regular insulin in 500 mL 20% dextrose infused over 1 hr. 44–88 mEq sodium bicarbonate IV. 20 mg furosemide IV.	Calcium stabilizes myocardium, but response lasts only 20–30 min. Insulin/glucose facilitates K movement into cellular compartment; reduces serum K by 1 mEq/L for 1 to 2 hr. Do not give with calcium or calcium carbonate precipitate may result. Diuresis can enhance urinary K excretion.
Hyperkalemia with ECG changes and circulatory compromise	10 mL calcium chloride (10%) IV in 3 min.	$CaCl_2$ contains three times more elemental calcium per gram than calcium gluconate.
AV block refractory to calcium treatment	Insulin and dextrose, as above. Transvenous pacemaker.	
Digitalis cardiotoxicity	2 g magnesium sulfate IV bolus. Administer antidigitalis Fab antibodies.	Do not administer calcium for hyperkalemia of digitalis toxicity.
Renal failure with hyperkalemia	Urgent hemodialysis.	The most effective treatment for severe hyperkalemia with minimal renal function is dialysis.

K, potassium; AV, atrioventricular. Adapted from Marino PL. *The ICU Book*, 3rd Ed. Philadelphia, PA: Lippincott Williams & Wilkins, 2007:620; and Hollander-Rodriguez JC, Calvert JF. Hyperkalemia. *Am Fam Physician.* 2006;73:283–290.

transfusion, chronic renal failure, pancreatitis, some drugs (e.g., aminoglycosides, heparin), and sepsis.

- **Clinical findings** include hyperreflexia, paresthesias, tetany, seizures, hypotension, cardiac arrhythmias, heart block, and ventricular tachycardia.
- **Management** is directed toward diagnosis and correction of the underlying condition. Symptomatic hypocalcemia or ionized calcium <0.65 mmol/L should be immediately corrected with calcium chloride or calcium gluconate IV, preferably through a central vein.
- **Hypercalcemia** is defined as total serum calcium higher than 10.5 mg/dL or ionized serum calcium higher than 1.3 mmol/L. In 90% of cases the underlying cause is hyperparathyroidism or malignancy; severe hypercalcemia (i.e., total calcium >14 mg/dL or ionized calcium >3.5 mmol/L) is associated with neoplasm. Other causes include thyrotoxicosis, thiazide diuretics, and lithium treatment. The most common mechanism of hypercalcemia in gynecologic oncology patients is increased osteoclastic bone resorption without direct bone metastases.
  - **Clinical findings** are nonspecific, but can include gastrointestinal (e.g., nausea, constipation, ileus, abdominal pain, pancreatitis), cardiovascular (e.g., hypovolemia, hypotension, hypertension, shortened QT interval), renal (e.g., polyuria, nephrolithiasis), and neurologic (e.g., lethargy, confusion, coma) abnormalities. Symptoms are usually present when total serum calcium exceeds 12 mg/dL.
  - **Acute management** aims to increase excretion and storage of calcium and adjust the ionized level closer to a physiologic concentration.
    - Hydration with **isotonic saline** promotes renal natiuresis and thereby increases calcium excretion.
    - Diuresis with **furosemide** (40 to 80 mg IV every 2 hr) with a goal of 100 to 200 mL urine output per hour further promotes urinary calcium excretion. Urine output, stimulated by hydration or pharmacologic diuresis, should be replaced with isotonic saline to prevent hypovolemia.
    - **Calcitonin** (salmon calcitonin 4 U/kg SQ or IM every 12 hr) rapidly inhibits bone resorption and may decrease serum calcium levels, though the effect is not profound.
    - **Hydrocortisone** (200 mg IV daily divided into three doses) inhibits some lymphoid neoplastic growth, decreasing bone calcium release.
    - **Pamidronate disodium** (90 mg IV over 2 hr) or zoledronate are effective for severe hypercalcemia, with peak effect in 2 to 4 days.
    - **Dialysis** is appropriate for patients with severe renal failure.

Acid-Base Disorders

- **Evaluation of acid-base disorders** requires arterial blood gas interpretation and should be considered within the entire clinical picture. A stepwise approach for basic analysis is outlined here (see Table 3-7).
  - First, **assess the pH and Pa_{CO_2}**. If either the pH or Pa_{CO_2} is abnormal, a disorder is present.
    - A primary metabolic disorder is present if the pH is abnormal and changes in pH and Pa_{CO_2} are in the same direction.
      - In **primary metabolic acidosis**, the pH is <7.36 and the Pa_{CO_2} is decreased. The primary defect is decreased bicarbonate.
      - In **primary metabolic alkalosis**, the pH is higher than 7.44 and the Pa_{CO_2} is increased. The primary defect is increased bicarbonate.

TABLE 3-7	Normal Values and Expected Changes in Various Acid-Base Disorders

Primary Disorder	Expected Result
Metabolic acidosis	Expected $Pa_{CO_2} = (1.5 \times HCO_3) + (8 \pm 2)$
Metabolic alkalosis	Expected $Pa_{CO_2} = (0.7 \times HCO_3) + (21 \pm 2)$
Acute respiratory acidosis	$\Delta pH = 0.008 \times \Delta Pa_{CO_2}$
	Expected $pH = 7.40 - [0.008 \times (Pa_{CO_2} - 40)]$
Acute respiratory alkalosis	$\Delta pH = 0.008 \times \Delta Pa_{CO_2}$
	Expected $pH = 7.40 + [0.008 \times (40 - Pa_{CO_2})]$
Chronic respiratory acidosis	$\Delta pH = 0.003 \times \Delta Pa_{CO_2}$
	Expected $pH = 7.40 - [0.003 \times (Pa_{CO_2} - 40)]$
Chronic respiratory alkalosis	$\Delta pH = 0.003 \times \Delta Pa_{CO_2}$
	Expected $pH = 7.40 - [0.003 \times (40 - Pa_{CO_2})]$

Normal values: pH = 7.36–7.44; P_{CO_2} = 36–44 mm Hg; HCO_3 = 22–26 mEq/L
Normal in
pregnancy: pH = 7.40–7.45; P_{CO_2} = 27–32 mm Hg; HCO_3 = 19–25 mEq/L

ΔpH, change in arterial pH; ΔPa_{CO_2}, change in arterial CO_2; HCO_3, serum bicarbonate. Adapted from Marino PL. *The ICU Book*, 3rd Ed. Philadelphia, PA: Lippincott Williams & Wilkins, 2007:535.

- A primary respiratory disorder is present if the Pa_{CO_2} is abnormal and changes in pH and Pa_{CO_2} are in opposite directions.
    - In **primary respiratory acidosis**, the Pa_{CO_2} is higher than 44 mm Hg and the pH is decreased. The primary defect is increased Pa_{CO_2}.
    - In **primary respiratory alkalosis**, the Pa_{CO_2} is <36 mm Hg and the pH is increased. The primary defect is decreased Pa_{CO_2}.
- A mixed disorder is present if either the pH or the Pa_{CO_2} is normal. Compensatory responses never completely correct the primary acid-base disturbance, so equal and opposite processes are occurring.
- Next determine the compensatory response to a primary acid-base disorder.
    - If there is a primary metabolic acidosis or alkalosis, determine the expected Pa_{CO_2} (see Table 3-7) and compare with the measured Pa_{CO_2}.
        - If the measured and expected Pa_{CO_2} are equal, the disorder is **fully compensated**.
        - If the measured Pa_{CO_2} is higher than expected, there is a **superimposed respiratory acidosis**.
        - If the measured Pa_{CO_2} is lower than expected, there is a **superimposed respiratory alkalosis**.
    - If there is a primary respiratory acidosis or alkalosis, determine the expected pH (see Table 3-7) and compare with the measured pH.
        - In *acute (uncompensated) respiratory acidosis* or *alkalosis,* the change in pH is 0.008 times the change in P_{CO_2}.
        - In *chronic (fully compensated) respiratory acidosis* or *alkalosis,* the change in pH is 0.003 times the change in P_{CO_2}.

- In *partially compensated respiratory acidosis or alkalosis*, the change in pH is 0.003 to 0.008 times the change in P_{CO_2}.
- If the change in pH is more than 0.008 times the change in P_{CO_2}, then a superimposed metabolic disorder is present (i.e., *a superimposed metabolic acidosis in the setting of a primary respiratory acidosis*).

- Finally, calculate the anion gap to help diagnose a metabolic acidosis using the formula anion gap = $[Na^+ + K^+] - [Cl^- + HCO_3^-]$ (normal range is 10 to 14 mEq/L).
  - **Causes of normal anion gap acidosis** (mnemonic **USEDCAR**) include: **U**rinary diversion (ureterosigmoidostomy), **S**aline administration (in the face of renal dysfunction), **E**ndocrine disorder (Addison's disease; primary hyperparathyroidism), **D**iarrhea/**D**rugs (spironolactone, triamterene, amiloride, amphotericin), **C**arbonic anhydrase inhibitors (acetazolamide, methazolamide, topiramate), **A**mmonium chloride/hyper**A**limentation, and **R**enal tubular acidosis.
  - **Causes of increased anion gap acidosis** (mnemonic **MUDPILES**) include: **M**ethanol, **U**remia, **D**iabetes (ketoacidosis)/**D**rugs (metformin), **P**araldehyde, **I**soniazid/**I**nfection/**I**schemia, **L**actic acidosis, **E**thylene glycol, **S**alicylates/**S**tarvation.
- **Treatment** is based on the severity and diagnosis. Typically is it only necessary to treat the underlying cause(s). In patients with profound disturbances (i.e., pH <7.2 or bicarbonate levels <10 mEq/L), bicarbonate infusion may be warranted.

Renal Function

Oliguria is frequently encountered in patients with critical illness and after surgery. A traditional definition is <400 mL urine output per 24 hr, but more convenient hourly calculations are usually used.

- **Minimum adequate urine output** should be 0.5 mL/kg ideal body weight per hour; clinicians often use 25 to 30 mL/hr as a routine approximation.
  - **Ideal body weight** for women = 45 kg + (2.3 kg/inch × height above 5 feet in inches).
- **Acute oliguric renal failure** (AORF) is classified by the RIFLE criteria, determined from lab values and estimated GFR calculated from the MDRD equation (Modified Diet in Renal Disease; calculator online http://www.nkdep.nih.gov/professionals/gfr_calculators). The severity of renal failure correlates well with overall mortality.
  - **R**isk = Serum creatinine increased 1.5-fold *OR* GFR decreased 25% *OR* urine output <0.5 mL/kg/hr × 6 hr.
  - **I**njury = Serum creatinine increased 2.0-fold *OR* GFR decreased 50% *OR* urine output <0.5 mL/kg/hr × 12 hr.
  - **F**ailure = Serum creatinine acutely increased >0.5 mg/dL to ≥4 mg/dL or increased 3.0-fold above baseline *OR* GFR decreased 75% *OR* urine output <0.3 mL/kg/hr × 24 hr *OR* anuria for 12 hr.
  - **L**oss = Persistent AORF with loss of renal function for >4 weeks.
  - **E**nd-stage kidney disease = Loss of renal function for >3 months.
- The **differential diagnosis** of AORF is classified anatomically.
  - A **prerenal disorder** causing decreased kidney perfusion is the etiology in approximately 40% of AORF cases. In gynecology, the most common causes are volume depletion from hemorrhage, third-spacing of fluids (e.g., with preeclampsia), or inadequate fluid resuscitation. Other common causes include hypotension, heart failure, renal vasoconstriction (e.g., from NSAIDs), and reduced glomerular filtration pressure (e.g., from ACE inhibitors).

- ○ A prerenal disorder is suggested by elevated urine specific gravity, decreased fractional excretion of sodium (FE_{Na}) of <1%, blood, BUN:creatinine ratio >20, and urine sodium <20 mEq/L.
- ○ An **intrinsic renal disorder** from direct injury/dysfunction of the kidney is the etiology in up to 50% of AORF cases in ICU patients. Causes include ischemia/hypoperfusion injury, inflammation, sepsis, radiocontrast dye, myoglobinuria, and other drugs/toxins. These can result in three types of renal pathology: acute tubular necrosis (ATN), acute glomerulonephritis, and acute interstitial nephritis.
  - **ATN** is the most common cause of intrinsic renal dysfunction, resulting from sepsis, shock, and toxins (e.g., contrast dye, aminoglycosides, amphotericin, cyclosporin, tacrolimus, cisplatin, acyclovir, sulfa drugs, pigments, uric acid). The renal tubules and parenchyma are damaged but glomeruli are usually intact. Injured tubular epithelial cells are shed, blocking the proximal tubular lumen and reducing net GFR.
  - ATN is suggested by FE_{Na} >2%, fractional excretion of urea >50%, urine sodium > 40 mmol/L, urine osmolarity <350 mOsm/L, and granular casts on microscopy.
- ○ A **postrenal disorder** results from obstruction of the urinary tract distal to the kidney and rarely leads to oliguria unless there is a single kidney or the condition is bilateral (e.g., advanced cervical cancer). The obstruction may occur in the collecting system (e.g., papillary necrosis), ureters (e.g., compression, calculus, tumor, papillary sloughing, clot/hematoma), bladder (e.g., calculus, neurogenic bladder, carcinoma, clot/hematoma), and urethra (e.g., calculus, stricture, clot/hematoma). Assessment includes bladder catheterization, urinary tract ultrasound/imaging, and laboratory evaluation for prerenal and intrarenal diseases. Early treatment can prevent permanent kidney damage. Significant postobstructive diuresis occurs with resolution of bilateral obstruction, leading to electrolyte abnormalities and volume contraction. Decompression of an overly distended bladder can reveal capillary bleeding with hematuria or even frank hemorrhage.
- **Clinical assessment** of the patient with oliguria is the first step in diagnosis.
  - Assess for mechanical problems with the urinary drainage (e.g., displaced bulb, obstruction that may be cleared by flushing the catheter). Consider an overfilled bladder (from catheter obstruction or postoperative urinary retention) in patients with postoperative hypertension.
  - Evaluate signs and symptoms that suggest hypovolemia (e.g., dizziness, chest pain, shortness of breath, palpitations, tachycardia, orthostatic hypotension), infection (e.g., fever, focal infection), and obstruction (e.g., pain, bloating, hypertension).
  - Calculate total fluid input and output. Oliguria with a negative fluid balance (input < output) may suggest hypovolemia. Oliguria with a positive fluid balance (input > output) may suggest cardiac dysfunction, massive third spacing of fluid, or postrenal obstruction. Serum and urine laboratory testing should be performed before initiating therapy if possible.
- **Laboratory assessment** of renal function is based upon patient history and clinical findings.
  - The **urine specific gravity** (range: 1.003 to 1.030) is elevated in the setting of dehydration, reflecting the concentrating ability of the kidney. False elevations can occur with mannitol, glucose, and radiocontrast dye.
  - **Urine microscopy** helps distinguish intrinsic disorders; it is not useful for prerenal diagnoses. Tubular epithelial cells and granular casts are pathognomonic for ATN. Leukocyte casts suggest interstitial nephritis (pyelonephritis). Red cell casts suggest glomerulonephritis. Pigmented casts suggest myoglobinuria. Sloughed

papillae from papillary necrosis may be seen in postrenal disorders involving the renal collecting system.
- A **24-hr urine specimen** is collected by discarding the first void and then collecting all subsequent voids for 24 hr. The specimen should be refrigerated throughout collection.
- The **urine sodium level (urine$_{Na}$)** is best assessed with a 24-hr urine specimen, but a random 10 mL specimen may also be used. Urine$_{Na}$ <20 mEq/L suggests a prerenal disorder; renal hypoperfusion leads to increased sodium reabsorption and decreased excretion. Urine$_{Na}$ >40 mEq/L suggests impaired sodium reabsorption from an intrinsic renal disorder, though it does not rule out coexisting prerenal disorders and may not be useful if diuretics have been administered or in elderly patients with obligatory urinary sodium loss.
  - Fractional excretion of sodium (FE$_{Na}$) is the fraction of sodium filtered at the glomerulus that is ultimately excreted in the urine. It is normally <1%. Calculation of this value in the setting of oliguria is one of the most reliable tests for distinguishing prerenal causes from intrarenal causes of AORF.
  - Urine sodium (urine$_{Na}$) and creatinine (urine$_{Cr}$) are measured in a random urine specimen at the same time that a blood sample is taken for sodium (plasma$_{Na}$) and creatinine (plasma$_{Cr}$) levels.
  - FE$_{Na}$ is calculated by the formula:

$$[(Urine_{Na}/plasma_{Na})/(urine_{Cr}/plasma_{Cr})] \times 100$$

  - FE$_{Na}$ <1% suggests a prerenal disorder and a FE$_{Na}$ >2% suggests an intrinsic renal disorder. It is not a useful test for nonoliguric renal dysfunction.
- **Fractional excretion of urea (FE$_{urea}$)** may be useful in patients on diuretics; urea transport is not altered. It is calculated from urine and blood using the formula:

$$[(Urine_{urea}/Plasma_{urea})/(Urine_{urea}/Plasma_{urea})] \times 100$$

A value <35% indicates prerenal disorders, while FE$_{urea}$ >50% suggests an intrarenal cause.
- **Creatinine clearance (Cl$_{Cr}$)** is best assessed with a 24-hr urine collection. The formula is:

$$Cl_{Cr} \text{ (mL/min)} = [Cr_{urine} \text{ (mg/dL)} \times \text{volume of urine (mL)}]/[Cr_{serum} \text{ (mg/dL)} \times \text{time (min)}]$$

where Cr$_{urine}$ and Cr$_{serum}$ are the urine and serum creatinine level, respectively. Normal Cl$_{Cr}$ for women is 72 to 110 mL/min at our institution. Renal impairment is considered at a Cl$_{Cr}$ level of 50 to 70 mL/min, renal insufficiency at a level of 20 to 50 mL/min, and renal failure at a level of 4 to 20 mL/min. Note that serum creatinine level of 1.2 mg/dL in a pregnant patient indicates >50% reduction in GFR.
- **Management** of acute oliguria should optimize central hemodynamics and increase glomerulotubular flow.
  - In patients with invasive hemodynamic monitoring, base the management on cardiac filling pressures (CVP and PCWP), cardiac output (using CI), and blood pressure (BP).
  - If CVP is <4 mm Hg and PCWP is <8 mm Hg, volume should be infused to reach CVP of 6 to 8 mm Hg and PCWP of 12 to 15 mm Hg.
    - The goal for CI is >3 L/min/m^2. If cardiac output is low, volume should be infused until CVP is 10 to 12 mm Hg and PCWP is near 20 mm Hg. If cardiac output remains low, inotropic support is indicated.

◦ If BP is normal, dobutamine infusion starting at 5 mg/kg/min can be initiated to improve inotropy. If BP is low, dopamine starting at 5 mg/kg/min can be initiated for inotropic and pressure support (see Table 3-3).

◦ If oliguria persists after these measures, the cause is probably an intrinsic disorder.

◦ There is no evidence that low "renal dose" dopamine or furosemide treatments are beneficial. Dopamine may increase risk for bowel ischemia.

◦ Furosemide drip (1 to 9 mg/hr) may be more helpful to remove fluid than boluses in patients with CHF or borderline low BP. The diuretic may assist in fluid management but will not influence the outcome of renal failure and may merely convert oliguric renal failure to nonoliguric renal failure.

• Rarely, a "lasix-dependent" patient is encountered who requires diuretic to maintain adequate urine output. This is very uncommon, however, and most postoperative patients with oliguria are simply hypovolemic. Volume status and cardiac output should be optimized before proceeding with pharmacologic management.

• Special attention should be given to urine output in postoperative gynecologic oncology patients who have had malignant ascites removed. The fluid tends to reaccumulate in the abdominal cavity quickly after drainage and may require massive ongoing fluid replacement.

SUGGESTED READINGS

American Society of Anesthesiologists Task Force on Pulmonary Artery Catheterization. Practice guidelines for pulmonary artery catheterization: an updated report. *Anesthesiology* 2004;99:988–1014.

Centers for Disease Control and Prevention. Guideline for Hand Hygiene in Healthcare Settings: Recommendations of the Healthcare Infection Control Practices Advisory Committee and the HICPAC/SHEA/APIC/IDSA Hand Hygiene Task Force. *Morb Mortal Wkly Rep* 2002;51 (No. RR-16).

De Backer D, Biston P, Devriendt J, et al. Comparison of dopamine and norepinephrine in the treatment of shock. *N Engl J Med* 2010;362(9):779–789.

Devereaux PJ, Beattie WS, Choi PTL, et al. How strong is the evidence for the use of perioperative beta blockers in non-cardiac surgery? Systematic review and meta-analysis of randomised controlled trials. *Br Med J* 2005; doi:10.1136/bmj.38503.623646.8F.

Fan E, Needham DM, Stewart TE. Ventilator management of acute lung injury and acute respiratory distress syndrome. *JAMA.* 2005; 294: 2889–2896.

Ricci Z, Cruz D, Ronco C. The RIFLE criteria and mortality in acute kidney injury: A systematic review. *Kidney Int* 2008;73(5):538–546.

Shafiee MAS, Bohn D, Hoorn EJ, et al. How to select optimal maintenance intravenous fluid therapy. *Q J Med* 2003;96:601–610.

The National Heart, Lung, and Blood Institute ARDS Clinical Network. Higher versus lower positive end-expiratory pressures in patients with acute respiratory distress syndrome. *N Engl J Med* 2004;351:327–336.

The Safe Study Investigators. A comparison of albumin and saline for fluid resuscitation in the intensive care unit. *N Engl J Med* 2004;350:2247–2256.

Yeomans ER, Gilstrap LC. Physiologic changes in pregnancy and their impact on critical care. *Crit Care Med* 2005;33(10; suppl):S256–S258.

Zeeman GG. Obstetric critical care: a blueprint for improved outcomes. *Crit Care Med* 2006;34(9 Suppl):S208–S214.

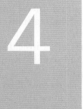

4 Preconception Counseling and Prenatal Care

Jessica B. Russell, Elizabeth Wood Denne, and David Schwartz

PRECONCEPTION CARE AND COUNSELING

Preconception care and counseling are important because they may identify women who can benefit from early intervention and may help to reduce birth defects. This education and planning can be incorporated into any visit with a woman of child-bearing age. The risk of major birth defects in the general population is about 3%. Optimizing maternal health and nutritional status prior to pregnancy and early in gestation is important because organogenesis begins just 17 days after fertilization. The following areas may be addressed in preconception care.

Reproductive History
- Diagnosis and treatment of conditions such as genital infections, maternal medical disease, and uterine malformations may lessen the risk of recurrent pregnancy loss. Recording the menstrual history provides an opportunity to evaluate a woman's knowledge of menstrual physiology and offer counseling about how she might plan a pregnancy.

Family History
- **Carrier screening** for hereditary disease is based on family history or the ethnic background of the couple and allows counseling before the first potentially affected pregnancy. Early recognition of carrier status informs patients of their risks outside of the emotional context of pregnancy, and facilitates educated decisions about reproductive goals and a plan for testing during or after pregnancy (see Table 4-1 for carrier screening guidelines).
- **Genetic disease testing.** Screening can suggest increased risks for specific diseases, such as Muscular dystrophy, Fragile X syndrome, or Down syndrome, for which genetic counseling should be offered. Information about diagnostic tests, such as chorionic villus sampling (CVS) or amniocentesis can be explained. In some instances, genetic counseling may result in a decision to forgo pregnancy or to use assisted reproductive technologies that can obviate risk.

Medical Assessment (Table 4-2)
Preconception care should include an assessment of medical problems and risks, for both fetus and mother. Obtaining consultation and ongoing close collaboration with other specialists may be indicated. General risk assessment includes the following:

TABLE 4-1   **Recommendations for Ethnicity-Based Carrier Screening**

Disease	Carrier Frequency
Ashkenazi Jewish	
Tay-Sachs	1/30
Canavan	1/40
Cystic fibrosis	1/29
Familial dysautonomia	1/30
Mediterranean	
Thalassemia	1/20–1/50
Sickle cell anemia	1/30–1/50
European Caucasian	
Cystic fibrosis	1/25–1/29
African American	
Sickle cell anemia	1/10
Thalassemia	1/30–1/75
Cystic fibrosis	1/65
Asian	
Thalassemia	1/20–1/50
Cystic fibrosis	1/90
Hispanic	
Cystic fibrosis	1/46
Sickle cell anemia	1/30–1/200
Thalassemia	1/30–1/75
French Canadian	
Tay-Sachs	1/15
Cystic fibrosis	1/29

- **Infectious disease screening**
  - Preconception screening for anti-rubella IgG identifies **Rubella** nonimmune women who should then be offered vaccination. No case of congenital rubella syndrome has ever been reported after rubella immunization within 3 months before or after conception.
  - Universal screening of pregnant women for **Hepatitis B virus (HBV)** has been recommended by the Centers for Disease Control and Prevention since 1988. Women with social or occupational risks for exposure to HBV should be counseled and offered vaccination.
  - Patients at risk for **tuberculosis** should be tested with subcutaneous purified protein derivative (PPD) challenge; if the patient has a history of bacillus Calmette-Guerin (BCG) vaccination, the PPD screen should still be used unless they have known positive skin testing. Preconception treatment for latent TB infection can be ordered as indicated.
  - **Cytomegalovirus (CMV)** screening should be offered to women who work in neonatal ICUs, child care facilities, or dialysis units.
  - **Parvovirus B19** IgG testing may be offered preconceptually to school teachers and child care workers.

TABLE 4-2	Preconception Risk Assessment: Laboratory Testing
Recommended for All Women	**Recommended for Some Women**

Hemoglobin level or hematocrit
Rh factor
Rubella factor
Urine dipstick testing (protein
  and sugar)
Pap smear test (for cervical cancer)
Gonococcal/chlamydial screen
Syphilis test
HBV screen
HIV screen
Illicit drug screen (offer)
	Tuberculosis screen
	Rubella IgG screen
	Varicella IgG screen
	Toxoplasmosis IgG screen
	CMV IgG screen
	Parvovirus B19 IgG screen
	Genetic carrier screening for
	  hemoglobinopathies, Tay-Sachs
	  disease, Canavan's disease, or
	  other genetic diseases
	Screening for parental karyotype for
	  habitual spontaneous abortion

HBV, hepatitis B virus; HIV, human immunodeficiency virus; CMV, cytomegalovirus; IgG, immunoglobulin. Adapted from U.S. Department of Health and Human Services. *Caring for our Future: The Content of Prenatal Care. A Report of the PHS Export Panel*. Washington, DC: U.S. Department of Health and Human Services, 1989, with permission.

- **Toxoplasmosis** is of concern in cat owners and women who eat or handle raw meat, but routine testing without risk factors is not recommended. Routine toxoplasmosis screening to determine antibody status before conception mainly provides reassurance to those who are already immune; patients' cats can also be tested.
- Screening for **varicella** IgG should be performed if a positive history cannot be obtained. The varicella zoster virus vaccine is now recommended for all nonimmune adults. It is a live virus vaccine that should be given prior to conception. Nonimmune individuals can be counseled regarding postexposure prophylaxis during pregnancy.
- Universal **human immunodeficiency virus (HIV)** counseling and testing should be offered routinely to all women. The CDC has recommended an "opt out" strategy to increase screening compliance.
- Testing for *Neisseria gonorrhea, Chlamydia trachomatis,* and *Treponema pallidum* is often performed routinely in sexually active patients.
- **Evaluation of exposure to medications** includes both over-the-counter and prescription drugs, herbs, and supplements. In general, FDA pregnancy Category X and D medications should be avoided. For other medications, maternal and fetal risk-benefit should be assessed.
- **Isotretinoin (Accutane)**, an oral treatment for severe cystic acne, is highly teratogenic, causing craniofacial defects (microtia, anotia). It should be discontinued prior to pregnancy.
- **Warfarin (Coumadin)**, an anticoagulant, and related vitamin K antagonists have been associated with warfarin embryopathy. Because heparins (both unfractionated and low molecular weight) do not cross the placenta, women requiring anticoagulation should be encouraged to switch to heparin therapy before conception.
- The offspring of women treated with **antiepileptic drugs (AED)** are at increased risk for congenital malformations, particularly when these drugs are used in the

first trimester. **Valproic acid** is associated with neural tube defects (NTDs) as well as craniofacial, limb, and cardiac abnormalities. **Carbamazepine** exposure has been associated with facial dysmorphism and fingernail hypoplasia. Data on second generation AEDs are still limited. It may be appropriate to discontinue anticonvulsants in women who have not had seizures for at least 2 years; preconception planning with referral to neurology may be warranted. For women who must continue with AEDs, regimens that have less teratogenicity may be attempted. A detailed fetal anatomy sonogram, maternal serum alpha-fetoprotein (MSAFP), and fetal echocardiogram may provide useful information for these patients.

- Use of **psychiatric medications** during pregnancy is of concern for teratogenesis; however, untreated psychiatric illness is also associated with poor pregnancy outcomes, including premature birth, low birthweights, and fetal growth restriction. Treatment of bipolar disorder with **lithium** has been associated with increased incidence of heart defects, and should be continued based upon the severity and frequency of illness. Fetal echocardiogram is recommended for women taking lithium in the first trimester. Most **selective serotonin reuptake inhibitors (SSRIs)** are considered safe; however, paroxetine early in pregnancy has been associated with increased risk of heart defects, and an FDA advisory notes an association between late-term SSRI use and persistent pulmonary hypertension in the newborn. SSRI use in pregnancy should be individualized, balancing the risks of maternal depression and potential fetal effects.

- No evidence indicates teratogenicity from **oral contraceptive** or **contraceptive implant** use.

- **Vaginal spermicides** are not teratogenic, but should be discontinued when a woman becomes pregnant.

- Assistance in answering questions about **reproductive toxicology** is available through the online database REPROTOX (http://reprotox.org). The Reproductive Toxicology Center at Columbia Hospital for Women Medical Center, one of the sponsors of REPROTOX, also offers a clinical inquiry program. Many states have teratogen hotlines or state-funded programs; the Organization of Teratology Information Specialists (OTIS) is a good source for information about these programs and offers other resources (www.otispregnancy.org).

Nutritional Assessment

- The **body mass index (BMI)**, defined as (weight in kilograms/[height in meters]^2), is the preferred indicator of nutritional status. Very overweight (BMI above 30) and very underweight women (BMI <20) are at risk for poor pregnancy outcomes.

- **Eating habits**, such as fasting, pica, eating disorders, and the use of megavitamin supplementation, should be discussed. Excess use of multivitamin supplements containing **Vitamin A** should be avoided because the estimated dietary intake of Vitamin A for most women in the United States is sufficient. Vitamin A is teratogenic in humans at dosages of more than 20,000 to 50,000 IU daily, producing fetal malformations like those seen with isotretinoin. Women with a history of anorexia or bulimia may benefit from both nutrition and psychologic counseling before conception.

- **Folic acid** supplementation reduces the risk of NTDs. The U.S. Public Health Service recommends daily supplementation with 0.4 mg of folic acid for all women capable of becoming pregnant. Unless contraindicated by the presence of pernicious anemia, women who have previously carried a fetus with a NTD should take 4.0 mg of folic acid daily.

Social Assessment

- A social and lifestyle history should be obtained to identify potentially risky behaviors and exposures that may compromise a good reproductive outcome and to identify social, financial, and psychological issues that could affect pregnancy planning.
- All patients should be asked about **alcohol, tobacco**, and **recreational substance** use. Alcohol is a known teratogen, and a clear dose-response relationship exists between alcohol use and fetal effects. Cocaine has been identified as a teratogen, as well as a cause of prematurity, abruptio placentae, and intrauterine growth restriction (IUGR). Tobacco use has been identified as the leading preventable cause of low birth weight. If substance addiction is present, structured recovery programs are needed to effect behavioral change. The preconception interview allows timely education about drug use and pregnancy, informed decision making about the risks of using these substances at the time of conception, and the introduction of interventions for women who need treatment.
- Victims of **domestic violence** should be identified before they conceive. They are more likely to be abused during pregnancy than at other times. Approximately 37% of abused women are assaulted during their pregnancy, resulting in possible abruptio placentae, antepartum hemorrhage, fetal fractures, rupture of the internal organs, and preterm labor. Information about community, social, and legal resources should be made available to women who are abused and a plan devised for dealing with the abusive partner. See Chapter 30.
- The preconception interview is an appropriate time to discuss insurance coverage and **financial difficulties**. Many women and couples do not know the eligibility requirements or amount of maternity coverage provided by their insurance carriers, or may lack medical insurance coverage altogether. Referral for medical assistance programs should be part of preconception planning.

GENETIC COUNSELING AND TESTING

Genetic Counseling

- Genetic counseling, risk assessment, and intervention are based on the family history of the biologic mother and father, maternal age, ethnicity, drug or environmental exposures, and medical and obstetric history (see Tables 4-1 and 4-3). Information on hereditary birth defects is best assessed with a three generation pedigree. Table 4-4 describes major modes of inheritance.
- Assisted reproductive technologies, such as donor egg and sperm, sperm sorting, and preimplantation genetic diagnosis (PGD), may obviate the risk in specific cases. Adoption and avoidance of pregnancy represent other choices. CVS and amniocentesis permit early diagnosis, facilitate preparation for the care of an affected child, and give the option for pregnancy termination.
- In general, prenatal screening involves three groups: the general pregnant population, patients with a specific ethnic background or positive family history for a genetic disorder, and patients with a fetal anomaly. The National Society of Genetic Counselors (NSGC) urges caution regarding prenatal testing for adult-onset conditions unless there are treatments or preventive measures that can be initiated during pregnancy or in early childhood.

Prenatal Screening

- Normally, 46 chromosomes (23 pairs) are found in every somatic cell of the body. **Aneuploidy** refers to the condition in which there is an abnormal number

TABLE 4-3	Indications for Genetic Counseling

Mother 35 y or older at her estimated date of delivery
Fetal anomalies detected via ultrasonography
Abnormal first trimester serum/nuchal translucency screening
Abnormal triple/quad screening or abnormal alpha-fetoprotein test results
Parental exposure to teratogens
   Drugs
   Radiation
   Infection
Family history of genetic disease (includes chromosome, single gene, and
   multifactorial disorders)
   Birth defects
   Mental retardation
   Cancer, heart disease, hypertension, diabetes, and other common conditions
     (especially when onset occurs at an early age)
Membership in ethnic group in which certain genetic disorders are frequent
   when appropriate screening for or prenatal diagnosis of the disease is
   available (e.g., sickle cell anemia, Tay-Sachs disease, Canavan's disease,
   thalassemia)
Consanguinity
Reproductive failure
   Infertility
   Repeated spontaneous abortions
   Stillbirths and neonatal deaths
Infant, child, or adult with the following:
   Dysmorphic features
   Developmental and/or growth delay
   Ambiguous genitalia or abnormal sexual development

of chromosomes. Regardless of the maternal age, aneuploidy screening should be offered to all women before 20 weeks' gestation. Women who do not seek prenatal care until the second trimester should be offered quadruple screening and ultrasound assessment. Women seen in the first trimester should be offered first trimester serum and nuchal translucency screening or an integrated approach combining first and second trimester screening.

- **Down syndrome**, the most common aneuploid condition in liveborns, is the result of an extra chromosome 21. Trisomy 21 most often results from meiotic nondisjunction during maternal chromosomal replication and division and is characterized by mental retardation, cardiac defects, hypotonia, and characteristic facial features. Although its incidence increases with maternal age (Table 4-5), 70% of cases occur in women younger than 35 years since most pregnancies occur in these younger women.
- **Trisomy 13 and 18** are more severe disorders which cause profound mental retardation and severe multiorgan birth defects. Few babies with trisomies 13 or 18 survive more than a few months. The risk of trisomy recurrence for a chromosomally normal couple is often cited to be 1%.

First Trimester Screening
- **First trimester screening,** performed between 11 and 14 weeks, includes maternal age, nuchal translucency, maternal serum free beta-human chorionic gonadotropin

TABLE 4-4	Major Modes of Inheritance		
Inheritance	**Risk of Recurrence**	**Properties**	**Conditions**
Autosomal dominant	If parent has gene: 50% for child	Multiple generations Both genders affected equally	Achondroplasia Acute intermittent porphyria Adult polycystic kidney dz BRCA1–BRCA2 breast Ca Familial hypercholesterolemia Familial hypertrophic cardiomyopathy Hemorrhagic telangiectasia Hereditary spherocytosis Huntington chorea Marfan syndrome Myotonic dystrophy Neurofibromatosis type 1 Nonpolyposis colon cancer Osteogenesis imperfecta Polyposis of the colon Tuberous sclerosis von Willebrand Waardenburg syndrome
Autosomal recessive	If both parents are carriers: 25% for child	Often seen in only one generation Both genders affected equally Consanguinity may be present between parents of an affected child Parents of an affected child are asymptomatic carriers	Albinism Canavan disease Congenital adrenal hyperplasia Cystic fibrosis Galactosemia Familial dysautonomia Friedreich's ataxia Hemochromatosis Homocystinuria Maple syrup urine disease Phenylketonuria Sickle cell disease Tay-Sachs disease Thalassemia Wilson's disease
X-linked recessive	If mother is carrier: 50% affected sons, 50% carrier daughters	No male-to-male transmission Heterozygous females usually unaffected, but may express	Duchenne muscular dystrophy Glucose-6-phosphate dehydrogenase deficiency Hemophilia A Hemophilia B

(Continued)

TABLE 4-4	Major Modes of Inheritance (Continued)		
Inheritance	**Risk of Recurrence**	**Properties**	**Conditions**
	If father is affected: 0% affected sons, 100% carrier daughters	condition (variable severity) due to skewed X-inactivation. A large proportion of isolated cases are due to new mutations.	Lesch-Nyan syndrome Menkes syndrome
X-linked dominant	If mother is affected: 50% of sons and 50% of daughters are affected. If father is affected: 0% affected sons, 100% affected daughters	No male-to-male transmission Often lethal in males Homozygous affected females may have more severe disease	Hypophosphatemic rickets Incontinentia pigmenti, type 2
Mitochondrial	Recurrence in males and females is variable due to heteroplasmy of mitochondria	Mitochondrial DNA inherited exclusively through females Variations in severity	Leber optic neuropathy MELAS Myoclonic epilepsy

BRCA1, breast cancer 1 gene; BRCA2, breast cancer 2 gene; MELAS, mitochondrial myopathy, encephalopathy, lactic acidosis, and stroke syndrome.

(free β-hCG), and pregnancy-associated plasma protein-A (PAPP-A). The detection rate for Down syndrome and trisomy 18 is about 89% and 95%, respectively, with a 5% false positive rate. First trimester screening with ultrasound assessment of the nasal bone (absent in about 70% of Trisomy 21 fetuses) improves the detection rate for Down syndrome to approximately 95% with a 5% false positive rate. First trimester screening does not screen for open NTDs.

Second Trimester Screening
• **Second trimester quad screening** is performed between 15 and 20 weeks and estimates risk for Down syndrome, open NTDs, and trisomy 18. It uses MSAFP, β-hCG, unconjugated estriol (uE3), and dimeric inhibin A (DIA), combined with maternal age. The detection rate for trisomy 21 is approximately 75% for women younger than 35 years old and 90% for those older than 35. Additionally, abnormal

TABLE 4-5	Chromosomal Abnormalities in Liveborns[a]	
Maternal Age	Risk of Down Syndrome	Total Risk of Chromosomal Abnormalities[a]
20	1:1,667	1:526
21	1:1,667	1:526
22	1:1,429	1:500
23	1:1,429	1:500
24	1:1,250	1:476
25	1:1,250	1:476
26	1:1,176	1:476
27	1:1,111	1:455
28	1:1,053	1:435
29	1:1,000	1:417
30	1:952	1:385
31	1:909	1:385
32	1:769	1:322
33	1:602	1:286
34	1:485	1:238
35	1:378	1:192
36	1:289	1:156
37	1:224	1:127
38	1:173	1:102
39	1:136	1:83
40	1:106	1:66
41	1:82	1:53
42	1:63	1:42
43	1:49	1:33
44	1:38	1:26
45	1:30	1:21
46	1:23	1:16
47	1:18	1:13
48	1:14	1:10
49	1:11	1:8

[a]Karyotype 47, XXX was excluded for ages 20 to 32 years (data not available). Adapted from Hook EB, Cross PK, Schreinemachers DM. Chromosomal abnormality rates at amniocentesis and in live-born infants. *JAMA* 1983;249:2034–2038, with permission; and Hook EB. Rates of chromosomal abnormalities at different maternal ages. *Obstet Gynecol* 1981;58:282–285, with permission.

values on this screening (elevated AFP and/or hCG) correlate with an increased risk of perinatal complications.

Combined Screening
- **Combined screening**, including integrated and sequential, uses combined first and second trimester screening to adjust a woman's age-related risk for a fetus with Down syndrome. **Integrated screening** uses nuchal translucency and PAPP-A from the first trimester screening, and MSAFP, estriol, hCG, and inhibin-A from the second trimester screening. Results are reported only after *both* screening tests are completed. The detection rate for this method is 94% to 96% with 5% false positives;

this is equivalent to first trimester screening when nasal bone is included in the risk assessment. In **sequential screening**, the patient is given the first trimester results. If at high risk, patients are given the option for invasive testing, while those at low risk can still undergo second trimester screening to achieve a higher detection rate.

Screening for Neural Tube Defects
- **NTDs** result from a failure of the neural tube to close or attain its normal musculoskeletal coverings in early embryogenesis. Among the most common major congenital malformations with an incidence of 1 to 2 in 1,000 live births, NTDs include the fatal condition of anencephaly as well as spina bifida (meningomyelocele and meningocele); most have the potential for surgical correction.
  - Family history of NTD increases risk. If one partner has an NTD, the recurrence risk is 2% to 3%. In a couple with a previously affected child, the risk of recurrence is also 2% to 3%. Ninety percent of NTDs, however, occur in families without such histories. All pregnant women should be offered NTD screening.
  - MSAFP is a fetal glycoprotein synthesized sequentially in the embryonic yolk sac, GI tract, and liver. Normally, AFP crosses the placenta to appear in the mother's blood. In addition, a small amount of AFP enters the amniotic fluid via fetal urination, GI secretions, and transudation from exposed blood vessels. The concentration of AFP in amniotic fluid (AFAFP) is highest at the end of the first trimester and slowly declines during the remainder of pregnancy. MSAFP concentrations, on the other hand, rise until approximately 30 weeks' gestation. With an open fetal NTD or an abdominal wall defect, increased AFP more than 2.5 MoM (Multiples of the Median) will be detected in amniotic fluid in over 95% of cases, and in the mother's blood in about 80% of cases. Elevated MSAFP levels can also occur with incorrect pregnancy dating, multiple pregnancies, congenital nephrosis, Turner's syndrome with cystic hygroma, fetal bowel obstruction, teratomas, IUGR, and fetal death. Closed defects are not associated with abnormal AFP findings.
  - Women who elected to undergo first trimester screening or have a normal result from CVS should still be offered NTD screening with a MSAFP in the second trimester.
  - Diagnostic ultrasonography should be performed on patients with elevated MSAFP screening results to confirm gestational age, as well as to visualize the placenta, detect multiple pregnancies, and detect any fetal anomalies. Assignment of incorrect gestational age may lead to incorrect interpretation of AFP levels, because both MSAFP and AFAFP levels change in relation to gestational age. Maternal smoking is also associated with false positive elevations in MSAFP.

Diagnostic Procedures
- **CVS** uses either a catheter (transcervically) or a needle (transabdominally) to biopsy placental tissue derived from the same fertilized egg as the fetus. CVS is usually performed at 10 to 13 weeks' gestation but transabdominal CVS may be performed throughout the second or third trimester. CVS offers the psychological and medical advantages of early diagnosis and possibility for first trimester termination.
  - When adjusted for confounding factors, such as gestational age and early spontaneous miscarriage rate, the CVS-related miscarriage rate is not statistically different from that for second trimester amniocentesis.
  - Unsensitized Rh-negative women are given Rh immunoglobin after CVS.
  - Cytogenetically ambiguous results caused by maternal cell contamination or mosaicism are reported more often after CVS than after amniocentesis. In such

instances, follow-up amniocentesis may be required to clarify results, which increases both the total cost of testing and the risk of miscarriage.

- Reports of infants born with limb defects after CVS were first published in 1991. This outcome is associated with gestational age and therefore CVS is not generally recommended before 9 weeks' gestation.
- **Amniocentesis** aspirates a small amount of amniotic fluid, containing cells that are shed from the fetal bladder, skin, GI tract, and amnion. These cells can be used for karyotyping or other genetic testing. Amniocentesis is most commonly performed at 15 to 18 weeks' gestation.
  - In the United States, the current standard of care is to offer CVS or amniocentesis to women who will be 35 years or older when they give birth. Patients with an obstetric history of NTD should be counseled about their 2% to 3% risk of recurrence and offered second trimester amniocentesis for AFAFP testing as well as detailed ultrasonographic evaluation of fetal anatomy at 18 to 20 weeks' gestation.
  - The amniocentesis site should be selected carefully, avoiding the placenta if possible as contamination with fetal blood will falsely elevate the AFAFP. False-positive results due to contamination with fetal blood can be identified by acetylcholinesterase testing (absent in pregnancies for which the elevated AFAFP can be explained by contamination with fetal blood).
  - The miscarriage rate from mid-trimester (16 to 20 week) amniocentesis is estimated to be 1 in 200 to 500. Other complications such as vaginal spotting or amniotic fluid leakage occur infrequently; most are transient. Unsensitized Rh-negative women are given Rh-immune globulin after amniocentesis.
- **Mid-trimester ultrasonographic evaluation** at 18 to 22 weeks' gestation should include a systematic fetal anatomy survey and growth assessment.
  - Ultrasound screening for Down syndrome, also called **age-adjusted ultrasound risk assessment** (AAURA), utilizes likelihood ratios associated with specific markers to adjust a woman's *a priori* risk. AAURA screening includes: thickened nuchal fold, echogenicity of the fetal bowl, short humerus and femur lengths, dilated renal pyelectasis, and intracardiac echogenic focus. Although helpful, an ultrasound cannot rule out Down syndrome. Assessment of the fetal karyotype (by amniocentesis or CVS) is necessary for definitive diagnosis. Ultrasonography is better at detecting aneuploidies other than Down syndrome, such as trisomy 18 or trisomy 13, which are associated with a higher incidence of major structural anomalies.

PRENATAL CARE (Table 4-6)

Gestational Dating

- **Pregnancy dating:** The average duration of human pregnancy is 280 days from the first day of the last menstrual period (LMP) until delivery. The 40-week gestational period is based on menstrual weeks (not weeks since conception), assuming ovulation and conception on the 14th day of a 28-day cycle.
- **Clinical dating.** Using Nägele's rule, the estimated date of delivery is calculated by subtracting 3 months from the 1st day of the LMP then adding 1 week. Doppler ultrasonography allows detection of fetal heart tones by 11 to 12 weeks' gestation. A fetoscope can enable detection of heart tones at 19 to 20 weeks' gestation. Quickening (maternal detection of fetal movement) is noted at approximately 19 weeks in the first pregnancy; in subsequent pregnancies, it is usually noted approximately 2 weeks earlier.
- **Ultrasonographic dating** is most accurate from 7 to 11-6/7 weeks of pregnancy. If LMP dating is consistent with ultrasonographic dating within the established range

TABLE 4-6	Routine Prenatal Testing
Timing	**Tests**
Initial obstetric visit	Blood type, Rh type, antibody screen, CBC, rubella, STS/RPR, HBsAg, HIV, Hgb electrophoresis, urine culture and sensitivity, pap smear, gonorrhea and chlamydia testing; dating sonogram, if questionable dating criteria for first trimester screening
16–18 weeks' gestation	MSAFP/quad screen (range: 15–20 wk)
16–20 weeks' gestation	Sonogram to rule out abnormalities
28 weeks' gestation	Blood type, Rh type, antibody screen, CBC, STS/RPR, glucose screen. If high-risk patient, repeat HBsAg, HIV, gonorrhea, and chlamydia testing
36 weeks' gestation	Group B streptococci culture

CBC, complete blood cell count; HBsAg, hepatitis B surface antigen; Hgb, hemoglobin; HIV, human immunodeficiency virus; MSAFP, maternal serum alpha-fetoprotein; RPR, rapid plasma reagin; STS, serologic test for syphilis.

of accuracy for ultrasonography (Table 4-7), the estimated date of delivery is based on LMP.

Nutrition and Weight Gain

- Pregnant women require 15% more **calories** than nonpregnant women, usually 300 to 500 kcal more per day, depending on the patient's weight and activity.
- Dietary allowances for most **vitamins and minerals** increase with pregnancy, and are adequately supplied in a well-balanced diet. Increased **iron**, however, is needed for both the fetus and the mother. Consumption of iron-containing foods should be encouraged, and iron supplements may be prescribed. The 30-mg daily elemental

TABLE 4-7	Accuracy of Pregnancy Dating by Ultrasonography According to Gestational Age	
Gestational Age (wk)	**Ultrasonographic Measurements**	**Accuracy**
<8	Sac size	±10 d
8–12	CRL	±7 d
12–14	CRL or BPD	±14 d
15–20	BPD/HC/FL/AC	±10 d
20–28	BPD/HC/FL/AC	±2 wk
>28	BPD/HC/FL/AC	±3 wk

AC, abdominal circumference; BPD, biparietal diameter; CRL, crown-rump length; FL, femur length; HC, head circumference; d, day(s); wk, week(s).

ferrous iron supplement is contained in approximately 150 mg of ferrous sulfate, 300 mg of ferrous gluconate, or 100 mg of ferrous fumarate.
- Prenatal **calcium** requirement is 1,200 mg/day.
- The **recommended weight gain** for pregnancy is based on the prepregnancy BMI. The total weight gain recommended is 25 to 35 pounds for women with a normal BMI. Underweight women may gain 40 pounds or more, and overweight women should limit weight gain to <25 pounds or less. Three to 6 pounds are gained typically in the first trimester and 0.5 to 1.0 pound/week is gained in the last two trimesters of pregnancy. If a patient has not gained 10 pounds by midpregnancy, her nutritional status should be evaluated carefully. Inadequate weight gain is associated with an increased risk of low birth weight in infants. Patients should be warned against weight loss during pregnancy. Total weight gain in an obese patient can be as low as 15 pounds, but weight gain of <15 pounds is associated with a lack of expansion of plasma volume and risk of IUGR.

Exercise
- In the absence of obstetric or medical complications, moderate physical activity can maintain cardiovascular and muscular fitness throughout pregnancy and the postpartum period. No data suggest that moderate aerobic exercise is harmful to the mother or fetus.
- The following conditions are **contraindications** to exercise during pregnancy: gestational hypertension, preterm rupture of membranes, preterm labor during a previous pregnancy or the current pregnancy, incompetent cervix or cerclage, persistent second- or third-trimester bleeding, and IUGR. Women with certain other conditions, including chronic hypertension or active thyroid, cardiac, vascular, or pulmonary disease, should be carefully evaluated to determine whether an exercise program is appropriate.

Smoking Cessation
- At least 11% of pregnant women in the United States smoke. Carbon monoxide and nicotine are believed to be the main ingredients in cigarette smoke that are responsible for adverse fetal effects. Smoking is associated with increases in the following:
  - Spontaneous abortion (1.2 to 1.8 times greater in smokers than in nonsmokers)
  - Abortion of a chromosomally normal fetus (39% more likely in smokers than in nonsmokers)
  - Abruptio placentae, placenta previa, and premature rupture of membranes
  - Preterm birth (1.2 to 1.5 times greater in smokers than in nonsmokers)
  - Low infant birth weight
  - Sudden infant death syndrome
- **Smoking cessation** during pregnancy improves the birth weight of the infant, especially if use stops before 16 weeks' gestation.
- Prospective randomized controlled clinical trials have shown that **intensive smoking reduction programs**, with frequent patient contact and close supervision, aid in smoking cessation and result in increased infant birth weights. Successful interventions emphasize ways to stop smoking rather than merely providing mandates to stop smoking.
- **Nicotine replacement therapy** (chewing gum or transdermal patch) carry warnings about the adverse effects of nicotine on mother and fetus. However, nicotine is only one of the toxins in tobacco smoke. Smoking cessation with nicotine replacement reduces fetal exposure to carbon monoxide and other toxins, and may improve outcomes. For

women who are unable to reduce their smoking otherwise, it may be reasonable to advise nicotine replacement as an adjunct to counseling even during pregnancy.

Alcohol Consumption

- Recent data show around 10% of pregnant women have consumed alcoholic beverages within the prior month and slightly <1% admit to heavy drinking.
- Ethanol freely crosses the placenta and the fetal blood–brain barrier, and is a known teratogen. Fetal ethanol toxicity is dose-related but without a defined lower threshold of exposure. The exposure time of greatest risk is the first trimester. Fetal brain development may be affected throughout gestation, however. Although an occasional drink during pregnancy has not been shown to be harmful, patients should be counseled that the threshold for adverse effects is unknown.
- **Fetal alcohol syndrome** is characterized by growth retardation (prenatally, postnatally, or both), facial abnormalities, and central nervous system (CNS) dysfunction. Facial abnormalities include shortened palpebral fissures, low-set ears, midfacial hypoplasia, a smooth philtrum, and a thin upper lip. CNS abnormalities of fetal alcohol syndrome include microcephaly, mental retardation, and behavioral disorders, such as attention deficit disorder. Skeletal abnormalities and structural cardiac defects are also seen with greater frequency in the children of women who abuse alcohol during pregnancy than in those who do not. The most common cardiac structural anomaly is ventricular septal defect, but several others occur.

Illicit Drug Use

- Recent data show about 4% of pregnant women use some illicit substance in pregnancy.
- **Marijuana.** No evidence exists that marijuana is a significant teratogen in humans. Cannabinoid metabolites can be detected in the urine of users for days to weeks after use, much longer than for alcohol and most other illicit drugs. The presence of cannabinoid metabolites in the urine may identify patients who are likely to be current users of other illicit substances as well.
- **Cocaine.** Adverse maternal effects include profound vasoconstriction, leading to malignant hypertension, cardiac ischemia, and cerebral infarction. Cocaine may have a direct cardiotoxic effect, leading to sudden death. Complications of cocaine use in pregnancy include spontaneous abortion, fetal death in utero, premature rupture of membranes, preterm labor and delivery, IUGR, meconium-staining of amniotic fluid, and abruptio placentae. Cocaine is teratogenic, and its use has been associated with cases of in utero fetal cerebral infarction, microcephaly, and limb reduction defects. Genitourinary malformations have been reported with first trimester cocaine use. Infants born to women who use cocaine are at risk for neurobehavioral abnormalities and impairment in orientation, motor, and state-regulation neurobehaviors.
- **Opiates.** Opiate use is associated with increased rates of stillbirth, fetal growth restriction, prematurity, and neonatal mortality, perhaps due to risky behaviors in opiate substance abusers. Opiates are not known to be teratogenic. Methadone treatment is associated with improved pregnancy outcomes. The newborn narcotic addict is at risk for a severe, potentially fatal, narcotic withdrawal syndrome. Although the incidence of clinically significant withdrawal is slightly lower among methadone-treated addicts, its course can be just as severe. Neonatal withdrawal is characterized by a high-pitched cry, poor feeding, hypertonicity, tremors, irritability, sneezing, sweating, vomiting, diarrhea, and, occasionally, seizures. Frequent sharing

of needles has resulted in high rates of HIV infection (>50%) and hepatitis among intravenous narcotic addicts.

- **Amphetamines.** Crystal methamphetamine, a potent stimulant that is inhaled, injected, or snorted, has been associated with decreased fetal head circumference and increased risk of abruptio placentae, IUGR, and fetal death in utero. However, no proven teratogenicity exists.
- **Hallucinogens.** No evidence proves that lysergic acid diethylamide (LSD) or other hallucinogens cause chromosomal damage, as was once reported. Few studies exist on the possible deleterious effects of maternal hallucinogen use during pregnancy. No proven teratogenicity to LSD exists.

Prenatal Care for the Substance Abuser
- Intensive prenatal care with a multidisciplinary team of health and social service providers reduces both maternal and neonatal complications. As long as the patient continues with substance abuse, it should be discussed at each appointment. The risks of preterm delivery, fetal growth restriction, fetal death, and long-term neurobehavioral effects for the child should be explained. Periodic urine toxicologic testing should be offered to encourage abstinence, though its reliability is limited by the rapid clearance of most substances. Overaggressive urine testing may be perceived as threatening and lead to decreased compliance. Early ultrasonographic confirmation of gestational age is necessary, because growth restriction is a frequent finding among fetuses of substance abusers. A fetal anatomic survey is indicated to evaluate for structural anomalies. Antepartum testing is appropriate when fetal compromise is suggested (e.g., decreased fetal movement, suspected growth restriction). When normal growth and an active fetus are present, no evidence shows that regular antepartum testing is associated with improved perinatal outcome in substance-abusing patients. All patients should be screened for substance abuse (including use of alcohol and tobacco) at the time of their first prenatal visit. Several screening questionnaires have been developed to detect problem drinking with the T-ACE and TWEAK screens validated in female populations.

Immunizations

- Preconception immunization of women to prevent disease in their offspring is preferred to vaccination of pregnant women; only live-virus vaccines, however, carry any risk to the fetus.
- All women of childbearing age should be immune to measles, rubella, mumps, tetanus, diphtheria, poliomyelitis, and varicella through childhood natural or vaccine-conferred immunization.
- All pregnant women should be screened for hepatitis B surface antigen. Pregnancy is not a contraindication to the administration of an HBV vaccine or hepatitis B immune globulin. Women at high risk of HBV infection who should be vaccinated during pregnancy include those with histories of the following: intravenous drug use, acute episode of any sexually transmitted disease, multiple sexual partners, occupational exposure in a health care or public safety environment, household contact with an HBV carrier, occupational exposure or residence in an institution for the developmentally disabled, occupational exposure or treatment in a hemodialysis unit, or receipt of clotting factor concentrates for bleeding disorders.
- Combined tetanus and diphtheria toxoids are the only immunobiologic agents routinely indicated for susceptible pregnant women.

- No evidence of fetal risk exists from inactivated virus vaccines, bacterial vaccines, or tetanus immunoglobulin, and these agents should be administered, if appropriate.
- Measles, mumps, and rubella single-antigen vaccines, as well as the combined vaccine, should be given at a preconception or postpartum visit. Despite theoretic risks, no evidence has been reported of congenital rubella syndrome in infants born to women inadvertently given rubella vaccine while pregnant. Women who undergo immunization should be advised not to become pregnant for at least 4 weeks afterward. There is no evidence for transmission from vaccinated family members.
- Immune globulin or vaccination against poliomyelitis, yellow fever, typhoid, or hepatitis may be indicated for travelers to areas where these diseases are endemic or epidemic.
- Influenza vaccination is indicated for all pregnant women during flu season, especially those who work at chronic care facilities that house patients with chronic medical conditions or who themselves have cardiopulmonary disorders, are immunosuppressed, or have diabetes mellitus. H1N1 influenza is disproportionately severe in pregnant women; therefore, H1N1 influenza vaccine should be offered to pregnant women when this strain of influenza is anticipated to be endemic. Consult current CDC and ACOG guidelines.
- Pneumococcal vaccine is recommended for women with special conditions that put them at high risk of infection.
- Immune globulin or a specific immune globulin may be indicated after exposure to measles, hepatitis A or B, tetanus, chickenpox, or rabies.
- Varicella zoster immune globulin (VZIG) should be administered to any newborn whose mother developed chickenpox within 5 days before or 2 days after delivery. No evidence shows that administration of VZIG to mothers reduces the rare occurrence of congenital varicella syndrome. VZIG can be considered for treating a pregnant woman to try to prevent the maternal complications of chickenpox.
- Recombinant vaccine for HPV viruses is not currently recommended for use in pregnant women.

Sexual Intercourse

- Generally, no restriction of sexual activity is necessary for pregnant women. Patients should be instructed that pregnancy may cause changes in physical comfort and sexual desire. Increased uterine activity after intercourse is common. For women at risk of preterm labor, those with placenta previa that persists into the third trimester, or vasa previa, avoiding sexual activity may be advised.

Employment

- Most patients are able to work throughout their entire pregnancy, though heavy lifting and excessive physical activity should be avoided. Modification of occupational activity is rarely needed, unless the job involves physical danger. Patients should discontinue an activity that causes discomfort. Jobs that involve strenuous physical exercise, standing for prolonged periods, operating industrial machinery, or adverse environmental exposure should be modified.

Travel

- Prolonged immobility (i.e., sitting) should be avoided because of the increased risk of venous thrombosis and thrombophlebitis during pregnancy. Patients should drive a maximum of 6 hr a day and should stop at least every 2 hr and walk for 10 minutes. Support stockings should be worn for prolonged sitting in cars or airplanes. A seat belt should always be worn; the belt should be placed under the abdomen as the pregnancy advances.

Carpal Tunnel Syndrome

• In pregnancy, weight gain and edema can compress the median nerve, producing carpal tunnel syndrome. The syndrome consists of pain, numbness, or tingling in the thumb, index finger, middle finger, and radial side of the ring finger on the palmar aspect. Compressing the median nerve and percussing the wrist and forearm with a reflex hammer (Tinel's maneuver) often exacerbates the pain. The syndrome most often occurs in primigravidas over age 30 during the third trimester and usually resolves within 2 weeks of delivery. Conservative treatment with wrist splints at night or local steroid injections for more severe cases may be helpful.

Back Pain

• Back pain may be aggravated by excessive weight gain. Exercises to strengthen back muscles and loosen the hamstrings can help alleviate back pain. Many pregnant women find pregnancy support belts or maternity girdles helpful in alleviating low back pain. Pregnant women should maintain good posture and wear low-heeled shoes.

Round Ligament Pain

• These very sharp groin pains are caused by spasm of round ligaments associated with movement. The spasms are generally unilateral and are more frequent on the right side than on the left because of the usual dextroversion of the uterus. Patients sometimes awaken at night with round ligament pain after having suddenly rolled over in their sleep. No treatment is necessary and the patient should be reassured that they are a common and benign complaint in pregnancy.

Hemorrhoids

• **Hemorrhoids** are varicose veins of the rectum, and may become swollen and painful during pregnancy.
• Patients with hemorrhoids should avoid constipation, because straining during bowel movement aggravates hemorrhoids. Good hydration and increased fiber consumption may help soften the stool. Patients should avoid prolonged sitting. Hemorrhoids often regress after delivery but usually do not disappear completely.

SUGGESTED READINGS

Bennett RL, Motulsky AG, Bittles A, et al. Genetic counseling and screening of consanguineous couples and their offspring: recommendations of the National Society of Genetic Counselors. *J Gen Couns* 2002;11(2):97–119.

Clinical management guidelines for obstetrician-gynecologists: Use of psychiatric medications during pregnancy and lactation. ACOG Practice Bulletin Number 92. American College of Obstetricians and Gynecologists. *Obstet Gynecol* 2008;111(4):1001.

Jack B, Atrash HK, eds. Preconception health and health care: the clinical content of preconception care (Supplement). *Am J Obstet Gynecol.* 2008 Dec; 199(6 Suppl B): 257–395.

Screening for fetal chromosomal abnormalities. ACOG Practice Bulletin Number 77. American College of Obstetricians and Gynecologists. *Obstet Gynecol* 2007;109(1):217–227.

Spencer K. Aneuploidy screening in the first trimester. *Am J Med Gent Part C* 2007;145C: 18–32.

II Obstetrics

5 Normal Labor and Delivery, Operative Delivery, and Malpresentations

Frank Aguirre and Betty Chou

Definition: Labor is defined as repetitive uterine contractions of sufficient frequency, intensity, and duration to cause progressive cervical effacement and dilation.

STAGES AND PHASES OF LABOR (Table 5-1)

- The **first stage** begins with the onset of labor and ends with full cervical dilation. It is divided into latent and active phases.
  - The **latent phase** begins with regular contractions and ends when there is an increase in the rate of cervical dilation (usually at 3 to 4 cm of dilation).
  - The **active phase** is characterized by an increased rate of cervical dilation and descent of the presenting fetal part. It ends with complete cervical dilation, and is further subdivided into:
    - **Acceleration Phase.** A gradual increase in the rate of dilation initiates the active phase and marks a change to rapid dilation.
    - **Phase of maximum slope.** The period of active labor with the greater rate of cervical dilation.
    - **Deceleration Phase.** During the terminal portion of the active phase, the rate of dilation may slow until full cervical dilation.
- The **second stage** of labor is the interval between full cervical dilation and delivery of the neonate.
- The **third stage** is the interval between delivery of the infant and delivery of the placenta.
- The **fourth stage**, or puerperium, follows delivery and concludes with resolution of the physiologic changes of pregnancy, usually by 6 weeks postpartum. During

TABLE 5-1	Stages and Phases of Labor	
Parameter	Nulliparous	Multiparous
Latent phase of first-stage labor		
Mean	6 hr	5 hr
Fifth percentile	21 hr	14 hr
First stage of labor (total)		
Mean	10 hr	8 hr
Fifth percentile	25 hr	19 hr
Second stage of labor		
Mean	33 min	9 min
Fifth percentile	118 min	47 min
Prolonged (without epidural)	2 hr	1 hr
Prolonged (with epidural)	3 hr	2 hr
Third stage of labor		
Mean	5 min	5 min
Prolonged	30 min	30 min
Rate of maximal dilation		
Mean	3.0 cm/hr	5.7 cm/hr
Fifth percentile	1.2 cm/hr	1.5 cm/hr
Rate of descent		
Mean	3.3 cm/hr	6.6 cm/hr
Fifth percentile	1.0 cm/hr	2.0 cm/hr

Adapted from Liao JB, Buhimschi CS, Norwitz ER. Normal labor: mechanism and duration. *Obstet Gynecol Clin N Am* 2005;32(2):145–164; American College of Obstetricians and Gynecologists. Dystocia and augmentation of labor. ACOG Practice Bulletin Number 49. *Obstet Gynecol* 2003;102: 1445–1454.

this time, the reproductive tract returns to the nonpregnant state, and ovulation may resume.

MECHANISM OF LABOR

The cardinal movements of labor refer to the changes in position of the fetal head during passage through the birth canal in vertex presentation:
- **Engagement** is descent of the biparietal diameter of the fetal head below the plane of the pelvic inlet. Clinically, if the lowest portion of the occiput is at or below the level of the maternal ischial spines (station 0), engagement has occurred. Engagement can occur before the onset of true labor, especially in nulliparous patients.
- **Descent** of the fetal head to the pelvic floor is an important event of labor. The highest rate of descent occurs during the deceleration phase of the first stage and during the second stage of labor.
- **Flexion** of the fetal head is a passive movement that permits the smallest diameter of the fetal head (suboccipitobregmatic diameter) to pass through the maternal pelvis.

- **Internal Rotation.** The fetal occiput rotates from its original position (usually transverse) toward the symphysis pubis (occiput anterior) or, less commonly, toward the hollow of the sacrum (occiput posterior).
- **Extension.** The fetal head is delivered by extension from the flexed position as it travels beneath the symphysis pubis.
- **External Rotation.** The fetus resumes its face-forward position, with the occiput and spine lying in the same plane.
- **Expulsion.** Further descent brings the anterior shoulder of the fetus to the level of the symphysis pubis. After the shoulder is delivered under the symphysis pubis, the rest of the body is usually expelled quickly.

MANAGEMENT OF NORMAL LABOR AND DELIVERY

Initial Assessment

History
- Onset, strength, and frequency of contractions
- Leakage of fluid
- Vaginal bleeding
- Fetal movement
- Maternal allergies
- Medications
- Last oral intake
- Review of prenatal lab tests and history including gestational age, parity, and size of infants previously delivered vaginally.

Physical Exam
- Maternal vital signs (pulse, blood pressure, respiration, temperature)
- Fetal heart rate (assessment of fetal well-being)
- Frequency and intensity of contractions
- Fetal presentation and estimated fetal weight (via **Leopold's maneuvers**, confirmed by ultrasound)
  - Leopold step No. 1: Palpate the fundus to ascertain a fetal pole and obtain fundal height.
  - Leopold step No. 2: Palpate the lateral walls of the uterus to determine fetal lie (vertical vs transverse) and the location of fetal spine and extremities.
  - Leopold step No. 3: Grasp and palpate the upper and lower poles to determine presentation, assess mobility and fetal weight, and to estimate the amniotic fluid volume.
  - Leopold step No. 4: Palpate the presenting part from lateral to medial to assess engagement in the maternal pelvis, the location of the fetal brow, and the degree of flexion.
- **Sterile speculum exam**
  - Vulvar, vaginal, cervical inspection (especially noting lesions or scars)
  - Vaginal pooling and bleeding evaluation
  - Nitrazine/ferning (for leakage of amniotic fluid)
  - Wet mount, gonorrhea/chlamydia DNA probe or culture, group B strep (GBS) culture, if indicated
- **Sterile vaginal (digital) exam**—defer if estimated gestational age is <34 weeks with ruptured membranes.
  - **Cervical dilatation** is the estimated diameter of the internal os in centimeters. Ten centimeters corresponds to complete dilation.

- **Cervical effacement** is the length of the cervix, expressed as the percent change from full length (0% or "long" means not shortened at all, while 100% means only a paper thin rim of cervix is detected). Some providers prefer to describe effacement directly in centimeters (e.g., 4 cm *long*).
- **Fetal station** describes the distance in centimeters between the presenting *bony* part and the plane of the ischial spines. Station 0 defines the level of the spines. Below the spines is +1 cm to +5 at the perineum. Station above the spines is –1 cm to –5 at the level of the pelvic inlet.
- **Clinical pelvimetry**: Evaluation of the maternal pelvis by vaginal exam.
  - **Diagonal conjugate** is the distance between the sacral promontory and the posterior edge of the pubic symphysis. A measure of at least 11.5 cm suggests a sufficiently adequate pelvic inlet for an average weight fetus.
  - Estimate the **transverse diameter** by placing a closed fist between the ischial tuberosities at the perineum. An intertuberous diameter of at least 8 cm suggests an adequate pelvic outlet, average is 10 cm.
- The **pelvic type** can be classified into four types based on general shape and bony characteristics. Gynecoid and anthropoid types are most amenable to successful vaginal birth.

Standard Admission Procedures
- For patients without prenatal care, hepatitis B surface antigen, human immunodeficiency virus, ABO blood group and antibody screen, urine culture and toxicology, rubella IgG, complete blood count (CBC), and syphilis screening should be sent.
- Patients with prenatal laboratory results on record and an uncomplicated prenatal course require only urine testing (for protein and glucose), CBC, and a blood bank specimen for cross-matching if needed.
- Intravenous access (heplock or continuous infusion) is recommended. Decisions regarding showers and positioning during labor and delivery should coincide with the wishes of the patient and her family. Informed consent for management of labor and delivery should be obtained.

Management of Labor
- The quality and frequency of uterine contractions should be assessed regularly by palpation, tocodynamometer, or intrauterine pressure catheter (if indicated).
- The fetal heart rate should be assessed by intermittent auscultation, continuous electronic Doppler monitoring, or fetal scalp electrode (if indicated).
- Cervical examinations should be kept to the minimum required to detect abnormalities in the progression of labor.
- The lithotomy position is most frequently assumed for vaginal delivery in the United States, although alternative birthing positions, such as the lateral or Sim's position or the partial sitting or squatting positions, are preferred by some patients, physicians, and midwives.

Induction of Labor
- **Indications.** Induction is indicated when the benefits of delivery (for mother or fetus) outweigh the benefits of continued pregnancy. Induction should not be initiated if vaginal delivery is contraindicated (see Table 5-2). Consideration of **fetal lung maturity** is necessary before elective induction of labor prior to 39 weeks' gestation. Amniocentesis is not necessary if the induction is medically indicated and the risk of continuing the pregnancy is greater than the risk of delivering before lung maturity.

TABLE 5-2	Induction of Labor: Indications and Contraindications

Indications

- Abruptio placentae, chorioamnionitis, gestational hypertension
- Premature rupture of membranes, postterm pregnancy, preeclampsia, eclampsia
- Maternal medical conditions (e.g., diabetes mellitus, renal disease, chronic pulmonary disease, chronic hypertension)
- Fetal compromise (e.g., severe fetal growth restriction, isoimmunization)
- Fetal demise
- Elective inductions for gestational age >39 wk for logistical issues such as remote access to care, psychosocial reasons, and history of rapid deliveries. Typically only considered if cervix is favorable.

Contraindications

- Vasa previa or complete placenta previa
- Transverse fetal lie
- Infection—active HSV, high viral load HIV
- Pelvic structural deformities
- Umbilical cord prolapse
- Advanced cervical cancer

Adapted from American College of Obstetricians and Gynecologists. Induction of Labor. ACOG Practice Bulletin Number 107. *Obstet Gynecol* 2009;114:386–397.

- The state of the cervix at the time of induction is related to the success of labor induction. When the **Bishop score** (Table 5-3) exceeds 8, the likelihood of vaginal delivery after induction is similar to that with spontaneous labor. Induction with a lower Bishop score has been associated with a higher rate of failure, prolonged labor, and cesarean delivery.
  - **Cervical ripening** may be used to soften the cervix before induction if the Bishop score is low. Spontaneous cervical ripening usually precedes spontaneous labor at term. In many postterm pregnancies, the cervix remains unripe. Acceptable methods for cervical ripening include:

TABLE 5-3	Components of the Bishop Score			
	Rating			
Factor	**0**	**1**	**2**	**3**
Dilation	Closed	1–2 cm	3–4 cm	5+ cm
Effacement	0%–30%	40%–50%	60%–70%	80%+
Station	−3	−2	−1, 0	>+1
Consistency	Firm	Medium	Soft	—
Position	Posterior	Mid position	Anterior	—

Adapted from Bishop EH. Pelvic scoring for elective induction. *Obstet Gynecol* 1964;24:267.

- **Pharmacologic Methods**
  - Low-dose **oxytocin** may be used with or without mechanical dilators.
  - **Prostaglandin E$_2$** is superior to placebo in promoting cervical effacement and dilation, and may enhance sensitivity to oxytocin.
    - **Prepidil** (prostaglandin E$_2$) gel contains 0.5 mg of dinoprostone in a 2.5-mL syringe; the gel is injected into the cervical canal every 6 hr for up to three doses in a 24-hr period.
    - **Cervidil** (prostaglandin E$_2$) is a vaginal insert containing 10 mg of dinoprostone. It provides a lower rate of release of medication (0.3 mg/hr) than the gel but has the advantage that it can be removed if hyperstimulation occurs.
  - **Prostaglandin E$_1$** is also effective in stimulating cervical ripening
    - **Cytotec (misoprostol)** (prostaglandin E$_1$) is administered as 25 to 50 µg every 3 to 6 hr intravaginally. The use of misoprostol for cervical ripening is off-label.
  - **Side Effects.** The major complication with prostaglandin induction is uterine hyperstimulation, which is usually reversible with administration of a beta-adrenergic agonist (e.g., terbutaline sulfate). Maternal systemic effects, such as fever, vomiting, and diarrhea, are also possible.
  - **Contraindications** to prostaglandin induction include history of uterine surgery or prior cesarean delivery, allergy to the medication, or active vaginal bleeding. Caution should be exercised when using prostaglandin E$_2$ in patients with glaucoma or severe hepatic or renal impairment.
- **Mechanical methods of labor induction and cervical ripening**
  - Membrane stripping
  - Amniotomy
  - 24 French transcervical Foley balloon with 30-mL bulb
  - Hygroscopic dilators (laminaria)
  - Double-balloon (Atad Ripener) device

Oxytocin Administration

- **Indications.** Oxytocin is used for both induction and augmentation of labor. Augmentation should be considered for protraction or arrest disorders of labor, or the presence of a hypotonic uterine contraction pattern. A range of opinions regarding the dosage of oxytocin exist. In general, starting dosages of 0.5 to 4 mIU/min, with incremental increases of 1 to 2 mIU/min every 20 to 30 minutes, are reasonable. Cervical dilation of at least 1 cm/hr in the active phase indicates that oxytocin dosing is adequate. If an intrauterine pressure catheter is in place, 180 Montevideo units (MVU) per 10-minute period is considered adequate. However, some practitioners use a threshold of 250 to 275 MVU with increased success of induction and minimal adverse consequences.
- **Complications.** Adverse effects of oxytocin are primarily dose related. The most common complication is uterine tachysystole which may result in uteroplacental hypoperfusion. Uterine tachysystole is usually reversible when oxytocin infusion is decreased or discontinued. If necessary, a beta-adrenergic agent may be administered. Prolonged use of oxytocin increases the risk of postpartum uterine atony and hemorrhage. Rapid infusion of oxytocin can result in hypotension. Prolonged infusion can result in water intoxication and hyponatremia because oxytocin structurally resembles antidiuretic hormone.

Labor Progress Assessment

- Friedman's studies on normal labor resulted in widely used guidelines for normal labor progress (see Table 5-1).
- Abnormal labor progression is identified when the patient falls below the fifth percentile of expected cervical change and fetal descent.

- **Latent phase prolongation** is somewhat controversial, as measurement of this phase is difficult and inexact. Generally speaking, without induction, this phase is considered prolonged if it exceeds 20 hr in a nulliparous patient and 14 hr in a multiparous patient.
- The **active phase** is considered protracted if the rate of cervical change is <1.2 cm/hr for the nulliparous patient and <1.5 cm/hr in the multiparous patient. Arrest of dilation occurs when there is no apparent cervical change over a 2-hr period despite adequate contractions (180 to 250 MVU).
- The **second stage** of labor is considered protracted after 2 hr of pushing in nulliparous patients or 1 hr in parous patients. An additional hour may be allowed if epidural anesthesia is used. Arrest of descent occurs when there is no apparent descent of the presenting part over a 1-hr period of pushing during the second stage.
- The **third stage** averages 10 minutes and is considered prolonged if it lasts longer than 30 minutes.
- Patients undergoing induction or augmentation of labor may not necessarily follow the Friedman curve for normal labor progression. Their individual labor curves need to be evaluated, and more liberal definitions of progress applied.
- **Abnormal labor** may be due to:
  - Inadequate uterine contractions or maternal expulsive effort (**power**)
  - Large fetus or abnormal proportions (**passenger**)
  - Small pelvis relative to the other two categories (**passage**)
- **Risk factors** for abnormal labor could be any medical condition or clinical situation that affects the categories above.
  - **Risks for an abnormal first stage of labor**: increased maternal age, diabetes, hypertension, premature rupture of membranes, macrosomnia, epidural anesthesia, chorioamnionitis, a history of previous complications like perinatal death, and amniotic fluid abnormalities.
  - **Risks for an abnormal second stage of labor**: an increased first stage, occiput posterior position, epidural anesthesia, nulliparity, short maternal stature, increased birth weight, and high station at complete cervical dilation.

Interventions for Abnormal Labor

- **Analgesia/anesthesia**: The data on prolongation of labor by epidural anesthesia are mixed. In most cases there is no reason that patients should not be offered adequate pain control.
- **Amniotomy:** There is good evidence that amniotomy may enhance progress for a patient who is in active labor, though it does increase the risk for chorioamnionitis.
- **Augmentation of labor via oxytocin**: Oxytocin has been shown to decrease the time of active labor in nulliparous women. In addition, some studies have shown that it decreases the rate of cesarean section for failure to progress.
- **Uterine contraction monitoring**: Placement of an intrauterine pressure catheter provides information about the frequency and strength of contractions and may be useful for titrating oxytocin to maximize the chance for successful vaginal delivery.

FETAL HEART RATE EVALUATION

Guidelines for fetal heart rate interpretation are given in Table 5-4.
- **Baseline rate:** Lasts for at least 2 minutes during a 10-minute section.
- **Normal rate:** 110 to 160 beats per minute (bpm).

TABLE 5-4	Fetal Heart Tracing Interpretation, Categories, and Criteria

Three-Tiered Fetal Heart Rate Interpretation System

Category I
- Category I FHR tracings include all of the following:
- Baseline rate: 110–160 beats/min
- Baseline FHR variability: moderate
- Late or variable decelerations: absent
- Early decelerations: present or absent
- Accelerations: present or absent

Category II
Category II FHR tracings includes all FHR tracings not categorized as Category I or Category III. Category II tracings may represent an appreciable fraction of those encountered in clinical care. Examples of Category II FHR tracings include any of the following:
Baseline rate
- Bradycardia not accompanied by absent baseline variability
- Tachycardia
Baseline FHR variability
- Minimal baseline variability
- Absent baseline variability with no recurrent decelerations
- Marked baseline variability
Accelerations
- Absence of induced accelerations after fetal stimulation
Periodic or episodic decelerations
- Recurrent variable decelerations accompanied by minimal or moderate baseline variability
- Prolonged deceleration more than 2 min but less than 10 min
- Recurrent late decelerations with moderate baseline variability
- Variable decelerations with other characteristics such as slow return to baseline, overshoots, or "shoulders"

Category III
Category III FHR tracings include either
- Absent baseline FHR variability and any of the following:
  - Recurrent late decelerations
  - Recurrent variable decelerations
  - Bradycardia
- Sinusoidal pattern

FHR, fetal heart rate. From Macones GA, Hankins GD, Spong CY, et al. The 2008 National Institute of Child Health and Human Development workshop report on electronic fetal monitoring update on definitions, interpretation, and research guidelines. *Obstet Gynecol* 2008;112:661–666.

- **Bradycardia** is a baseline rate <110 bpm. Causes of bradycardia range from fetal head compression or hypoxemia to maternal hypothermia. The clinical picture is as important as the heart rate in interpreting fetal bradycardia.
- **Tachycardia** is defined for baseline heart rate above 160 bpm. The most common cause is maternal fever or infection. Other, less common causes of fetal

tachycardia are fetal arrythmias or maternal administration of parasympatholytic or sympathomimetic drugs.
- **Variability** is the presence of instantaneous variation in the heart rate from beat to beat. It is most reliable when measured with a fetal scalp electrode.
  - **Absent:** Undetectable variation in heart rate
  - **Minimal:** Detectable variation ≤5 bpm
  - **Moderate:** Variation from 6 to 25 bpm
  - **Marked:** Variation >25 bpm
- **Accelerations:** For GA >32 weeks, acceleration is an increase in fetal heart rate (FHR) of at least 15 bpm that lasts for at least 15 seconds. For gestational age (GA) <32 weeks, the increase only needs to be >10 bpm for 10 seconds.
- A fetal heart tracing is **reactive** if it shows two accelerations within 10 minutes.
- A **sinusoidal** fetal heart tracing (FHT) is a persistent smooth undulating pattern with a frequency of 3 to 5 cycles/min. It is concerning and requires further evaluation. Fetal anemia, analgesic drugs such as morphine, meperidine, alphaprodine, and butorphanol, and chronic fetal distress should be considered.
- **Decelerations:** The fetal CNS is very sensitive to hypoxia. In some instances, the pattern of deceleration of the fetal heart rate can be used to identify the cause.
  - **Variable decelerations** may start before, during, or after the uterine contraction starts (hence the designation variable). They usually show an abrupt onset and return, which gives them a characteristic V-shape. The decrease is >15 bpm lasting >15 seconds but <2 minutes. Variable decelerations may be caused by umbilical cord compression.
  - **Early decelerations** are shallow, symmetric, and reach their nadir at the peak of the contraction. They are caused by vagus nerve–mediated response to fetal head compression.
  - **Late decelerations** are U-shaped decelerations of gradual onset and gradual return, reach their nadir after the peak of the contraction, and do not return to the baseline until after the contraction is over. They may result from uteroplacental insufficiency and relative fetal hypoxia. Recurrent late decelerations can be an ominous sign.
  - **Prolonged deceleration:** Lasts longer than 2 minutes but <10 minutes.
  - **Recurrent decelerations:** Occur with >50% of uterine contractions in any 20-minute span.
  - **Intermittent decelerations:** Occur with <50% of uterine contractions in any 20-minute span.

Overall Assessment
- **Category I FHT** have only reassuring components.
- **Category II FHT** are those that cannot be classified in the other categories.
- **Category III FHT** have concerning findings such as minimal variability, recurrent variable or late decelerations, bradycardia, or sinusoidal pattern. Consideration for delivery should be given.

Management of Nonreassuring Fetal Heart Rate Patterns
- Nonreassuring fetal heart rate patterns do not necessarily predict adverse events, and though electronic fetal heart monitoring has resulted in increased cesarean deliveries, there has not been a decrease in long-term adverse neurologic outcomes such as cerebral palsy. Nevertheless, the known relationships between fetal hypoxemia/acidemia and abnormal heart rate patterns make fetal heart tracing (FHT) interpretation a critical part of labor management.

Noninvasive Management
- **Oxygen.** Supplemental oxygen to the mother often results in improved fetal oxygenation, assuming adequate placental exchange and circulation.
- **Maternal position.** Left lateral positioning releases vena cava compression by the gravid uterus, promoting increased venous return, increased cardiac output, increased BP, and improved uterine blood flow.
- **Discontinue oxytocin** until the fetal heart rate and uterine activity become normal.
- **Vibroacoustic stimulation (VAS)** or fetal scalp stimulation may be used to induce accelerations when the fetal heart rate lacks variability for a long period of time. Heart rate acceleration in response to these stimuli indicates the absence of acidosis and correlates with a mean pH value of about 7.3. Conversely, a 50% chance of acidosis exists in a fetus who fails to respond to VAS in the setting of a nonreassuring heart rate pattern.

Invasive Management
- **Amniotomy.** If the fetal heart rate cannot be monitored adequately externally, an amniotomy should be performed to place internal monitors, unless these are contraindicated by the clinical situation. Cervical examination verifies that the cord is not prolapsed.
- **Fetal scalp electrode.** Direct application of a fetal scalp electrode records the fetal electrocardiogram (ECG) and may allow closer evaluation of the fetal heart rate.
- **Intrauterine pressure catheter and amnioinfusion.** A catheter is inserted into the chorioamnionic sac and attached to a pressure gauge. Pressure readings provide quantitative data on the strength and duration of contractions. Amnioinfusion of room temperature normal saline can be used to replace amniotic fluid volume to relieve recurrent variable decelerations in patients with oligohydramnios. Care should be used to avoid overdistention of the uterus.
- **Tocolytic agents.** Beta-adrenergic agonists (e.g., terbutaline, 0.25 mg subcutaneously or 0.125 to 0.25 mg IV) can be administered to decrease uterine activity in the presence of uterine tachysystole. Potential side effects of beta-adrenergic agonists include elevated serum glucose levels and increased maternal and fetal heart rates.
- **Management of maternal hypotension.** Maternal hypotension, as a complication of the sympathetic blockade associated with epidural anesthesia or from compression of the vena cava, can lead to decreased placental perfusion and fetal heart rate decelerations. IV fluid bolus, left uterine displacement, and ephedrine administration may be appropriate.
- **Fetal scalp blood pH.** Determination of fetal scalp blood pH can clarify the acid-base state of the fetus. A pH value of 7.25 or higher is normal. A pH range of 7.20 to 7.24 is a preacidotic. A pH of <7.20 on two collections 5 to 10 minutes apart may indicate sufficient fetal acidosis to warrant immediate delivery.

ASSISTED SPONTANEOUS VAGINAL DELIVERY

The goals of assisted spontaneous vaginal delivery are reduction of maternal trauma, prevention of fetal injury, and initial support of the newborn.
- **Episiotomy** is an incision into the perineal body to enlarge the outlet area and facilitate delivery. Episiotomy may occasionally be necessary in cases of vaginal soft tissue dystocia or as an accompaniment to forceps or vacuum delivery. Prophylactic episiotomy increases the risk of higher degrees of perineal tears.

- An incision is made vertically in the perineal body (midline episiotomy) or at a 45-degree angle off the midline (mediolateral episiotomy). The incision should be approximately half the length of the perineal body. The incision should extend into the vagina 2 to 3 cm. Excessive blood loss can result from performing the episiotomy too early. The episiotomy can be performed either before or after the application of forceps or a vacuum.
- Midline episiotomies are associated with increased risk of extension to 3rd- or 4th-degree laceration when compared with mediolateral episiotomy or no episiotomy. Mediolateral episiotomies may require more postpartum analgesia.
- The goal of assisted **delivery of the head** is to prevent excessively rapid delivery. If extension of the head does not occur easily, a modified Ritgen's maneuver can be performed by palpating the fetal chin through the perineum and applying pressure upward. After delivery of the head, external rotation is possible, which brings the occiput in line with the fetal spine. If a nuchal cord is present, it is reduced over the head or double-clamped and cut. Mucous and amniotic fluids are aspirated from the infant's mouth and nose using bulb suction.
- **Delivery of the shoulders and body.** After the fetal airway has been cleared, the fetus is directed posteriorly until the anterior shoulder has passed beneath the pubic bone. The fetus is then directed anteriorly until the posterior shoulder passes the perineum. After the shoulders are delivered, the fetus is grasped with one hand supporting the head and neck, and the other hand along the spine.

OPERATIVE VAGINAL DELIVERY

Operative vaginal delivery can be an effective alternative to cesarean section for women in the second stage of labor who meet specific criteria.

Forceps Delivery

- Classification is by station of the fetal head at the time that the forceps are applied
  - **Mid forceps.** Head is engaged (but above +2 station).
  - **Low forceps.** Station is +2 or lower.
  - **Outlet forceps.** Scalp is visible without separating the labia, skull has reached pelvic floor, head is at or on perineum, and the occiput is either directly anterior-posterior in alignment or does not require more than 45 degrees of rotation.
- **Indication:** None are absolute, but they include
  - prolonged second stage of labor
  - maternal exhaustion
  - inadequate maternal expulsive effort
  - fetal intolerance of labor
  - a maternal condition requiring a shortened/passive second stage
- **Prerequisites:** Before operative vaginal delivery is attempted, the following criteria should be met:
  - The fetal head must be engaged in the pelvis.
  - The cervix must be fully dilated.
  - The bladder should be empty.
  - The exact station and position of the fetal head should be known.
  - Maternal pelvis must be adequate.
  - If time permits, the patient should be given adequate anesthesia.
  - If forceps delivery is done for nonreassuring fetal status, someone who is able to perform neonatal resuscitation should be available.

- The operator should have knowledge about, and experience with, the appropriate instrument, its proper application, and the possible complications.
- **Maternal complications:** Uterine, cervical, or vaginal lacerations, extension of the episiotomy, bladder or urethral injuries, and hematomas.
- **Fetal complications.** Cephalohematoma, bruising, lacerations, facial nerve injury, and, rarely, skull fracture and intracranial hemorrhage.

Soft Cup Vacuum Delivery

- Indications, contraindications, and complications are largely the same as for forceps delivery.
- The suction cup is applied in the midline on the sagittal suture about 1 to 3 cm anterior to the posterior fontanelle (the "flexion point").
- Maximum vacuum suction of 0.7 to 0.8 kg/cm^2 (500 to 600 mm Hg) is applied, then one hand maintains fetal flexion and supports the vacuum cup while the other applies sustained traction to assist delivery of the vertex.
- Traction is applied, without rocking or twisting, only during contractions.
- Vacuum pressure can be released between contractions and should not be maintained for longer than 30 minutes.
- Vacuum use should be avoided in fetuses <34 weeks' gestational age or with known thrombocytopenia, hemophilia, or von Willebrand's disease.

SHOULDER DYSTOCIA

Shoulder dystocia occurs in 0.15% to 1.70% of all vaginal deliveries and is defined as impaction of the fetal shoulder after delivery of the head. It is associated with increased fetal morbidity and mortality secondary to brachial plexus injuries and asphyxia. The diagnosis should be considered when the application of gentle, downward traction of the fetal head fails to accomplish delivery.

- **Macrosomia** is strongly associated with shoulder dystocia. Compared to average-sized infants, the risk of shoulder dystocia is 11 and 22 times greater for infants weighing more than 4,000 and 4,500 g, respectively. Up to 50% of cases, however, occur in infants weighing <4,000 g. Postterm and macrosomic infants are at risk because the trunk and shoulder growth is disproportionate to growth of the head in late pregnancy.
- Other **risk factors** include maternal obesity, previous macrosomic infant, diabetes mellitus, and gestational diabetes. Shoulder dystocia should be suspected in cases of prolonged second stage of labor or prolonged deceleration phase of first stage of labor.

Management

- Anticipation and preparation are important. Help should be available; extra hands may be needed during the delivery. A pediatrician should be notified. If available, an anesthesiologist should also be informed.
- The time should be marked when the dystocia is called, and the total time till delivery recorded in the notes. Once shoulder dystocia is identified, no significant traction should be applied to the head until the shoulders are delivered. Fundal pressure should *never* be applied; it only exacerbates the shoulder impaction.
- **McRoberts' maneuver** is performed by hyperflexion and abduction of the maternal hips, flattening the lumbar spine, and rotating the pelvis to increase the posterior

outlet diameter. **Suprapubic pressure** is applied in a vector chosen to anteriorly rotate the anterior fetal shoulder and dislodge the shoulder from the symphysis.

- Other measures in combination are chosen for the specific clinical situation based on clinician experience. There is no "right order" in which the maneuvers described below should be performed. If additional room is needed, a generous **episiotomy** should be performed without hesitation. The anterior fetal shoulder can be rotated obliquely with a vaginal hand (**Rubin's manuever**). The **Wood's corkscrew** maneuver is performed by rotating the posterior shoulder 180 degrees with a vaginal hand. The **posterior arm** can be flexed and swept across the fetal chest to deliver it first and create more room for the anterior shoulder. **Clavicles can be fractured** deliberately with the thumb applying outward pressure, to avoid lung or subclavian injury.
- In extreme cases, the **Zavanelli maneuver** (in which the fetal head is flexed and pushed back up into the uterus as preparations for emergent cesarean section are made) or **symphysiotomy** (performed by laterally displacing the urethra using the index and middle fingers placed against the posterior aspect of the symphysis and incising the cartilaginous portion of the symphysis) could be performed.

CESAREAN SECTION

- **Fetal indications** for C-section include:
  - Nonreassuring fetal heart tracing
  - Nonvertex presentation
  - Fetal anomalies, such as hydrocephalus, that would make successful vaginal delivery unlikely
  - Umbilical cord prolapse
  - Conjoined twins
- **Maternal indications** for C-section include
  - Obstruction of the lower genital tract (e.g., large condyloma)
  - Previous cesarean section (if vaginal birth after cesarean [VBAC] is declined or not appropriate)
  - Previous uterine surgery involving the contractile portion of the uterus (i.e., classical cesarean, transmural myomectomy)
  - History of severe pelvic floor injury from a prior vaginal delivery
  - Abdominal cerclage
- **Maternal and fetal indications** include
  - Abruptio placentae
  - Active maternal herpes simplex virus infection
  - Labor dystocia or cephalopelvic disproportion
  - Placenta previa or known vasa previa (absolute indication)
- The patient should be counseled regarding standard **risks of surgery**, such as pain, bleeding that may require transfusion, infection, damage to nearby organs, and a small but increased risk of death when compared to vaginal delivery.

VAGINAL BIRTH AFTER CESAREAN SECTION (VBAC)

- Provided there are no contraindications to vaginal delivery, a patient may be counseled and offered VBAC. Success rates are higher for patients with nonrecurring conditions, such as malpresentation or fetal intolerance of labor (60% to 85%) than for those with a prior diagnosis of dystocia (15% to 30%).

- **Contraindications** include previous classical, inverted T-shaped incision, transfundal uterine surgery, history of uterine rupture, contracted pelvis, and medical or obstetric contraindications to vaginal delivery. A history of two or more C-sections without any successful vaginal deliveries may preclude offering VBAC as well.
- Epidural anesthesia and oxytocin may be used with VBAC. The delivery hospital must have facilities and staffing for emergency cesarean delivery. Blood products should be readily available. The most common sign of uterine rupture is a nonreassuring fetal heart rate pattern with variable decelerations evolving into late decelerations, bradycardia, and undetectable fetal heart rate. Other findings include uterine or abdominal pain, loss of station of the presenting part, vaginal bleeding, and hypovolemia.

MALPRESENTATIONS

Normal presentation is defined by longitudinal lie, cephalic presentation, and flexion of the fetal neck. All other presentations are malpresentations. Occurring in approximately 5% of all deliveries, malpresentations may lead to abnormalities of labor and increased risk for mother or fetus.
- **Risk factors** for malpresentation are conditions that decrease the polarity of the uterus, increase or decrease fetal mobility, or block the presenting part from the pelvis.
  - **Maternal factors** include grand multiparity, pelvic tumors, uterine fibroids, pelvic contracture, and uterine malformations.
  - **Fetal factors** include prematurity, multiple gestation, polyhydramnios or oligohydramnios, macrosomia, placenta previa, hydrocephaly, trisomy, anencephaly, and myotonic dystrophy.
- **Breech** presentation occurs when the cephalic pole is in the uterine fundus. Major congenital anomalies occur in 6.3% of term breech presentation infants compared to 2.4% of vertex presentation infants.
  - The **incidence of breech** presentation is 25% of pregnancies at <28 weeks' gestation, 7% of pregnancies at 32 weeks' gestation, and 3% to 4% of term pregnancies in labor.
  - The **three types** of breech presentation are:
    - **Frank** breech (48% to 73%) occurs when both hips are flexed and both knees are extended.
    - **Complete** breech (5% to 12%) occurs when the fetus is flexed at the hips and flexed at the knees.
    - **Incomplete,** or footling breech (12% to 38%), occurs when the fetus has one or both hips extended (see Fig. 5-1).
- **Risks** of breech presentation include cord prolapse (15% in footling breech, 5% in complete breech, and 0.5% in frank breech), head entrapment, and spinal cord injury (with neck hyperextension).
- Fetuses in a complete or frank breech presentation may occasionally be considered for vaginal delivery with appropriate selection and counseling.
- Cesarean section poses risk of increased maternal morbidity and mortality.
- Vaginal breech delivery poses increased risk of fetal asphyxia, cord prolapse, birth trauma, spinal cord injury, and mortality. Planned vaginal breech delivery is not routinely offered, but with careful selection and evaluation, may be permitted.

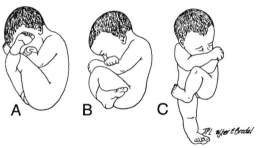

Figure 5-1. Breech presentations. (**A**) Frank breech. (**B**) Complete breech. (**C**) Incomplete breech, single footling. (From Beckmann CR, Ling FW, Herbert WN, et al. *Obstetrics and Gynecology*, 2nd Ed. Baltimore, MD: Williams & Wilkins, 1995:194, with permission.)

- For patients in advanced labor with a breech fetus for whom delivery is imminent, a trial of labor may be attempted if
  - The breech is frank or complete
  - The estimated fetal weight is <3,800 g
  - Pelvimetry suggests an adequate pelvis
  - The fetal head is flexed
  - Anesthesia is immediately available
  - The fetus is continuously monitored
  - A pediatrician is available
  - And an obstetrician who is experienced with vaginal breech delivery can attend
- In breech presentation, the fetus usually emerges in the sacrum transverse or oblique position. As crowning occurs (the bitrochanteric diameter passes under the symphysis), an episiotomy should be considered.
- When the umbilicus appears, one may place fingers medial to each thigh and press out laterally to deliver the legs (Pinard maneuver). The fetus should then be rotated to the anterior sacrum position, and the trunk can be wrapped in a towel for traction.
- When the scapulas appear, fingers should be placed over the shoulders from the back. The humerus should be followed down, and each arm rotated across the chest and out (Lovsett's maneuver). To deliver the *right* arm, the fetus is turned in a *counterclockwise* direction; to deliver the *left* arm, the fetus is turned in a *clockwise* direction.
- If the head does not deliver spontaneously, the head may be flexed by placing downward traction and pressure on the maxillary ridge (Mauriceau-Smellie-Veit maneuver). Direct vertical suprapubic pressure may also be applied. Piper forceps may be used to assist in delivery of the head.
- For delivery of a breech second twin, ultrasonography should be available in the delivery room. The operator reaches into the uterus and grasps both feet, trying to keep the membranes intact. The feet are brought down to the introitus, then amniotomy is performed. The body is delivered to the scapula by applying gentle traction on the feet. The remainder of the delivery is the same as that described earlier for a singleton breech.

- **Head entrapment** during breech vaginal delivery may be managed by one or more of the following procedures:
  - **Dührssen's incisions** are made in the cervix at the 2, 6, and 10 o'clock positions. Either two or three incisions can be made. The 3 and 9 o'clock positions should be avoided due to the risk of entering the cervical vessels and causing hemorrhage.
  - Relaxation agents (nitric oxide or nitroglycerine) may release the entrapped head, enable proper head flexion, and vaginal delivery.
  - Cephalocentesis can be performed if the fetus is not viable. The procedure is performed by perforating the base of the skull and suctioning the cranial contents.
- **External cephalic version**
  - **Indication** is persistent breech presentation at term. The version is performed to avoid breech presentation in labor.
  - **Risks** include cord accident, placental separation, fetal distress, fetal injury, premature rupture of membranes, and fetomaternal bleeding (overall incidence is 0% to 1.4%). The most common "risk" is failed version.
  - **Success rate** for external cephalic version ranges from 35% to 86%, but in 2% of cases the fetus reverts back to breech presentation.
  - **Technique.** A gestational age of at least 36 weeks, reactive nonstress test, and informed consent must be obtained. Version is generally accomplished by applying a liberal amount of lubrication then transabdominally grasping the fetal head and fetal breech, and manipulating the fetus through a forward or backward roll. Ultrasonographic guidance is an important adjunct to confirm position and monitor fetal heart rate. Tocolysis and spinal or epidural anesthesia may improve success rates. After the procedure, the patient should be monitored continuously until the fetal heart rate is reactive, no decelerations are present, and no evidence of regular contractions exists. Rh-negative patients should receive Rh_O (D) immune globulin (RhoGAM) after the procedure because of the potential for fetomaternal bleeding.
  - **Factors associated with failure** include obesity, oligohydramnios, deep engagement of the presenting part, a partial uterine septum, and fetal back posterior. Nulliparity and an anterior placenta may also reduce the likelihood of success.
  - **Contraindications** to external cephalic version include conditions in which labor or vaginal delivery would be contraindicated. Version is not generally recommended in cases of ruptured membranes, third trimester bleeding, oligohydramnios, multiple gestations, or after labor has begun.
- **Abnormal lie**
  - "Lie" refers to the alignment of the fetal spine in relation to the maternal spine. Longitudinal lie is normal, whereas oblique and transverse lies are abnormal. Abnormal lie is associated with multiparity, prematurity, pelvic contraction, and disorders of the placenta.
  - **Incidence** of abnormal lie is 1 in 300 term pregnancies. At 32 weeks' gestation the incidence is <2%.
  - **Risk.** The greatest risk of abnormal lie is cord prolapse, because the fetal parts do not fill the pelvic inlet.
  - **Management.** If abnormal lie persists beyond 35 to 38 weeks, external version may be attempted. An ultrasonographic examination should be performed to rule out major anomalies and abnormal placentation. If an abnormal axial lie persists, mode of delivery should be cesarean section. An intraoperative cephalic version may be attempted. A vertical uterine incision may be prudent in cases with back down transverse or oblique lie with ruptured membranes or poorly developed lower uterine segment.

- **Abnormal attitude and deflexion.** Full flexion of the fetal neck is considered normal. Abnormalities range from partial deflexion to full extension:
  - **Face presentation** results from extension of the fetal neck. The chin is the presenting part.
    - **Incidence** is between 0.14% and 0.54%. In 60% of cases, face presentation is associated with a fetal malformation. Anencephaly accounts for 33% of all cases.
    - **Diagnosis.** Face presentation may be diagnosed by vaginal examination, ultrasonography, or palpation of the cephalic prominence and the fetal back on the same side of the maternal abdomen when performing Leopold's maneuvers.
    - **Risk.** Perinatal mortality ranges from 0.6% to 5.0%.
    - **Management.** The fetus must be mentum (chin) anterior for a vaginal delivery to be successful.
  - **Brow presentation** results from partial deflexion of the fetal neck.
    - **Incidence** is 1 in 670 to 1 in 3,433 pregnancies. Causes of brow presentation are similar to those of face presentation.
    - **Risks.** Perinatal mortality ranges from 1.28% to 8.00%.
    - **Management.** The majority of cases spontaneously convert to a flexed attitude. A vaginal delivery should be considered only if the maternal pelvis is large, the fetus is small, and labor progresses adequately.
- **Compound presentation** occurs when an extremity prolapses beside the presenting part.
  - **Incidence** is 1 in 377 to 1 in 1,213 pregnancies and is associated with prematurity.
  - **Risks.** Fetal risks are cord prolapse in 10% to 20% of cases and birth trauma including neurologic and musculoskeletal damage to the involved extremity.
  - **Management.** The prolapsing extremity should not be manipulated. Continuous fetal monitoring is recommended because compound presentation can be associated with occult cord prolapse. Spontaneous vaginal delivery occurs in 75% of vertex/upper extremity presentations. Cesarean section is indicated in cases of nonreassuring fetal heart tracing, cord prolapse, and failure of labor to progress.

SUGGESTED READINGS

Cunningham FG, Leveno KJ, Bloom SL, et al. (Normal labor and delivery) and 18 (Intrapartum assessment). *Williams Obstetrics*, 23rd Ed. New York: McGraw-Hill, 2009.

Halpern SH, Leighton BL, Ohlsson A, et al. Effect of epidural versus parenteral opioid analgesia on the progress of labor: a meta-analysis. *JAMA* 1998;280(24):2105–2110.

Vaginal birth after previous cesarean delivery. ACOG Practice Bulletin Number 54. American College of Obstetricians and Gynecologists. *Obstet Gynecol* 2004;104(1):203–212.

Fetal Assessment

Melissa L. Russo, Janice Henderson, and
Kathleen A. Costigan

The primary goal of **antenatal fetal surveillance** is to prevent perinatal demise. In order to accomplish this, it is necessary to identify high-risk pregnancies and closely monitor those fetuses to circumvent fetal hypoxemia, acidemia, and death. A secondary goal is to prevent fetal asphyxia and neurological damage. Antenatal fetal testing is used for multiple purposes including reassurance of fetal well-being, guidance of future management, and determination of the necessity for admission to the hospital or for imminent delivery.

METHODS OF FETAL ASSESSMENT

There are numerous methods to assess fetal well-being, and there is no single test that is superior to the other methods. Each test has its own individual merits, and combinations of these tests create an overall picture of the fetal state and can help to identify fetal compromise (Table 6-1).

Fetal Movement
- **Maternal assessment of fetal movement (kick counts)**
  - This is the simplest test of fetal surveillance.
  - It is the least expensive and least invasive fetal assessment test.
  - **Purpose:** It can be used for screening and reassurance in healthy pregnancies where a mother is concerned about the perception of decreased fetal movement. It can also be used as a first method of surveillance in some higher risk pregnancies, for example, in women with a prior history of stillbirth.
  - **Method of testing:** This method relies on the mother to count the number of fetal movements in a finite period of time. To optimize the success of reassurance of fetal well-being, the mother should perform this test lying on her left side to improve blood flow to the fetus and should eat prior to starting the test, to stimulate the fetus.
    - The Cardiff technique involves the mother counting fetal movements when she first gets up in the morning and recording the time required for the fetus to move ten times. On average this process should only take 2 to 3 hr; longer time periods should prompt the mother to call her physician for further fetal testing.
    - The Sadovsky technique involves the mother counting fetal movements over the course of 1 hr. This test is usually performed after meals, lying in the left lateral position. To be considered "reassuring," four or more fetal movements should be observed over the course of the hour. If four movements have not been felt over the first hour, a second hour monitoring should be attempted. If, after 2 hr, four fetal movements have not been felt, the mother should contact her doctor for further recommendations of fetal testing.
  - **Management after abnormal results:** After the observation of decreased fetal movement, the next sequential test to evaluate fetal well-being is a nonstress test (NST).

TABLE 6-1	Comparison of Antenatal Fetal Tests		
Antenatal Tests	**Strengths**	**Limitations**	**Influential Factors**
Kick counts	• Inexpensive • Noninvasive • Simple	• Need maternal participation • No supervision of physician	
Nonstress test (NST)	• Noninvasive • Simple	• Limited value <32 wk • Low sensitivity • High false positive rate	• Smoking • Other maternal medications • Illicit drug use • Magnesium sulfate • Sleep cycle • Prematurity
Vibroacoustic stimulation (VAS)	• Noninvasive • Prevents some false positive results from NST	• Limited value <32 wk • Low sensitivity	
Contraction stress test (CST)	• Highest specificity	• Contraindications: preterm labor, ruptured membranes, placenta previa, extensive uterine surgery • Cannot use in premature infants • Labor intensive	
Biophysical profile (BPP)	• Useful in premature fetuses	• High false positive rate	• Betamethasone • Maternal hypoglycemia
Uterine artery Doppler ultrasound	• Predicts fetal compromise earlier than other tests	• Only useful in specific conditions	

Fetal Heart Monitoring

- **Nonstress test**
  - **Method of testing:** The NST is performed using cardiotocography to record the fetal heart rate and uterine activity. The fetal heart rate is monitored with an external cardioechometer. The external cardioechometer uses ultrasound to evaluate fetal heart motion, giving an average of fetal heart beats. Uterine activity is monitored with an external tocodynamometer. This is a simple method of fetal assessment and is relatively noninvasive.

- **Criteria for test results:** A "reactive" NST demonstrates at least two accelerations of the fetal heart rate over a 20-minute period. Each of the two accelerations must be 15 seconds in duration and must reach a peak of 15 beats above the baseline level (Fig. 6-1). If the fetal heart rate is "nonreactive" after 20 minutes, the fetal heart rate should be observed for an additional 20 minutes to account for the possibility that the fetus could have been in quiet sleep during the initial 20-minute observation period. There are many other factors that can influence the fetal heart rate tracing (see below).
- **Strengths and limitations:** A "reactive" NST is highly predictive of a low risk of fetal morality in the subsequent 72 hr, 96 hr, or a week depending on the indication for fetal testing. The negative predictive value of an NST is >90%. The positive predictive value is only 50% to 70%. Therefore, the NST is better suited to rule out rather than predict fetal compromise. It has a high false positive rate and a "nonreactive" NST should be followed by more extensive testing such as biophysical profile (BPP), vibroacoustic stimulation (VAS), or contraction stress test (CST).
  - Before 32 weeks' gestational age, 50% of normal fetuses will have a "nonreactive" NST secondary to immaturity of the fetal sympathetic and parasympathetic innervation. However, there are modified criteria of two accelerations of 10 minutes in duration and 10 beats above baseline levels that are defined as a reactive tracing.

Contraction Stress Test

- **Contraction stress test** or **oxytocin challenge test (OCT)**
  - **Purpose:** The CST is designed to assess fetal response to the stress of induced uterine contractions causing relative uteroplacental insufficiency.
  - **Method of testing:** The mother is placed in the left lateral tilt position, and external monitors are applied. Contractions are induced either by having the patient stimulate her nipples or by infusing a dilute solution of oxytocin until three contractions occur in a 10-minute time period. Many institutions have their own defined protocol for titration of pitocin and the starting dose for this test.

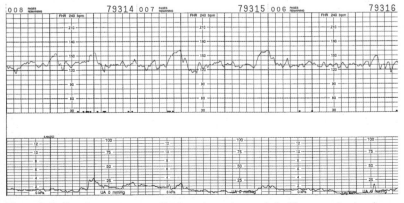

Figure 6-1. Reactive nonstress test. Fetal monitor strip records fetal heart rate (**top**) and uterine contractile activity (**bottom**). Several accelerations are evident.

- **Criteria for test results:** A "positive" CST is one in which late decelerations occur with more than 50% of contractions (Fig. 6-2). Late decelerations are decelerations that reach their nadir after the peak of the contraction. A "negative" CST is one in which no late decelerations occur. A CST with nonrepetitive late decelerations is considered equivocal, and further evaluation of the pregnancy is performed. An "inadequate" or "unsatisfactory" CST is one in which adequate contractions are not achieved. If hyperstimulation occurs, an abnormal fetal response may be the result of the testing technique alone and should be repeated or another form of testing should be done.
- **Strengths and limitations:** CST is one of the most labor-intensive methods of fetal surveillance, but has the highest specificity for detecting the compromised fetus. It has a negative predictive value of >99%. Relative contraindications to CST include preterm labor, preterm premature rupture of membranes (PPROM), placenta previa, and high risk for uterine rupture. Previous low transverse cesarean section is not a contraindication.

Vibroacoustic Stimulation

- **Vibroacoustic stimulation test (VAS)**
  - **Purpose**: VAS is a useful adjunct to a nonreactive NST. This test will decrease false positive results of nonreactive NST if the cause of the abnormal test is fetal sleep.
  - **Method of testing:** This test is performed by placing an auditory source, such as an artificial larynx, on the maternal abdomen. The sound device is placed halfway between the pubic symphysis and umbilicus, and it delivers a short burst of sound to the fetus for 5 seconds. The procedure stimulates the fetus to move and shortens the time necessary to produce fetal heart rate accelerations. It is important to avoid stimulating the fetus when it is experiencing stress from a contraction because this may cause the fetus to have a drop in heart rate.
  - **Criteria for test results:** The VAS is used in conjunction with the NST and is interpreted similarly to the NST. See above.

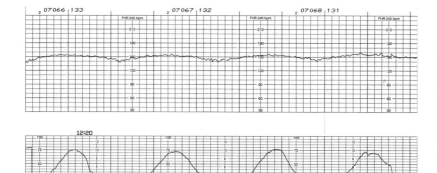

Figure 6-2. Fetal heart tracing with late decelerations. Following each contraction (**bottom tracing**) is a slight depression of the fetal heart rate (**top tracing**), suggesting uteroplacental insufficiency. (Original fetal monitor strip from Dr. Janice Henderson, Johns Hopkins Hospital, Department of Gynecology and Obstetrics, Division of Maternal Fetal Medicine.)

Biophysical Profile

- **Biophysical profile (BPP)**
  - **Purpose:** The BPP was developed to help predict acute and chronic tissue hypoxia. It has excellent negative predictive value for fetal mortality in the 72 to 96 hr after the test. It has been shown to reduce perinatal morbidity and mortality.
  - **Method of testing:** The BPP has five components: the NST, fetal breathing, fetal movement, fetal tone, and amniotic fluid assessment determined by ultrasound. Two points are awarded for each observed parameter. The maximum score is 10. The specific criteria of these components are listed in Table 6-2. All of the sonographic criteria must be observed within a 30-minute period.
  - **Criteria for test results:** A score of 8 or 10 is reassuring, and routine surveillance and expectant obstetric management may continue. A score of 6 raises concern, and the BPP should be repeated in 6 to 24 hr, especially in fetuses over 32 weeks' gestation. If the score does not improve, delivery should be considered, depending on gestational age and individual circumstances. Scores of 4 or below are worrisome, and delivery should be considered, again depending on gestational age and clinical context. It is important to consider that fetal breathing can be reduced in preterm fetuses <34 weeks' gestation, and this may affect interpretation.

Modified BPP
- **Modified BPP**
  - **Purpose:** This test is also known as the **NST and amniotic fluid index (AFI)**. In the third trimester, an AFI and NST are often used together to assess fetal well-being. The AFI is the sum of the maximum vertical pockets of umbilical cord-free amniotic fluid in each of the four quadrants of the uterus. In general, the AFI reflects fetal perfusion, and, if decreased, raises suspicion for placental insufficiency.
  - **Criteria for test results:** A normal test has a reactive NST and an AFI >5. An abnormal test lacks one or both of these findings.

TABLE 6-2	Biophysical Profile	
Biophysical Variable	**Normal (Score = 2)**	**Abnormal (Score = 0)**
Fetal breathing movements	One episode of fetal breathing 30 s	Less than 30 s of fetal breathing; absent breathing
Fetal movements	Three discrete body/limb movements	Two or fewer body/limb movements
Fetal tone	One episode of active extension, with return to flexion of fetal limbs or trunk	Extended position with no or slow return to flexion; absent movement
Nonstress test	Reactive	Nonreactive
Amniotic fluid volume	One pocket of fluid at least 2 cm in two perpendicular planes	No amniotic fluid or pocket <2 cm in size

Doppler Velocimetry

- **Doppler velocimetry**
  - **Purpose**: Doppler velocimetry is a noninvasive method of assessing fetal vascular impedance (see Fig. 6-3).
  - **Method of testing:** Umbilical artery flow can be documented using real-time sonography. A free floating loop of umbilical cord is identified, and continuous or pulsed wave Dopplers are used to identify arterial flow. The waveform pattern is recorded and analyzed. The most common method of analysis is the systolic/diastolic (S/D) ratio. The presence of diastolic flow has greater clinical significance than the S/D ratio. The normal values vary depending on gestational age. Significant elevations in the S/D ratio have been associated with intrauterine growth retardation, fetal hypoxia or acidosis or both, and higher rates of perinatal morbidity and

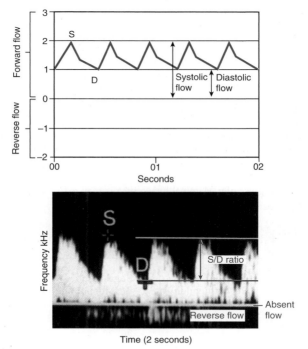

Figure 6-3. Evaluation of umbilical artery flow by Doppler velocimetry. **Top panel** illustrates the findings for a normal umbilical artery. **Bottom image** is a typical normal Doppler recording. Ratio of flow during systole and diastole (S/D ratio) reflects placental bed resistance. S, systole; D, diastole. (Adapted from Druzin ML, Gabbe SG, Reed KL. Antepartum fetal evaluation. In Gabbe SG, Niebyl JR, Simpson JL, eds. *Obstetrics: Normal and Problem Pregnancies*, 4th Ed. New York, NY: Churchill Livingstone, 2001:334 and from MacDonald MG, Mullet MD, Seshia MMK. *Avery's Neonatology Pathophysiology & Management of the Newborn*, 6th Ed. Philadelphia, PA: Lippincott Williams & Wilkins, 2005.)

mortality. Absent and reversed end-diastolic flow are the more extreme examples of abnormal S/D ratio and may prompt delivery in some situations.

- **Strengths and limitations:** Abnormal umbilical artery blood flow patterns are reported to precede abnormal FHR patterns by a median of 7 days. For this reason, it is used in conjunction with other tests for pregnancies complicated by intrauterine growth restriction (IUGR), preeclampsia, or chronic hypertension.
- **Indications for use:** Umbilical artery doppler should not be used as a screening tool in the general population. It has been shown to be useful in pregnancies complicated by IUGR and in pregnancies complicated by hypertension/preeclampsia.

CONFOUNDING FACTORS IN FETAL ASSESSMENT

- **Sleep cycles:** The fetus may have sleep cycles 20 to 80 minutes in duration. During these periods, the long-term variability of the fetal heart rate is decreased, and the tracing is likely to be nonreactive. To rule out sleep cycle as a cause for a nonreactive NST, prolonged monitoring is often required (longer than 80 minutes at times).
- **Medications:** Certain medications taken by the mother cross the placenta and can have an effect on the fetal heart rate, movement, and amniotic fluid volume. There are a number of medications administered in the management of labor and complications of labor that can have an influence on the tests for fetal well-being. Glucocorticosteroids given for the purpose of maturing premature fetal lungs have been shown to influence BPP scores by decreasing the AFI, decreasing fetal movement, and decreasing breathing motion. Magnesium sulfate can decrease the fetal heart rate variability. Other medications, such as narcotics, sedatives, and beta-blockers have been shown to decrease fetal heart rate variability and reactivity.
- **Maternal smoking and illicit drugs:** The maternal use of illicit drugs and smoking results in a transient decrease in fetal heart rate variability.
- **Maternal hypoglycemia:** Maternal hypoglycemia may reduce fetal heart rate variability as well as fetal movement and fetal breathing.

TABLE 6-3	Recommendations for Antenatal Fetal Assessment: Diabetes		
Indication	**Recommended Tests**	**Suggested Gestational Age for Commencement**	**Frequency of Testing**
Pregestational diabetes	US and fetal echo	18–20 wk	Once
	Kick counts	26–28 wk	Daily
	US fetal growth	28 wk	q4wk
	NST/BPP	32 wk	2×/wk
Gestational diabetes Class A1	Kick counts	28 wk	Daily
Gestational diabetes Class A2	Kick counts	26–28 wk	Daily
	US fetal growth	28 wk	q4–6wk
	NST/BPP or modified BPP	32 wk	1–2×/wk

TABLE 6-4	Recommendations for Antenatal Fetal Testing: Fetal Conditions		
Indication	Recommended Tests	Suggested Gestational Age for Commencement	Frequency of Testing
Intrauterine growth restriction	Umbilical Dopplers NST AFI BPP	Time of diagnosis	Weekly or Twice weekly Weekly to daily Weekly Weekly to Daily
Postterm Pregnancy	NST	41 wk	2–3×/wk
Isoimmunization	MCA Doppler for fetal anemia	16–18 wk	Weekly
Preterm premature rupture of membranes (PPROM)	NST BPP	At time of PPROM	Daily to 2×/wk
Cholestasis of pregnancy	NST	28–32 wk	2×/wk
Oligohydramnios	AFI	Time of diagnosis	Weekly
History of prior stillbirth	Kick counts NST, AFI, BPP	26–28 wk 32 wk or 1–2 wk prior to GA of previous stillbirth	Daily weekly to 2×/wk

INDICATIONS FOR FETAL TESTING

- **Maternal conditions and complications of pregnancy:** There are numerous maternal medical conditions, complications of pregnancy, and fetal conditions that confer increased risk of adverse fetal outcomes. Therefore, antenatal fetal surveillance is recommended in these high-risk pregnancies in an attempt to prevent fetal morbidity and mortality. Tables 6-3 and 6-4 outline some of the maternal and fetal indications for antenatal fetal surveillance, the methods of testing to be employed for fetal assessment, the gestational age to begin testing, and the frequency of monitoring. Other indications for fetal testing are: chronic hypertension, preeclampsia, maternal renal disease, lupus, maternal hemoglobinopathies, antiphospholipid syndrome, chronic abruption, and monoamnionic monochorionic twins.
- **Commencement and frequency of testing:** Each maternal and fetal indication for fetal surveillance has its own recommendations for the commencement and frequency of testing based on the underlying etiology of disease and the perceived risk to the fetus. These are outlined in Tables 6-3 and 6-4.

SUGGESTED READINGS

Antepartum fetal surveillance. Practice Bulletin Number 9. American College of Obstetricians and Gynecologists. *Int J Gynaecol Obstet* 2000;68(2):175–185.

Devoe LD. Antenatal fetal assessment: contraction stress test, nonstress test, vibroacoustic stimulation, amniotic fluid volume, biophysical profile, and modified biophysical profile—an overview. *Semin Perinatol* 2008;32:247–252.

Nageotte M. Antenatal testing: diabetes mellitus. *Semin Perinatol* 2008;32:269–270.

Turan S, Miller J, Baschat A. Integrated testing and management in fetal growth restriction. *Semin Perinatol* 2008;32:194–200.

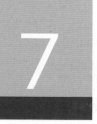

7 Complications of Labor and Delivery

Elizabeth Purcell and Jessica L. Bienstock

POSTPARTUM HEMORRHAGE (PPH)

PPH is defined as
- Estimated blood loss (EBL) >500 mL for a vaginal delivery or >1,000 mL for a cesarean delivery; or
- Ten percent drop in hematocrit between admission and the postpartum period; or
- Any bleeding sufficient to cause symptoms or require erythrocyte transfusion.
  - Although traditionally 500 mL has been used to define PPH for vaginal delivery, that is probably close to the normal average blood loss, given visual underestimation of EBL.

Incidence
- PPH is the leading cause of maternal death, accounting for at least 25% of maternal deaths worldwide. It is the second leading cause of pregnancy-related death in the United States, accounting for 17% of maternal mortality.

Etiology and Management (see Table 7-1)
- Patients often tolerate loss of up to 20% of blood volume before symptoms of hypovolemia develop. Prompt, even anticipatory, action is crucial. Blood flow to the gravid uterus is 600 mL/min; patients can become unstable rapidly.
- Establish large bore intravenous (IV) access. Initiate IV fluid resuscitation. Administer supplemental oxygen, and order cross-matched blood. After these initial steps, examine the patient to determine the underlying cause and address the problem expeditiously.
- Blood transfusion should be considered after 1 to 2 L EBL. Coagulation factors (fresh frozen plasma [FFP] and coprecipitate) and platelets should be repleted with massive blood loss. One unit of FFP is given for every 4 to 6 units of packed red blood cells to reduce dilutional and citrate coagulopathy. Consider platelet transfusion as the platelet count drops below 50,000/μL.

Uterine Atony
- **Uterine atony** (postpartum uterine contraction inadequate for hemostasis) is the most common cause of PPH.
- Normally, uterine contraction after delivery compresses uterine vessels, thereby reducing blood loss. Atony permits continuous brisk bleeding.
- Risk factors include uterine overdistention (as with fetal macrosomia, polyhydramnios, or multiple gestation); prolonged, augmented, or precipitous labor; chorioamnionitis; grand multiparity; and use of tocolytic agents.
- Initial management is **bimanual massage** of the uterus to stimulate contraction and evacuation of clot from the lower uterine segment to remove a distending mass. Along with oxytocin administration, this is sufficient in most cases.
- **Procontractile agents** can be administered if atony persists (Table 7-2). Oxytocin, methylergonovine, and prostaglandins are appropriate. Rectal misoprotol (800 to 1,000 μg) is often used to stimulate sustained uterine contraction.

TABLE 7-1	Etiology of PPH
Early (<24 hr Postpartum)	**Late (24 hr to Several Months Postpartum)**
Uterine atony	Infection
Retained placental fragments	Placental site subinvolution
Lower genital tract lacerations	Retained placental fragments
Uterine rupture	Hereditary coagulopathy
Uterine inversion	Preexisting uterine pathology
Hereditary coagulopathy	
Placenta accreta	

Adapted from American College of Obstetricians and Gynecologists. Postpartum hemorrhage. ACOG Practice Bulletin Number 76. *Obstet Gynecol* 2006;108:1039–1047, with permission.

- If atony continues, **blunt curettage** may be performed to remove retained products of conception. Using large "banjo" curettes under ultrasound guidance may reduce the risk of uterine perforation.
- Selective **uterine arterial embolization** may be considered, if the patient is stable for transport and this resource is available.
- When these more conservative interventions are unsuccessful, **surgical exploration** through a vertical midline incision should be considered. Depending on the patient's desire for future childbearing, the extent of hemorrhage, and the experience of the surgeon, several approaches may be used:
- **B-Lynch compressive sutures** can be effective for uterine atony (Fig. 7-1).
- **O'Leary bilateral uterine artery ligation** effectively reduces blood loss (Fig. 7-2). After identifying the ureter, ascending branches of the uterine arteries are ligated at the level of the vesicouterine peritoneal reflection. The suture is placed through the lateral lower uterine segment, close to the cervix, and then passed through an avascular area of the broad ligament lateral to the uterine vessels. Utero-ovarian vessels (near the cornua) and infundibulopelvic vessels may also be ligated if needed.
- **Internal iliac artery ligation** (anterior division of the internal iliac/hypogastric artery) significantly decreases uterine pulse pressure, promoting hemostasis. The artery is carefully isolated and ligated with permanent suture such as silk approximately 2 cm distal to the origin of the posterior branch; this placement prevents gluteal ischemia and improves hemostasis by limiting collateral flow to the uterus. Take care to avoid injuring the fragile hypogastric vein or ligating the nearby external iliac artery. This procedure is not always successful (<50% effective), requires a high level of surgical expertise, and carries significant risk of morbidity.
- **Hysterectomy** is the definitive procedure for intractable uterine bleeding and should not be delayed when needed. Intensive care monitoring may be required after peripartum hysterectomy due to massive blood loss and large postoperative fluid shifts.

Lacerations and Hematomas
- Suspect **uterine**, **vaginal**, or **cervical laceration** if the uterine fundus is well contracted but bleeding persists, particularly if operative delivery or episiotomy was performed. Adequate visualization is mandatory to investigate a laceration. Administer adequate analgesia and perform your inspection with excellent light and exposure.

TABLE 7-2 Medical Management of PPH with Uterotonic Agents

Agent	Dose	Comments and contraindications
Oxytocin (*Pitocin*)	10–40 U/L IV at 120 mL/hr or 10 units IM	Do not give undiluted IV bolus. Antidiuretic effect with prolonged infusion or high dose; can cause volume overload.
Methylergonovine maleate (*Methergine*)	0.2 mg IM every 2–4 hr. May give additional doses of 0.2 mg PO every 6 hr. Do not start PO until 4 hr after last parenteral dose.	Avoid in patients with hypertension, preeclampsia, or Raynaud's phenomenon. May cause nausea and vomiting.
15-methyl prostaglandin F$_2\alpha$ analogs (carboprost tromethamine [*Hemabate*])	0.25 mg IM (skeletal or myometrium) every 15–90 min to a maximum of 8 doses	Avoid in patients with asthma. Renal, hepatic, and cardiac disease are relative contraindications. May cause nausea/vomiting, tachycardia, diarrhea, pyrexia.
Prostin E$_2$ (dinoprostone)	20 mg vaginal or rectal suppository every 2 hr.	Avoid in hypotensive patients. Commonly causes fever.
Prostaglandin E$_1$ analog (misoprostol [*Cytotec*])	800–1,000 µg rectal suppository	Caution in renal disease and cardiac disease.

Adapted from American College of Obstetricians and Gynecologists. Postpartum Hemorrhage. ACOG Practice Bulletin Number 76. *Obstet Gynecol* 2006;108:1039–1047.

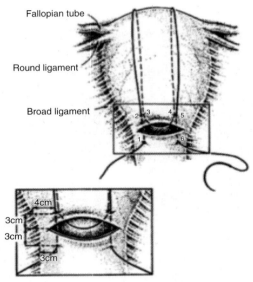

Figure 7-1. B-Lynch suture. (From Dildy GA. Postpartum hemorrhage: new management options. *Clin Obstet Gynecol* 2002;45:330–344.)

The cervix, entire vagina, and perineum should be evaluated systematically. Moving to the operating room often facilitates this process.

- Occult bleeding in **vulvar and vaginal hematomas** is identified mainly by hypotension and pelvic pain. Stable hematomas may be managed conservatively, but expanding hematomas should be evacuated. Perform a generous incision, irrigate copiously, and ligate the bleeding vessels. Layered closure is recommended to assist

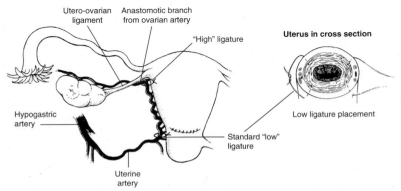

Figure 7-2. O'Leary uterine artery ligation. (From *TeLinde's Operative Gynecology*, 10th Ed. Philadelphia, PA: Lippincott Williams & Wilkins, 2008. With permission from *Contemp Obstet Gynecol* 1984;24:70 and *Surgical Obstetrics.* Philadelphia, PA: WB Saunders, 1992:272.)

hemostasis and eliminate dead space. Vaginal packing (for 12 to 18 hr) may be helpful. Broad-spectrum antibiotics should be administered.

- **Retroperitoneal hematoma** is potentially life threatening. It may present as hypotension, cardiovascular shock, or flank pain. Stable retroperitoneal bleeding can be managed conservatively. The pressure from the expanding hematoma will tamponade vessels and stop blood loss. Continued expansion necessitates surgical exploration.

Retained Products of Conception

- **Retained products of conception** can cause PPH.
- Risk factors include accessory placental lobes, abnormal placentation, placenta accreta, chorioamnionitis, and very preterm delivery.
- In *placenta accreta*, the normal plane of separation between uterus and placenta is absent (see Chapter 10). If the third stage of labor lasts longer than 30 minutes, consider abnormal placentation. Manual extraction and uterine exploration are performed. Blunt curettage may be required. It may be impossible to remove the entire placenta without damaging the uterus. If bleeding is controlled with uterotonic agents, conservative management may be sufficient.
- Balloon catheter (Bakri Balloon) can be placed in the uterus and inflated to tamponade bleeding from abnormal placentation. It may provide complete hemostasis or simply give time to stabilize the patient and arrange additional care, such as uterine artery embolization. The balloon catheter may be left in place for 12 to 24 hr.
- Laparotomy and peripartum hysterectomy are the definitive procedures for bleeding due to *placenta accreta*.

Coagulopathy

- **Coagulopathy** can cause PPH.
- Risk factors include severe pre-eclampsia, abruptio placentae, idiopathic/autoimmune thrombocytopenia, amniotic fluid embolism (AFE), disseminated intravascular coagulation, and hereditary coagulopathies (e.g., von Willebrand's disease).
- If bleeding is due to coagulopathy, surgical treatment will only increase the hemorrhage. Replete coagulation factors and platelets as needed.

UTERINE DEHISCENCE OR RUPTURE

Dehiscence is defined as lower uterine scar separation that does not breach the serosa; it rarely causes significant bleeding. **Rupture** is defined as complete separation of the uterine wall and may lead to fetal distress and significant maternal hemorrhage.

Incidence

- Uterine rupture occurs in 0.2% to 1% of patients with a previous low segment transverse cesarean section and in 4% to 9% of patients with a prior uterine active segment incision (classical cesarean or T-incision). One third of prior classical cesarean scar rupture occurs before the onset of labor.

Etiology

- Risk factors include prior uterine surgery, cesarean section, myomectomy, previous resection of a cornual ectopic pregnancy, and prior uterine perforation.
- Prostaglandin induction of labor with history of prior cesarean increases risk.
- Internal version or extraction, operative delivery, and trauma increase the risk for uterine rupture.

Diagnosis and Management

- Fetal bradycardia is clinically manifested in 33% to 70% of cases. Fetal distress may be the initial presentation in catastrophic uterine rupture.
- In milder cases, the initial presentation may be a simple rise in fetal station or change in the position for fetal heart monitor placement.
- Maternal signs and symptoms include hypotension, uterine tenderness, a change in uterine shape, or constant abdominal pain.
- When uterine rupture is suspected, proceed to emergent laparotomy with delivery of the infant and repair of the uterine rupture.

UTERINE INVERSION

In **uterine inversion**, the uterus is turned inside out, with the fundus protruding through the cervical os into or out of the vagina. It is classified as *incomplete* if the corpus travels partially through the cervix, *complete* if the corpus travels entirely through the cervix, and *prolapsed* if the corpus travels beyond the vaginal introitus.

Incidence

- Occurs in approximately 1 in 2,500 deliveries, usually with a fundal placenta.

Etiology and Management

- Risk factors include multiparity, long labor, short umbilical cord, abnormal placentation (i.e., accreta), connective tissue disorders, short umbilical cord, and excessive traction on the cord.
- Establish additional IV access, begin fluid resuscitation, and prepare for massive PPH.
- Attempt to replace the uterus manually.
  - In the *Johnson's maneuver*, the inverted fundus is grasped and pushed cephalad through the cervix into the normal position. Leaving the placenta in place may reduce blood loss; it can be removed manually after normal anatomy is restored. However, if the placenta prevents replacement of the uterus, it should be removed quickly before attempting to push the fundus into place.
  - If the maneuver is unsuccessful or a contracted ring of uterine tissue prevents access, uterine-relaxing agents can be administered. The preferred agent is nitroglycerin (up to three doses of 50 to 100 μg IV or sublingual spray); it has a rapid onset of about 30 seconds and a short half-life. Other uterine relaxants such as terbutaline sulfate or halogenated general anesthetics (e.g., halothane, isoflurane) could also be used.
- Administer uterotonics as soon as normal uterine anatomy is restored.
- Laparotomy is indicated if manual restoration fails. Vaginal elevation, upward traction on the round ligaments, or a posterior vertical incision on the lower uterine segment can all facilitate replacement of the uterus.

AMNIOTIC FLUID EMBOLISM

AFE is a rare complication. Fetal fluid, tissue, or debris enters the maternal circulation via the placental bed and triggers acute anaphylaxis.

Incidence

- Approximately 1 in 20,000 singleton pregnancies is complicated by AFE.
- Mortality is around 25% in the United States, much lower than the typically reported 60% to 80%. AFE accounts for 10% of maternal deaths in the United

States. Irreversible neurologic deficits occur in over 80% of survivors. Neonatal survival is reported at 70%.

Etiology and Diagnosis

- The term *embolism* is a misnomer because the clinical findings are probably a result of anaphylactic shock rather than pulmonary embolism.
- Risk factors include induced labor, advanced maternal age, multiparity, uterine rupture, abdominal trauma, placental abruption, diabetes, and operative delivery.
- AFE is primarily a clinical diagnosis of exclusion, made when a woman acutely presents with profound shock and cardiovascular collapse during or immediately after labor. Cyanosis, hemorrhage, coma, and disseminated intravascular coagulation rapidly ensue.
- The differential diagnosis includes other acute events such as pulmonary embolism, hemorrhage, drug reaction, anaphylaxis, sepsis, and myocardial infarction.
- Useful laboratory data include arterial blood gas, serum electrolytes, calcium and magnesium levels, coagulation profile, and complete blood count.
- Definitive diagnosis is made only at autopsy, when amniotic fluid debris (e.g., fetal squamous cells or hair) are found in the maternal pulmonary vasculature. This debris may be present in the maternal circulation of women without AFE, however, so this finding is not pathognomonic.

Management

- Approximately 65% of AFE occurs before delivery. Emergent delivery is required for both fetal and maternal benefits.
- The patient should be intubated and aggressively resuscitated.
- Administer IV fluids, inotropic agents, and pressors to maintain adequate blood pressure. Packed red blood cells and FFP should be available, as there is a high risk for disseminated intravascular coagulation. Despite all efforts, maternal morbidity and mortality are high.

CHORIOAMNIONITIS

Chorioamnionitis is infection/inflammation of the placenta, chorion, and amnion.

Incidence

- Occurs in 1% to 2% of term and 5% to 10% of preterm deliveries.

Etiology and Diagnosis

- Risk factors include nulliparity, prolonged labor, prolonged ruptured membranes, use of internal monitors, maternal bacterial vaginosis, and multiple vaginal examinations.
- Chorioamnionitis is an ascending polymicrobial infection. The most common pathogens are *Ureaplasma urealyticum, Mycoplasma hominis, Bacteroides bivius, Gardnerella vaginalis,* Group B streptococci, and *Escherichia coli.*
- The diagnosis is clinical. Signs and symptoms include maternal fever 38.0°C or higher without other obvious infection, maternal or fetal tachycardia, uterine tenderness, foul-smelling amniotic fluid or frankly purulent discharge, and leukocytosis (typically >15,000 with a left shift).
- If the diagnosis is uncertain and the clinical situation warrants, amniocentesis may be performed. Positive amniotic fluid culture gives definitive diagnosis. Other helpful amniotic fluid tests include glucose level, Gram stain, and IL-6 levels.

- Suspect chorioamnionitis in any patient with preterm labor that is unresponsive to tocolysis and inform the pediatrics team of your diagnosis.

Management

- Definitive treatment is delivery and evacuation of uterine contents. Antibiotics are administered during labor for fetal benefit. When the diagnosis of chorioamnionitis is made, labor should be induced; often a rapidly progressing preterm delivery will ensue without assistance.
- Acceptable antibiotic regimens include:
  - Ampicillin (2 g IV every 6 hr) plus gentamicin sulfate (2 mg/kg IV to load then 1.5 mg/kg IV every 8 hr) until delivery. If cesarean delivery is performed, clindamycin or metronidazole may be added for anaerobic coverage.
  - For nonanaphylactic penicillin allergy, substitute cefazolin (1 g IV every 8 hr) for ampicillin.
  - For severe penicillin allergy, substitute clindamycin (900 mg IV every 8 hr) or vancomycin (500 mg every 6 hr) for ampicillin.
  - Single drug regimens have also been used: Ampicillin/Sulbactam (Unasyn, 3 g IV every 6 hr), piperacillin/tazobactam (Zosyn, 3.375 g IV every 6 hr), and ticarcillin/clavulanate (Timentin, 3.1 g every 6 hr) have been used.
  - No data suggest that one regimen is better than another.
  - At delivery, obtain membrane culture by carefully peeling the amnion and chorion apart and swabbing between the layers. The placenta should be sent to pathology for histologic examination.
  - Unless the patient remains febrile, antibiotics are not needed after delivery.
  - After cesarean section with chorioamnionitis, broad coverage should be continued for 24 to 48 hr after the last recorded temperature of 38.0°C or higher. Triple coverage with ampicillin, gentamicin, and clindamycin (or metronidazole) is typical.

POSTPARTUM ENDOMYOMETRITIS

Postpartum endomyometritis is infection of the endometrium, myometrium, and parametrial tissues.

Incidence

- About 5% of vaginal deliveries and 10% of cesarean deliveries are affected by postpartum uterine infection. Rates are significantly higher in women of lower socioeconomic status.

Etiology and Diagnosis

- Risk factors include cesarean section, maternal diabetes mellitus, manual removal of the placenta, and all of the risks for chorioamnionitis.
- Endomyometritis, like chorioamnionitis, is an ascending polymicrobial infection caused by normal vaginal flora.
- May develop immediately to several days after delivery.
- Diagnosis is clinical: fever 38.0°C or greater, uterine tenderness, tachycardia, purulent vaginal discharge, and associated findings such as dynamic ileus, pelvic peritonitis, pelvic abscess, and bowel obstruction.
- Endometrial cultures are unnecessary; they are typically contaminated by normal flora. Blood culture is indicated only for the most severe cases with concern for sepsis.

Management

- Acceptable broad-spectrum antibiotic regimens include
  - Triple therapy with ampicillin, gentamicin, and clindamycin (or metronidazole) until 24 to 48 hr afebrile.
  - Alternate single agent therapies include ertapenem, ceftriaxone, cefotetan, Unasyn, Zosyn, or Timentin. The aim is broad polymicrobial coverage.
  - Gentamicin is administered every 8 hr before delivery. For postpartum treatment, however, several studies show 5 to 7 mg/kg daily dosing is safe, efficacious, and cost-effective. Drug levels are not monitored for daily dosing.
- Endomyometritis typically resolves with 48 hr of antibiotic treatment. If fever persists, additional workup should be considered including urine and blood cultures; chest and abdominal radiographs; pelvic examination; and possibly pelvic/abdominal ultrasound, CT, or MRI.
- Oral antibiotics are not necessary after full treatment with IV antibiotics.

SEPTIC PELVIC THROMBOPHLEBITIS

Septic pelvic thrombophlebitis (SPT) exists in two forms: **ovarian vein thrombosis/thrombophlebitis** and **deep pelvic septic thrombophlebitis**. SPT occurs in 1 in 2,000 to 1 in 3,000 deliveries, most commonly after cesarean section.

Diagnosis and Etiology

- Consider SPT in patients with persistent spiking fevers despite 3 days of antibiotic treatment for endometritis. The patient usually appears well between febrile episodes, and pain is minimal. Thrombi form in the deep pelvic veins as a result of pregnancy-induced hypercoagulability and venous congestion; they may become infected, releasing septic emboli which travel to the lungs. When other causes of postpartum fever have been excluded, pelvic ultrasound and pelvic/abdominal computed tomography (CT) or magnetic resonance imaging (MRI) helps diagnose abscess or large thrombus. A negative result, however, does not rule out SPT, which is largely a diagnosis of exclusion. Blood cultures are typically negative.

Management

- Treat SPT with broad-spectrum antibiotics (typically gentamicin plus clindamycin ± ampicillin; or broad-spectrum single agent ertapenem/imipenem), and consider heparin or enoxaparin anticoagulation.
- Heparin theoretically terminates embolic showers that may cause the spiking fever. Give a 5,000 unit heparin bolus, then a continuous infusion (usually 16 to 18 μm/kg/hr) with an activated partial thromboplastin time ratio (aPTTr) goal of 1.5 to 2.0 times normal. Low molecular weight heparin is also acceptable.
- Antibiotics are administered until the patient is 24 to 48 hr afebrile. The duration of anticoagulation is somewhat controversial, with recommendations ranging from 24 hr to 2 weeks after the last fever. If imaging clearly detects a deep vein or pulmonary thrombus, 6 months of anticoagulation with warfarin or enoxaparin are indicated.

UMBILICAL CORD PROLAPSE

Umbilical cord prolapse occurs when the umbilical cord slips beyond the presenting fetal part and passes through the open cervical os (overt) or descends alongside the presenting part (occult). The fetal blood supply is compromised when the cord is compressed against the cervix. The overall incidence is 1 to 6 per 1,000 births. The incidence in breech deliveries is slightly higher than 1%, while for footling breech, it may be as high as 10% to 15%.

Etiology

- Risk factors include ruptured membranes, unengaged fetal presenting part, malpresentation (breech, transverse, oblique), prematurity, multiple gestation (second twin), multiparity, and polyhydramnios.

Diagnosis

- Cord prolapse usually causes severe prolonged fetal bradycardia or persistent moderate-to-severe variable decelerations. Vaginal exam may confirm overt prolapse; the cord will be palpable.

Management

- If the cord is felt on vaginal examination, elevate the presenting part to relieve pressure on the cord, call for help, and move to the operating room for emergent cesarean section.
- Appropriate anesthesia should be administered in the operating room and the viability of the fetus confirmed before proceeding with cesarean section.
- If a patient presents with a prolapsed cord occurring prior to arrival, fetal viability must be established before proceeding with cesarean section.
- Placing the patient in Trendelenburg or knee-chest position may relieve cord compression with prolapse, but the vaginal hand should continue to elevate the presenting part.
- Neonatal outcomes are generally good. The interval between cord prolapse and delivery is the major predictor of newborn status.

MECONIUM ASPIRATION

Meconium staining of the amniotic fluid complicates 7% to 20% of all live births. It increases the risk of neonatal respiratory disorders.

Etiology and Complications

- Fetal acidosis, fetal heart rate abnormalities, and low Apgar scores are associated with meconium-stained fluid. Fetal stress and hypoxia stimulate meconium passage. The majority of pregnancies complicated by meconium-stained amniotic fluid, however, result in normal healthy newborns.
- Two to nine percent of fetuses with meconium staining will aspirate meconium before or during delivery. Those neonates are at risk for **meconium aspiration syndrome**, with subsequent mortality risk of 12%.
- Aspiration has three major pulmonary effects: (a) airway obstruction, (b) surfactant dysfunction, and (c) chemical pneumonitis.
- Risk factors for meconium aspiration syndrome include moderate or thick meconium, nonreassuring fetal heart rate tracing, meconium below the cords, and low Apgar scores.

Management

- **Amnioinfusion** is no longer used for all cases of meconium. A large multicenter trial showed that amnioinfusion for thick meconium did not reduce the risk of moderate or severe meconium aspiration syndrome, perinatal death, or other major neonatal complications.

- The most recent Neonatal Resuscitation Program guidelines advise against routine intrapartum suctioning for infants with meconium-stained fluid. Again, a large multicenter trial showed that deep suctioning before delivery of the shoulders did not reduce the rate of intubation, meconium aspiration syndrome, the need for mechanical ventilation, or overall mortality. The infant should be passed after delivery to the pediatric team with minimal stimulation. Endotracheal suctioning is performed only for nonvigorous infants, per Neonatal Resuscitation Program guidelines.

SUGGESTED READINGS

Conde-Agudelo A, Romero R. Amniotic fluid embolism: an evidence-based review. *Am J Obstet Gynecol* 2009;201:445.e1–445.e13.

French LM, Smaill FM. Antibiotic regimens for endometritis after delivery. *Cochrane Database Syst Rev* 2004;4:CD001067.

Mousa HA, Alfirevic Z. Treatment for primary postpartum haemorrhage. *Cochrane Database Syst Rev* 2007;1:CD003249. Update of 2003 review.

Tomacruz RS, Bristow RE, Montz FJ. Management of pelvic hemorrhage. *Surg Clin N Am* 2001;81(4):925–948.

Vain NE, Szyld EG, Prudent LM, et al. What (not) to do at and after delivery? Prevention and management of meconium aspiration syndrome. *Early Hum Develop* 2009;85:621–626.

Xu H, Hofmeyr J, Roy C, et al. Intrapartum amnioinfusion for meconium-stained amniotic fluid: a systematic review of randomised controlled trials. *BJOG* 2007;114:383–390.

You WB, Zahn CM. Postpartum hemorrhage: abnormally adherent placenta, uterine inversion, and puerperal hematomas. *Clin Obstet Gynecol* 2006;49:184–197.

Gestational Complications

Valerie A. Jones and Janice Henderson

This chapter reviews several common **antenatal complications**:
- Amniotic fluid disorders (including oligohydramnios, polyhydramnios)
- Intrauterine growth restriction (IUGR)
- Cervical insufficiency (CI)
- Multiple gestation
- Postterm pregnancy
- Fetal demise in utero (FDIU)

AMNIOTIC FLUID DISORDERS

- **Amniotic fluid volume (AFV)** represents the balance between production and removal of fetal fluids.
  - In early gestation, fluid is produced from the fetal surface of the placenta, from transfer across the amnion, and from embryonic surface secretions.
  - In mid to late gestation, fluid is produced by fetal urination and alveolar transudate. By 16 weeks, there is about 250 mL of fluid, increasing to approximately 800 mL by 34 to 36 weeks' gestation.
  - Fluid is removed by fetal swallowing and absorption at the amnion-chorion interface.
  - The most accurate measurement of AFV is by dye dilution techniques or direct measurement at the time of hysterotomy. Ultrasound provides a standard noninvasive tool to estimate AFV (see Table 8-1).
- **Polyhydramnios** is the pathologic accumulation of amniotic fluid defined as more than 2,000 mL at any gestational age, more than the 95th percentile for gestational age, or an amniotic fluid index (AFI) >25 cm at term.
  - The incidence of polyhydramnios in the general population is about 1%. Mildly increased AFV is usually clinically insignificant. Markedly increased AFV is associated with increased perinatal morbidity due to preterm labor, cord prolapse upon membrane rupture, underlying comorbidities, and congenital malformations.
  - Abruptio placentae is associated with polyhydramnios and rupture of membranes due to rapid decompression of the overdistended uterus. Increased maternal morbidity also results from postpartum hemorrhage due to uterine overdistention leading to atony.
  - The **etiology** of most polyhydramnios is idiopathic (Fig. 8-1). More specific causes include:
    - **Fetal structural malformations.** In cases of acrania or anencephaly, polyhydramnios occurs from an impaired swallowing mechanism, low antidiuretic hormone causing polyuria, and possibly transudation across the exposed fetal meninges. GI tract anomalies may also lead to polyhydramnios by either direct physical obstruction or decreased absorption. Ventral wall defects increase AFV from transudation across the peritoneal surface or bowel wall.

TABLE 8-1	Methods of Amniotic Fluid Assessment	
Diagnostic Method	**Interpretation**	**Clinical Value**
Single deepest pocket (SDP)—measure vertical dimension of SDP	Oligo ≤2 cm Normal = 2.1–8 cm Poly ≥8 cm	• 94% concordant with dye-determined normal pregnancies • Less accurate for low AFV • Useful predictor of adverse events
Amniotic fluid index (AFI)—measurement and summation of deepest pocket in each of four quadrants	Oligo ≤5 cm Normal = 5.1–25 cm Poly ≥25 cm	• 71%–78% concordant with dye-determined normals • Abnormal not highly predictive of adverse events • High false-positive rate
Two-diameter pocket—multiply vertical and horizontal dimensions from deepest single pocket	Oligo ≤15 cm Normal = 15.1–50 cm Poly ≥50 cm	• 80%–90% concordant with dye-determined normals • High error rate; accuracy not superior to AFI
Subjective assessment—performed by experienced sonographer	Subjective result	• 65%–70% concordant with dye-determined normals • Very poorly identifies abnormal volumes
2 × 2 cm pocket—sonographic survey to verify at least one 2 × 2 cm fluid pocket	Evaluates for presence or absence of 2 × 2 cm pocket	• 98% concordant with dye-determined normals • Found in <10% of oligo

Adapted and expanded from Moore TR. Clinical assessment of amniotic fluid. *Clin Obstet Gynecol* 1997;40(2):303–313.

- **Chromosomal and genetic abnormalities.** As many as 35% of fetuses with polyhydramnios (>23 cm AFI) have chromosomal abnormalities. The most common are trisomy 13, 18, and 21.
- **Neuromuscular disorders.** Impaired fetal swallowing can increase AFV.
- **Diabetes mellitus.** Maternal diabetes mellitus is a common cause of polyhydramnios, especially with poor glycemic control or associated fetal malformations. Fetal hyperglycemia can increase fluid transudation across the placental interface and cause fetal polyuria.
- **Alloimmunization.** *Hydrops fetalis* can increase AFV.

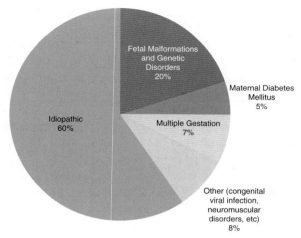

Figure 8-1. Causes of polyhydramnios.

- ° **Congenital infections.** In the absence of other factors, polyhydramnios warrants screening for congenital infections, such as toxoplasmosis, cytomegalovirus, and syphilis. These are, however, rare causes of polyhydramnios.
- ° **Twin-to-twin transfusion syndrome (TTTS).** The recipient twin develops polyhydramnios and occasionally *hydrops fetalis*, while the donor twin develops growth restriction and oligohydramnios.
- **Ultrasound** quantifies AFV, identifies multiple gestations, and detects fetal abnormalities. **Amniocentesis** for karyotype is offered if any anomalies are diagnosed.
- **Treatment** is aimed at the underlying cause. Mild to moderate polyhydramnios can be managed expectantly until the onset of labor or spontaneous rupture of membranes. If the patient develops dyspnea, abdominal pain, or difficulty ambulating, treatment becomes necessary.
  - ° **Amnioreduction** can alleviate significant maternal symptoms. Amniocentesis is performed, and fluid is removed. Frequent removal of smaller volumes (total 1,500 to 2,000 mL or until the AFI is <8 cm) is less associated with preterm labor than removal of larger volumes. Amnioreduction is repeated every 1 to 3 weeks as needed. Antibiotic prophylaxis is unnecessary.
  - ° **Pharmacologic treatment** reduces fetal urine production. Fetal renal blood flow and glomerular filtration rate (GFR) are sensitive to prostaglandins. The cyclooxygenase inhibitor indomethacin (25 mg PO every 6 hr) can decrease fetal renal blood flow and urination. Premature closure of the fetal ductus arteriosus is a potential complication of indomethacin that requires close AFV and ductus diameter monitoring. Discontinue therapy if there is any suggestion of ductus closure. The risk of complications is low if the total daily dose of indomethacin is <200 mg, the treatment is limited to pregnancies <32 weeks, and the duration of therapy is <48 hours.
- **Oligohydramnios** is defined as an AFI less than the fifth percentile for gestational age or ≤5 cm at term. It is associated with increased perinatal morbidity and mortality at any gestational age, but the risks are particularly high during the second trimester when perinatal mortality approaches 80% to 90%. Pulmonary hypoplasia can result from insufficient fluid filling the terminal air sacs. Prolonged oligohydramnios

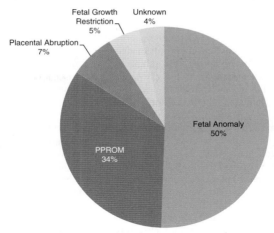

Figure 8-2. Causes of oligohydramnios. (Adapted from Shipp TD, Bromley B. Outcome of singleton pregnancies with severe oligohydramnios in the second and third trimesters. *Ultrasound Obstet Gynecol* 1996;7(2):108–113.)

in the second and third trimester leads to cranial, facial, or skeletal abnormalities in 10% to 15% of cases.

- The **etiology** of oligohydramnios includes ruptured membranes, fetal urinary tract malformations, postterm pregnancy, and placental insufficiency. Rupture of membranes must be considered at any gestational age. Renal agenesis or urinary tract obstruction often becomes apparent during the second trimester of pregnancy, when fetal urine flow begins to contribute significantly to AFV. Placental insufficiency can cause both oligohydramnios and IUGR. The cause of oligohydramnios in postterm pregnancies may be deteriorating placental function (Fig. 8-2).

- **Ultrasound** is used to diagnose oligohydramnios. Rupture of membranes should be evaluated, and in cases of preterm gestation with uncertain membrane status, a tampon dye test can be performed (see Chapter 9).

- **Treatment** for oligohydramnios is limited. Maternal intravascular fluid status appears to be closely tied to that of the fetus; maternal hydration may improve the AFV. In cases of obstructive genitourinary defects, in utero surgical diversion has produced some promising results. For optimal benefit, urinary diversion must be performed before renal dysplasia develops and early enough in gestation to permit normal lung development. Until near term, oligohydramnios is managed with frequent fetal surveillance. Indications for induction of labor include term gestation or nonreassuring fetal testing after 34 weeks. Oligohydramnios is not a contraindication to labor.

INTRAUTERINE GROWTH RESTRICTION

Intrauterine growth restriction (IUGR) is suggested when the estimated fetal weight falls below the 10th percentile for gestational age. Approximately 70% of so-called IUGR is merely constitutional. The incidence of pathologic IUGR is between 4% to 8%

of gestations in developed countries and 6% to 30% in developing countries. Fetuses with IUGR have a two- to six-fold increase in perinatal morbidity and mortality.

* The **etiology** of IUGR includes both maternal and fetal causes:
  * **Constitutionally small mothers and inadequate weight gain.** Women who weigh <100 pounds at conception have double the risk for a small-for-gestational-age newborn. Inadequate or arrested weight gain after 28 weeks of pregnancy is also associated with IUGR. Underweight women should be encouraged to reach ideal body weight and gain an additional 20 to 25 pounds (total of 25 to 40 pounds) during pregnancy.
  * **Chronic maternal disease.** Multiple medical conditions of the mother, including chronic hypertension, cyanotic heart disease, pregestational diabetes, malnutrition, and collagen vascular disease, can cause growth restriction. Preeclampsia and smoking can also lead to IUGR.
  * **Fetal infection.** Viral causes including rubella, CMV, hepatitis A, Parvovirus B19, varicella, and influenza are among the best-known infectious antecedents of IUGR. In addition, bacterial (listeriosis), protozoal (toxoplasmosis), and spirochetal (syphilis) infections may be causative.
  * **Congenital malformations and chromosomal abnormalities.** Chromosomal abnormalities, such as trisomy 13, 18, and Turner's syndrome, and severe cardiovascular malformations are often associated with IUGR. Trisomy 21 usually does not cause significant growth restriction.
  * **Teratogen exposure.** Any teratogen can produce fetal growth restriction. Anticonvulsants, tobacco, illicit drugs, and alcohol can impair fetal growth.
  * **Placental abnormalities.** Any placental abnormality can cause growth restriction due to decreased blood flow to the fetus.
  * **Multiple gestation** is complicated by growth impairment of at least one fetus in 12% to 47% of cases.
* **Diagnosis** is made by sonographic assessment (Table 8-2). Gestational age must be established with certainty, preferably in the first trimester, to assess fetal growth accurately. A lag in fundal height of more than 3 cm from gestational age after 20 weeks should prompt sonographic evaluation. Oligohydramnios frequently precedes fetal growth restriction.
* **Management** generally depends on gestational age. In general, growth restriction less than the third percentile diagnosed before 32 weeks prompts amniocentesis or fetal blood sampling for karyotype and viral studies. Even when termination is not considered, the information gained from these tests may be important for parents, obstetricians, and pediatricians planning the delivery and newborn care. Other management includes:
  * **IUGR ≥37 weeks:** Deliver.
  * **IUGR at 34 to 36 weeks:** Deliver if no fetal growth has been documented in the preceding weeks.
  * **IUGR remote from term:** Attempt conservative management. Restrict physical activity, ensure adequate nutrition, and initiate fetal surveillance. Fetal assessment includes daily kick counts, serial fetal growth ultrasounds every 3 to 4 weeks, and nonstress test or biophysical profile once or twice per week. Umbilical artery Doppler velocimetry showing elevated systolic-to-diastolic ratios or absent or reversed end-diastolic flow suggests fetal compromise (see Chapter 6).
* The decision to **deliver** an IUGR infant remote from term weighs the risk of preterm birth against continued exposure to the intrauterine environment. Vaginal delivery is not contraindicated, but there is an increased risk of fetal intolerance of labor. Growth-restricted newborns are susceptible to hypothermia and other

TABLE 8-2	Sonographic Measurements Used to Assess Fetal Growth	

Sonographic Measurement	Advantages	Disadvantages
Abdominal circumference	• Best correlates with fetal weight • High sensitivity for IUGR	• Cannot determine asymmetric vs symmetric IUGR • Subject to variability due to sonographer and fetal position changes
Transverse cerebellar diameter	• Correlates with gestational age up to 24 wk • Not significantly affected by growth restriction	• Correlates best up to 24 wk • Status as a predictor is variable
Head circumference (HC):Abdominal circumference (AC) ratio	• More accurate at diagnosing growth restriction related to placental insufficiency	• Not specific • Not all scans with increased HC/AC ratio are confirmed to have IUGR
Umbilical Artery Dopplers	• Can help distinguish between constitutionally small versus IUGR • Useful for evaluating pregnancies at risk for adverse events	• Not beneficial in low-risk pregnancies • Not useful as a screening tool

For additional information see Platz E, Newman R. Diagnosis of IUGR: traditional biometry. *Semin Perinatol* 2008;32:140–147, and Turan S, Miller J, Baschat AA. Integrated testing and management in fetal growth restriction. *Semin Perinatol* 2008;32:194–200.

metabolic abnormalities, such as severe hypoglycemia. Some data show that fetal growth restriction has long-term negative effects on cognitive function, independent of other variables.

CERVICAL INSUFFICIENCY

Cervical Insufficiency (CI), or cervical incompetence, occurs in 1 in 50 to 1 in 2,000 gestations. Risk factors include prior cervical laceration, history of cervical conization, multiple terminations with mechanical cervical dilation, intrauterine diethylstilbestrol exposure, and congenital cervical anomaly.

• The epidemiology is as imprecise as the various, sometimes controversial, criteria used to diagnose CI. One reasonable definition is recurrent painless cervical dilation in the absence of infection, placental abruption, uterine contractions, or uterine anomaly. Since CI is a diagnosis of exclusion, alternate diagnoses must be rigorously sought. *Prophylactic cervical cerclage has only been shown to be effective after **three or more** second-trimester pregnancy losses due to CI,* though patient concerns and provider judgement rarely tolerate waiting so long before proceeding with elective preventive treatment (i.e., cerclage). Cervical funneling on ultrasound is not adequate justification for cerclage placement, though serial cervical ultrasound of *high-risk* women starting at 16 to 20 weeks may identify early those pregnancies requiring additional management. Admittedly, diagnosis of CI and selection of patients for elective cervical cerclage are as much art as science.

- Pelvic rest, bedrest, pessary placement, and cervical cerclage have been suggested to prevent repeated pregnancy loss from CI, but the evidence for their effectiveness is mixed. A careful review of maternal history and prior pregnancy losses, complete counseling on the risks and benefits of cerclage (e.g., PPROM, chorioamnionitis, preterm birth, cervical laceration), and early screening for aneuploidy and congenital anomalies (see Chapter 12) should be offered *before* proceeding with cerclage placement.

  - McDonald or Shirodkar cerclages are placed vaginally, usually at 12 to 14 weeks' gestation; selection of technique depends on the available cervical length and surgeon experience/preference. Prophylactic antibiotics and postoperative tocolysis have not been shown to affect outcome but are often employed. The risk of iatrogenic pregnancy loss ranges from 1% to nearly 20% for elective cases. Rescue cerclage for CI/bulging membranes is associated with >50% risk of complications. Abdominal cerclage is placed at laparotomy in rare instances for women who have minimal to no residual cervical length (often due to large cone biopsies or trachelectomy) and who will subsequently be delivered by cesarean section.

  - Cerclage is removed when the patient begins to labor (with contractions, vaginal bleeding), when membranes rupture, if there is evidence of uterine infection, or if the patient reaches 36 weeks' gestation.

MULTIPLE GESTATION

Multiple gestation occurs in approximately 3% of all births in the United States and is increasing annually due to assisted reproductive technologies (ART). The incidence of monozygotic twins is constant at approximately 4 in 1,000 gestations. The incidence of dizygotic twins varies widely and is higher in some families, in individuals of African descent, with ovulation induction, and with increasing maternal age, parity, weight, and height. In the absence of fertility drugs, triplet pregnancies occur in 1 of 8,000 gestations. Higher order births are much rarer. Multiple gestation increases morbidity and mortality for both mother and fetus. Perinatal mortality rates in developed countries range from 50 to 100 per 1,000 births for twins and from 100 to 200 per 1,000 births for triplets.

- **Diagnosis** is confirmed by sonogram. Suspect multiple gestation if uterine size is greater than expected for gestational age, multiple fetal heart rates are detected, multiple fetal parts are felt, the human chorionic gonadotropin (hCG) and maternal serum alpha-fetoprotein levels are elevated for gestational age, or the pregnancy is a result of ART.
- **Zygosity, placentation, and mortality**
  - **Dizygotic dichorionic/diamnionic twins** (70% to 80% of all twins) result from the fertilization of two ova. Each fetus has its own placenta and a complete and separate amnion-chorion membrane.
  - **Monozygotic twins** (20% to 30% of all twins) result from cleavage of a single, fertilized conceptus. The timing of cleavage determines the placentation.

- **Dichorionic/diamnionic monozygotic twins** (8% of all twins) are produced by cleavage in the first 3 days after fertilization. They will have separate amnions and chorions, just like dizygotic twins. They have the lowest perinatal mortality rate (<10%) of all monozygotic twins.
- **Monochorionic/diamnionic twins** (14% to 20% of all twins) are produced by cleavage between days 4 and 8 after fertilization. They share a single placenta, but separate amnionic sacs. The mortality rate for monochorionic/diamnionic twins is approximately 25%.
- **Monochorionic/monoamnionic twinning** (<1% of cases) occurs after the 8th day. The fetuses share a single placenta and a single amnionic sac because both amnion and chorion were formed before cleavage. Later cleavage is even rarer and results in conjoined fetuses. Monoamnionic gestations have a 50% to 60% mortality rate, usually occurring before 32 weeks.
- **Higher-order multiples** have more frequent placental anomalies. Monochorionic and dichorionic placentation may both be present.
- **Complications** are more common in multiple gestations.
- **Miscarriage** is at least twice as common in multiple gestations, compared with singleton pregnancies. Fewer than 50% of twin pregnancies diagnosed by ultrasonography in the first trimester result in live birth of twins.
- **Congenital anomalies and malformations** are about twice as common in dizygotic twins and three times more common in trizygotic triplets compared to singletons. Monozygotic twins have a 2% to 10% risk of developmental defects, about twice the rate for dizygotic twins. Because the risk of chromosomal anomalies increases with each additional fetus, we encourage amniocentesis at 33 years for twins and at 28 years for triplets.
- **Nausea and vomiting** are often worse in multiple gestations. Although the etiology is unclear, higher levels of hCG may be the cause.
- **Preeclampsia** is more common, occurs earlier, and is more severe in multiple gestations. Approximately 40% of twin pregnancies and 60% of triplet pregnancies are affected.
- **Polyhydramnios** occurs in 5% to 8% of multiple pregnancies, particularly with monoamnionic twins. Acute polyhydramnios before 28 weeks' gestation has been reported in 1.7% of twin pregnancies. The perinatal mortality in those cases approaches 90%.
- **Preterm delivery** approaches 50% in twin gestations. The average gestational age at delivery is 36 to 37 weeks for twins and 32 to 33 weeks for triplets. Twin gestations account for 10% of all preterm deliveries and 25% of all preterm perinatal deaths. Most neonatal deaths in multiple premature births are associated with gestations <32 weeks and birth weight under 1,500 g (see Chapter 9).
- **IUGR** is common, and low birth weight has an additive effect with prematurity on neonatal morbidity and mortality.
- **Discordant twin growth** is defined as a discrepancy of more than 20% in the estimated fetal weights. It is calculated as a percentage of the larger twin's weight. Causes include TTTS, chromosomal or structural anomalies in either twin, discordant viral infection, and unequal division of the placenta mass. When discordance exceeds 25%, the fetal and neonatal death rates increase 6.5-fold and 2.5-fold, respectively.
- The risk of uterine atony and **postpartum hemorrhage** is significantly increased in multiple pregnancies.

- **Intrapartum complications** including malpresentation, cord prolapse, cord entanglement, dysfunctional labor, fetal distress, and urgent cesarean delivery are more common for multiple gestations compared with singletons.
- **TTTS** occurs in 20% to 25% of monochorionic twin pregnancies. Fifty to seventy-five percent of monochorionic twin placentae have vascular anastomoses. When anastomoses are not balanced, one fetus "donates" blood to the other, leading to hypervolemia, heart failure, and hydrops in the recipient twin and hypovolemia, oligohydramnios, and growth restriction in the donor twin.
  - Rapid uterine growth between 20 and 30 weeks' gestation from polyhydramnios of the recipient twin is common. TTTS can be diagnosed when sonography suggests a single chorion, discordant fetal growth, polyhydramnios around the larger twin, and oligohydramnios around the smaller fetus ("stuck twin" sign or "poly-oli" syndrome). The severity and timing of growth discrepancy depend on the degree of arteriovenous shunting. Fetal hydrops is usually an ominous sign.
  - If extreme prematurity prevents immediate delivery, management includes serial amnioreduction for the recipient twin, intrauterine blood transfusion for the donor twin, selective fetal reduction, or fetoscopic laser ablation of placental anastomoses.
- **Antenatal management of multiple gestations** includes adequate nutrition (300 additional calories per day per fetus), more frequent prenatal visits, periodic ultrasound assessment of fetal growth and well-being, and prompt hospital admission for preterm labor or obstetric complications. No evidence supports bed rest or prophylactic tocolytics for preterm labor in multiple gestations.
  - **Ultrasonographic assessments** should be conducted every 3 to 4 weeks from 23 weeks' gestation to monitor fetal growth and detect discordance. Monochorionic placentation may warrant ultrasonography every 2 weeks to evaluate for evidence of TTTS.
  - **Fetal surveillance** with nonstress testing (NST) is not indicated for dizygotic twins unless clinical or ultrasonographic data suggest IUGR or discordance. When NSTs are discordant, additional testing may be necessary. The use of contraction stress testing is controversial and rarely used as it might precipitate preterm delivery.
  - **Amniocentesis** should be performed for both fetuses, if indicated, for prenatal diagnosis of genetic disorders or alloimmunization. One to five mL of indigo carmine is injected into the first sac, following fluid aspiration to ensure that both sacs are sampled. To establish lung maturity, amniotic fluid evaluation from one fetal sac is adequate. For discordant twins, amniotic fluid should be obtained from the larger twin, which usually reaches pulmonary maturity later.
  - **Multifetal pregnancy reduction** may be offered to reduce risk in higher-order pregnancies. Because the presence of three or more fetuses is associated with such increased maternal and perinatal mortality and morbidity, fetal reduction may be appropriately offered. The risk of subsequent pregnancy loss is 5% to 10%. **Selective termination** refers specifically to the termination of one or more specific fetuses with structural or chromosomal anomalies.
  - **Management for fetal demise** is based on gestational age and the condition of the surviving fetus. Until the surviving twin develops lung maturity, weekly fetal surveillance and maternal coagulation profile testing should be performed. Consider delivery when fetal lung maturity is demonstrated, if fetal status deteriorates, or if disseminated intravascular coagulation (DIC) develops in the mother. In TTTS, one fetal demise should prompt consideration for delivery, particularly after 28 weeks.

- The optimal **route of delivery** for twins remains controversial and should be assessed on a case-by-case basis. Decisions about delivery must consider the presentations, gestational age, maternal or fetal complications, the experience of the obstetrician, and the availability of anesthesia and neonatal intensive care support.
  - **Vertex/vertex** (43%) presentation can have a successful vaginal delivery in 70% to 80% of cases. Surveillance of twin B between deliveries is advised.
  - **Vertex/nonvertex** (38%) presentation can have a vaginal delivery if estimated fetal weights are within 20% concordant. External cephalic version or podalic version and breech extraction of twin B may be attempted. Vaginal delivery of twin B in nonvertex presentation may be considered for infants with an estimated weight between 1,500 and 3,500 g. Success rates are more than 96%. There is insufficient data to advocate a specific route of delivery for a second twin weighing <1,500 g.
  - **Nonvertex presenting twins** (19%) are typically delivered by cesarean for both fetuses.
  - **Locked twins** is a rare condition occurring with breech/vertex twins, when the body of twin A delivers, but the chin "locks" behind the chin of twin B. Hypertonicity, monoamnionic twinning, or reduced amniotic fluid may contribute to interlocking fetal heads.

POSTTERM PREGNANCY

Postterm Pregnancy is defined as 294 days or 42 *completed* weeks since the 1st day of the last menstrual period (LMP). Perinatal morbidity and mortality increase *after* 42 weeks' gestation, as does the incidence of congenital anomalies. The incidence of postterm pregnancy ranges between 7% and 12% of all pregnancies. Approximately, 4% of all pregnancies extend beyond 43 weeks. About 30% to 40% of women with a prior postterm pregnancy will have prolonged gestation in subsequent pregnancies.

- **Diagnosis** of postterm pregnancy is based upon accurate estimation of gestational age. Obstetric dates should be validated by two or more of the following: certain LMP, positive urine pregnancy test within 6 weeks of LMP, fetal heart tone detected with Doppler testing at 10 to 12 weeks' gestation, fundal height at the umbilicus at 20 weeks' gestation, pelvic examination consistent with LMP before 13 weeks' gestation, and ultrasonographic dating by crown–rump length between 6 and 12 weeks' gestation or by biparietal diameter before 26 weeks' gestation. The best estimate of gestational age is confirmed by as many criteria as possible.
- The **etiology** is usually incorrect dating. Risk factors for postterm pregnancy may include primiparity, previous postterm pregnancy, placental sulfatase deficiency, fetal anencephaly, family history, and fetal male sex.
- **Complications** of postterm pregnancy include:
  - **Postmaturity syndrome** exhibiting subcutaneous wasting, intrauterine growth failure, meconium staining, oligohydramnios, absent *vernix caseosa* and lanugo hair, and peeling newborn skin. Such findings are described in only 10% to 20% of true postterm newborns.
  - **Macrosomia** is more common in postterm pregnancies. Twice as many postterm fetuses weigh more than 4,000 g compared to term infants. Birth injuries caused by shoulder dystocia and delivery complications are increased postterm.

- **Oligohydramnios** is more common in postterm pregnancies, probably due to decreasing uteroplacental function. Low AFV is associated with increased intrapartum fetal distress and cesarean delivery.
- **Meconium**-stained amniotic fluid and meconium aspiration syndrome increase in postterm gestation.
- **Management** after 40 completed weeks' gestation (e.g., at 41 weeks) includes daily fetal movement assessment (kick counts), semiweekly fetal testing (NST), and AFV testing (AFI). Whether the patient who reaches 41 to 42 weeks' gestation with an unripe cervix is better managed by cervical ripening and induction or by continued testing is debated.
- **Induction of labor** at 41 weeks or fetal surveillance until induction at 42 weeks' gestation are both acceptable.

FETAL DEMISE IN UTERO

FDIU, also called intrauterine fetal demise (IUFD), is the antenatal diagnosis of a stillborn infant after 20 weeks' gestation. Approximately 50% of perinatal deaths are stillbirths. Of all fetal deaths in the United States, over two thirds occur before 32 weeks' gestation, 20% occur between 36 and 40 weeks' gestation, and approximately 10% occur beyond 41 weeks' gestation.

- FDIU is suspected with any maternal report of more than a few hours of absent fetal movement. Definitive diagnosis is by absent fetal cardiac activity on real-time ultrasonography.
- Fetal deaths can be categorized by occurrence during the antepartum period or during labor (intrapartum stillbirth). The antepartum fetal death rate in an unmonitored population is approximately 8 in 1,000 and represents 86% of fetal deaths.
- The etiology of antepartum fetal death can be divided into broad categories: chronic hypoxia of diverse origin (30%), congenital malformation or chromosomal anomaly (20%), complications of pregnancy such as Rh alloimmunization (<1%), abruptio placentae (20% to 25%), fetal infection (<5%), and idiopathic/unexplained (25% or more).
- **Antepartum fetal assessment** may not prevent but can significantly reduce the frequency of antenatal fetal deaths. Inclusion criteria for antepartum fetal assessment are uteroplacental insufficiency, postterm pregnancy, diabetes mellitus requiring medication, hypertension requiring medication, previous stillbirth, IUGR, decreased fetal movement, and Rh disease.
- Both expectant and active **management** are acceptable after fetal demise. Spontaneous labor occurs within 2 to 3 weeks in 80% of cases. In cases of prolonged demise, induction of labor should be offered due to emotional burden and the risk of chorioamnionitis and DIC with prolonged demise. Dilation and evacuation early in the second trimester is an option. Testing to determine the cause of the loss is usually negative but can include chromosomes, infection evaluation (TORCH), maternal thyroid screening, and fetal autopsy.

SUGGESTED READINGS

Creasy RK, Resnik R, Iams JD, et al., eds. Biology of twinning (Ch. 4), Multiple gestation (Ch. 25), Postterm pregnancy (Ch. 32), Embryonic and fetal demise (Ch. 33), and Intrauterine growth restriction (Ch. 34). In *Maternal-Fetal Medicine: Principles and Practice,* 6th Ed. Philadelphia, PA: Saunders Elsevier, 2009.

Intrauterine growth restriction. ACOG Practice Bulletin Number 12. American College of Obstetricians and Gynecologists. *Obstet Gynecol* 2000 (reaffirmed 2008);95(1).

Management of postterm pregnancy. ACOG Practice Bulletin Number 55. American College of Obstetricians and Gynecologists. *Obstet Gynecol* 2004;104:639–646.

Robyr R, Quarello E, Ville Y. Management of fetofetal transfusion syndrome. *Prenat Diagn* 2005;25:786.

Silver RM, Varner MW, Reddy U. Workup of stillbirth: A review of the evidence. *Am J Obstet Gynecol* 2007;196(5):433–444.

Snijders RJ, Nicolaides KH. Fetal biometry at 14–40 weeks' gestation. *Ultrasound Obstet Gynecol* 1994;4:34.

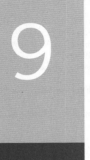

Preterm Labor and Preterm Premature Rupture of Membranes

Abigail E. Dennis and Janyne E. Althaus

PRETERM LABOR

Preterm Labor (PTL) is defined as
- Regular uterine contractions, with
- Cervical change, at
- Gestation <37 weeks. *Extreme PTL* occurs before 28 weeks' gestation.

Incidence and Significance
- PTL is the leading cause of neonatal morbidity in developed countries (Fig. 9-1).
- PTL accounts for 40% to 50% of preterm births. Rupture of membranes, placental abruption, and indicated deliveries also lead to preterm birth.
- Short-term neonatal morbidity includes respiratory distress syndrome (RDS), hypothermia, hypoglycemia, jaundice, intraventricular hemorrhage, necrotizing enterocolitis, bronchopulmonary dysplasia, sepsis, and patent ductus arteriosus.
- Long-term morbidity includes cerebral palsy, mental retardation, and retinopathy of prematurity.

Etiology
Risk factors include
- **Previous preterm delivery (PTD)**
  - Most significant risk factor for PTL.
  - With history of prior spontaneous PTD, recurrence rate is 17% to 30%.
- **Infection**
  - Systemic or local infections including urinary tract infections, pyelonephritis, bacterial vaginosis.
  - Chorioamnionitis affects 25% of preterm deliveries.
    ○ Pathogens include *Ureaplasma urealyticum, Mycoplasma hominis, Gardnerella vaginalis, Peptostreptococci,* and *Bacteroides* species.
    ○ Release of cytokines from endothelial cells, including interleukin-1, interleukin-6, and tumor necrosis factor-α, stimulates a cascade of prostaglandin production that stimulates uterine contractions.
- **Uterine overdistension:** Multiple gestation, polyhydramnios.
- **Uterine malformations:** Bicornuate uterus, leiomyomata, uterine didelphys.
- **Second or third trimester vaginal bleeding:** Placenta previa, placental abruption.

Prevention
- Educate patients about the early signs of PTL.

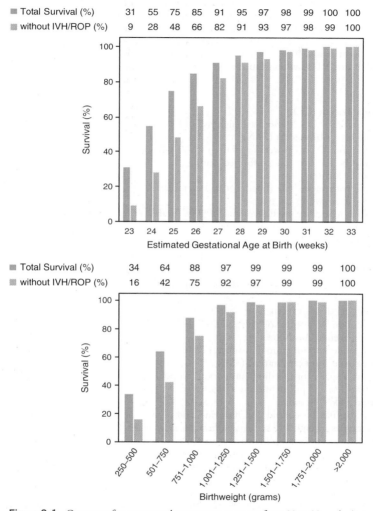

Figure 9-1. Outcomes for nonanomalous preterm neonates from 23 to 33 weeks (**top panel**) and from 250 to 2,000 g (**bottom panel**) are shown. Prognosis is affected by many factors other than gestational age and birthweight and is evaluated on an individual basis. Intraventricular hemorrhage (IVH) and retinopathy of prematurity (ROP) are only two possible major complications of prematurity. Adapted from Pediatrix/Obstetrix Medical Group outcomes data at: www.pediatrix.com/body_university.cfm?id=596 (accessed August 14, 2010).

- Treat infections promptly, especially urinary tract infections and lower genital tract infections.
- Most important risk factor (prior preterm delivery) cannot be modified.
  - Weekly injections (250 mg) of 17-alpha-hydroxyprogesterone caproate or daily progesterone vaginal suppositories (100 to 200 mg) beginning at 16 to 20 weeks' gestation reduce the recurrence of preterm delivery. Although there is no evidence to support progesterone therapy for patients with *active* PTL, it is sometimes initiated during PTL and continued until near term.

Screening
- **Cervical length (CL)**
  - Patients with CL <20 mm have high risk of PTL/PTD.
- **Vaginal fetal fibronectin (FFN)**
  - Collect from 24 to 34 weeks' gestation with signs and symptoms of PTL.
  - Should be the first test performed during exam. The sample is taken from the posterior fornix.
  - Invalid with vaginal bleeding, ruptured membranes, or a history of intercourse or vaginal exam within 24 hr.
  - FFN has a negative predictive value of 99% for delivery within 7 days.
  - The positive predictive value for delivery within 7 days is as low as 14%; use the test to rule out PTL.

Evaluation
- Establish best dating for gestational age using last menstrual period, fundal height, ultrasound data, and prenatal records if available.
- Obtain vital signs. A temperature ≥38°C or fetal or maternal tachycardia may indicate an underlying infection. Hypotension with fetal or maternal tachycardia may suggest placental abruption.
- Fundal tenderness on exam may suggest chorioamnionitis or placental abruption.
- **Sterile speculum examination (SSE)**
  - Inspect visually for bleeding, amniotic fluid pooling, advanced dilation, bulging membranes, and purulent cervical discharge.
  - Perform FFN if desired.
  - Swab vaginal pool fluid for nitrazine and fern tests to evaluate rupture of membranes. Membrane status significantly alters management, so this testing is mandatory even in the absence of symptoms.
    - Normal vaginal pH is <5.5, amniotic fluid pH is usually 7.0 to 7.5. A pH >6.5 is consistent with rupture of membranes.
    - False-positive tests can be observed when blood, semen, *Trichomonas*, cervical mucus, or urine contaminates the sample.
    - Ferning may be falsely negative in the presence of blood. Cervical fluid can also produce misleading ferning results.
  - For pooling, have the patient cough or valsalva to see whether apparent amniotic fluid accumulates in the vagina.
  - Obtain Group B streptococci (GBS) anovaginal culture.
  - Obtain cervical cultures for *Chlamydia trachomatis* and *Neisseria gonorrhea*.
  - Evaluate wet mount for bacterial vaginosis, *Trichomonas*, and yeast.
- After ruling out PPROM, perform **digital examination** for dilation, effacement, and station.

- Obtain **laboratory studies** including a complete blood count, urinalysis with microscopic evaluation, and all cultures obtained in the SSE. Obtain cultures before antibiotics are given.
- Perform **ultrasound** to assess fetal presentation, estimated fetal weight (EFW), gestational age, placental location, amniotic fluid index, and fetal or uterine anomalies. Cervical length can also be examined.
- Initiate continuous fetal heart monitoring and tocodynamometry. Fetal tachycardia or nonreassuring fetal heart tracing may indicate chorioamnionitis, abruption, or cord compression.

Management

- The **goals** of PTL management are the following:
  - To delay delivery by reducing or stopping contractions if infection and maternal/fetal indications for delivery have been ruled out; and
  - To optimize fetal well-being with the administration of steroids and GBS prophylaxis per guidelines.
- **Oral or intravenous hydration** can be used as an initial approach to preterm contractions due to dehydration; however, randomized trials show that hydration does not reduce the incidence of preterm birth. Clinical experience will guide the initial treatment.
- **Strict bed rest** is usually recommended on admission to the hospital, with gradual liberalization of activity over the next few days to weeks.
  - Maintain strict bed rest in certain patient populations (e.g., funic presentation, advanced cervical dilation).
  - Initiate thromboembolic prophylaxis and consider a physical therapy consultation in all patients with activity limitations.
  - Limited evidence suggests that prolonged standing, strenuous activity, and sexual activity are associated with PTL.
  - Randomized trials of bed rest for the prevention or treatment of preterm delivery in multiple gestation show either no benefit or increased risk of preterm birth.
- **Group B streptococcus prophylaxis** is continued until cervical exam is stable and risk for PTD is lower.
- **Administer corticosteroids** between 24 and 34 weeks' gestation.
  - Give two doses of betamethasone (12 mg IM) 24 hr apart or four doses of dexamethasone (6 mg IM) 12 hr apart.
  - Corticosteroid administration reduces risk for RDS, intraventricular hemorrhage, necrotizing enterocolitis, and neonatal death.
  - No studies to date show any benefit from multiple courses of steroids. Repeated or extended courses have been linked to increased neonatal necrotizing enterocolitis. Rescue dose steroid administration at 28 to 34 weeks after earlier administration for extreme PTL is under investigation.
  - Corticosteroids increase maternal white blood cell count and serum glucose, so exercise caution in interpreting those lab values.
- **Tocolysis** is used to give time for transport to tertiary centers for extreme PTL and to allow time for the full course and maximum efficacy of steroid treatment (see Table 9-1).
  - No study to date shows that tocolysis beyond 48 hr improves fetal or maternal outcomes.
  - Contraindications to tocolysis include the following: nonreassuring fetal status, chorioamnionitis, eclampsia or severe preeclampsia, fetal demise, fetal maturity, and maternal hemodynamic instability.

TABLE 9-1 Common Tocolytic Agents for Preterm Labor

Drug	Mechanism of Action	Dosing Regimen	Contraindications	Side Effects	Notes
Indomethacin	Prostaglandin synthetase inhibitor → prevents production of prostaglandin $F_{2\alpha}$, which normally stimulates uterine contractions	Loading dose: 50–100 mg orally or per rectum Maintenance dose: 25–50 mg orally or per rectum q4–6hr × 72 hr	Peptic ulcer disease Renal disease Hepatic dysfunction Coagulopathy Oligohydramnios	Oligohydramnios Nausea GERD/gastritis Emesis Platelet dysfunction (rare)	First-line agent in gestations <32 wk. Avoid at >32 weeks' gestation (associated with premature closure of fetal ductus arteriosus). Avoid using for >72 hr (associated with oligohydramnios).
Nifedipine	Calcium channel blocker → inhibits myometrial calcium entry	10–20 mg orally q6hr	Hypotension Congestive heart failure Aortic stenosis	Hypotension Flushing Lightheadedness Dizziness Nausea	First-line agent

Terbutaline	β-sympathomimetic → causes uterine smooth muscle relaxation	0.25 mg SC injection every 20–30 min, as needed	Cardiac disease Hypertension Digitalis use Hyperthyroidism Poorly controlled diabetes mellitus	Tachycardia Pulmonary edema Elevated blood sugar levels Cardiac arrhythmias Myocardial ischemia Heart failure	β_2-adrenergic agonists can reduce contractions, but no improvement in perinatal outcome or rate of preterm birth has been reported.
Magnesium	Competes for myome-trial calcium entry, thereby decreases uterine contractility	Loading dose: 4–6 g IV or 10 g IM Maintenance: Infusion of 2–4 g/hr Therapeutic levels are between 6 and 8 mg/dL	Myasthenia gravis Heart block Renal failure	Respiratory depression Pulmonary edema Cardiac arrest Nausea/vomiting Flushing Muscle weakness Hypotension Hyporeflexia	Systematic review found no evidence that magnesium helps to prevent PTD. One gram of calcium gluconate is the antidote for $MgSO_4$ toxicity

- First-line tocolytics are nifedipine and, in pregnancies <32 weeks, indomethacin.
- Use of multiple tocolytics concurrently should be avoided given the risk of pulmonary edema (excluding indocin).
- There is no uniform standard for **fetal monitoring**.
  - Maintain external fetal monitoring/tocodynamometry until active PTL resolves (i.e., no cervical change and minimal contractions).
  - Once PTL resolves, there is no need for further continuous monitoring. On our inpatient unit, we check fetal doptones one to two times daily with vital signs and perform a fetal nonstress test one to three times per week.
- The recommended **route of delivery varies by gestational age**.
  - If <26 weeks or EFW <750 g, offer vaginal delivery, regardless of presentation. There is no significant benefit to cesarean delivery at this early gestation.
    - Discuss the risks and benefits of C-section for fetal distress given the increased maternal morbidity and poor neonatal prognosis. Discuss risks and future implications of classical cesarean section. Document your discussion carefully in the chart, and revisit the issue as gestation progresses.
  - If >26 weeks or EFW is >1,000 g, offer vaginal delivery only for vertex presentation.
    - Offer C-section for breech presentation given the risk of head entrapment.
- **Criteria for discharge** include acontractile, stable cervical exam (without advanced cervical dilation [>4 cm], bulging membranes, or significant effacement), no vaginal bleeding, no suspicion of ruptured membranes, reasonable hospital access with appropriate level of neonatology support, ability to comply with activity recommendations (modified bed rest and complete pelvic rest), and reassuring fetal status (we typically do a nonstress test on the day of discharge).

PRETERM PREMATURE RUPTURE OF MEMBRANES

Preterm premature rupture of membranes (PPROM) can be defined as spontaneous rupture of the amnion and chorion membranes before the onset of labor (**Premature Rupture of Membranes, PROM**) or PROM before 37 weeks' gestation (**PPROM**). The latency period is the time from PROM or PPROM to onset of labor. At term, latency is 1 to 12 hr.

Incidence and Significance

- PROM occurs in 3% to 19% of pregnancies; it accounts for 30% of preterm deliveries.
- Fifty percent of patients with PPROM before 26 weeks will labor within 1 week.
- Fifty percent of patients with PPROM between 28 and 34 weeks will labor within 24 hr, and 80% to 90% will labor within 1 week.

Etiology

- Risk factors include intrauterine infection, prior history of PPROM, trauma, amniocentesis, and polyhydramnios.

Evaluation

- Perform the evaluation described for PTL (above), and make careful note of the circumstances, character, and timing of rupture of membranes (ROM), and the consistency of the fluid.
- Only a SSE should be performed. Avoid digital cervical exam unless delivery is imminent. Digital examination decreases the latency period and increases the risk of neonatal sepsis.

- When clinical suspicion of PROM is high despite negative ferning, nitrazine, and pooling, retest after prolonged recumbency (several hours).
  - Consider ultrasound-guided amnioinfusion of indigo carmine for a "tampon test." A tampon or packing is placed in the vagina, and dye is injected into the amniotic fluid via the amniocentesis needle. After some time, the tampon is examined to see whether blue-stained fluid has leaked through the cervix.

Management

Management for PRROM and PTL is similar.
- The **goals** are to screen for underlying chorioamnionitis or placental abruption and move toward delivery if these conditions are identified. Otherwise, prolonging the latent period is desired, depending on gestational age.
  - If the fetal vertex is not well applied to the cervix, **strict bed rest** should be maintained to avoid cord accident.
- Before 34 weeks in the absence of chorioamnionitis initiate **latency antibiotics**, which delay the onset of PTL.
  - The standard latency regimen is: Intravenous ampicillin 2 g IV and erythromycin 250 mg IV every 6 hr for 48 hr, followed by oral amoxicillin 250 mg and erythromycin 330 mg every 8 hr (or 250 mg erythromycin every 6 hr) for five additional days. The entire latency course is 7 days.
- Tocolysis is generally contraindicated in PPROM except for extreme prematurity to allow corticosteroid administration. If chorioamnionitis is suspected, do not tocolyze.
- Once the patient and fetus are stable, **monitor fetal heart tones** every 8 hr and perform daily fetal testing.
- At <32 weeks' gestation, manage PRROM as outlined above with latency antibiotics and steroids.
- At 32 to 34 weeks' gestational age, consider delivery with documented fetal pulmonary maturity.
- At >34 weeks augment labor for delivery or proceed to cesarean section depending on the fetal presentation and obstetric indications.
- Evidence of chorioamnionitis or nonreassuring fetal status warrants prompt delivery.
- Continue inpatient management for PPROM until delivery unless membranes reseal, as documented by negative blue dye tampon test.

SUGGESTED READINGS

Berghella V, Hayes E, Visintine J, et al. Fetal fibronectin testing for reducing the risk of preterm birth. *Cochrane Database Syst Rev* 2008;(4):CD006843.

Doyle LW, Crowther CA, Middleton P, et al. Antenatal magnesium sulfate and neurologic outcome in preterm infants: a systematic review. *Obstet Gynecol* 2009;113(6):1327–1333.

Gilstrap LC, Christensen R, Clewell WH, et al. Effect of corticosteroids for fetal maturation on perinatal outcomes. NIH Consensus Development Panel on the Effect of Corticosteroids for Fetal Maturation on Perinatal Outcomes. *JAMA* 1995;273(5):413–418.

Goldenberg RL, Culhane JF, Iams JD, et al. Epidemiology and causes of preterm birth. *Lancet* 2008;371(9606):75–84.

Haas DM, Imperiale TF, Kirkpatrick PR, et al. Tocolytic therapy: a meta-analysis and decision analysis. *Obstet Gynecol* 2009;113(3):585–594.

Meis PJ. Prevention of recurrent preterm delivery by 17 alpha-hydroxyprogesterone caproate. *N Engl J Med* 2003;348(24):2379–2385.

Mercer BM, Miodovnik M, Thurnau GR, et al. Antibiotic therapy for reduction of infant morbidity after preterm premature rupture of the membranes. A randomized controlled trial. National Institute of Child Health and Human Development Maternal-Fetal Medicine Units Network. *JAMA* 1997;278(12):989–995.

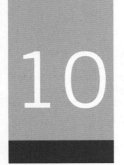

10 Third-Trimester Bleeding

Natalia A. Colón Guzmán and Cynthia Holcroft Argani

Third-trimester bleeding, ranging from spotting to massive hemorrhage, occurs in 2% to 6% of all pregnancies. The differential diagnosis includes bloody show from labor, abruptio placentae (AP), placenta previa (PP), vasa previa (VP), cervicitis, postcoital bleeding, trauma, uterine rupture, and carcinoma. AP, PP, and VP can lead to significant maternal and fetal morbidity and mortality.

ABRUPTIO PLACENTAE

AP is the premature separation of the normally implanted placenta from the uterine wall due to maternal/uterine bleeding into the *decidua basalis*.

Epidemiology

- One third of all antepartum bleeding is due to AP, with an incidence of 1 in 75 to 1 in 225 births.
- AP recurs in 5% to 17% of pregnancies after one prior episode and up to 25% after two prior episodes.
- There is a 7% incidence of stillbirth in future pregnancies after AP leading to fetal death.

Etiology

- Bleeding does not correlate with abruption size and may vary from scant to massive.
- Blood in the *basalis* layer stimulates forceful, classically tetanic, uterine contractions leading to ischemic abdominal pain.
- AP is associated with maternal hypertension, advanced maternal age, multiparity, cocaine use, tobacco use, chorioamnionitis, and trauma. Many cases are idiopathic.
- Patients with chronic hypertension, superimposed preeclampsia, or severe pre-eclampsia have fivefold increased risk of severe abruption compared to normotensive women. Antihypertensive medications do not reduce the risk of abruption for chronic hypertension.
- Cigarette smoking increases the risk of stillbirth from AP by 2.5-fold. The risk increases by 40% for each pack per day smoked.
- Rapid changes in intrauterine volume can lead to abruption, such as in rupture of membranes or therapeutic amnioreduction with polyhydramnios or during delivery of multiple gestations.
- Abruption occurs more frequently when the placenta implants on abnormal uterine surfaces as with submucous myomas or uterine anomalies.
- Hyperhomocysteinemia, Factor V Leiden, and prothrombin 20210 mutations (thrombophilias) are associated with an increased risk of abruption.

Complications

- Massive maternal blood loss may lead to **hemorrhagic shock** (see Chapter 3).
- Maternal **disseminated intravascular coagulation (DIC)** can occur and is found in 10% to 20% of AP with stillbirth.
- Extravasation of blood directly into the uterine muscle (Couvelaire's uterus) can lead to **uterine atony** and massive postpartum hemorrhage.
- **Fetal hypoxia** may occur, leading to acute fetal distress, hypoxic-ischemic encephalopathy, premature delivery, and fetal death. Milder chronic abruption may lead to growth restriction, major malformations, or anemia.

Diagnosis

History and Physical Examination

- Classically presents late in pregnancy with vaginal bleeding and acute severe constant abdominal pain. Even slight clinical suspicion should prompt rapid investigation and close monitoring.
- Maternal vital signs, fetal heart rate assessment, and uterine tone should be evaluated immediately.
- Mark or record the fundal height to follow expansion of concealed hemorrhage. Blood may be sequestered between the uterus and placenta when the placental margins remain adherent. Membranes or the fetus itself may obstruct the cervical os and prevent accurate assessment of blood loss.
- Defer digital cervical exam until PP and VP have been ruled out. Ultrasound is insensitive in diagnosing AP, but large abruptions may be seen as hypoechoic areas underlying the placenta.
- Perform a speculum exam to evaluate vaginal or cervical lacerations and the amount of bleeding. If discharge or signs of cervicitis are noted, obtain a wet prep, potassium hydroxide slide (KOH), and cervical swabs for gonorrhea and chlamydia testing.

Laboratory Tests

- **Complete blood cell count** with hematocrit and platelets (<100,000 plts/µL suggests severe abruption)
- Blood **type and screen** (cross-match should be strongly considered)
- **Prothrombin/activated partial thromboplastin time**
- **Fibrinogen** (<200 mg/dL suggests severe abruption)
- **Fibrin split-products**
- Consider holding a whole blood specimen at the bedside while lab work is pending. If a clot does not form within 6 minutes or forms and lyses within 30 minutes, DIC may be present.
- The **Apt test** can be performed to evaluate whether vaginal blood is from the mother or the fetus. The blood is collected and lysed in water to release hemoglobin. Sodium hydroxide is mixed with the supernatant. Fetal hemoglobin is resistant to the base and will remain pink, while maternal hemoglobin will oxidize and turn brown. In theory, this qualitative test could be used to identify bleeding from VP, but the short time to fetal distress after a ruptured umbilical vessel and the sensitivity of fetal heart monitoring make the test largely unnecessary.
- The Kleihauer-Betke test for fetal hemoglobin in the maternal circulation is not valuable in diagnosing AP.

Management

- Large-bore **intravenous access** should be obtained.

- **Fluid resuscitation** should be initiated and a **Foley catheter** placed to monitor urine output (more than 0.5 mL/kg/hr or at least 30 mL/hr should be observed).
- Close monitoring of **maternal vital signs** and continuous **fetal monitoring** should be maintained.
- **Rh D immunoglobulin** should be administered to Rh-negative individuals.
- Further management depends on the gestational age and hemodynamic status of both mother and fetus.

Term Gestation, Hemodynamically Stable
- Plan for vaginal delivery with cesarean section for usual indications and initiate induction of labor.
- Follow serial hematocrit and coagulation studies.
- Consider fetal scalp electrode for accurate and continuous fetal monitoring and intrauterine pressure catheter to assess resting uterine tone.

Term Gestation, Hemodynamic Instability
- Aggressively fluid resuscitate.
- Transfuse packed red blood cells, fresh frozen plasma, and platelets as needed. Maintain fibrinogen level >150 mg/dL, hematocrit more than 25%, and platelets over 60,000/μL.
- Once the mother is stabilized, proceed to urgent cesarean section, unless vaginal delivery is imminent.

Preterm Gestation, Hemodynamically Stable
- Eighty-two percent of patients with evidence of AP at <20 weeks' gestation will progress to term. Only 27% of patients who present after 20 weeks' gestation, however, will have a term delivery.
- *In the absence of labor,* preterm AP should be followed closely with serial ultrasound evaluation of fetal growth from 24 weeks and regular antepartum testing. Steroids should be given to promote fetal lung maturity. If maternal instability or fetal distress arises, delivery should be performed as above. Otherwise, labor can be induced at term.
- *For preterm AP with labor* and completely stable hemodynamics and reassuring fetal signs, tocolysis may be used in selected rare cases. Magnesium sulfate tocolysis at <32 weeks' gestation may delay delivery, giving time to administer a course of corticosteroids. Magnesium is preferred over terbutaline or nifedipine as it may be less likely to obscure signs of shock. Indomethacin is avoided because of its effect on platelet function. If maternal or fetal compromise arises, delivery should be performed after appropriate resuscitation.

Preterm Gestation, Hemodynamic Instability
- Delivery should be performed after appropriate resuscitation.

PLACENTA PREVIA

PP is the presence of placental tissue over or near the internal cervical os. It can be classified into four types based on the location relative to the cervical os:
- **complete** or **total previa**, in which the placenta covers the entire cervical os;
- **partial previa**, in which the margin of the placenta covers part but not all of the internal os;

- **marginal previa,** in which the edge of the placenta lies adjacent to the internal os; and
- **low-lying placenta,** in which the placenta is located near (within 2 cm) but not on the internal os.

Epidemiology

- In general, the incidence of PP is 1 in 200 to 1 in 390 pregnancies over 20 weeks' gestational age. The frequency varies with parity, however, giving an incidence of 0.2% in nulliparas and as high as 5% in grand multiparas.
- The placenta covers the cervical os in 5% of pregnancies in the second trimester. Usually the placenta will migrate away from the cervical os as the uterus grows with gestational age and the upper third of the cervix develops into the lower uterine segment.

Etiology

- The most important risk factor for PP is a previous cesarean section. PP occurs in 1% of pregnancies after a single cesarean section. The incidence after four or more cesarean sections increases to 10% and 40-fold increased risk compared with no cesarean section.
- Other risk factors include increasing maternal age (especially after age 40), multi-parity, smoking, residing at higher elevations, male fetus, multiple gestation, and previous uterine curettage.
- These risk factors suggest two explanations for PP development:
  - Endometrial scarring in the upper portion of the uterus promotes implantation in the lower uterine segment; and
  - Reduced uteroplacental oxygen exchange favors increased placental surface area and thereby previa formation.

Complications

- Bleeding occurs with the development of the lower uterine segment in the third trimester in preparation for labor. The placenta separates and the thinned lower segment cannot contract sufficiently to stop blood flow from the exposed uterine vessels. Cervical exams or intercourse may also cause separation of the placenta from the lower uterine segment. Bleeding can range from spotting to massive hemorrhage.
- PP increases the risk for other abnormalities of placentation:
  - **Placenta accreta.** The placenta adheres directly to the uterus without the usual intervening *decidua basalis.* The incidence in patients with previa who have not had previous uterine surgery is approximately 4%, increasing to as many as 25% of patients who have had a previous cesarean section or uterine surgery.
  - **Placenta increta.** The placenta invades the myometrium but does not cross the serosa.
  - **Placenta percreta.** The placenta penetrates the entire uterine wall, potentially growing into bladder or bowel.
- PP is associated with double the rate of fetal congenital malformations, including anomalies of the CNS, GI tract, cardiovascular system, and respiratory system. No specific syndrome has been identified.
- PP is also associated with fetal malpresentation, preterm premature rupture of membranes, intrauterine growth restriction, velamentous cord insertion, and VP.

Diagnosis

History and Physical Exam

- Seventy to 80% of PP presents with the acute onset of painless vaginal bleeding with bright red blood.
- The first bleeding episode is usually around 34 weeks. About one third of patients develop bleeding before 30 weeks, while another third present after 36 weeks and 10% go to term. The number of bleeding episodes is unrelated to the degree of PP or the prognosis for fetal survival.
- A thorough medical, obstetric, and surgical history should be obtained along with documentation of previous ultrasound examinations. Other causes of vaginal bleeding must also be ruled out, such as placental abruption.
- Maternal vital signs, abdominal exam, uterine tone, and fetal heart rate monitoring should be assessed.
- Vaginal sonography is the gold standard for diagnosis of previa. The placenta must be within 2 cm of the cervical os to make the diagnosis and may be missed by a transabdominal scan, especially if the placenta lies in the posterior portion of the lower uterine segment where it is poorly visualized. Having the patient empty her bladder may help in identifying anterior PP. Trendelenburg position may be useful in diagnosing posterior PP.
- *If PP is present or suspected, digital examination is contraindicated.* A gentle speculum exam can be used to evaluate the presence and quantity of vaginal bleeding, but in most cases, this can be assessed adequately by inspecting the perineum and thereby avoid exacerbating the hemorrhage.

Laboratory Studies

- **Complete blood cell count**
- **Type and cross-match**
- **Prothrombin time** and **activated thromboplastin time**
- **Kleihauer-Betke test** to assess for fetomaternal hemorrhage in Rh-negative unsensitized patients. Not useful for the diagnosis of PP.
- **Apt test** (as described above for abruption).

Management

- In general, patients diagnosed with PP but *without* bleeding in the third trimester should have ultrasound confirmation of persistent previa. They should maintain **strict pelvic rest** (i.e., nothing in the vagina, including intercourse or pelvic exams) and avoid strenuous activity or exercise. They should receive advice about when to seek medical attention and be scheduled for fetal growth **ultrasounds** every 3 to 4 weeks.
- In general, patients with PP, who *are* bleeding, should be hospitalized for hemodynamic stabilization and continuous **maternal and fetal monitoring**. **Laboratory studies** should be ordered as described. **Steroids** are administered to promote lung maturity for gestations between 24 and 34 weeks, and **Rh D immunoglobulin** should be administered to Rh-negative mothers.
- Management of placenta accreta, or its variants, can be challenging. In patients with PP and a prior history of cesarean section, cesarean hysterectomy may be required. In cases where uterine preservation is highly desired and no bladder invasion has occurred, bleeding might be successfully controlled with selective arterial embolization or packing of the lower uterine segment, with removal of the pack through the vagina in 24 hr. The Bakri balloon catheter has also been used to help control bleeding from the placental bed.

- Specific management of PP is based on gestational age and assessment of the maternal and fetal status:

Term Gestation, Hemodynamically Stable
- Patients with **complete previa** at term require cesarean section.
- Patients with **partial or marginal previa** at term may deliver vaginally, with thorough consent regarding risks for blood loss and need for transfusion. The staff and facilities for immediate emergent Cesarean section must be available. If maternal or fetal stability is compromised at any point in labor, urgent cesarean section is performed.

Term Gestation, Hemodynamic Instability
- Stabilize the mother with fluid resuscitation and blood products
- Delivery via cesarean section is indicated for nonreassuring fetal heart monitoring, life-threatening maternal hemorrhage, or bleeding after 34 weeks with documented fetal lung maturity. If the mother is stable and intrauterine fetal loss occurs or the fetus is <24 weeks' gestational age, vaginal delivery can be considered.

Preterm Gestation, Hemodynamically Stable
- Patients at 24 to 37 weeks' gestation with PP *in the absence of labor can be* managed expectantly until term or fetal lung maturity is documented.
- There is no evidence-based consensus on management of bleeding PP without hemodynamic compromise. In general, once a patient has been hospitalized for three separate episodes of bleeding, she should remain in the hospital until delivery. For each bleeding episode, the following are recommended:
  - Hospitalization until stabilized on bed rest with bathroom privileges.
  - Periodic assessment of maternal hematocrit and maintenance of an active type and screen.
  - Red blood cell transfusion as needed to maintain hematocrit above 30% for slight but continuous bleeding.
  - Corticosteroids and Rhogam as indicated.
  - Fetal testing and growth ultrasounds to assess for intrauterine growth restriction.
  - Tocolysis is not warranted unless to administer a course of steroids in an otherwise stable patient.
  - Amniocentesis can be used to assess fetal lung maturity.
- After initial hospital management, outpatient care may be considered if bleeding stops for >48 hr, no other complications exist, and the following criteria are met:
  - The patient can maintain bed rest at home and is adherent to medical care.
  - There is a responsible adult present at all times who can assist in an emergency.
  - The patient lives near the hospital with dependable transportation.
- For preterm gestations with PP *and contractions*, it can be difficult to diagnose labor. Cervical exams are contraindicated and twenty percent of patients with PP show some uterine activity. If the patient and fetus are stable, tocolysis may be considered with magnesium sulfate. As with AP, terbutaline, nifedipine, and indomethacin should be avoided.

Preterm Gestation, Hemodynamic Instability
- Appropriate stabilization and resuscitation are initiated with rapid delivery by cesarean section.

VASA PREVIA

VP occurs when the umbilical cord inserts into the membranes, instead of the central placental disc. When the vessels traverse the membranes near the internal os in advance of the fetal presenting part, they are at risk of rupture, causing fetal hemorrhage. VP can also occur when a velamentous cord insertion or vessels for an accessory lobe are located near the cervical os. Velamentous cord insertion is much more common in multiple gestations.

Epidemiology

- The incidence of VP is between 1/1,000 and 1/5,000 pregnancies.
- Fetal mortality may be as high as 60% with intact membranes and 75% when membranes rupture.

Etiology

- The cause of VP is unknown. Because of the association between velamentous cord insertion, multiple gestations, and VP, one theory suggests that it develops due to trophoblastic growth and placental migration toward the more vascular uterine fundus. The initial cord insertion at the center of the placenta becomes more peripheral as one portion of the placenta actively grows and another portion does not.

Complications

- Even small amounts of fetal hemorrhage can result in morbidity and possible death, due to the small total fetal blood volume.
- Rupture of the membranes can result in rapid exsanguination of the fetus.

History

- The patient usually presents with acute onset vaginal bleeding after rupture of membranes.
- The bleeding is associated with an acute change in fetal heart pattern. Typically, fetal tachycardia occurs, followed by bradycardia with intermittent accelerations. Short-term variability is often maintained. Occasionally, a sinusoidal pattern may be seen.

Diagnosis

- **Transvaginal ultrasound**, in combination with color Doppler ultrasonography, is the most effective tool in antenatal diagnosis.
- In one study, there was a 97% survival rate in cases diagnosed antenatally compared to a 44% survival rate in those without prenatal diagnosis.

Management

- Third-trimester bleeding caused by VP is often accompanied by acute and severe fetal distress. **Emergency cesarean section** is indicated.
- If VP is diagnosed antenatally, **planned cesarean section** should be scheduled at 36 to 38 weeks under controlled circumstances and before the onset of labor, to reduce fetal mortality. Earlier delivery can be considered with documented fetal lung maturity.

SUGGESTED READINGS

Love CD, Wallace EM. Pregnancies complicated by placenta praevia: what is appropriate management? *Br J Obstet Gynecol* 1996;103(9):864–867.

Magann EF, Cummings JE, Niederhauser A, et al. Antepartum bleeding of unknown origin in the second half of pregnancy: a review. *Obstet Gynecol Surv* 2005;60(11):741–745.

McCormack RA, Doherty DA, Magann EF, et al. Antepartum bleeding of unknown origin in the second half of pregnancy and pregnancy outcomes. *BJOG* 2008;115(11):1451–1457.

Oyelese Y, Smulian JC. Placenta previa, placenta accreta, and vasa previa. *Obstet Gynecol* 2006;107(4):927–941.

Perinatal Infections

Hindi Stohl and Andrew J. Satin

CYTOMEGALOVIRUS

Epidemiology

- **Cytomegalovirus (CMV)** is the most common congenital viral infection, with intrauterine infection occurring in 0.2% to 2.5% of live births. CMV is a ubiquitous DNA herpes virus; about 50% of the US population has antibodies to CMV. Transmission occurs through direct contact with infected saliva, semen, cervical and vaginal secretions, urine, breast milk, or blood products. Vertical transmission can occur transplacentally, during delivery, or postpartum. An estimated 40,000 infants are born with CMV infection in the United States annually.

Clinical Manifestations

- **Maternal infection.** In immunocompetent adults, CMV infection is typically silent. Symptoms, however, can include fever, malaise, swollen glands, and rarely hepatitis. After the primary infection, the virus becomes dormant, with periodic episodes of reactivation and viral shedding.
- **Congenital (fetal) infection.** Most fetal infections are due to recurrent maternal infection and rarely lead to congenital abnormalities. Previously acquired maternal immunity confers protection from clinically apparent disease by maternal antibodies. Mothers determined to be seronegative for CMV before conception or early in gestation have a 1% to 4% risk of acquiring the infection during pregnancy and 40% to 50% rate of fetal transmission after seroconversion.
  - Approximately 90% of infants with congenital CMV infection will be asymptomatic at birth. Ten to fifteen percent of these may later develop symptoms including developmental delay, hearing loss, and visual and dental defects. Unlike recurrent infection, primary maternal infection during pregnancy can often lead to serious neonatal sequelae with neonatal mortality as high as 30%. Fetuses infected earlier in gestation have higher risk of sequelae than those infected in the third trimester.
  - Fetal ultrasound may demonstrate microcephaly, ventriculomegaly, intracranial calcifications, oligohydramnios, and intrauterine growth restriction. Nonimmune hydrops has also been reported. The most common clinical findings at birth include the presence of petechiae, hepatosplenomegaly or jaundice, and chorioretinitis. These symptoms constitute fulminant cytomegalic inclusion disease. Infants show signs of respiratory distress, lethargy, and seizures. Long-term sequelae include mental retardation, motor disabilities, and hearing and visual loss.

Diagnosis

- **Maternal** CMV screening is not routine. Only women at high risk, such as day care workers and health care providers, should be offered serum antibody testing (both IgG and IgM). IgM immunoblot may be performed to help determine whether an infection is recurrent or primary. Screening is of limited value since there is no CMV vaccine, and we cannot predict accurately the severity of fetal sequelae.

• **Fetal** ultrasonography may detect characteristic anomalies. Amniocentesis and cordocentesis for PCR DNA testing have also been used to diagnose intrauterine infection.

Management

• There is no effective in utero therapy for CMV. Because it is difficult to predict the severity of sequelae, counseling patients appropriately about pregnancy termination is problematic. Most infected fetuses do not suffer serious problems. Breast-feeding is discouraged in women with active infection.

Prevention

• CMV transmission requires close personal contact or contact with contaminated bodily fluids. Preventive measures include transfusing only CMV-negative blood products, safe sex practices, and frequent hand-washing.

VARICELLA ZOSTER VIRUS

Epidemiology

• **Primary varicella infection** is estimated to affect only 1 to 5 of every 10,000 pregnancies. **Herpes zoster** is also uncommon in women of childbearing age.
• The major mode of transmission is respiratory, although direct contact with vesicular or pustular lesions may also result in disease. In the past, nearly all persons were infected before adulthood, 90% before age 14. Since the advent of varicella vaccine, most people in the United States have vaccine-induced immunity.
• Varicella outbreaks occur most frequently during the winter and spring. The incubation period is 10 to 21 days. Infectivity is greatest 24 to 48 hr before the onset of rash and lasts 3 to 4 days into the rash. The virus is rarely isolated after the lesions have crusted over.

Clinical Manifestations

• **Maternal.** Primary varicella infection tends to be more severe in adults than in children, and is especially severe in pregnancy. The risk of varicella pneumonia is increased in pregnancy, starting several days after the onset of the characteristic rash. Maternal mortality with varicella pneumonia may reach 40% in the absence of antiviral therapy, so early signs and symptoms should be managed aggressively. In contrast, herpes zoster infection (reactivation of varicella) is more common in older and immunocompromised patients and poses little risk to the fetus.
• **Congenital.** Fetal infection with varicella zoster can lead to one of three major outcomes: intrauterine infection, which infrequently causes congenital abnormalities; postnatal disease, ranging from typical varicella with a benign course to fatal disseminated infection; and shingles, appearing months or years after birth. The risk of congenital malformation after fetal exposure to primary maternal varicella before 20 weeks' gestation is estimated to be <2%.
    • The abnormalities are diverse, including cutaneous scars, limb-reduction anomalies, malformed digits, muscle atrophy, growth restriction, cataracts, chorioretinitis, micro-ophthalmia, cortical atrophy, microcephaly, and psychomotor retardation.
    • Infection after 20 weeks' gestation may lead to postnatal disease. If maternal infection occurs within 5 days of delivery, hematogenous transplacental viral transfer may cause significant infant morbidity and neonatal mortality rates as high as

25%. Sufficient transplacental antibody transfer to confer fetal immunity requires at least 5 days after the onset of the maternal rash. Women who develop chickenpox, especially near term, should be observed. Delay in delivery may offer the fetus the benefit of passive immunity. Neonatal therapy with immunoglobulin is also important when a mother develops signs of chickenpox within 3 days postpartum. Herpes zoster infection during pregnancy is not associated with fetal sequelae due to maternal antibody transfer.

Diagnosis

- **Clinical.** The diagnosis of acute varicella zoster in the mother usually can be established by the characteristic cutaneous manifestations described as chickenpox. The generalized vesicular rash usually appears on the head and ears, and then spreads to the face, trunk, and extremities. Mucous membrane involvement is common. Lesions in different areas will be in different stages of evolution. Vesicles and pustules evolve into crusted lesions, which then heal and may scar. Herpes zoster, or shingles, demonstrates a unilateral vesicular eruption in a dermatomal distribution.
- **Laboratory.** Confirmation of the diagnosis may be obtained by examining scrapings of vesicular lesions that will reveal multinucleated giant cells. For rapid diagnosis, varicella zoster antigen may be demonstrated in exfoliated cells from lesions by immunofluorescent antibody staining.
- **Ultrasonography.** Detailed ultrasonographic examination is the best means for assessing a fetus for major limb abnormalities or growth disturbances associated with varicella infection. PCR testing of amniotic fluid can diagnose intrauterine infection.

Management

- **Varicella exposure during pregnancy.** An IgG titer should be obtained within 24 to 48 hr of exposure to a person with noncrusted lesions. The presence of IgG reflects prior immunity, while absence of varicella IgG indicates susceptibility.
- **Varicella zoster immune globulin (VZIG)** may be administered to susceptible women (i.e., women without detectable varicella IgG) within 72 hr of exposure to reduce the severity of maternal infection. VZIG is administered intramuscularly at a dose of 125 U/10 kg to a maximum of 625 U. Maternal administration of VZIG, however, does not ameliorate or prevent fetal infection.
- Usually, the disease course is similar in pregnant and nonpregnant patients; only **supportive care** with fluids and analgesics is needed. If evidence of pneumonia or disseminated disease appears, the patient should be admitted to the hospital for treatment with intravenous (IV) acyclovir. Acyclovir administered to pregnant women with varicella pneumonia during the second or third trimester decreases maternal morbidity and mortality. The dosage of acyclovir is 10 to 15 mg/kg IV every 8 hr for 7 days, or 800 mg by mouth (PO) five times per day. Tocolytics are generally avoided in women with varicella pneumonia, though induction should only be performed for obstetric indications.

Prevention

- An **attenuated live vaccine** was approved by the FDA in 1995. One dose is recommended for all children between ages 1 and 12. Two doses, given 4 to 8 weeks apart, are recommended for adolescents and adults without history of varicella infection. The seroconversion rate after vaccination is approximately 82% in adults and 91% for children. Use of the vaccine during pregnancy is not recommended but is appropriate for breast-feeding mothers.

PARVOVIRUS B19

Epidemiology

- **Parvovirus B19 infection**, commonly known as *erythema infectiosum* or *fifth disease,* occurs in school-aged children. By adulthood, 30% to 60% of women have acquired immunity to the virus. Parvovirus B19 is a single-stranded DNA virus passed primarily by respiratory secretions. Outbreaks usually occur in the midwinter to spring months.

Clinical Manifestations

- **Maternal.** Adults may present with typical clinical features: a red, macular rash and facial erythroderma, which gives a characteristic "slapped cheek" appearance. The rash may also cover the trunk and extremities. Infected adults often have acute joint swelling, usually with symmetric involvement of peripheral joints. The arthritis may be severe and chronic. Some adults have a completely asymptomatic infection. Parvovirus B19 may cause aplastic crisis in patients with chronic anemia (e.g., sickle cell disease or thalassemia). The course of the infection is unchanged in pregnancy.
- **Congenital.** Approximately one third of maternal infections are associated with fetal infection via transplacental transfer of the virus. Infection of fetal red blood cell precursors can result in fetal anemia, which, if severe, leads to nonimmune hydrops fetalis. The likelihood of severe fetal disease is increased if maternal infection occurs during the first 18 weeks of pregnancy, but the risk of hydrops fetalis persists even when infection occurs in the late third trimester. Fetal immunoglobulin M (IgM) production after 18 weeks' gestation probably contributes to the resolution of infection in fetuses who survive. The overall risk of fetal death after maternal infection before 20 weeks is 6% to 11%, and after 20 weeks' gestation is <1%.

Diagnosis

- The illness may be suspected if a regional outbreak is ongoing or if family members are affected. Children are the most common vectors for parvovirus B19 transmission. Usual presentation includes fever, malaise, myalgia, and headaches as well as a confluent, indurated facial rash that imparts the characteristic appearance of fifth disease. The rash spreads to other areas over 1 to 2 days, especially exposed surfaces, such as the arms and legs and is usually macular and reticular in appearance.
- A pregnant woman who has been exposed to a child with fifth disease and presents with an unexplained morbilliform or purpuric rash, or who has a known history of chronic hemolytic anemia and presents with an aplastic crisis, should be evaluated with parvovirus B19 immunoglobulin titers. Parvovirus B19 IgM appears 3 days after the onset of illness, peaks in 30 to 60 days, and may persist for 3 to 4 months. Parvovirus B19 IgG is usually detected by the 7th day of illness and persists for years. PCR of amniotic fluid can be used to detect fetal infection in a woman who was recently exposed or has ultrasound findings of fetal hydrops.

Management

- No specific antiviral therapy exists for parvovirus B19 infection. IV gamma globulin may be administered on an empiric basis to immunocompromised patients with known exposure to parvovirus B19 and should be used for treatment of women in aplastic crisis with viremia.

- Parvovirus B19 can infect the fetal bone marrow, which may lead to severe fetal anemia. Therefore, when maternal infection is confirmed, serial screening sonograms should be performed to assess for signs of fetal anemia such as hydrops and elevated fetal middle cerebral artery (MCA) Dopplers. Hydrops fetalis usually develops within 6 weeks but can develop as late as 10 weeks after maternal infection. Weekly or biweekly ultrasonographic scans can be useful to follow patients.
- Intrauterine blood transfusion is a successful therapeutic intervention for correcting fetal anemia and hydrops in several small studies. Single or serial intrauterine transfusions may be undertaken.

Prevention

- Usual conscientious hand-washing and avoiding known infected contacts are advised.

RUBELLA VIRUS

Epidemiology

- Despite widespread immunization programs in the United States, the CDC reports 10% to 20% of adults remain susceptible to **rubella**. The annual number of reported cases in the United States, however, remains extremely low, with fewer than ten cases of congenital rubella occurring annually. Transmission results from direct contact with the nasopharyngeal secretions of an infected person. The disease is communicable for 1 week before and for 4 days after the onset of the rash, with the most contagious period occurring a few days before the onset of the maculopapular rash. The incubation period ranges from 14 to 21 days.

Clinical Manifestations

- **Maternal.** Rubella usually presents as a maculopapular rash that persists for 3 days, generalized lymphadenopathy (especially postauricular and occipital), which may precede the rash, transient arthritis, malaise, and headache. Rubella, typically, follows the same mild course in pregnancy and may be asymptomatic. The majority of women with affected infants report no history of a rash during their pregnancies.
- **Congenital.** Maternal viremia leads to fetal infection in 25% to 90% of cases. Fetal sequela are dependant on gestational age, with 90% of first trimester exposures resulting in clinical signs, 54% at 13 to 14 weeks, and 25% by the end of the second trimester. Congenital rubella syndrome involves multiple organs. The most common manifestations are sensorineural hearing loss, developmental delay, growth retardation, and cardiac and ophthalmic defects.
  - As many as one third of asymptomatic exposed infants may develop late manifestations, including diabetes mellitus, thyroid disorders, and precocious puberty. The extended rubella syndrome (progressive panencephalitis and type 1 diabetes mellitus) may develop as late as the second or third decade of life.

Diagnosis

- Infection is confirmed by serology. Viral isolation is technically difficult and tissue culture results may take up to 6 weeks. Specimens should be obtained as soon as possible after exposure, 2 weeks later, and if necessary, 4 weeks after exposure. Serum specimens from both acute and convalescent phases should be tested; a fourfold or greater increase in titer or seroconversion indicates acute infection. If the patient is IgG-seropositive on the first titer, no risk to the fetus is apparent. Primary rubella confers lifelong immunity. Reinfection with rubella is usually subclinical, rarely associated with viremia, and infrequently results in a congenitally infected infant.

- Prenatal diagnosis is made by identification of rubella-specific IgM antibody in fetal blood samples obtained at 22 weeks' gestation or later. IgM does not cross the placenta, and therefore its presence indicates fetal infection.

Management

- If a pregnant woman is exposed to rubella, serologic evaluation is recommended. If primary rubella is diagnosed, the mother should be informed about the implications of the infection for the fetus including the high rate of fetal infection and the option for termination discussed. Women electing to continue the pregnancy may be given immune globulin because it may modify clinical rubella in the mother. Immune globulin, however, does not prevent infection or viremia and affords no protection to the fetus.

Prevention

- Pregnant women should undergo rubella serum evaluation as part of routine prenatal care. A clinical history of rubella is unreliable. If the patient is nonimmune, she should receive rubella vaccine after delivery. The rubella vaccine is a live attenuated virus, so should be avoided in pregnancy due to the theoretic risk of teratogenicity. The CDC maintains a registry to monitor fetal effects of vaccination, and there have been no reported cases of congenital rubella syndrome after vaccination. Nonetheless, the CDC recommends contraception for 28 days after vaccination.

HEPATITIS A VIRUS

Epidemiology

- An estimated 200,000 cases of **hepatitis A virus (HAV)** infection occur annually in the United States. HAV is transmitted primarily through fecal-oral contamination and typically is not excreted in urine or other bodily fluids. Epidemics frequently result from contaminated food or water supplies. The incubation period ranges from 15 to 50 days, with a mean of about 30 days. The duration of viremia is short. Obstetric patients at highest risk of developing HAV infection are those who have emigrated from or traveled to countries where the virus is endemic (e.g., Southeast Asia, Africa, Central America, Mexico, and the Middle East). It affects approximately 1:1,000 pregnant American women.

Clinical Manifestations

- **Maternal.** Symptoms of HAV infection include malaise, fatigue, anorexia, nausea, and abdominal pain, typically right upper quadrant or epigastric. Physical findings include jaundice, upper abdominal tenderness, and hepatomegaly. Serious complications are uncommon, and, unlike other hepatitides, a chronic carrier state does not exist.
- **Congenital.** Perinatal transmission of HAV has not been documented.

Diagnosis

- A complete travel history suggests the diagnosis in a jaundiced patient. Laboratory studies may reveal a transaminitis (elevated ALT and AST) as well as hyperbilirubinemia. Abnormal coagulation studies and hyperammonemia may suggest more significant

TABLE 11-1	Interpretation of Hepatitis Serology Results						
Significance	Anti-HAV IgM	HBsAg	HBeAg	Anti-HBcAg IgG	Anti-HBcAg IgM	Anti-HBsAg IgG	Anti-HCV IgG/IgM
Acute HAV infection	+	–	–	–	–	–	–
Acute HBV infection	–	+	+	–	+	–	–
Chronic HBV infection, active replication	–	+	+	+	–	–	–
Chronic HBV infection, quiescent	–	+	–	+	–	–	–
HBV infection, resolved	–	–	–	–	–	+	–
Post-HBV vaccine	–	–	–	–	–	+	–
Acute or chronic HCV infection	–	–	–	–	–	–	+

HAV, hepatitis A virus; HBcAg, hepatitis B core antigen; HBeAg, hepatitis B envelope antigen; HBsAg, hepatitis B surface antigen; HBV, hepatitis B virus; HCV, hepatitis C virus; IgG, immunoglobulin G; IgM, immunoglobulin M; +, positive; –, negative.

liver injury. The presence of IgM antibody to HAV confirms the diagnosis. IgG antibody will persist in patients with a history of exposure (Table 11-1).

Management

- Individuals with close personal or sexual contact with an affected individual may receive HAV immune globulin in a single IM dose. This treatment is 80% to 90% effective in preventing infection but ineffective if given >2 weeks after exposure. HAV immune globulin is safe in pregnancy.
- Treatment of HAV is supportive. There is no antiviral therapy. Activity level should be decreased, and upper abdominal trauma should be avoided. Patients with hepatitis-induced encephalopathy or coagulopathy and debilitated patients should be hospitalized.

Prevention

- The HAV vaccine (inactivated virus vaccine) may be used in pregnancy. The vaccine is recommended for individuals traveling to endemic areas and is administered in two injections 4 to 6 months apart.

HEPATITIS B VIRUS

Epidemiology

- In North America, **hepatitis B virus (HBV)** transmission occurs most commonly via parenteral exposure or sexual contact. Approximately 200,000 persons in the United States are newly diagnosed each year, with an estimated 1.25 million chronic carriers. Acute HBV occurs in 1 to 2 per 1,000 pregnancies and chronic HBV in 5 to 15 per 1,000. Mother-to-child transmission (MTCT) is an important cause of chronic HBV infection worldwide. Transmission can occur prenatally, during delivery, or postpartum and is highest in women who are HBeAg-positive. The vertical transmission rate in these women is as high as 90% in the puerperium if prophylaxis is not given to their neonates.
- **Natural history.** HBV contains three principal antigens: HBV surface antigen (HBsAg), HBV core antigen (HBcAg), and HBV envelope antigen (HBeAg). HBsAg is detectable in serum during acute and chronic infection. HBcAg compromises the central nucleocapsid of the virus; it is found only in hepatocytes during active viral replication and is not detected in serum. HBeAg is a secretory product that is processed from the precore protein; it is a marker of active HBV replication and increased infectivity. The presence of HBeAg is usually associated with high levels of HBV DNA in serum and higher rates of HBV transmission. Circulating antibodies against these viral antigens develop in response to infection.

Clinical Manifestations

- **Maternal.** The clinical manifestations of HBV during pregnancy are similar to those for the nonpregnant patient. HBV infection presents with nonhepatic prodomal symptoms, including rash, arthralgia, myalgia, and occasionally frank arthritis. Jaundice occurs in a minority of patients. In adults, between 95% and 99% of acute infections resolve completely, and the patient develops protective levels of antibody. The remaining 1% to 5% of patients become chronically infected. These patients are clinically asymptomatic and usually have normal liver function tests. They nonetheless have detectable levels of HBsAg. The incidence of cirrhosis in a chronic HBV carrier is 8% to 20% over 5 years. Acute hepatitis B carries a 1% risk of maternal mortality.
- **Fetal infection.** Maternal-fetal transmission can occur at any time during pregnancy but most commonly occurs at the time of delivery. In women who are seropositive for both HBsAg and HBeAg (indicating active replication), the vertical transmission rate approaches 90%. However, in a woman who is HBsAg-positive and anti-HepB surface antibody–positive with an undetectable hepatitis B viral load (carrier state), the risk of transmission drops to 10% to 30%. The frequency of vertical transmission is also affected by the timing of maternal infection. When maternal infection occurs in the first trimester, 10% of neonates are seropositive; when it occurs in the third trimester, 80% to 90% of neonates are infected. Whether infection occurs in utero or intrapartum, the presence of HBeAg in the neonates carries an 85% to 90% likelihood of progression to chronic HBV infection and the associated hepatic sequelae. Fetal malformation, intrauterine growth restriction, spontaneous abortion, or stillbirth is not associated with HBV infection.

Diagnosis

- Diagnosis is confirmed by serology (see Table 11-1).
  - HBsAg appears in the serum 1 to 10 weeks after an acute exposure prior to the onset of clinical symptoms, then becomes undetectable in 4 to 6 months in

patients who eventually recover. Persistence of HBsAg for >6 months implies chronic infection.

- The disappearance of HBsAg is followed by the appearance of anti-HBs. In most patients, anti-HBs persists for life, conferring long-term immunity.
- HBeAg is detected during active viral replication. The disappearance of HBeAg and the appearance of anti-HBeAg IgG signal a decrease in infectivity. The presence of anti-HBsAg IgG indicates immunity or recovery.
- If a patient is tested during the period in which results for HBsAg are negative, HBV can be identified by the presence of anti-HBsAg IgM.

Management

- Patients with acute hepatitis B infection may require hospitalization and supportive care. The disease is generally self-limited, and symptoms resolve within 1 to 2 weeks. Administration of alpha interferon has been shown to alter the natural history of acute HBV infection but has multiple side effects (myelosuppression, autoantibody formation, thyroid disturbances, and possible cardiotoxicity). The safety of alpha interferon during pregnancy is unknown.
- Current CDC recommendations include universal screening of all pregnant women for HBV at the first prenatal visit. Serum transaminase levels should be measured in seropositive patients to assess active chronic hepatitis.
- Women exposed to HBV should receive passive immunization with HBV immune globulin (HBIG) and receive recombinant HBV vaccine, preferably in the contralateral arm. HBIG is 75% effective in preventing maternal HBV infection.
- HBIG should be administered to the neonate of an infected mother within the first 12 hr of life. HBIG is followed immediately by the standard three-dose HBV immunization series. The combination of HBIG and HBV vaccine prevents vertical transmission in 85% to 90% of cases.
- Invasive intrapartum fetal monitoring (fetal scalp electrodes or fetal scalp blood sampling) should be avoided if maternal infection is known.

Prevention

- Vaccination for Hepatitis B is recommended for all women of reproductive age, preferably during preconception or routine gynecologic care but is also safe to use during pregnancy.

HEPATITIS C VIRUS

Epidemiology

- Transmission of the **hepatitis C virus (HCV)** is similar to that of HBV but occurs via percutaneous blood contamination and rarely through sexual contact. An increased incidence of HCV is noted among intravenous drug abusers and recipients of blood products. Mass screening of the blood supply for HCV has markedly decreased the risk of HCV infection to <1 per 1,000,000 screened units of blood.

Clinical Manifestations

- **Maternal.** Acute HCV infection presents after an incubation period of 30 to 60 days. Asymptomatic infection occurs in 75% of patients, and at least 50% of infected individuals progress to chronic infection, regardless of the mode of acquisition or severity of initial infection. Of these patients, approximately 20% subsequently develop chronic active hepatitis or cirrhosis. Concomitant infection with

HIV may accelerate the progression and severity of hepatic injury. Unlike HBV antibodies, antibodies to HCV are not protective. HCV causes acute hepatitis in pregnancy but may go undetected if liver function tests and HCV antibody tests are not performed.

- **Congenital.** Vertical transmission is proportional to the maternal serum HCV viral RNA titer. Transmission is approximately 4% to 7% in women with HCV viremia and is four to five times more likely in the setting of maternal coinfection with HIV. Currently, there is no method or technique to prevent prenatal transmission. If transmission occurs transplacentally, the neonate is at increased risk of acute hepatitis and of probable chronic hepatitis or carrier status. To date, no teratogenic syndromes associated with HCV have been defined. During labor, invasive procedures such as a fetal scalp electrode or fetal scalp blood sampling should be avoided. According to CDC guidelines, maternal infection with hepatitis C is not an absolute contraindication to breast-feeding.

Diagnosis

- Anti–Hepatitis C antibody is detected in serum, but may take up to 1 year from exposure to test positive. HCV viral RNA can be detected by PCR assay of serum soon after infection and in chronic disease and can be used to quantify active viral replication (see Table 11-1).

Management

- Because there is no prophylaxis for transmission, primary prevention of maternal infection is the mainstay of management. Treatment with alpha interferon in pregnant women has not been well studied and is generally considered contraindicated.

Prevention

- Avoiding contaminated needle injections, including occupational hazards such as needle sticks, is advised.

TOXOPLASMA

Epidemiology

- In the United States, the incidence of acute **toxoplasmosis** infection in pregnancy is estimated at 0.2% to 1.0%. Congenital toxoplasmosis occurs in 1 to 8:1,000 live births. Transmission occurs primarily by eating undercooked or raw meat containing cysts, ingesting food or water contaminated by the feces of an infected cat, inhaling aerosolized oocysts from cat litter, or handling material contaminated by the feces of an infected cat. Approximately one third of American women carry antibodies to *Toxoplasma*.

Clinical Manifestations

- **Maternal.** Up to 90% of acute toxoplasmosis infections are asymptomatic. A mononucleosis-like syndrome, including fatigue, malaise, cervical lymphadenopathy, sore throat, and atypical lymphocytosis, may occur. Placental infection and subsequent fetal infection occur during the spreading phase of the parasitemia. The overall risk of fetal infection is estimated to be 30% to 40%, and the rate of transmission increases with gestational age.
- **Congenital.** The rate of transmission is approximately 15% in the first trimester, 30% in the second trimester, and 60% in the third trimester. Fetal morbidity and

mortality rates are higher after early transmission, with 11% risk of perinatal death from infection in the first trimester, 4% in the second trimester, and 0% in the third trimester. Infected neonates often exhibit low birth weight, hepatosplenomegaly, icterus, and anemia. Sequelae such as vision loss and psychomotor and mental retardation are common. Hearing loss is demonstrated in 10% to 30% and developmental delay in 20% to 75%. Up to 90% of infants with congenital toxoplasmosis are asymptomatic at birth.

Diagnosis

- Screening for toxoplasmosis is not routine in the United States. Because most women with acute toxoplasmosis are asymptomatic, the diagnosis is not suspected until an affected infant is born. For women who do present with symptoms of acute infection, both IgM and IgG titers should be measured as soon as possible (Table 11-2).
  - Negative IgM excludes acute or recent infection, unless the serum has been tested so early that an immune response has not yet been mounted. A positive test is more difficult to interpret because IgM may be elevated for more than a year after infection. Seroconversion of IgG on repeat testing can be useful as well.
  - PCR testing for toxoplasma DNA can be performed on amniotic fluid. This is the best method for confirming congenital infection.
  - Sonographic findings include dilated cerebral ventricles, intracranial and intrahepatic lesions, and placental hyperdensities. Occasionally, pericardial and pleural effusions are observed.

Management

- For women who elect to continue their pregnancies after a diagnosis of toxoplasmosis, therapy should be started immediately and continued in the infant for 1 year or more to decrease risk for developmental sequelae. Antibiotics decrease the risk permanent deficits by 50%.
  - **Spiramycin** reduces the incidence but not necessarily the severity of fetal infection. Spiramycin is recommended for the treatment of acute maternal infections diagnosed before the third trimester and should then be continued for the duration of the pregnancy. If amniotic fluid PCR results for *Toxoplasma* are negative, spiramycin is used as a single agent; if results are positive, pyrimethamine and sulfadiazine should be added. Spiramycin dosing is 500 mg PO five times daily, or 3 g/day in divided doses.

TABLE 11-2		Interpretation of *Toxoplasma* Serology Results
IgM[a]	**IgG**	**Interpretation**
+	−	Possible acute infection; IgG titers should be reassessed in several weeks
+	+	Possible acute infection
−	+	Remote infection
−	−	Susceptible; uninfected

[a]IgM titers may remain elevated for up to 1 year.
IgG, immunoglobulin G; IgM, immunoglobulin M; +, positive; −, negative.

- **Pyrimethamine and sulfadiazine.** Patients with documented *Toxoplasma gondii* infection of the fetus may be offered treatment with Pyrimethamine 25 mg PO daily and sulfadiazine PO 1 g four times daily for 28 days. Folinic acid, 6 mg IM or PO, is administered three times per week to prevent toxicity. During the first trimester, pyrimethamine is not recommended due to teratogenic risk. Sulfadiazine is omitted from the regimen at term.

Prevention

- Pregnant women should eat only fully cooked meats, wash their hands after preparing meat for cooking, wash fruits and vegetables well, and avoid contact with cat litter boxes.

HERPES SIMPLEX VIRUS (HSV)

Epidemiology

- Type 1 **HSV** is responsible for most nongenital herpetic infections and up to 50% of genital lesions. Type 2 HSV is usually recovered from the genital tract. Approximately 1:7,500 live-born infants contract HSV perinatally. Whether pregnancy alters the rate of recurrence or frequency of cervical shedding of virus is debated. The incidence of asymptomatic shedding in pregnancy is 10% after a first episode and 0.5% after a recurrent episode.
- Primary maternal infection with HSV results from direct contact, generally sexual, with mucous membranes or skin infected with the virus.
- Fetal infection with HSV can occur transplacentally, as an ascending infection from the cervix, or most commonly through direct contact with infectious maternal genital lesions during delivery.

Clinical Manifestations

- **Maternal.** Primary infections range from mild or asymptomatic to severe. Vesicles appear on the cervix, vagina, or vulva from 2 to 10 days after exposure. Swelling, erythema, pain, and regional lymphadenopathy are common. The lesions persist for 1 to 3 weeks with concomitant viral shedding. Reactivation occurs in 50% of patients within 6 months of the initial outbreak and subsequently at irregular intervals. Symptoms of recurrent outbreaks are generally milder, with viral shedding lasting less than a week. In pregnancy, primary outbreaks are not associated with spontaneous abortion but may increase the incidence of preterm labor in the latter half of pregnancy.
- **Fetal** infection is usually the result of primary maternal infection. Transmission from a recurrent maternal infection is rare, accounting for <1% of fetal infections. Transfer of maternal IgG is believed to account for the low rate. Overall, congenital infections are very rare, and few are asymptomatic. The majority ultimately produce disseminated or CNS disease. Localized infection is usually associated with a good outcome, but infants with disseminated infection have a mortality rate of 60%, even with treatment. At least half of infants surviving disseminated infection develop serious neurologic and ophthalmic sequelae.

Diagnosis

- When HSV is suspected, a swab specimen may be obtained from the lesion for culture and immunofluorescent or PCR studies. Seven to ten days must be allowed for isolation of the virus via tissue culture, but the sensitivity is 95% and specificity is also high. Serology is of limited value in diagnosis because a single antibody titer is not predictive viral shedding and IgG will be positive indefinitely after the primary outbreak. Smears of scrapings from the bases of vesicles may be stained using Tzanck or Papanicolaou techniques may reveal multinucleated giant cells, but that only suggests viral infection and may not differentiate HSV from other cervical infections such as CMV. Immunofluorescent detection of viral antigens in the scraped sample is rapid but less sensitive. PCR for HSV DNA is sensitive and rapid.

Management

- Patients with a history of genital herpes should undergo a careful perineal examination at the time of delivery. Vaginal delivery is permitted if no signs or symptoms of HSV are present. Active genital HSV in patients in labor or with ruptured membranes at or near term is an indication for cesarean section, regardless of the duration of rupture. Evidence shows that HSV recurrences in the regions of the buttocks, thighs, and anus are associated with low rates of cervical virus shedding. Lesions in these areas should not preclude a vaginal delivery; however, it is recommended that the lesion(s) be covered for delivery. Acyclovir may be used to treat HSV infection in pregnancy; however, valacyclovir hydrochloride (Valtrex) has been shown to be more effective and is more easily tolerated due to a twice-daily dosing schedule. Third trimester suppression with valacyclovir, 500 mg PO daily or twice daily, should be considered in women with frequent outbreaks during their pregnancies.

Prevention

- Barrier contraception can be recommended to avoid primary maternal infection as part of routine safer sex counseling.

GROUP B *STREPTOCOCCUS*

Epidemiology

- **Group B *Streptococcus* (GBS)** (*Streptococcus agalactiae*), a Gram-positive bacteria, can be isolated from the vagina and/or rectum in 5% to 40% of pregnant women in the United States. Neonatal colonization may occur as a result of ascending infection from the maternal genital tract or during passage of the fetus through the birth canal during a vaginal delivery. The vertical transmission rate may be as high as 72%, but invasive disease in term neonates is rare. In preterm infants, however, invasive disease is more common and is accompanied by significant morbidity and mortality.

Clinical Manifestations

- **Maternal**. GBS is a common urinary pathogen in pregnant women. GBS is isolated in 5% to 29% of cases of asymptomatic bacteriuria and in 1% to 5% of cases of acute cystitis during pregnancy. When inadequately treated, both asymptomatic bacteriuria and acute cystitis can progress to pyelonephritis, necessitating hospitalization. Maternal GBS infection has also been associated with premature rupture of membranes, preterm labor, chorioamnionitis, bacteremia, puerperal endometritis, and postoperative wound infections after cesarean section.

- **Congenital.** Neonatal colonization with GBS results from contamination from the mother's genital tract in 75% of cases. One to 2% of colonized infants will develop early-onset GBS infection (infection occurring within the first 7 days of life), with a case fatality of 11% to 50%. Preterm and/or low-birth-weight infants are at higher risk than term neonates. Maternal risk factors that predispose a neonate to early-onset GBS infection include preterm delivery, prolonged rupture of membranes (>18 hr), intrapartum temperature of at least 38°C or 100.4°F, or a prior infant who had GBS infection.
- Late-onset GBS infection, which occurs 7 days or more after birth, affects 0.5 to 1.8 per 1,000 live births. It may result from maternal-neonatal transmission or nosocomial or community contacts. Mortality for late-onset disease is approximately 10%.
- Meningitis occurs in 85% of all affected neonates, but infants may also present with bacteremia without localizing symptoms. Other clinical syndromes include pneumonia, osteomyelitis, cellulitis, and sepsis. Neurologic sequelae develop in 15% to 30% of meningitis survivors.

Diagnosis

- Group B streptococcal colonization can be detected by culture or rapid DNA-based testing. Anorectovaginal culture remains the gold standard and can be performed in a single swab of the areas. Samples must be inoculated immediately into Todd-Hewitt broth or onto selective blood agar to inhibit the growth of competing organisms. The predominant limitation of culture is time. Results are not available for 24 to 48 hr, making management difficult if delivery is imminent. Rapid-diagnostic tests are available that detect specific polysaccharide antigens. They are easy to perform, generally less expensive than a culture, and produce results within a short period of time (usually 1 hr). The tests are highly sensitive in patients who are heavily colonized with GBS; however, their lower sensitivity and higher false-negative rate compared with those of cultures prevent their widespread clinical application. Rapid DNA-based testing is also available with excellent sensitivity.

Management

- Treatment of uncomplicated GBS lower urinary tract infection is with amoxicillin or penicillin. Hospitalization is required for cases of pyelonephritis, and patients should be treated with an appropriate regimen until afebrile and asymptomatic for 24 to 48 hr. She may then be discharged to complete a total of 10 days of antibiotics.
- The American College of Obstetricians and Gynecologists recommends universal screening for GBS at 35 to 37 weeks' gestation with a swab of the lower vagina and rectum. Women with a positive screen, a previous infant with GBS infection, urine colonization or infection with GBS during the current pregnancy, labor before 37 weeks with unknown GBS status, rupture of membranes >18 hr at term with unknown GBS status, or signs of chorioamnionitis should receive intrapartum antibiotics. Treatment is typically with penicillin 5-million-U IV loading dose followed by 2.5 million U IV every 4 hr. For patients with a penicillin allergy, genital culture results should be evaluated for sensitivity to clindamycin and erythromycin. If sensitivities are unknown, vancomycin should be administered.

SEQUELAE OF PERINATAL INFECTIONS

- Table 11-3 summarizes the **sequelae of the perinatal infections** discussed above.

TABLE 11-3 Maternal and Fetal Manifestations of Perinatal Infections

Infection	Maternal Disease	Fetal Sonographic Findings	Congenital Disease
Toxoplasmosis	Usually asymptomatic; may include mononucleosis-like syndrome	Nonspecific but may include intracranial calcification or ventricular dilatation	Usually asymptomatic at birth. Triad of congenital toxoplasmosis: chorioretinitis, hydrocephalus, and intracranial calcifications
Rubella	Maculopapular rash, generalized lymphadenopathy, low-grade fever, malaise.	Increased risk of spontaneous abortion, stillbirth, intrauterine growth restriction. No specific sonographic findings	Sensorineural deafness, cataracts, glaucoma, patent ductus arteriosus, peripheral pulmonary artery stenosis, mental retardation, growth restriction. Classic purpuric skin lesions at birth called "blueberry muffin" lesions
CMV	May be asymptomatic or may include fever, malaise, and lymphadenopathy. Rarely includes hepatitis	May present with microcephaly, hepatosplenomegaly, and intracranial calcification. Normal ultrasound does not exclude infection	Up to 90% are asymptomatic at birth. Symptomatic infection includes petechiae, hepatosplenomegaly, jaundice, chorioretinitis, and seizures
HSV	Usually localized vesicular lesions on cervix, vagina, or vulva. Disseminated disease is uncommon.	None	Most neonates appear normal at birth. Disease subsequently develops in one of three patterns: localized lesions on skin, eyes, mouth; localized CNS disease; disseminated multiorgan disease

(Continued)

TABLE 11-3 Maternal and Fetal Manifestations of Perinatal Infections *(Continued)*

Infection	Maternal Disease	Fetal Sonographic Findings	Congenital Disease
Varicella	Prodromal symptoms include fever, malaise, and myalgia followed by "chicken pox" vesicular rash. Risk of varicella pneumonia increased in pregnancy	May include hypoplastic limbs, malformed digits, clubbed feet, microcephaly, intrauterine growth restriction	Dermatomal scarring, cataracts, chorioretinitis, Horner syndrome, microphthalmos, nystagmus, low birth weight, cortical atrophy, mental retardation, and hypoplastic limbs
Parvovirus B19	Facial macular rash with "slapped cheek" appearance, arthritis, and rarely, aplastic anemia.	Fetal anemia, which may lead to nonimmune hydrops fetalis. May also cause fetal hydrocephaly, cleft lip and palate, cardiomyopathy, and ocular defects when infection present in first trimester.	No specific congenital syndrome
GBS	Usually asymptomatic but may cause urinary tract infection	None	Early-onset disease may present as generalized sepsis, pneumonia, or meningitis. Late-onset disease most often presents as bacteremia without a focus.

CMV, cytomegalovirus; HSV, herpes simplex virus; GBS, group B streptococcus.

SUGGESTED READINGS

Centers for Disease Control and Prevention (CDC). Perinatal group B streptococcal disease after universal screening recommendations—United States, 2003–2005. *MMWR Morb Mortal Wkly Rep* 2007;56(28):701–705.

Corey L, Wald A. Maternal and neonatal herpes simplex virus infections. *N Engl J Med* 2009;361(14):1376–1385.

Lin K, Vickery J. Screening for hepatitis B virus infection in pregnant women: evidence for the U.S. Preventive Services Task Force reaffirmation recommendation statement. *Ann Intern Med* 2009;150(12):874–876.

Malm G, Engman ML. Congenital cytomegalovirus infections. *Semin Fetal Neonatal Med* 2007;12(3):154–159 [Epub 2007 Mar 6].

Perinatal viral and parasitic infections. ACOG Practice Bulletin Number 20, September 2000 (Replaces educational bulletin number 177, February 1993). American College of Obstetricians and Gynecologists. *Int J Gynaecol Obstet* 2002;76(1):95–107.

Sharma D, Spearman P. The impact of cesarean delivery on transmission of infectious agents to the neonate. *Clin Perinatol* 2008;35(2):407–420.

Winn HN. Group B streptococcus infection in pregnancy. *Clin Perinatol* 2007;34(3):387–392.

Congenital Anomalies

Valerie A. Jones and Maria Palmquist

Congenital anomalies are among the most common causes of neonatal morbidity and mortality. They occur in 3% to 4% of live births and account for 25% of all pediatric hospital admissions. Birth defects may be isolated or multiple and may involve one or more organ systems. The causes of congenital anomalies are both genetic and nongenetic.

ETIOLOGY AND OVERVIEW

- **Genetic etiologies** include the following: chromosomal disorders such as Down syndrome; monogenic disorders such as cystic fibrosis, Fragile X syndrome, and hemophilia; and multifactorial disorders such as isolated congenital heart disease, cleft lip and palate, and clubbed foot, which result from interactions of several genes and environmental factors.
- **Nongenetic etiologies** include the following: teratogens such as ethanol, certain medications, and some illicit drugs; maternal medical conditions such as diabetes; and maternal infections such as CMV or rubella.
- Ninety percent of infants with congenital anomalies are born to women with no risk factors. Causes may be idiopathic, multifactorial, familial, or chromosomal; hence, obtaining a thorough family history and screening low-risk populations are important.
- Given the significant morbidity and mortality of congenital defects, all patients should be offered screening for fetal chromosomal abnormalities and an anatomy ultrasound at 18 to 22 weeks. High-risk patients should have a detailed anatomy scan regardless of serum testing (Table 12-1). Detailed ultrasonography by an experienced technician can detect up to 80% of fetal anomalies, allowing the full range of management options: expectant management, in utero therapy, further workup (e.g., karyotyping and viral studies), and pregnancy termination.
- Management should take into consideration the fetus, the mother, and the family. Treatment and prognosis should be discussed in detail with the entire family. A multidisciplinary approach may include counseling from many specialists, including maternal-fetal medicine specialists, genetic counselors, neonatologists, pediatric surgeons, urologists, and neurosurgeons. Social work and bereavement counseling can also be offered. Coordination of care must be timely, unbiased, and sensitive to the concerns of the patient and her family.

SCREENING AND EVALUATION

Methods of evaluation and **screening regimens** for aneuploidy include maternal serum screening (Table 12-2), ultrasound, and amniocentesis or chorionic villus sampling (CVS).

TABLE 12-1	Factors Associated with Increased Risk for Congenital Abnormalities

Maternal age ≥35 at the time of birth
Pregestational diabetes
Exposure to a known teratogen
History of having a child with birth defect
Personal or family history of a known genetic abnormality (e.g., balanced translocation, mutation, or aneuploidy)
Abnormal serum screening
Multiple gestation

- **First-trimester screening** for Down syndrome with biochemical and ultrasound evaluation allows earlier decisions, greater privacy, and safer management for those who select termination.
  - Pregnancy-associated plasma protein (PAPP-A) and human chorionic gonadotropin (β-hCG) are the **serum markers** most commonly used in first trimester screening for Down syndrome. Affected fetuses have lower PAPP-A (0.38 multiples of the mean [MoM]) and higher β-hCG (1.83 MoM).
  - **Nuchal translucency** (NT) on early ultrasound quantifies the amount of fluid at the dorsum of the fetal neck. It is best evaluated at 12 to 13 weeks' gestation. Increased NT correlates with an increased risk of Down syndrome and improves screening detection when combined with serum marker testing. NT is also useful for Down syndrome screening in multiple gestation when serum screening is not as accurate.

TABLE 12-2	Down Syndrome Screening and Detection Rates

Screening Test or Scheme	Detection Rate (%)
First trimester	
NT measurement	64–70
NT measurement, PAPP-A, free or total beta-hCG	82–87
Second trimester	
Triple screen	69
(MSAFP, hCG, unconjugated estriol)	
Quadruple screen	81
(MSAFP, hCG, unconjugated estriol, inhibin A)	
First plus second trimester	
Integrated (NT, PAPP-A, quad screen)	94–96
Serum integrated (PAPP-A, quad screen)	85–88
Stepwise sequential	95

NT, nuchal translucency; PAPP-A, pregnancy-associated plasma protein A; hCG, human chorionic gonadotropin; MSAFP, maternal serum alpha-fetoprotein. Data from Malone FD, Canick JA, Ball RH, et al. for the First- and Second-Trimester Evaluation of Risk (FASTER) Research Consortium. First-trimester or second trimester screening or both for Down syndrome. *N Engl J Med* 2005;353:2001–2011.

○ Increased NT >99th percentile or >3.5 mm, with normal chromosomes is an indication for fetal echocardiography and targeted second trimester ultrasound as these fetuses are at higher risk for congenital heart defects, abdominal wall defects, diaphragmatic hernias, skeletal dysplasias, and other genetic syndromes. First trimester testing should only be offered if CVS is available as follow-up or as a part of integrated/sequential screening.

- **Second-trimester serum screening** is often the screening test used; it is performed between 15 and 21 weeks' gestation. Generally, detection rates are standardized for a false-positive rate of 5%. The patient should be counseled about the meaning of a *screening test* and the risk of false-positive and false-negative results. If a patient has no interest in invasive testing, serum screening may not be indicated.
  - Elevated **maternal serum alpha-fetoprotein (MSAFP)** suggests neural tube or ventral wall defect, congenital nephrosis, or fetal skin lesions. It is also associated with increased fetal wastage, premature delivery, low birth weight, gestational hypertension, and other high-risk conditions. The pregnancy should be monitored closely. Low MSAFP, in conjunction with maternal age, detects about 55% of Down syndrome.
  - **The triple screen** combines unconjugated estriol (uE3), hCG, and AFP. It detects 69% of Down syndrome fetuses with decreased AFP, decreased estriol, and elevated hCG. Trisomy 18 fetuses typically have all three markers reduced. An extremely low estriol level (<0.3 MoM) prompts consideration for Smith-Lemli-Opitz syndrome.
  - **The quadruple screen** adds inhibin A to the triple screen and increases the Down syndrome detection rate to 81%. Levels of inhibin A are increased at 1.77 MoM in Down syndrome pregnancies.
  - **Integrated screening** uses both first and second trimester screening to report Down syndrome risk after all tests are completed. It has the highest detection rate and lowest false-positive rate. However, the delay between initial first trimester screening and final result in the second trimester may produce unacceptable confusion or anxiety for parents.
  - **Sequential screening** does inform the patient of her first trimester screening results. Those at high risk may opt for early diagnostic testing while those at low risk can continue with second trimester screening to obtain increased sensitivity.
- **Ultrasonography** can be used to diagnose many major anomalies, confirm the actual gestational age, define placental location and quality, measure amniotic fluid volume, and evaluate fetal growth.
  - Detailed anatomy scan is indicated with abnormal serum screening or high suspicion for congenital anomaly (e.g., diabetic mother).
  - Optimal timing for the anatomic survey is between 18 and 20 weeks. By that time, organogenesis is complete, bony ossification does not yet obscure sonography, and structures are large enough for accurate assessment but still small enough to visualize within a single ultrasound window. There is still time to work up any detected anomalies and proceed with genetic termination if desired.
  - The structures that are assessed in the anatomy screen include the following:
    ○ **Head.** The biparietal diameter and head circumference are measured, both in the same view at the level of the thalamus and cavum septum pellucidum. The intracranial contents, ventricular structures, cerebellar diameter, and cisterna magna should be evaluated.
    ○ **Spine.** Sagittal, transverse, and coronal views are obtained at all levels to screen for neural tube defects (NTDs).

- ° **Heart.** Four-chamber view and visualization of left and right outflow tracts are required. If an abnormality is suspected, fetal echocardiogram should be performed.
- ° **Abdomen.** The stomach and umbilical vein should be visualized in the same plane for the abdominal circumference measurement. Abdominal wall defects are ruled out by verifying normal cord insertion and the absence of bowel loops in the amniotic fluid. The kidneys, renal pelves, and bladder should be evaluated.
- ° **Limbs.** The four limbs should be imaged to their distal ends and the humerus and femur measured. The hands should be seen to open and close and the feet examined for normal positioning and appearance.
- **Amniocentesis** and **chorionic villous sampling (CVS)** can collect fetal cells for karyotyping and other genetic evaluation.
  - Amniocentesis collects amniotic fluid for AFP and acetylcholinesterase testing, chromosome analysis, and viral culture.
  - In certain circumstances, late gestation fetal blood sampling may be necessary to provide more rapid diagnosis.
  - Fetal skin biopsy may be necessary to evaluate mosaicism.
  - Amniocentesis is usually performed between 16 and 20 weeks, while CVS is performed at 10 to 12 weeks.
  - Miscarriage occurs after about 1 in 300 amniocenteses. The risk for CVS is slightly higher. Rarely, CVS at <9 weeks' gestation or with excessive tissue removal causes limb reduction defects.

COMMON CHROMOSOMAL ABNORMALITIES

Trisomy 21

- **Trisomy 21 (Down syndrome)** is the most common genetic disorder, with a frequency of 1:660 to 1:800 births. Trisomic disorders have an extra copy or extra portion of a chromosome. Aberrant distribution of chromosomes leading to Down syndrome increases with maternal age.
  - Different types of Down syndrome can occur:
    - ° Full or primary trisomy 21 (94%)
    - ° Trisomy 21 mosaicism (2% to 3%)
    - ° Chromosome 21 translocation (3% to 4%)
  - Ultrasound markers for Down syndrome include short femur, short humerus, echogenic intracardiac focus, echogenic bowel, pyelectasis, and increased NT. These adjust a patient's *a priori* age-related risk or *a priori* serum markers risk for Down syndrome.
  - Neonatal features consistent with Down syndrome include hypotonia, flat facial profile, excess dorsal nuchal skin, upslanting palpebral fissures, epicanthal folds, single palmar crease, and small ears.

Trisomy 13 and 18

- **Trisomy 13** is usually due to meiotic primary nondisjunction giving rise to a 47 +13, XX or XY genotype. Trisomy 13 is invariably fatal; approximately 50% of newborns die in the first month of life.
  - Anomalies include the following: holoprosencephaly, microphthalmia, cleft lip and palate, low-set ears, and rocker-bottom feet. Cardiac anomalies and severe mental retardation are common.
- **Trisomy 18** is most commonly due to meiotic primary nondisjunction giving rise to a 47 +18, XX or XY genotype. Life expectancy for these infants is usually very limited.

- The most common anomalies are cardiac and renal. Characteristic features include: microcephaly, low-set ears, micrognathia, overlapping fingers, and rocker-bottom feet. Mental retardation is severe.

Turner Syndrome

- **Turner syndrome** (also called Ullrich-Turner syndrome or gonadal dysgenesis) is usually 45, X genotype although it can also involve deletion of the p arm of one X chromosome. Some individuals are mosaic, with both 45, X and 46, XX cell lines.
  - Characteristics of the Turner syndrome phenotype include: low hairline, webbed neck, shield chest, wide-spaced hypoplastic nipples, and short stature. Functional anomalies include gonadal dysgenesis, congenital heart disease (particularly coarctation of the aorta), renal anomalies, and learning disabilities. Cystic hygroma is common on prenatal ultrasounds.

Triploidy

- **Triploidy** (also known as partial mole) has one entire extra haploid set (i.e., 69 chromosomes). Sonographic findings include the following: early and severe IUGR, ventriculomegaly, syndactyly, and abnormal cystic placenta (see Chapter 46).

SPECIFIC ANOMALIES

Specific congenital anomalies include the following:
- **NTDs** result from failure of the neuropores to close during the 3rd to 4th weeks' gestation. The main forms of NTD are anencephaly and spina bifida (Table 12-3).
  - **Spina bifida** can be closed, in which the unfused vertebral arches are covered, or open, in which the neural canal is exposed. Closed defects are not detectable by AFP screening. NTD risk factors include family history of NTD, poorly controlled diabetes, seizure medications, and poor nutritional status or low folate stores.

TABLE 12-3	Types of Neural Tube Defects	
	Anencephaly	**Spina Bifida**
Affected neuropore	Caudal	Rostral
Findings	Absent cranial vault, absent telencephalon and encephalon	Vertebral schisis, with or without overlying soft tissue; frontal cranial narrowing ("lemon sign"); convex cerebellum ("banana sign"); hydrocephalus
Associations	Polyhydramnios	Arnold-Chiari type II malformation
Outcomes	Fatal	Dependent on level; worse with high defects or hydrocephalus; consider in utero treatment.

- **Diagnosis** is by serum screening and prenatal ultrasound. Amniotic fluid AFP and acetylcholinesterase can help to diagnose NTDs as well.
- **Prevention** with preconception folate supplementation (0.4 mg/day) significantly lowers the incidence of NTDs. For women with a previously affected pregnancy, a higher dose of 4.0 mg of daily folate is recommended.
- **Hydrocephalus** results in ventriculomegaly. Causes include obstruction, inability to reabsorb cerebrospinal fluid (CSF), congenital infection such as CMV, X-linked hydrocephalus, and aneuploidy.
  - **Diagnosis** is by recognition of enlarged ventricles on ultrasound. A useful rule of thumb is that the transverse diameter of the atrium of the nondependent lateral ventricle should not measure >1 cm at any gestational age.
  - **Management** options include karyotyping, viral studies, counseling/consultation with neurosurgery, and termination. Hydrocephalic infants should be delivered at a tertiary care center where neurosurgical intervention is available. In cases where the head becomes macrosomic, cesarean delivery should be considered.
  - **Prognosis** for hydrocephalus depends on the etiology, severity, and interventions. Except in extreme circumstances, prognosis cannot be determined by the size of the ventricle or the degree of cortical compression alone. Asymmetric ventriculomegaly increases the suspicion for infection, hemorrhage, and ischemia. Amniotic fluid cultures and workup for neonatal alloimmune thrombocytopenia (NAIT) should be offered.
- **Congenital diaphragmatic hernia** occurs when the embryologic sections of the diaphragm fail to fuse properly, allowing abdominal contents to herniate into the thoracic cavity. The perinatal morbidity and mortality are due to the mass effect of the herniated abdominal contents. The mass prevents expansion of the developing lungs, causing pulmonary hypoplasia.
  - **Diagnosis** is by ultrasound. Herniated abdominal contents (stomach, bowel, and/or liver) are seen in the thorax and the mediastinum may be shifted. Hernias are more often unilateral, posterolateral, and left sided. Associated anomalies are common.
  - **Management** includes karyotyping, and termination should be discussed. Pediatric surgery and genetics consultations can clarify the prognosis and outline the associated syndromes and treatment plan. Delivery should be performed at a tertiary center that has extracorporeal membrane oxygenation (ECMO) available.
  - **Prognosis** has improved significantly in recent years related to improved techniques for ventilation and with the use of ECMO. Overall survival now exceeds 80%.
- **Congenital cystic adenomatoid malformation (CCAM)** is a congenital lung malformation that is diagnosed more frequently after birth than by prenatal ultrasound. Affected individuals have cystic lung lesions (usually on the right side and involving one lobe or segment).
  - If detected, prenatal diagnosis is by ultrasound. These lesions are divided into three types based on the size and number of cysts. Cysts >5 mm are called *macrocystic* and have a better prognosis.
- **Pulmonary sequestration** and CCAM are both in the differential for fetal lung malformations. Sequestered lung is separated from the normal pulmonary blood supply and bronchial tree. Finding the systemic blood supply with color Doppler is key.
  - Sequestered lung is usually left sided, and intralobar or extralobar. Five percent of extralobar lesions are intra-abdominal. Mediastinal shift and hydrops may be present. Associated anomalies are common.

- **Management** of CCAM/pulmonary sequestration includes pediatric surgery consultation, plan for delivery at a tertiary center, and close fetal surveillance. Hydrops is associated with poor prognosis, and delivery should be considered if pulmonary maturity is likely.
- **Congenital heart abnormalities** are among the most common birth defects (Table 12-4). Maternal diabetes, teratogen exposure, and genetic causes are linked to heart anomalies. About 25% of fetuses with a detected fetal heart anomaly will have an associated chromosomal abnormality. The likelihood of a cardiac defect exceeds 50% for Down syndrome and is 90% for trisomies 13 and 18.
- **Diagnosis** is by ultrasound. Any irregularity of the standard heart views should be referred for fetal echocardiogram. Any infant at high risk (e.g., diabetic mother) should be referred as well.
  - The finding of an echogenic intracardiac focus is not an indication for a fetal echocardiogram but should initiate a search for other markers of Down syndrome.
  - The functional consequences of cardiac anomalies are usually not evident until conversion from fetal to neonatal circulation after birth. Many common defects, therefore, such as ventriculoseptal and atrioseptal defects and coarctation, are frequently missed even by experienced sonographers.

TABLE 12-4	Most Common Congenital Cardiac Defects	
Name	**Findings**	**Percentage of Cardiac Defects[a]**
Hypoplastic left heart syndrome	Small left ventricle, aortic atresia, hypoplastic mitral valve	2%–4%
Endocardial cushion defect/ atrioventricular septal defect	Missing "crux" of the heart in four-chamber view	2%–7%
Ventricular septal defect (VSD)	Abnormal communication between left and right ventricles, causing shunt	20%–40%
Persistent truncus arteriosus	Single overriding arterial trunk	1%–2%
Complete transposition of great arteries	Aorta arises from right ventricle, and pulmonary artery from left.	2.5%–5%
Double outlet right ventricle	Both great arteries arise from right ventricle.	1%–2%
Tetrology of fallot	VSD, overriding aorta, pulmonary artery stenosis, right ventricular hypertrophy	3%–7%

[a]Does not add to 100%; minor cardiac defects are not listed. Adapted from Woodward PJ, Kennedy A, Roya S, et al., eds. *Diagnostic Imaging: Obstetrics*, 1st Ed. Salt Lake City, UT: Amirsys/Elsevier, 2005.

- **Management** depends on the specific lesion. Hydrops in utero is a poor prognostic sign. Offer karyotyping, genetic counseling, and appropriate surgical consultation. Most cardiac defects can be corrected surgically but may require multiple procedures. Discuss termination. Delivery in a tertiary center is crucial because therapy to maintain fetal circulation may need to be started immediately.
- **Intestinal obstruction** includes **atresia**, which occurs usually in the esophagus and duodenum, and **obstruction**, which occurs elsewhere in the small bowel and large intestine. Surgical management is required.
- **Abdominal wall defects** include **gastroschisis** and **omphalocele** (Table 12-5). Both are detected by prenatal ultrasound. Gastroschisis has no covering membrane, with the abdominal contents directly exposed to the amniotic fluid. Omphalocele appears as a mass of abdominal contents covered by a thin membrane. Both disorders are associated with increased MSAFP levels and require postnatal surgical correction. IUGR and oligohydramnios are associated with gastroschisis.
- **Renal agenesis** may be unilateral or bilateral. Bilateral renal agenesis is diagnosed when kidneys and bladder are not seen on ultrasound and is lethal. Severe oligohydramnios or anhydramnios is present, causing severe pulmonary hypoplasia. Fetal kidneys do not contribute the majority of amniotic fluid until after 18 weeks, so early sonograms may show normal amniotic fluid volume. Unilateral agenesis has a normal prognosis. The single kidney may hypertrophy.
- **Multicystic dysplastic kidney disease (MCKD)** is a form of dysgenesis characterized by increased renal size and with numerous large noncommunicating cysts alternating with areas of increased echogenicity on ultrasound. Bilateral multicystic dysplasia is associated with severe oligohydramnios and is fatal. Infants may survive with unilateral disease as long as the unaffected kidney has normal function. Pediatric urology consultation is recommended.

TABLE 12-5	Omphalocele and Gastroschisis	
	Omphalocele	**Gastroschisis**
Relationship to cord insertion	Umbilical cord enters into the hernia sac.	Normal umbilical cord insertion
Physical findings	Defect covered by amnioperitoneal membrane; size variable; may contain bowel loops only or entire abdominal contents	Defect has no covering membrane; small bowel usually herniates; other organs may herniate also.
Additional anomalies	Common; occur in up to 45%	No significant association
Chromosomal anomalies	Occur in up to 30%; association with Beckwith-Wiedemann	No significant association
Long-term prognosis	Dependent on presence of other anomalies	Excellent after surgical repair

TABLE 12-6	Skeletal Dysplasias	
Type of Dysplasia	**Description**	**Outcome**
Thanatophoric	Cloverleaf skull, thoracic deformity, extreme shortening of limbs	Usually lethal
Camptomelic	Short, bowed limbs, cervical spine anomalies, airway instability	Usually lethal
Diastrophic dwarfism	Severe limb shortening, scoliosis, hitchhiker thumbs	Problems with feeding, walking
Osteogenesis imperfecta	Bone fragility and fractures due to mutation in COL1A1 or COL1A2 gene, affecting type I collagen	Severity depends on type

- **Infantile polycystic kidney disease** or autosomal recessive polycystic kidney disease is characterized by large echogenic kidneys, absent bladder, and oligohydramnios. Again, ultrasound after 16 to 18 weeks is recommended if the fetus is at risk. Autosomal dominant polycystic kidney disease is occasionally diagnosed in the fetus.
- **Ureteropelvic junction obstruction** is the most common congenital urinary tract abnormality and results in mild dilation of the renal pelvis (pyelectasis) or hydronephrosis when calyceal dilation is present. Pyelectasis is a weak marker for Down syndrome, and it should prompt investigation for other markers and serum screening.
- Outlet obstructions include **posterior urethral valve (PUV)** syndrome (most common), **urethral atresia**, and **cloacal abnormalities**. Ultrasound of affected fetuses shows bilateral hydronephrosis, hydroureter, and megacystis. With PUV, the bladder may have a characteristic keyhole appearance. Urinary diversion may be helpful, but there is often severe irreversible renal impairment. Pediatric urology consultation should be offered.
- **Skeletal dysplasias** come in several types (Table 12-6). Ultrasonographic limb length measurements must be compared with gestational nomograms. Abnormalities of the calvarium, face, spine, and thorax are common. Fractures and hypomineralization are seen with osteogenesis imperfecta.

SUGGESTED READINGS

Barboza, JM, Dajani NK. Prenatal diagnosis of congenital cardiac anomalies: a practical approach using two basic views. *Radiographics* 2002;22:1125–1138.

Cuckle HS, Malone FD, Wright D, et al. Contingent screening for Down syndrome—results from the FaSTER trial. *Prenat Diagn* 2008;28(2):89–94.

Cunningham FG, Leveno K, Bloom SL, et al. Preconceptional counseling (Chapter 7) and Tetralogy (Chapter 14). *Williams Obstetrics*, 23rd Ed. New York, NY: McGraw Hill, 2001.

Laurence KM, James N, Miller MH, et al. Double blind randomized controlled trial of folate treatment before conception to prevent recurrence of neural tube defects. *JAMA* 1988;260:3141–3145.

Leschot NJ, Verjaal M, Treffers PE. Risks of midtrimester amniocentesis: assessment in 3000 pregnancies. *Br J Obstet Gynaecol* 1985;92:804–807.

Rhoads GG, Jackson LG, Schlesselman SE, et al. The safety and efficacy of chorionic villus sampling for early prenatal diagnosis of cytogenetic abnormalities. *N Engl J Med* 1989;320:609–617.

Taipale P, Hiilesmaa V, Salonen R, et al. Increased nuchal translucency as a marker for fetal chromosomal defects. *N Engl J Med* 1997;337:1654–1658.

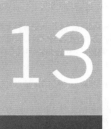

13 Endocrine Disorders of Pregnancy

Alexandre Buckley de Meritens, K. Joseph Hurt, and Lorraine A. Milio

DIABETES MELLITUS

Diabetes mellitus (DM) is the most common medical complication of pregnancy in the United States. As the incidence of type 2 DM increases, cases of **gestational diabetes mellitus (GDM)** have grown also.

- Diabetes in pregnancy can be classified as Type 1, Type 2 (Table 13-1), or GDM.
- Four to five percent of pregnancies are complicated by diabetes.
- In 90% of diabetic pregnancies, the cause is GDM.
- One half to one percent of pregnancies are complicated by pregestational DM (diagnosed prior to pregnancy).
- **Carbohydrate metabolism** changes during pregnancy to provide adequate nutrition for both the mother and the fetus.
  - In the fasting state, maternal serum glucose is lower in pregnancy than in the nonpregnant state (55 to 65 mg/dL), whereas free fatty acid, triglyceride, and plasma ketone concentrations are increased. A state of relative maternal starvation exists in pregnancy, during which glucose is spared for fetal consumption and alternate fuels are used by the mother.
  - GDM is similar to type 2 DM, in which increased pancreatic secretion cannot overcome decreased insulin sensitivity of maternal target tissues. Increased metabolism in pregnancy also increases insulin clearance. These changes are due to the effects of estrogen, progesterone, cortisol, prolactin, and human placental lactogen.

Diagnosis and Screening

- **Diagnosis** of type 1 and 2 DM before pregnancy is by standard criteria: two abnormal fasting glucose levels ≥126 mg/dL or a random glucose level of ≥200 mg/dL (Table 13-2). Classic symptoms are polydipsia, polyuria, and polyphagia. Clinical signs include weight loss, hyperglycemia, persistent glucosuria, and ketoacidosis.
- **Universal screening** for GDM is standard in the United States, whether by patient history, clinical risk factors, or laboratory testing. Testing is typically performed at 24 to 28 weeks, but if strong risk factors such as obesity, family history, or a personal history of GDM are present, screening can be performed at the first visit. Not all patients require screening via blood glucose testing (Table 13-3).
- For screening, a 50 g **oral glucose challenge** is consumed, followed by serum glucose measurement at 1 hr. No fasting or dietary preparation is required.
  - Serum glucose ≥140 mg/dL identifies 80% of GDM.
  - Serum glucose ≥130 mg/dL identifies over 90% of GDM.
  - Serum glucose ≥200 mg/dL diagnoses GDM without additional testing.
    - If the screening test is positive, then a diagnostic 3-hr **glucose tolerance test** (GTT) should be performed with 100 g oral glucose after at least 8 hr of fasting

TABLE 13-1	Comparison of Type 1 and Type 2 Diabetes Mellitus

Type 1	Type 2
Formerly known as juvenile-onset or insulin-dependent DM.	Formerly known as adult-onset or non–insulin-dependent DM.
Pathophysiology is absolute insulin deficiency.	Pathophysiology is tissue resistance to insulin.
Patients are at risk for severe hypoglycemia and DKA.	Patients may develop hyperosmolar coma. DKA is rare.
Increased risk for chronic microvascular disease at an early age.	Lower incidence of microvascular disease during reproductive age range.

(Table 13-4). With abnormal fasting or any other two abnormal values, the diagnosis of DM is confirmed. In patients at high risk for GDM with a normal GTT, a follow-up GTT can be performed at 32 to 34 weeks to identify later-onset diabetes.

○ The final classification of GDM depends on the management required to control blood glucose levels. White's classification Class A refers to GDM. Type A1 achieves euglycemia by dietary changes alone. Type A2 requires additional (i.e., medical) therapy.

Fetal Complications of DM

• **Fetal and neonatal complications** of DM in pregnancy are increased with both gestational and pregestational DM, but the incidence is much higher in pregestational DM and with poor glycemic control. Fetal glucose levels are similar to maternal blood glucose levels, and both fetal hyperglycemia and hypoglycemia have important effects.

TABLE 13-2	Diabetic Screening in the Nonpregnant Patient

	Fasting Glucose Level (mg/dL)	Glucose Level 2 hr After 75 g Load (mg/dL)	Management
Normal	<110	<140	Annual screening
Carbohydrate intolerant	110–125	140–199	Diet and exercise modification; annual screening
Diabetic	≥126	≥200	Treatment as indicated.

The fasting plasma glucose test is preferred. An initial abnormal value must be confirmed on a different day, by repeat fasting glucose level, plasma glucose level after glucose load, or random plasma glucose level if symptoms are present. Adapted from Position Statement: Standards In Medical Care in Diabetes. *Diabetes Care* 2009;32(S1):S13–S61.

TABLE 13-3	Gestational Diabetes Risk Assessment

Low Risk
Age younger than 25 years old
Not a member of an ethnic group with increased risk for type 2 DM (Hispanic, African, Native American, South or East Asian, or Pacific Islander ancestry)
BMI <25; normal weight at birth
No history of abnormal glucose tolerance
No history of poor obstetric outcomes
No first degree relatives with DM

High Risk
Severe obesity
Strong family history of type 2 diabetes
Previous history of GDM, impaired glucose metabolism, or glucosuria

Patients who meet all low-risk criteria and have no high-risk factors may forgo oral glucose challenge testing if appropriate. Adapted from Metzger BE, Buchanan TA, Coustan DR, et al. Summary and Recommendations of the Fifth International Workshop-Conference on Gestational Diabetes Mellitus. *Diabetes Care* 2007;30(2):S251.

- **Spontaneous abortion** ranges between 6% and 29% with pregestational DM and correlates with poor glucose control and an elevated hemoglobin A1C (HbA1C) around the time of conception. Type 1 and type 2 DM carry the same risk of pregnancy loss, but the main causes of fetal loss for type 1 DM are congenital anomalies and complications of prematurity while for type 2 DM they are stillbirth, birth asphyxia, and chorioamnionitis. There is no increased incidence of miscarriage in women with excellent preconception glucose control (i.e., HbA1C <6%).
- **Congenital malformations** are the most common cause of perinatal mortality in pregestational diabetic pregnancies and correlate with elevated HbA1C. Congenital anomalies account for 30% to 50% of perinatal mortality from diabetes. Though maternal hyperglycemia is probably the principal factor causing congenital

TABLE 13-4	Criteria for Diagnosis of Gestational Diabetes from Oral Glucose Tolerance Testing

Time Since 100-g Glucose Load (hr)	Modified O'Sullivan Scale	Carpenter and Coustan Scale
Fasting	≥105	≥ 95
1	≥190	≥180
2	≥165	≥155
3	≥145	≥140

Values are plasma glucose levels in mg/dL. Adapted from O'Sullivan JB, Mahan CM. Criteria for the oral glucose tolerance test in pregnancy. *Diabetes* 1964;13:278–285; and Carpenter MW, Coustan DR. Criteria for screening tests for gestational diabetes. *Am J Obstet Gynecol* 1982;144:768–773.

malformations, hypoglycemia and hyperketonemia are also suspected. Six to ten percent of infants of diabetic mothers have a major congenital anomaly (see Chapter 12).

- The most common congenital malformations in diabetic pregnancies are cardiovascular. Defects include **transposition of the great vessels, ventricular and atrial septal defects, hypoplastic left ventricle, situs inversus, aortic anomalies,** and **complex cardiac anomalies**. The rate of cardiac malformations is fivefold higher in diabetics.
- **Sacral agenesis/caudal regression** is highly suggestive of diabetic fetopathy. It is a rare malformation but diagnosed up to 400 times more frequently in diabetic mothers and nearly pathognomonic.
- There is a 10-fold increase in the incidence of CNS malformations in infants of diabetic mothers, including **anencephaly, holoprosencephaly, open spina bifida, microcephaly, encephalocele,** and **meningomyelocele.**
- GI system malformations, including **tracheoesophageal fistula, bowel atresia, and imperforate anus,** are also increased in diabetic gestations.
- Genitourinary system anomalies including **absent kidneys** (leading to Potter's syndrome)**, polycystic kidneys,** and **double ureter** are more common in pregnancies complicated by diabetes.
- **Polyhydramnios** occurs in 3% to 32% of diabetic pregnancies, 30 times the rate for nondiabetic gestations. Diabetes alone is the leading cause of polyhydramnios. Furthermore, diabetes-associated congenital anomalies of the central nervous and gastrointestinal systems can also lead to polyhydramnios. Mechanisms of polyhydramnios include increased fetal glycemic load resulting in polyuria, decreased fetal swallowing, and fetal GI obstructions. Higher perinatal morbidity and mortality rates are associated with polyhydramnios, attributed in part to the higher incidence of congenital anomalies and preterm delivery.
- **Macrosomia** is defined as an estimated fetal weight more than 4,000 to 4,500 g or the 90th percentile, depending on the authority. It occurs in 25% to 42% of diabetic versus 8% to 14% of euglycemic pregnancies, and maternal diabetes is the most significant single risk factor. Diabetic macrosomia is characterized specifically by a large fetal abdominal circumference and decreased head to abdominal circumference ratio because fetal hyperinsulinemia leads to abnormal fat distribution. Macrosomic fetuses have an increased mortality rate and higher risk for hypertrophic cardiomyopathy, vascular thrombosis, neonatal hypoglycemia, and birth trauma. They are more likely to be delivered by cesarean section and are at increased risk for fractured clavicles, facial paralysis, Erb's palsy, Klumpke's palsy, phrenic nerve injury, and intracranial hemorrhage.
- **Intrauterine growth restriction (IUGR)** may complicate pregnancy for diabetic women with microvascular disease. Placentae of diabetic pregnancies can be compromised and may exhibit pathohistologic changes, including fibrinoid necrosis, abnormal villus maturation, and proliferative endarteritis of fetal stem arteries. There is wide variation, but these observations occur even with good glucose control, suggesting that irreversible placental abnormalities occur very early in gestation.
- Poorly controlled diabetes increases risk for **fetal demise in utero** during the third trimester. Cord thrombosis and accelerated placental aging may be the cause.
- **Shoulder dystocia** is increased threefold in diabetic gestations and is of even greater concern when macrosomia is also present. If shoulder dystocia occurs, infants of diabetic mothers are more likely to have brachial plexus injury than infants of women without DM. In macrosomic infants of diabetic mothers, vaginal delivery carries a 2% to 5% risk of brachial plexus injury.

- Twenty-five to forty percent of infants of diabetic mothers develop **neonatal hypoglycemia**. The serum glucose nadirs at about 24 hr of life. Poor maternal glycemic control during pregnancy and elevated maternal glucose levels at delivery increase the risk. The pathogenesis is in utero stimulation of the fetal pancreas by maternal hyperglycemia leading to fetal islet cell hypertrophy and beta cell hyperplasia. When the maternal glucose source is eliminated, the continued overproduction of insulin leads to newborn hypoglycemia with cyanosis, convulsions, tremor, apathy, diaphoresis, and a weak or high-pitched cry. Severe or prolonged hypoglycemia is associated with neurologic sequelae and death. Treatment should be instituted when the infant's blood glucose drops below 40 mg/dL.
- **Neonatal hypocalcemia and hypomagnesemia** are common in infants of diabetic mothers and correlate with the degree of glycemic control.
- Thirty-three percent of infants born to diabetic mothers have **polycythemia** (hematocrit higher than 65%). Chronic intrauterine hypoxia increases erythropoietin production, resulting in vigorous hematopoiesis. Alternatively, elevated glucose may lead to early increased red blood cell destruction, followed by increased erythrocyte production.
- **Neonatal hyperbilirubinemia** and **neonatal jaundice** occur more commonly in infants of diabetic mothers than in infants of nondiabetic patients of comparable gestational age. Poor glycemic control delays fetal liver maturation.
- **Neonatal respiratory distress syndrome (RDS)** may occur more frequently in diabetic pregnancies as a result of delayed fetal lung maturation. Fetal hyperinsulinemia may suppress production and secretion of surfactant required for normal lung function at birth.
- The risk of fetal **cardiac septal hypertrophy** and **hypertrophic cardiomyopathy** is increased in diabetic pregnancies (up to 10% have hypertrophic changes). There is a strong correlation between cardiomyopathy and poor maternal glycemic control. As an isolated finding, cardiac septal hypertrophy is a benign neonatal condition. However, it increases the risk of morbidity and mortality in neonates with sepsis or congenital structural heart disease.

Maternal Complications of DM

- **Maternal complications** are increased with diabetes.
- **Diabetic ketoacidosis (DKA)** is a potentially life-threatening metabolic emergency for both mother and fetus. In pregnant patients, DKA can occur at lower blood glucose levels (i.e., <200 mg/dL) and more rapidly than in nonpregnant diabetics. Although maternal death is rare with proper treatment, fetal mortality rates from 10% to 30% are reported. About half of DKA cases are due to medical illness, usually infection; another 20% result from dietary or insulin noncompliance. In 30% of cases, no precipitating cause is identified. Antenatal steroids for fetal lung maturity and beta adrenergic tocolytics can precipitate or exacerbate DKA in pregestational diabetics.
  - The **pathophysiology** of DKA is relative or absolute insulin deficiency. The resulting hyperglycemia and glucosuria lead to osmotic diuresis, promoting urinary potassium, sodium, and fluid loss. Insulin deficiency also increases lipolysis and hepatic oxidation of fatty acids, producing ketones and eventually causing metabolic acidosis.
  - **Diagnosis** is by objective documentation of maternal hyperglycemia, acidemia, and serum ketosis. Signs and symptoms include abdominal pain, nausea and vomiting, polydipsia, polyuria, hypotension, rapid deep respiration, and impaired

TABLE 13-5   Initial Management of Diabetic Ketoacidosis

IV Fluid Hydration
- 1 L of normal saline (NS) administered in the first hour.
- 500 to 1,000 mL/hr for the next 2 to 4 hr followed by 250 mL/hr.
- Change fluids to D5 NS when blood sugar decreases to 250 mg/dL.

Insulin Infusion (Rapid-Acting Insulin)
- Loading dose of 0.2 to 0.4 U/kg.
- IV infusion of 2 to 10 U/hr (double the rate if glucose level does not decrease by 25% in first 2 hr).
- When blood sugar declines to 150 mg/dL, decrease infusion to 1 to 2 U/hr. Continue until urine ketones are cleared.
- When the patient is able to tolerate food, start their usual insulin regimen.

Potassium
- If initially normal or reduced, an infusion rate up to 15 to 20 mEq KCl/hr may be required; if elevated, wait until potassium levels decrease into the normal range, then add KCl to intravenous solution in a concentration of 20 to 30 mEq/L.

Bicarbonate
- Add one ampule bicarbonate (44 mEq) to 1 L of 0.45 normal saline, if pH is <7.1

From American College of Obstetricians and Gynecologists. Pregestational diabetes mellitus. ACOG Practice Bulletin No. 60. *Obstet Gynecol* 2005 (reaffirmed 2007);105:675–685.

mental status (ranging from mild drowsiness to profound lethargy). Acidosis can be defined as a plasma bicarbonate level <15 mEq/L or arterial pH <7.3. In the presence of hyperglycemia, ketosis is presumed and can be verified by serum testing. Because pregnancy is a state of physiologic respiratory alkalosis, profound DKA may occur at a higher pH.

- **Initial management** consists of vigorous IV hydration followed by IV insulin drip and frequent blood sugar checks to titrate dosing. Potassium and bicarbonate supplementation may be necessary. Check electrolytes every 4 hr and blood sugar hourly until DKA is resolved (Table 13-5).
- **Hypoglycemia** that is serious enough to require hospitalization may occur in up to 45% of mothers with type 1 DM. Patients with poorer glycemic control can have blunted autonomic responses and milder symptoms so they may present with more severe or prolonged episodes. Vomiting in early pregnancy also predisposes diabetics to low blood sugars. Severe hypoglycemia may be teratogenic in early gestation, but the effects on the developing fetus are not fully understood.
  - **Symptoms** include nausea, headache, diaphoresis, tremors, blurred or double vision, weakness, hunger, confusion, paresthesia, and stupor. **Diagnosis** is by careful history and review of symptoms and confirmed with a blood glucose measurement <60 mg/dL.
  - **Treatment** starts with 4 ounces of juice or a glucose tablet. Assess serum glucose after 15 to 20 minutes, and repeat feeding until blood sugar is >70 mg/dL. Then feed complex carbohydrates or the scheduled meal or snack. If the patient is unable to tolerate food and drink, an ampule of dextrose 10% can be given IV push followed by IV fluids containing 5% dextrose.

- The **Somogyi effect** is rebound hyperglycemia after hypoglycemia, secondary to counterregulatory hormone release. It usually occurs in the middle of the night but can happen after any hypoglycemic episode, manifesting as wide variations in blood glucose levels over a short period of time (e.g., between 2:00 and 6:00 A.M.). Diagnosis is by checking additional blood sugars (i.e., 3:00 A.M.) to identify unrecognized hypoglycemia. Treatment involves adding or modifying a nighttime snack or decreasing the overnight insulin dose in order to better match insulin needs with dietary intake.

- The **dawn phenomenon** is also an early morning increase in plasma glucose, possibly due to normal nighttime production of growth hormone (GH), catecholamines, and cortisol. It is also diagnosed by checking early morning (i.e., 3:00 A.M.) blood sugar level. If the patient is euglycemic overnight, she may require increased bedtime insulin dosing to cover the effect of normal morning hormones. Differentiating between the Somogyi effect and the dawn phenomenon helps tailor the insulin regimen and achieve optimal glucose control.

- **Rapid progression of microvascular and atherosclerotic disease** can occur in pregnant diabetics. Any evidence of **ischemic heart disease, heart failure, peripheral vascular disease, or cerebral ischemia** should be evaluated carefully. A pregestational diabetic over age 30 should have a baseline ECG. Maternal echocardiogram and cardiology consultation may be warranted. Preconception counseling is useful for these patients. For the most severe disease, it may be appropriate to offer termination in early pregnancy.

- **Nephropathy** complicates 5% to 10% of diabetic pregnancies. In advanced renal disease with creatinine >1.5mg/dL, pregnancy can worsen the prognosis and accelerate the progression to end-stage disease. Diabetic nephropathy increases the risk for maternal hypertensive complications, preeclampsia, preterm birth, fetal growth restriction, and perinatal death. A new diagnosis of diabetic nephropathy is made in pregnancy if persistent proteinuria >300 mg/day in the absence of urinary tract infection is detected prior to 20 weeks' gestation. Creatinine clearance <50 mL/min is associated with increased incidence of severe preeclampsia and fetal loss. Treatment with angiotensin-converting enzyme inhibitors (ACE-Is) *before* pregnancy has a prolonged maternal renal protective effect and improves outcomes. ACE-I are teratogenic, however, and should be discontinued at conception. Intensive maternal and fetal surveillance throughout gestation is required with renal disease but can result in fetal survival rates >90% (see Chapter 16).

- **Diabetic retinopathy** is the most common vascular manifestation of diabetes and a principal cause of adult-onset blindness in the United States. Proliferative retinopathy is believed to be a consequence of persistent hyperglycemia and directly related to the duration of disease. Pregnancy does not change the long-term prognosis, but an ophthalmologic evaluation is recommended in preconception counseling or at the time of the pregnancy diagnosis.

- The incidence of **chronic hypertension** is increased in patients with pregestational DM, especially those with nephropathy (see Chapter 14).

- **Preeclampsia** is two to four times more common in pregestational diabetics. The risk is increased with longer duration of disease, nephropathy or retinopathy, and chronic hypertension. Up to a third of women with long-standing diabetes (>20 years) will develop preeclampsia. The threshold for preeclampsia workup in these women should be very low (see Chapter 14).

- **Preterm labor and delivery** may be three to four times higher in patients with DM. Poor glycemic control, noncompliance with diabetic management, and nonreassuring fetal status result in many iatrogenic preterm deliveries.

- The choice of **tocolytics** for diabetic patients is limited. Sympathomimetics (e.g., terbutaline) act on hepatic β-adrenergic receptors, causing increased glycogenolysis leading to hyperglycemia. Indomethacin may be used only if maternal renal function is adequate. Magnesium sulfate or nifedipine may be acceptable alternatives.
- **Corticosteroids** should be administered as indicated for suspected preterm delivery before 34 weeks. Additional insulin or oral agents may be required for 5 to 7 days after administration.
- Diabetics also have increased maternal risk for adverse obstetric outcomes including **3rd and 4th degree perineal lacerations** and **wound infection**.

Management of Diabetes in Pregnancy

- Ideally, diabetic women desiring pregnancy should seek **preconception consultation** and maintain euglycemia before conception. The initial prenatal visit should include a detailed history and physical examination, an ophthalmologic examination, an electrocardiogram (for women older than age 30, smokers, or hypertensives), and 24-hr urine collection for protein and creatinine clearance. Echocardiography and cardiology consultation should be obtained for known or suspected cardiovascular disease. HbA1C is helpful in evaluating recent (8 to 12 weeks) glycemic control and assessing risk for fetal malformations. HgbA1C $\geq 9.5\%$ carries $>20\%$ risk of major fetal malformation. Strict glucose control (i.e., HgbA1C $\leq 6\%$) during organogenesis dramatically reduces embryopathy to nondiabetic levels. Early nutrition consult and counseling may be beneficial.
- **Blood glucose goals** in pregnancy are given in Table 13-6.
  - Patients should start or continue intensive glucose monitoring early in pregnancy using a home glucometer. They should record fasting and 1-hr (or 2-hr) postprandial blood sugar levels for each meal.
  - Postprandial glycemic control correlates best with risk for neonatal hypoglycemia, macrosomia, fetal death, and neonatal complications. Home monitoring records are reviewed every 1 to 2 weeks and therapy is optimized.

GDM Management

- **Management for GDM** initially consists of diet and exercise. If good glucose control is not achieved, oral hypoglycemic agents or insulin are then prescribed.
  - Women with newly diagnosed GDM are started on a diabetic diet of 1,800 to 2,400 kcal/day.

TABLE 13-6	Goals for Glycemic Control in Pregnancy
Goal Blood Sugar Values	
Fasting	60–90 mg/dL
Premeal	<100 mg/dL
1 hr postprandial	<140 mg/dL
2 hr postprandial	<120 mg/dL
Bedtime	<120 mg/dL
2:00–6:00 A.M.	60–90 mg/dL

From Metzger BE, et al. Summary and Recommendations of the Fifth International Workshop-Conference on Gestational Diabetes Mellitus. *Diabetes Care.* 2007;30(2):S251.

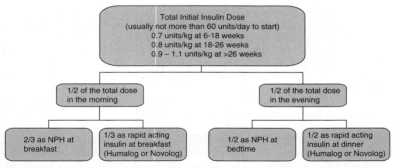

Figure 13-1. Calculation and dose distribution for initial insulin management in pregnancy. (Adapted from Gabbe SG. Management of diabetes mellitus complicating pregnancy. *Obstet Gynecol* 2003;102(4):857.)

- Moderate exercise can improve glycemic control in GDM. Patients are encouraged to maintain a consistent level of activity throughout pregnancy provided there are no complications (e.g., preterm labor).
- **Oral hypoglycemic agents** are acceptable GDM management when dietary efforts fail. Glyburide, for example, works by increasing tissue insulin sensitivity and has minimal placental transfer. The starting dose is usually 2.5 mg PO at bedtime or 2.5 mg PO twice daily, titrated to a maximum dose of 10 mg PO twice a day. Four to twenty percent of patients will need additional therapy with insulin, particularly if fasting blood sugars are high. Glyburide side effects include hypoglycemia, nausea, heartburn, and allergic skin reactions. Metformin is also safe and effective; about one half of patients on metformin will require insulin as well.
- **Insulin therapy** can improve glycemic control for GDM. Different types of insulin are combined to maintain even control through day and night (Fig. 13-1).
- Neutral Protamine Hagedorn (NPH) insulin is an intermediate-acting insulin given in the morning and at night, with peak activity at 5 to 12 hr.
- Rapid-acting insulin (e.g., Humalog or Novolog) is administered with meals because its onset is 5 to 15 minutes and peak activity occurs at 2 to 4 hr.
- **Fetal monitoring** is not required for GDM-A1 diabetics. They are not at increased risk for fetal demise before 40 weeks' gestation. Women with GDM-A2 (i.e., on medication) require antenatal testing similar to that recommended for pregestational DM (twice weekly NSTs or BPP from 32 to 34 weeks until delivery). Delivery by 40 weeks' gestation is recommended.

Pregestational DM Management
- **Management of Pregestational DM**
  - The recommended diet for pregnant diabetic women is 1,800 to 2,400 kcal daily, made up of 20% protein, 60% carbohydrates, and 20% fat. Carbohydrate counting, with 180 to 210 g of daily carbohydrates, is becoming more common and replacing caloric guidelines. Nutrition consult should be part of preconception or early pregnancy planning.
  - Patients are usually continued on their normal prepregnancy **insulin regimen** while initial blood sugar monitoring is performed. Monitoring and goals are the same for GDM and pregestational DM (Table 13-6).

○ The American Diabetes Association recommends insulin for pregnant women with DM and for women with DM considering pregnancy. Patients taking oral hypoglycemic agents (except glyburide) or a 70/30 (NPH/regular) mixed insulin regimen are switched to NPH and a rapid-acting insulin analog. Patients with type 1 DM usually require 50% to 100% increased insulin doses in the second half of pregnancy. Type 2 DM insulin dosing is frequently more than doubled in pregnancy.

○ Insulin pumps provide a continuous subcutaneous infusion. Pump dosing must be managed carefully, because the risk of severe hypoglycemia causing seizures and death is increased in pregnancy. Patients must be carefully selected.

• **Fetal assessment** and monitoring for pregestational diabetes varies according to gestational age.

  • **First trimester:** Obtain an early dating sonogram to confirm gestational age and document fetal viability.

  • **Second trimester:** Offer maternal serum AFP screening for neural tube defects (either alone or as part of aneuploidy screening if desired by the patient; see Chapter 12). Ultrasonography at 18 to 20 weeks is recommended for complete anatomy evaluation. Fetal echocardiography is also recommended at 19 to 22 weeks for pregestational diabetics.

  • **Third trimester:** Twice weekly antenatal testing should be initiated for all diabetic pregnancies starting at 32 to 34 weeks' gestation. Patients with comorbidities or very poor glycemic control may start assessment as early as 28 weeks. Serial ultrasonographic exams for fetal growth should be considered at 28 to 30 weeks and again at 34 to 36 weeks. Earlier assessment and umbilical artery Doppler velocimetry may be required to assess for IUGR in patients with microvascular disease (see Chapter 6).

Labor and Delivery in Diabetic Pregnancies

• **Timing of delivery** in an insulin-requiring diabetic patient should consider maternal glycemic control, maternal comorbidities, estimated fetal weight, antenatal testing, and amniotic fluid volume. In many patients with well-controlled DM, labor may be induced safely at 39 to 40 weeks.

  • Amniocentesis for fetal lung maturity is recommended before elective delivery for gestations of <39 weeks. Amniocentesis may need to be repeated until 39 weeks or fetal lung maturity is achieved, or until delivery for other obstetric indications (e.g., nonreassuring fetal testing).

  • Tests for fetal lung maturity include the following:

    ○ **Fluorescence polarization**. Maturity suggested by >55 mg surfactant/g albumin

    ○ **Lecithin/sphingomyelin ratio**. Maturity suggested by *L/S* ratio of ≥2.0

    ○ **Phosphatidylglycerol**. Maturity suggested by positive test.

• **Glucose control** during labor and delivery should maintain blood sugar ≤110 mg/dL. Continuous intravenous insulin and glucose infusions can titrate optimal glycemic control. With elective induction, the patient receives her usual insulin the prior evening but holds her morning dose. On admission, IV fluids are started along with serial glucose monitoring (every 1 to 2 hr). The infusion fluids are adjusted to maintain blood glucose levels between 70 and 110 mg/dL (Table 13-7). Short-acting insulin boluses may be required in addition to the IV drip.

TABLE 13-7	Low-dose Continuous Insulin Infusion for Labor and Delivery	
Blood Glucose (mg/dL)	Insulin Dosage (U/hr)[a]	Fluids (125 mL/hr)
<60	0	One ampule D50 or D5NS, by severity
60–100	0[a]	D5 NS
101–140	1.0[b]	D5 NS
141–180	1.5[b,c]	D5 NS
181–220	2.0[b,c]	D5 NS
>220	2.5[b,c]	Normal saline

[a]Type 1 diabetic patients need baseline insulin when blood glucose is >60 mg/dL; 0.5 units insulin/hr is reasonable to start. [b]Increase as needed. [c]Boluses of insulin may be required in addition to an increase in the insulin drip. D5NS, 5% dextrose in normal saline. Adapted from Rosenberg V, Eglinton GS, Rauch ER, et al. Intrapartum glycemic control in women with insulin requiring diabetes: a randomized clinical trial of rotating fluids versus insulin drip. *Am J Obstet Gynecol* 2006;195(5):1095–1099.

- **Route of delivery** is determined by usual obstetric indications. If fetal macrosomia >4,500 g is suspected, cesarean section is indicated, otherwise induction of labor is warranted.

Postpartum Care for Diabetics

- **Postpartum management** of diabetic mothers depends on the severity and type of DM.
- For GDM, no immediate postpartum testing is required. Most true gestational DM resolves rapidly after delivery, though these women are at increased risk for type 2 DM (20% to 50% within 10 years). Glucose tolerance testing is recommended for primary preventive care at 6 to 12 weeks postpartum (Table 13-8). GDM will recur in 30% to 50% of subsequent pregnancies.
- For type 1 DM, blood sugar can be monitored with nonpregnant regimen (i.e., before meals and at bedtime). The insulin dose is typically one half the dose at the end of pregnancy. Blood sugar testing every 4 to 6 hr for 24 hr after cesarean section,

TABLE 13-8	Postpartum Glucose Tolerance Test		
	No DM	Impaired Glucose Tolerance	Overt DM
8 hr Fasting	<100	100–125	≥126
2 hr after 75 g glucose load	<140	140–199	≥200

Values are plasma glucose levels in mg/dL. Adapted from Metzger BE, et al. Summary and Recommendations of the Fifth International Workshop-Conference on Gestational Diabetes Mellitus. *Diabetes Care* 2007;30(2):S251; and American Diabetes Association Standards of Medical Care in Diabetes—2010. *Diabetes Care* 2010;33:S11–S61.

with sliding scale insulin dosing, may be helpful until the patient can resume her normal routine. Keeping blood sugar <150 mg/dL can improve wound healing.
• For type 2 DM, insulin can be discontinued postpartum and oral hypoglycemic agent doses significantly decreased. Patients usually resume their prepregnant regimen.

THYROID DISORDERS

Thyroid disorders are common in women of reproductive age, occurring in 3% to 4% of pregnancies. Only about one in ten of those exhibit clinically important disease, however.

Thyroid Hormones in Pregnancy

• **Thyroid hormone levels** are altered in pregnancy (Table 13-9).
• **Total T3 and T4** increase due to hCG stimulation of thyroid-stimulating hormone (TSH) receptors. In the first trimester, total serum T4 can increase two- to three-fold and TSH may decrease, but no real hyperthyroidism is present since estrogen stimulates the liver to increase thyroxine-binding globulin (TBG), maintaining a constant proportion of active free T3 (fT3) and free T4 (fT4). Therefore, serum fT4 may offer better specificity for thyroid testing during pregnancy. The free T4 index (FTI) can be used as an indirect estimation of free T4, but direct fT4 measurement is preferred.

TABLE 13-9	Thyroid Function Test Results in Pregnancy Compared with Hyperthyroid and Hypothyroid Conditions		
Test	**Normal Pregnancy**	**Hyperthyroidism**	**Hypothyroidism**
Thyroid-stimulating hormone (TSH)	No change	Decreased	Increased
Thyroxine-binding globulin (TBG)	Increased	No change	No change
Total T_4 (T_4)	Increased	Increased	Decreased
Free T_4 (fT_4) or Free T4 Index (FTI)	No change	Increased	Decreased
Total triiodothyronine (T_3)	Increased	Increased or no change	Decreased or no change
Free T_3 (fT_3)	No change	Increased or no change	Decreased or no change
T_3 resin uptake (T_3RU)	Decreased	Increased	Decreased
Iodine uptake	Increased	Increased or no change	Decreased or no change

Adapted from American College of Obstetricians and Gynecologists. Thyroid disease in pregnancy. ACOG Practice Bulletin No. 37. *Obstet Gynecol* 2002 (reaffirmed 2008);100:387–396; and Rashid M, Rashid MH. Obstetric management of thyroid disease. *Obstet Gynecol Surv* 2007;62(10):680–688.

TABLE 13-10	Indications for Thyroid Function Testing in Pregnancy

Patient on thyroid therapy
Large goiter or thyroid nodularity
History of hyperthyroidism or hypothyroidism
History of neck irradiation
Previous infant born with thyroid dysfunction
Type 1 diabetes mellitus
Family history of autoimmune thyroid disease
Fetal demise in utero

Adapted from Mestman JH. Thyroid diseases in pregnancy other than Graves' disease and postpartum thyroid dysfunction. *Endocrinologist* 1999;9:294–307.

- The **serum TSH** level is more useful for diagnosing primary hypothyroidism than hyperthyroidism in pregnancy. TSH is not protein bound and does not cross the placenta. Normal TSH with low free T4 may suggest secondary hypothyroidism from a central hypothalamic-pituitary defect.
- The **thyroid gland** itself is moderately enlarged in normal pregnancy, though nodularity or clear thyromegaly should provoke thorough evaluation.
- There are few strong indications for **thyroid testing** during pregnancy (Table 13-10). Universal screening is not necessary.
  - Figure 13-2 outlines a thyroid testing algorithm.
  - Testing for anti-TSH receptor antibodies is indicated in certain circumstances (Table 13-11). IgG antibodies cross the placenta and can affect the fetal thyroid function. TSH-stimulating immunoglobulin (TSI) will stimulate while TSH receptor–blocking antibodies (TRAb) will inhibit fetal thyroid function. The presence of these antibodies in high titers can produce fetal or neonatal hyperthyroidism or hypothyroidism.

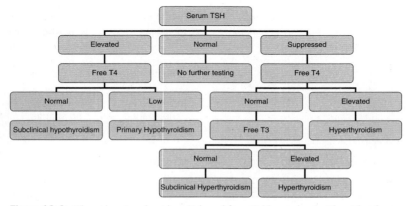

Figure 13-2. Thyroid testing algorithm. (Adapted from Gabbe, et al., eds. Thyroid and parathyroid diseases in pregnancy. In *Obstetrics: Normal and Problem Pregnancies.* Philadelphia, PA: Churchill Livingstone, 2007.)

TABLE 13-11	Indications for TSH Receptor Antibody Testing in Pregnancy

Graves' disease (TSI)
  Fetal or neonatal hyperthyroidism in previous pregnancy
  Euthyroid, postablation, in the presence of
    Fetal tachycardia
    IUGR
    Incidental fetal goiter on ultrasound
Incidental fetal goiter on ultrasound (TRAb)
Infant born with congenital hypothyroidism (TRAb)

TSI, TSH receptor–stimulating Immunoglobulin; TRAb, TSH Receptor–blocking Antibodies.
Adapted from Mestman JH. Hyperthyroidism in pregnancy. *Best Pract Res Clin Endocrinol Metab* 2004;18(2):267–288.

Hyperthyroid Conditions

- **Specific hyperthyroid conditions** include Graves' disease, hyperemesis gravidarum, gestational trophoblastic disease, struma ovarii, toxic adenoma, toxic multinodular goiter, subacute thyroiditis, TSH-producing pituitary tumor, metastatic follicular cell carcinoma, and painless lymphocytic thyroiditis. Thyrotoxicosis occurs in up to 1 in 500 pregnancies and increases risk for complications such as preeclampsia, thyroid storm, congestive heart failure, IUGR, preterm delivery, and stillbith.
  - **Clinical signs** of thyrotoxicosis include tachycardia, exophthalmos, thyromegaly, onycholysis, heat intolerance, pretibial myxedema, menstrual irregularities, and weight loss. Table 13-11 lists diagnostic test results for normal and hyperthyroid pregnancy.
- **Graves' disease** is the primary cause of thyrotoxicosis in pregnancy, accounting for 90% to 95% of cases. It is an autoimmune disease in which thyroid-stimulating antibodies (TSAs) or thyroid-blocking antibodies (TRAb) bind to the thyroid TSH receptors and activate or antagonize thyroid growth and function, respectively. The antibodies can also cross the placenta and affect the fetus. Up to 5% of affected fetuses can develop neonatal Graves' disease, which is unrelated to maternal thyroid function. Infants of women who have been treated previously with radioactive iodine or surgery may be at higher risk for neonatal complications since the mothers are not maintained on suppressive medications.
- **Hyperemesis gravidarum** with high hCG levels in early pregnancy can produce biochemical hyperthyroidism with low TSH and elevated fT4 that typically resolves by the mid second trimester. Hyperemesis is rarely associated with clinically important hyperthyroidism, and routine thyroid testing is not recommended in the absence of other findings.

Hyperthyroid Management

- **Medical management** is with propylthiouracil (PTU) or methimazole. Both cross the placenta and can potentially cause fetal hypothyroidism and goiter. Maintaining high normal range thyroid hormone levels with a minimum drug dosage is the goal.
  - **PTU** blocks iodide organification in the thyroid and the peripheral conversion of T4 to T3. It is traditionally preferred to methimazole, though placental transfer of

the two drugs is nearly equivalent. Both drugs have <0.5% risk of agranulocytosis and <1% risk of thrombocytopenia, hepatitis, and vaculitis. Breast-feeding is allowed for mothers taking PTU as only a small fraction passes into milk.

o Initial dose of PTU is 300 to 400 mg daily (divided into an 8 hr dosing schedule). fT4 should be checked regularly (every 2 to 4 weeks) and the PTU dose adjusted to a maximum of 1,200 mg daily to maintain fT4 levels in the normal range.

- **Methimazole** can also be used in pregnancy. The dose is 15 to 100 mg daily (divided into 8 hr schedule). The association of methimazole with fetal aplasia cutis has largely been refuted.
- **Beta-blockers** are used for symptom management in thyrotoxicosis until thyroid hormone levels are normalized with suppressive therapy. Propranolol hydrochloride is the most widely used. Adverse side effects include decreased ventricular function resulting in pulmonary edema. The dose of propranol is 20 to 80 mg orally every 4 to 6 hr to maintain heart rate below 100 bpm.
- **Iodine 131** thyroid ablation is contraindicated in pregnancy.
- **Surgical management** is reserved for severe cases that are unresponsive to medical therapy. Subtotal thyroidectomy may be performed at any time during pregnancy if required.
- **Thyroid storm** is a medical emergency occurring in <1% of pregnant patients with hyperthyroidism. Heart failure due to the long-term effects of increased T_4 is more frequent, and can be exacerbated during pregnancy by preeclampsia, anemia, or infection. Clinical signs include fever higher than 103°F, severe tachycardia, widened pulse pressure, and changes in mentation. Thyroid blood testing is sent, but treatment should be initiated immediately.
- Treatment by a standard series of medications is initiated immediately for thyroid storm. Bloodwork for free T3 and T4 and TSH is sent to confirm the diagnosis, but testing should not delay therapy. Oxygen, cooling blankets, antipyretics, and IV hydration are initiated. Fetal monitoring is performed when appropriate.
  o PTU 600 to 800 mg PO once then 150 to 200 mg PO every 4 to 6 hr blocks hormone synthesis and conversion.
  o Saturated potassium iodide solution two to five drops every 8 hr blocks thyroid hormone release.
  o Dexamethasone 2 mg IV or IM every 6 hr for 24 hr decreases hormone release and peripheral conversion.
  o Propranolol is given as above for symptoms.
  o Phenobarbital 30 to 60 mg every 6 to 8 hr can relieve extreme restlessness.

Hypothyroid Conditions

- **Hypothyroidism** in pregnancy is uncommon, because untreated hypothyroidism is associated with infertility. Common causes include Hashimoto's thyroiditis, subacute thyroiditis, prior radioablative treatment, and iodine deficiency.
- Type 1 diabetes is associated with 5% incidence of hypothyroidism during pregnancy and up to 25% incidence of postpartum thyroid dysfunction. Complications of hypothyroidism in pregnancy include preeclampsia, abruptio placentae, anemia, and postpartum hemorrhage. Fetal complications include IUGR, congenital cretinism (growth failure and neuropsychological deficits), and stillbirth. Infants of optimally treated hypothyroid mothers usually have no evidence of thyroid dysfunction.
- The most common etiology of hypothyroidism in the United States is Hashimoto's chronic autoimmune thyroiditis, resulting from thyroid antimicrosomal and

antithyroglobulin antibodies. Worldwide the most common cause of hypothyroidism is iodine deficiency.

- **Presentation** may be asymptomatic or include disproportionate weight gain, lethargy, weakness, constipation, carpal tunnel syndrome, cold sensitivity, hair loss, dry skin, and eventually myxedma. Table 13-11 lists test results for hypothyroid pregnancy.
- **Treatment** is initiated if thyroid function testing is consistent with hypothyroidism, regardless of symptoms. Thyroxine replacement is based on the patient's clinical history and laboratory test values and adjusted until TSH remains normal and stable.
  - The starting dose for levothyroxine is 50 to 100 µg daily. It may be several weeks before the full effect is obtained. TSH can be checked every 4 to 6 weeks initially. The dose may need to be increased in pregnancy. Stable patients can be tested every trimester.

Nodular Thyroid

- **Nodular thyroid disease** should be evaluated if detected. Thyroid cancer occurs in 1 in 1,000 pregnancies, and up to 40% of nodules will be malignant. Ultrasonography, fine-needle aspiration, or tissue biopsy can be performed in pregnancy. Surgical excision is the definitive treatment and should not be postponed because of pregnancy, while radiation treatment is deferred until after delivery.

PARATHYROID DISORDERS

Parathyroid disorders and calcium dysregulation are uncommon in pregnancy. Calcium requirements do increase during pregnancy, however, so 1,000 to 1,300 mg calcium and 200 IU vitamin D supplementation are recommended. Fetal calcium uptake, increased plasma volume, renal loss from increased glomerular filtration rate (GFR), and hypoalbuminemia lead to lower total maternal serum calcium levels, but ionized calcium remains fairly constant.

- **Serum calcium levels** are regulated by several hormones:
  - **Parathyroid hormone (PTH)** increases calcium mobilization from bone, calcium recovery in the kidney, and calcium absorption in the intestine (indirectly via activation of **vitamin D**). PTH increases throughout pregnancy until term, possibly to counteract the inhibitory effects of estrogen on bone.
  - **Parathyroid hormone related peptide (PTHrP)** is produced by the placenta and fetal parathyroid to activate active placental calcium transport and, like PTH, mobilize maternal calcium stores.
  - **Calcitonin** is produced in the parafollicular cells of the thyroid and acts to decrease serum calcium levels.

Hyperparathyroidism

- **Hyperparathyroidism** produces hypercalcemia. Clinical manifestations include hyperemesis, weakness, constipation, polyuria, polydipsia, nephrolithiasis, mental status changes, arrhythmias, and occasionally pancreatitis. Symptoms often improve during pregnancy, but hypercalcemic crisis is possible after delivery. Obstetric and fetal complications include preeclampsia, stillbirth, premature delivery, neonatal tetany, and neonatal death.
- The **differential diagnosis** of hypercalcemia includes thyrotoxicosis, hypervitaminosis A and D, familial hypocalciuric hypercalcemia, granulomatous disease, and malignancy.

- **Laboratory findings** include elevated free serum calcium and decreased phosphorus levels. Disproportionately high PTH relative to serum calcium may also be found. ECG abnormalities, including arrhythmias, may be present. Ultrasonography is recommended for localization. If radiation exposure is necessary to identify local disease, it should be kept to a minimum.
- Surgical **treatment** (e.g., excision) of a parathyroid adenoma is indicated in the second trimester. Conservative treatment with oral phosphates can be used for mild cases (1 to 1.5 g daily) or in preparation for surgery. Hypercalcemic crisis is corrected with IV hydration, furosemide, electrolyte correction, and calcitonin. Data are limited on the use of bisphosphonates in pregnancy.

Hypoparathyroidism

- **Hypoparathyroidism** is rare and usually occurs iatrogenically after neck surgery. It is the most common cause of hypocalcemia. Patients exhibit cramps, paresthesias, bone pain, hyperacute deep tendon reflexes, tetany, prolonged QT interval, arrythmias, and laryngospasm. Trousseau's sign (carpopedal spasm after BP cuff inflation above systolic pressure for several minutes) or Chvostek's sign (upper lip twitching after tapping of the facial nerve) may be present. Fetal skeletal demineralization, subperiosteal resorption, osteitis fibrosa cystica, growth restriction, and neonatal hyperparathyroidism can develop.
- The **differential diagnosis** of hypocalcemia includes prior parathyroidectomy or thyroid surgery, prior radioactive iodine or radiation treatment, vitamin D deficiency, hypomagnesemia or hypermagnesemia, autoimmune disorders (e.g., Addison's disease, chronic lymphocytic thyroiditis), eating disorders, renal failure, DiGeorge syndrome, and pseudohypoparathyroidism (i.e., PTH resistance).
- **Laboratory evaluation** shows low serum calcium, low PTH, and elevated serum phosphate levels. 1,25-dihydroxy vitamin D levels are decreased, and ECG changes include prolongation of the QT interval.
- **Treatment** is with vitamin D (50,000 to 150,000 IU/day) and calcium (1,000 to 1,500 mg/day) supplementation, and low phosphate diet. Doses may need to be increased during pregnancy and reduced postpartum. Maternal repletion with calcium gluconate during labor and delivery may prevent neonatal tetany. Acute symptomatic hypocalcemia is treated with IV calcium gluconate infusion.

PITUITARY DISORDERS

Pituitary disorders are not common in pregnancy; many pituitary hormone irregularities can cause anovulatory infertility.

- **Pituitary hormone** release is under hypothalamic control. The anterior pituitary (adenohypophysis) releases adrenocorticotropin (ACTH), TSH, prolactin, GH, follicle stimulating hormone (FSH), luteinizing hormone (LH), and endorphins. The posterior pituitary (neurohypophysis) contains the nerve terminals projecting from the hypothalamus that release oxytocin and antidiuretic hormone (ADH; also called arginine vasopressin [AVP]).
- During normal pregnancy, the pituitary gland may more than double in size. Lactotroph growth in response to estrogen leads to increased serum prolactin levels, while ACTH release increases in response to placental corticotropin releasing hormone (CRH). LH and FSH secretion are decreased in pregnancy. Pituitary GH and TSH decrease as placental GH and hCG rise, respectively. ADH secretion may

be increased in pregnancy, but placental vasopressinase increases degradation, leading to a lowered plasma osmolality setpoint (i.e., 5 to 8 mOsm/kg decrease).
- The **differential diagnosis** of pituitary dysfunction includes tumor, infarction, autoimmune/inflammatory disease, infection, infiltrative processes, head trauma, sporadic or familial genetic mutations, prior surgery or radiotherapy, hypothalamic lesions, and empty sella syndrome.

Prolactinoma

- **Prolactinoma** is the most common pituitary tumor of reproductive age women. Elevated prolactin can cause amenorrhea, anovulation, infertility, and galactorrhea. With increasing size and mass effect, prolactinoma can cause headaches, visual changes, and diabetes insipidus (DI).
- **Microadenomas** are classified as ≤10 mm and rarely (<2%) progress to **macroadenomas** (>10 mm) during pregnancy. Up to one third of previously untreated macroadenomas, however, may become symptomatic during pregnancy.
- **Initial diagnosis** is by history, physical exam, and CT or MRI of the head. Serum prolactin may not be useful during pregnancy, due to normal pregnancy–induced elevations. Patients with microadenomas can be monitored for symptoms at each prenatal visit, with visual field testing and MRI if visual symptoms develop. Patients with macroadenomas should have baseline visual field testing early in pregnancy and referral for endocrinology and ophthalmology consults can be considered.
- **Treatment** of symptomatic prolactinoma is with dopamine agonists, which mimic the prolactin-inhibiting factor activity of hypothalamic dopamine. Bromocriptine (drug of choice; 2.5 to 5 mg daily) or cabergoline (0.5 to 3 mg weekly) can shrink the adenoma and decrease serum prolactin levels. Patients taking these medications should stop them during pregnancy unless they have a symptomatic or large tumor. Trans-sphenoidal surgical resection of the macroadenoma is indicated for macroadenomas or high prolactin levels that are not controlled with medication. Radiotherapy can also be used to treat persistent disease. Radiologic evaluation and serum prolactin testing should be followed after treatment.

Acromegaly

- **Acromegaly** is caused by a GH-secreting pituitary adenoma. Symptoms include coarsened facial features, prominent chin, large feet, spade-like hands, irregular menses, headaches, visual changes, hyperhidrosis, arthralgias, and carpal tunnel syndrome. Usually these women are infertile, with hyperprolactinemia and anovulation. In the rare patient with acromegaly who becomes pregnant, there are no deleterious or teratogenic effects for the fetus. Carbohydrate intolerance, hypertension, and cardiac abnormalities may complicate pregnancy, however. Laboratory testing shows elevated serum insulin-like growth factor 1 (IGF-1) levels and nonsuppressed GH during glucose tolerance testing (100 g glucose load normally suppresses GH release). Diagnosis during pregnancy is complicated by placental GH secretion. Head CT or MRI can localize the tumor. Treatment is with surgical exicison, radioablation, or medical treatment with bromocriptine, somatostatin analogues (e.g., octreotide or lanreotide), or the newer GH receptor antagonist pegvisomant.

Diabetes Insipidus

- **Diabetes insipidus (DI)** results from abnormal water homeostasis. Central DI results from decreased ADH/vasopressin release due to pituitary tumor, metastases, granuloma, infection, trauma, Sheehan's syndrome, or lymphocytic hypophysitis. Nephrogenic DI is rare due to renal resistance to ADH hormone, and primarily found in males. Psychogenic DI is due to massive free water consumption. Subclinical DI may be identified during pregnancy when ADH/vasopressin metabolism is increased. Viral hepatitis, preeclampsia, HELLP syndrome, and acute fatty liver of pregnancy (AFLP) can also exacerbate or promote DI. Polyuria (>3 L/day) and polydipsia are the clinical hallmarks of DI.

- **Diagnosis** is by the water deprivation test, showing low urine osmolality and high plasma osmolality with fluid restriction. dDAVP injection corrects central DI and can be used with plasma osmolality testing to diagnose central DI. Head CT or MRI is used to identify pituitary lesions.
- **Treatment** is with synthetic ADH/vasopressin (i.e., DDAVP; L-deamino-1-D-arginine vasopressin) at 10 to 25 µg/day intranasally. Higher doses may be required during pregnancy.

Other Pituitary Disorders

- **Sheehan's syndrome** results from pituitary necrosis following massive obstetric blood loss or lymphocytic hypophysitis. Clinical findings include tachycardia, postural hypotension, hypoglycemia, agalactorhea, anorexia, nausea, lethargy, weakness, weight loss, decreased pigmentation, periorbital edema, normocytic anemia, and DI. Approximately 4% of patients with obstetric hemorrhage may have mild pituitary dysfunction, but frank Sheehan's syndrome can present up to 20 years later. Diagnosis requires laboratory testing for stimulated pituitary hormone secretion (i.e., after injecting hypothalamic releasing hormones). Random blood hormone levels are not useful.
- **Lymphocytic hypophysitis** is caused by autoimmune lymphocyte and plasma cell infiltration and destruction of the pituitary gland. Symptoms vary from mild pituitary dysfunction to headache and visual changes from mass effect. Laboratory data show modest prolactinemia and hypothyroidism. Head CT or MRI may reveal a pituitary mass. Up to 25% of patients have other autoimmune diseases (e.g., thyroiditis, adrenalitis). Hormone replacement is administered if needed and surgery is reserved for severe symptoms. The inflammatory process is typically self-limited.

ADRENAL DISORDERS

Adrenal disorders are not pregnancy induced but do persist during pregnancy. The adrenal gland is profoundly affected by pregnancy. CRH is secreted by the placenta, stimulating ACTH release from the pituitary that increases cortisol production in maternal adrenal glands. Cortisol clearance is also decreased, leading to more than twofold increase in total and free serum cortisol levels by the third trimester. Aldosterone production is stimulated by elevated renin/angiotensin II levels in pregnancy; renin activity peaks by the second trimester. Androgen levels are increased five- to eightfold, while dehydroepiandrosterone sulfate (DHEA-S) is decreased in pregnancy.

Cushing syndrome

- **Cushing syndrome** results from long-term exposure to glucocorticoids, either from exogenous steroid use (as in treatment of lupus erythematosus, sarcoidosis, or severe asthma) or from increased endogenous hormone production (from excessive pituitary ACTH production, adrenal hyperplasia, or adrenal neoplasia).

Corticotropin-independent causes of Cushing syndrome are more common in pregnancy (up to 50%).

- **Signs and symptoms** include moon facies, buffalo hump, truncal obesity, striae, fatigue, weakness, hirsutism, easy bruising, nephrolithiasis, mental status changes, and hypertension.
- **Diagnosis** is by laboratory testing, showing increased plasma cortisol levels or increased 24-hr urine free cortisol. It can be difficult to identify mild cases due to the normal pregnancy–induced changes in cortisol levels. The dexamethasone suppression test can be used to differentiate a pituitary cause (i.e., Cushing's disease) from adrenal or exogenous sources of the increased cortisol. Head or abdominal CT or MRI is recommended to localize tumors.
- **Treatment** of Cushing syndrome entails medical management of blood pressure and subsequent surgical excision of pituitary or adrenal adenoma. Medical management of the pregnant patient until delivery is usually preferred, though maternal morbidity may be higher with adrenal adenomas, prompting earlier surgical treatment. Metyrapone has been used to block cortisol secretion with adrenal hyperplasia, though it crosses the placenta and may affect fetal adrenal function. Ketoconazole and mifepristone are contraindicated in pregnancy.
- **Prognosis** is improved with early detection and close management, though these patients are at increased risk for maternal complications including hypertension, DM, preeclampsia, cardiac problems, and death. There is increased risk for perinatal complications including IUGR, preterm delivery, stillbirth, and neonatal death.

Hyperaldosteronism

- **Hyperaldosteronism** can result from adrenal aldosteronoma or carcinoma (about 75%) and bilateral adrenal hyperplasia (about 25%). Symptoms include hypertension, hypokalemia, and weakness. Laboratory testing shows increased serum or urine aldosterone and low plasma renin levels. MRI can be used to identify and localize an adrenal tumor. Definitive treatment is tumor resection, which can be performed laparscopically in the second trimester. Medical management is potassium supplementation and treatment of hypertension. Spironolactone is not used in pregnancy; calcium channel blockers or beta blockers are preferred for blood pressure control.

Pheochromocytoma

- **Pheochromocytoma** is a rare catecholamine-secreting tumor of chromaffin cells. Ninety percent arise in the adrenal medulla and 10% in sympathetic ganglia. Ten percent of tumors are bilateral. Ten percent are malignant. It is associated with medulary thyroid cancer and hyperparathyroidism in Multiple Endocrine Neoplasia (MEN) type 2 syndromes.
- When diagnosed during pregnancy, pheochromocytoma increases maternal mortality to approximately 10%. Fetal mortality increases to nearly 50%, even though the catecholamines do not cross the placenta or directly affect the fetus. IUGR is common, but there is no increased neonatal mortality after delivery. When the diagnosis is not made before delivery, postpartum maternal mortality increases to about 50%.
- **Signs and symptoms** of pheochromocytoma include paroxysmal or sustained hypertension, headaches, anxiety, chest pain, visual changes, palpitations, diaphoresis, nausea and vomiting, pallor or flushing, abdominal pain, and seizures. The **differential diagnosis** should include preeclampsia and other hypertensive disease.

- **Diagnosis** is by laboratory testing showing elevated catecholamines, metanephrines, and vanillylmandelic acid in a 24-hr urine specimen. Methyldopa should be discontinued before this test as it will give a false-positive result. Abdominal CT or MRI can be used for localizing the tumor in pregnancy; MIBI scan can identify extra-adrenal sites.
- Definitive **treatment** is adrenalectomy. Surgical intervention is recommended at gestational age <24 weeks or following delivery by cesarean section. Medical therapy includes alpha adrenergic blockers, phenoxybenzamine (10 to 30 mg PO two to four times daily), or phentolamine (for acute treatment IV). Beta adrenergic blockers are useful to treat tachycardia (e.g., propanolol 20 to 80 mg PO four times daily). Cesarean delivery is recommended to avoid the catecholamine surges of labor and delivery.

Adrenal Insufficiency

- **Adrenal insufficiency** may be primary (Addison's disease) or secondary to pituitary failure or adrenal suppression from exogenous steroid treatments. Primary adrenal failure presents only after destruction of more than 90% of the gland and results in depletion of all steroid hormones. Secondary adrenal failure results in significant losses of glucocorticoids. When treated, adrenal insufficiency is not associated with adverse fetal or neonatal outcomes.
- **Signs and symptoms** include hypotension, weakness, fatigue, anorexia, nausea and vomiting, weight loss, and hyperpigmentation of the skin. Pregnancy can exacerbate adrenal insufficiency resulting from Addison's disease.
- The **differential diagnosis** includes idiopathic autoimmune adrenalitis, tuberculosis, histoplasmosis, hemorrhagic necrosis, and infiltrative neoplasms. Other autoimmune disease may also be present, such as Hashimoto thyroiditis, premature ovarian failure, type 1 DM, and Graves' disease
- **Diagnosis** of primary adrenal insufficiency is by laboratory testing showing low plasma cortisol levels and an abnormal ACTH stimulation test in which injection of 0.25 mg ACTH fails to increase plasma cortisol within 1 hr.
- **Treatment** includes maintenance replacement of corticosteroids with hydrocortisone (20 mg PO each morning and 10 mg PO each evening) or prednisone (5 mg each morning and 2.5 mg each evening). Fludrocortisone (0.05 to 0.1 mg PO daily) is given for mineralocorticoid replacement. Patients should continue their usual regimen during pregnancy, with careful follow-up. Stress-dose steroids should be administered during labor and delivery (e.g., hydrocortisone 100 mg IV every 8 hr till delivery) at the time of major surgical procedures and for severe infection or other significant stress.

SUGGESTED READINGS

Gandhi RA. HbA1C during pregnancy: Its relationship to meal related glycemia and neonatal birth weight in patients with diabetes. *Eur J Obstet Gynecol Reprod Biol* 2008;138(1): 45–48.

Gestational diabetes. ACOG Practice Bulletin Number 30. American College of Obstetricians and Gynecologists. *Obstet Gynecol* 2001 (reaffirmed 2008);98:525–538.

Lindsay JR. Adrenal disorders in pregnancy. *Endocrinol Metab Clin N Am* 2006;35:1–20.

Molitch ME. Pituitary disorders during pregnancy. *Endocrinol Metab Clin N Am* 2006;35: 99–116.

Moore TR. Glyburide for the treatment of gestational diabetes. *Diabetes Care* 2007;30:209.

Neale DM, Cootauco AC, Burrow G. Thyroid disease in pregnancy. *Clin Perinatol* 2007; 34(4):543–557.

Pregestational diabetes mellitus. ACOG Practice Bulletin Number 60. American College of Obstetricians and Gynecologists. *Obstet Gynecol* 2005 (reaffirmed 2007);105:675–685.

Rowan JA. Metformin versus insulin for the treatment of gestational diabetes. *N Engl J Med* 2008; 358:2003.

Schnatz PF, Thaxton S. Parathyroidectomy in the third trimester of pregnancy. *Obstet Gynecol Surv* 2005;60(10):672–682.

Screening for gestational diabetes mellitus: U.S. Preventive Task Force Management Statement. *Ann Intern Med.* 2008;148(10):759.

The HAPO Study Cooperative Research Group. Hyperglycemia and adverse pregnancy outcomes. *NEJM* 2008;358:1991.

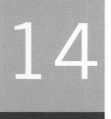

14 Hypertensive Disorders of Pregnancy

Catherine Eppes and Frank R. Witter

DEFINITIONS OF HYPERTENSIVE DISORDERS

Hypertensive disorders affect 5% to 10% of all pregnancies.

- **Hypertension** is defined as systolic blood pressure (BP) ≥140 mm Hg or diastolic BP ≥90 mm Hg on two separate occasions at least 6 hr but not more than 7 days apart.
- **Chronic hypertension** is high blood pressure diagnosed before pregnancy or before 20 weeks' gestation, or first recognized during pregnancy but persisting later than 42 days postpartum.
- **Gestational hypertension,** formerly known as pregnancy-induced or transient hypertension, is defined as BP ≥140/90 during pregnancy or within the first 24 hr postpartum without a history of chronic hypertension and without the signs and symptoms of preeclampsia. If the BP is ≥160/110 for more than 6 hr, the diagnosis is severe gestational hypertension.
- **Preeclampsia** is diagnosed by elevated BP and proteinuria after 20 weeks' gestation in a patient known to be previously normotensive. Trophoblastic disease or multiple gestation can present with preeclampsia before 20 weeks' gestation.
  - **Mild pre-eclampsia** is defined by the following criteria:
    - **BP** ≥140/90 mm Hg confirmed on two measures at least 6 hr but not more than 7 days apart, *and*
    - **Proteinuria** ≥300 mg on a 24-hr urine collection or two random urine dipstick results of at least 30 mg/dL ("1+"). Spot urine protein:creatinine ratios are used by some investigators instead of 24-hr urine collection and show excellent predictive value.
      - Preeclamptic patients often have wide variation in urine protein values over time, possibly from renal vasospasm. Discrepancies between the random urine dipstick and 24 hr urine collection measurements have been well described. The 24-hr urine collection, therefore, remains the preferred measure for diagnosing preeclampsia. The random protein to creatinine ratio is helpful primarily at the lower range of values.
  - **Severe preeclampsia** is classified by the following criteria:
    - **BP** during bed rest of ≥160 mm Hg systolic or ≥110 mm Hg diastolic; *or*
    - **Proteinuria** ≥5 g on a 24-hr urine collection even if BP is in the mild range. Persistent urine dipstick ≥3+ also qualifies; *or*
    - **Signs, symptoms, or lab values** of severe preeclampsia with any elevated BP.
      - **Oliguria** with 24-hr urine output <500 mL.
      - **Cerebral** or **visual disturbances** including altered consciousness, persistent headache, scotomata, or blurred vision.
      - **Pulmonary edema**

- **Epigastric** or **right upper quadrant pain** or **elevated serum liver transaminases** without a known cause.
- **Thrombocytopenia** with platelet count ≤100,000/μL.
- **Microangiopathic hemolytic anemia** with abnormal findings on peripheral smear, increased serum bilirubin, elevated serum lactate dehydrogenase (LDH), or decreased serum haptoglobin.
- **Intrauterine growth restriction.**
- **Preeclampsia superimposed on chronic hypertension** occurs in patients with preexisting high blood pressure. Differentiating chronic hypertension with superimposed preeclampsia from a gestational exacerbation of chronic hypertension can be difficult, especially if there is baseline proteinuria. In general, diagnosis requires a change from baseline proteinuria and hypertension.
- **Hemolysis, Elevated Liver Enzymes, and Low Platelets (HELLP) Syndrome** is a variant of preeclampsia defined by the following criteria:
  - **Hemolysis** identified by burr cells and schistocytes on an abnormal peripheral smear, an elevated serum bilirubin (>1.2 mg/dL) or LDH level (>600 IU/L), or a low serum haptoglobin.
  - **Thrombocytopenia** with platelets ≤100,000/μL is the most consistent finding in HELLP syndrome.
  - **Elevated liver function tests** (i.e., transaminases) greater than two times the upper limit of normal.
  - Note that hypertension may be absent (12% to 18% of cases), mild (15% to 50%), or severe (50%). Proteinuria may be absent as well (13%).
- **Eclampsia** is seizure or unexplained coma in a patient with preeclampsia. Eclampsia can present without hypertension (16%) or proteinuria (14%).

CHRONIC HYPERTENSION

Chronic hypertension carries increased risk for superimposed preeclampsia, preterm delivery, abruptio placentae, and IUGR. See Chapter 1 for general classification and treatment of hypertension.
- The **differential diagnosis** of chronic hypertension in pregnancy includes the following:
  - Essential hypertension, which causes 90% of hypertension outside of pregnancy.
  - Other common conditions, which can present with hypertension including kidney disease, adrenal disorders (e.g., primary aldosteronism, congenital adrenal hyperplasia, Cushing syndrome, pheochromocytoma), hyperthyroidism, new onset collagen vascular disease, systemic lupus erythematosus, aortic coarctation, chronic obstructive sleep apnea, and cocaine use.
  - Worsening chronic hypertension is difficult to distinguish from superimposed pre-eclampsia. If seizures, thrombocytopenia, pulmonary edema, unexplained hemolysis, or elevation in liver enzyme levels develops, superimposed preeclampsia should be diagnosed. Monitoring trends in blood pressure and urine protein may also be helpful.
    - A 24-hr urine calcium measurement may be useful. Urine calcium with pre-eclampsia is lower than in patients with hypertension alone.
      - A value <195 mg total urine calcium in 24 hr predicts preeclampsia with a sensitivity of 86% and specificity of 84%.
- Obtain **baseline information** early in pregnancy for chronic hypertension, including
  - History of first diagnosis, etiology, duration, and current and prior treatments.

- Complete medical history including cardiovascular risk factors (e.g., smoking, increased plasma lipid levels, obesity, diabetes mellitus) and complicating medical factors (e.g., headaches, history of chest pain, myocardial infarction, stroke, renal disease).
- Complete medication list including vasoactive over-the-counter drugs (e.g., sympathomimetic amines, nasal decongestants, diet pills).
- Baseline CBC and serum creatinine, urea nitrogen, uric acid, and calcium levels.
- Baseline electrocardiogram (ECG) if not documented within the prior 6 months.
- Baseline 24-hr urine protein.
- **Treatment** is tailored to the severity of illness and presence of comorbidities.
  - Mild hypertension often responds to conservative management.
    - Sodium restriction of ≤2.4 g/day. Dietary modifications with increased fruits and vegetables and decreased total and saturated fats can be encouraged.
    - Smoking and alcohol cessation.
    - Mild activity restrictions, due to concern for decreased uteroplacental blood flow increasing risk of preeclampsia.
    - Dieting and weight loss are not advised in pregnancy, even for obese women.
    - Serial fetal growth ultrasounds every 4 to 6 weeks starting after the anatomy scan at 18 to 20 weeks' gestation. More severe or worsening hypertension may require **drug therapy** and requires closer monitoring of fetal well being. Patients receiving antihypertensive agents should undergo antepartum fetal surveillance with nonstress test (NST) or biophysical profile (BPP) and a BP check one to two times per week starting at 28 weeks' gestation (earlier if severe hypertension or suspected IUGR).
  - Treatment for BP ≥160/105 mm Hg can include the following during pregnancy:
    - **Methyldopa** (Aldomet)—a centrally acting sympathetic outflow inhibitor that decreases systemic vascular resistance and is safe in pregnancy. Side effects include hepatic damage, therefore liver function tests should be monitored at least once per trimester. Starting dose is 250 mg PO three times daily with a maximum dose of 3 g/day. The dose may be adjusted at intervals of not less than every 2 days.
    - **Hydralazine**—a direct peripheral vasodilator that can be combined with methyldopa or a beta-blocker. It can cause a lupus-like syndrome but usually only at doses higher than 200 mg/day for an extended time. The starting oral dose is 10 mg four times a day and may be increased to a maximum of 200 mg/day.
    - **Labetalol**—an α_1 and nonselective β adrenergic antagonist that can be used as monotherapy or combined with hydralazine or a diuretic. The initial dose is 100 mg twice daily and may be increased in increments of 100 mg twice daily every 2 to 3 days, to a maximum of 2,400 mg daily. It is contraindicated in patients with greater than first-degree heart block. Chronic beta-blocker use in pregnancy has a mild association with IUGR.
    - **Nifedipine**—a calcium channel blocker used commonly in pregnancy that allows convenient daily dosing with the sustained release formulation. A multi-center prospective study of first-trimester drug exposure to calcium antagonists found no increased teratogenicity. The initial dose of nifedipine is 30 mg daily. The dose can be increased to 60 mg daily if adequate response is not seen in 7 days. The maximum daily dose is 90 mg. Exercise caution when magnesium treatment is started for patients on nifedipine as the combination can rarely lead to hypotension or neuromuscular blockade.
    - **Thiazide diuretics**—inhibit renal sodium and chloride reabsorption. A large meta-analysis found no adverse outcomes in pregnancy, however decreased plasma volume from diuresis carries a theoretic risk of placental insufficiency,

which deters its use as a first-line agent. The initial dose of hydrochlorothiazide (HCTZ) is 12.5 to 25 mg daily, titrated every 2 to 3 weeks to a maximum daily dose of 50 mg daily. Diuretics are not recommended in the setting of preeclampsia, uteroplacental insufficiency, or IUGR. Serum uric acid increases with thiazide diuretics, limiting diagnostic options for preeclampsia.

- **ACE inhibitors**—inhibit angiotensin I conversion to the vasoconstrictor angiotensin II. ACE inhibitors are *not recommended* in pregnancy due to severe fetal malformations and neonatal renal failure, pulmonary hypoplasia, and fetal death.

GESTATIONAL HYPERTENSION

Gestational hypertension is the most common etiology of hypertension in pregnancy, affecting 6% to 7% of nulliparous and 2% to 4% of parous women. The incidence increases with a history of preeclampsia and in multiple gestations. Earlier diagnosis of gestational hypertension increases the risk of preeclampsia; up to 50% of those with hypertension before 30 weeks will progress to preeclampsia.

- **Prognosis and management** depend on timing and severity.
  - **Mild Gestational Hypertension** after 37 weeks has a similar outcome to normotensive patients but an increased rate of labor induction and cesarean section.
    - If <37 weeks, monitor closely for progression to severe hypertension, preeclampsia, and fetal growth restriction.
    - If remote from term, manage expectantly as for mild preeclamptic patients.
    - If >37 weeks (full term), deliver if the cervix is favorable, otherwise close follow-up may be permitted.
  - **Severe gestational hypertension,** especially in early pregnancy, increases fetal and maternal morbidity even more than mild preeclampsia. Risks include placental abruption, preterm delivery, and small-for-gestational-age infants.
    - When BP is ≥160/110, antihypertensive therapy is indicated. The goal is to maintain uteroplacental perfusion, but gently reduce systolic and diastolic BP to the mild hypertensive range.
    - If the response to medical therapy is inadequate, the patient must be admitted to the antepartum service for close monitoring.

PREECLAMPSIA

Preeclampsia occurs in 2% to 7% of healthy nulliparous women and 1% to 5% of parous women. The incidence is higher in twin pregnancies (14%) and for women with a history of preeclampsia (18%). It is the third leading cause of maternal mortality, responsible for over 17% of maternal deaths, and a major cause of neonatal morbidity and mortality.

- **Risk factors** for preeclampsia include
  - Nulliparity
  - Multifetal gestation
  - Obesity
  - Chronic hypertension (15% to 50% of cases)
  - Systemic lupus erythematosus
  - Thrombophilia
  - Pregestational diabetes (10% to 36% of cases)
  - Kidney disease
  - History of preeclampsia or eclampsia

- Poor outcome in a previous pregnancy
- Family history of preeclampsia, eclampsia, or cardiovascular disease
- Molar pregnancy
- Conception via assisted reproductive technologies, and
- Abnormal uterine Doppler studies at 18 and 24 weeks.
- The **pathophysiology** of preeclampsia requires the presence of trophoblastic tissue but not necessarily a fetus (e.g., molar pregnancy). Proposed mechanisms include impaired trophoblastic differentiation and invasion, immunologic response to pregnancy, and placental or endothelial abnormalities. The temporal sequence and relative importance of these alterations are under investigation.
- The best **preventive** measures for preeclampsia are early evaluation, risk reduction, and optimizing maternal health. Women with preeclampsia in the second trimester have a recurrence rate as high as 65%. Supplementation with fish oil, calcium, or vitamin C and E, and early antihypertensive therapy are ineffective.
- **Diagnosis** of preeclampsia is by BP, signs, symptoms, and laboratory data.
  - **Symptoms** of preeclampsia may include the following: headache; visual symptoms (e.g., blurred vision, scotomata, and blindness from retinal detachment); epigastric, right upper quadrant, or constant low abdominal pain from liver dysfunction or from abruptio placentae; nausea and vomiting; dyspnea from pulmonary edema; decreased urine output, hematuria, or rapid weight gain >5 pounds in 1 week; and absent or decreased fetal movement.
  - **Physical findings** of preeclampsia may include the following:
    - Elevated BP measured in the sitting or semireclined position with the arm positioned roughly at heart level.
    - Nondependent or generalized edema.
    - Rales or crackles on lung examination.
    - Right upper quadrant tenderness secondary to hepatic edema.
    - Uterine tenderness or tetany secondary to placental abruption.
  - **Laboratory findings** of preeclampsia may include the following:
    - Diagnostic proteinuria (described above).
    - Decreased hematocrit secondary to severe hemolysis in HELLP syndrome.
    - Elevated hematocrit resulting from decreased intravascular volume secondary to third spacing of fluid.
    - Elevated serum uric acid level ≥5 mg/dL.
    - Elevated serum creatinine ≥1.2 mg/dL. Remember that creatinine normally decreases in pregnancy, so even slight increases warrant investigation.
    - Elevated serum transaminases (AST >70 IU/L).
    - Decreased platelet count ≤100,000/μL).
    - Prolonged prothrombin and partial thromboplastin times that may be due to primary coagulopathy, hepatic synthesis dysfunction, or abruptio placentae leading to disseminated intravascular coagulation.
    - Decreased fibrinogen, increased fibrin degradation products, or both, as a result of coagulopathy or abruptio placentae.
- Definitive **management** for gestational hypertension, preeclampsia, and eclampsia is delivery.
  - In general, **mild preeclampsia** (see definitions above) at term is treated by delivery.
    - Optimal treatment prior to 37 weeks is usually expectant management. The benefits of bed rest, antihypertensive medications, and hospitalization are not clearly established. There are no large, randomized trials on the management of mild pre-eclampsia.

- Close maternal and fetal observation is essential, but there is no standard protocol for testing or frequency. Most centers recommend at least weekly nonstress testing for mild preeclampsia.
- Fetal monitoring can include growth ultrasound and amniotic fluid assessment every 3 to 4 weeks, uterine artery Doppler velocimetry, and weekly or semiweekly NST or BPP.
- Maternal monitoring can include weekly or semiweekly BP check and evaluation, and periodic lab testing such as 24 hr urine protein, serum creatinine, platelet count, and serum transaminases to detect progression to severe preeclampsia.
- A gestational age of >34 weeks with progressive labor, abnormal fetal testing, or growth restriction should prompt delivery.
- The first priority in treating **severe preeclampsia** is to assess and stabilize the mother.
  - **At ≥34 weeks** delivery is indicated, although immediate cesarean section is not usually warranted.
    - Patients in labor, or with a favorable cervix, can deliver vaginally. Careful monitoring, at least hourly assessments, and strict intake/output recordings should be maintained.
  - **Between 24 and 34 weeks** expectant management is acceptable if BP is adequately controlled with antihypertensive agents, fetal testing is reassuring, and there is no evidence of IUGR.
    - Magnesium sulfate and IV antihypertensives may be given initially while betamethasone is administered.
    - Fluid status should be monitored.
    - CBC, platelets, and LFTs are checked daily.
    - Fetal surveillance with NST or BPP is performed at least weekly and patients are instructed regarding monitoring of fetal movement.
    - Delivery is indicated by the following: IUGR, nonreassuring fetal tracing, eclampsia, neurologic deficits, pulmonary edema, right upper quadrant/epigastric pain, oliguria <500 mL in 24 hr or creatinine >1.5, DIC, HELLP, placental abruption, or uncontrolled severe BP.
  - **At 24 weeks' gestation and earlier**, expectant management is associated with high maternal morbidity and limited perinatal benefit.
  - Expectant management of severe preeclampsia with intrauterine growth restriction has been associated with increased risk of fetal death (rate of perinatal death is 5.4%).
- **Seizure prophylaxis** during labor and for 24 hr postpartum is recommended for patients with preeclampsia. Some patients with severe persistent preeclampsia need seizure prophylaxis for longer periods *before and after* delivery.
  - **Magnesium Sulfate (MgSO$_4$)** is the agent of choice for eclamptic seizure prophylaxis. Magnesium sulfate has been shown to decrease the risk of eclampsia by more than 50%.
    - We use a loading dose of 6 g MgSO$_4$ IV administered over 15 to 20 minutes.
    - Maintenance dose is 2 g/hr IV (dose should be titrated down if the patient has poor urine output or an elevated serum creatinine).
    - If there is no IV access, the loading dose is 5 g MgSO$_4$ (50% solution) in each buttock (10 g total), with a maintenance dose of 5 g in alternating buttocks every 4 hr.
    - The therapeutic serum magnesium level for seizure prophylaxis is 4 to 6 mEq/L although it is our practice only to follow magnesium levels for patients in

whom we are unusually concerned for developing supratherapeutic levels For such patients, check serum magnesium level 4 hr after the loading dose, then every 6 hr as needed or if symptoms suggest magnesium toxicity

- Diuresis is a useful criterion for early cessation of seizure prophylaxis. Urine output exceeding ≥100 mL/hr for 2 hr suggests resolving preeclampsia with no or rare complications.
- Patients are monitored hourly for signs and symptoms of magnesium toxicity:
  - Loss of patellar reflexes at 8 to 10 mEq/L.
  - Respiratory depression or arrest at 12 mEq/L.
  - Mental status changes at >12 mEq/L followed by ECG changes and arrhythmias.
  - If magnesium toxicity develops, check the patient's vital signs, stop magnesium and check plasma levels, administer 1 g calcium gluconate IV over ≥3 minutes and consider diuretics (e.g., furosemide, manitol).

○ **Phenytoin (Dilantin)** is a secondary agent for eclamptic seizure prophylaxis. Magnesium was clearly superior in a large randomized clinical trial.
  - The loading dose is maternal weight based. For <50 kg, load 1,000 mg; for 50 to 70 kg, load 1,250 mg; and for >70 kg, load with 1,500 mg phenytoin.
  - The first 750 mg of the loading dose should be given at 25 mg/min and the rest at 12.5 mg/min. If the patient maintains normal cardiac rhythm and has no history of heart disease, ECG monitoring is not necessary at this infusion rate.
  - Check the serum phenytoin level at 30 to 60 minutes after infusion.
  - A therapeutic level is >12 μg/mL; recheck level in 12 hr.
  - If the level is <10 μg/mL, reload with 500 mg and check again in 30 to 60 minutes.
  - If the level is 10 to 12 μg/mL, reload with 250 mg and check again in 30 to 60 minutes.

- **Antihypertensive therapy** is indicated for patients with a diastolic BP of ≥105 mm Hg. Acute treatment aims to reduce BP in a controlled manner without compromising uteroplacental perfusion.
  ○ It is reasonable to reduce the patient's systolic BP to 140 to 155 mm Hg and the diastolic BP to 90 to 105 mm Hg. It is more important to decrease the diastolic pressure.
  ○ Useful antihypertensive agents for acute management include
    - **Hydralazine hydrochloride** has an onset of action within 10 to 20 minutes. The duration of action is 4 to 6 hr.
      - Begin with a 5 mg IV bolus, and repeat every 20 minutes to a maximum of 20 mg as needed.
    - **Labetalol hydrochloride** has an onset of action within 5 to 10 minutes and lasts for 3 to 6 hr. It is contraindicated in greater than first-degree maternal heart block.
      - Begin with a 20 mg IV loading dose, then continuous infusion or an escalating bolus protocol.
      - The escalating bolus protocol uses labetolol doses of 20, 40, 80, 80, and 80 mg given at 10-minute intervals, to a maximum of 300 mg/24 hr.
      - The continuous-infusion protocol starts at 0.5 mg/kg/hr and increases every 30 minutes by 0.5 mg/kg/hr to a maximum dose of 3 mg/kg/hr.

- **Fluid management.** Patients with preeclampsia are frequently hypovolemic due to third spacing from low serum oncotic pressure and increased capillary permeability. These same abnormalities also increase risk for pulmonary edema.

Diuretics may be used to treat pulmonary edema but should not be used otherwise in preeclamptic patients.

○ Oliguria is defined as urine output of <100 mL in 4 hr. It is treated with 500-mL crystalloid bolus if the lungs are clear. If there is no response, another 500-mL bolus can be administered. If there is no response after 1 L, central hemodynamic monitoring can be considered (see Chapter 3).

‒ Central venous pressure monitoring does not correlate well with pulmonary capillary wedge pressure. A Swan-Ganz catheter may be required to help guide fluid management and prevent flash pulmonary edema.

○ Patients usually begin to diurese well about 12 to 24 hr after delivery. In cases of severe renal compromise, it may take 72 hr or more for adequate diuresis to resume.

• **Maternal complications** of severe pre-eclampsia require a high index of clinical suspicion and include renal failure (acute tubular necrosis), acute cardiac failure, pulmonary edema, thrombocytopenia, disseminated intravascular coagulopathy, and cerebrovascular accidents.

• **Perinatal outcome.** There is a high perinatal morbidity and mortality in pregnancies complicated by severe preeclampsia. Fetal mortality rates range from 5% to more than 70%.

HELLP Syndrome

HELLP syndrome often presents with nonspecific complaints such as malaise, abdominal pain, vomiting, shortness of breath, or bleeding.

• The **differential diagnosis** for HELLP syndrome includes
  • Acute fatty liver of pregnancy (AFLP)
  • Thrombotic thrombocytopenic purpura (TTP)
  • Hemolytic uremic syndrome (HUS)
  • Immune thrombocytopenic purpura (ITP)
  • Systemic lupus erythematosus (SLE) flare
  • Antiphospholipid antibody syndrome
  • Cholecystitis
  • Fulminant hepatitis (of any cause)
  • Acute pancreatitis
  • Disseminated herpes zoster

• **Management** is the same as for severe pre-eclampsia. Short-term expectant management in order to allow for administration of steroids to enhance fetal well-being *may* be possible in a very select group of patients with HELLP prior to 34 weeks; however, there are no data suggesting improved perinatal outcomes with this approach.

ECLAMPSIA

Eclampsia should be the presumed diagnosis in obstetric patients with seizures and/or coma. The incidence of eclampsia is between 1 in 2,000 and 1 in 3,500 pregnancies in developed countries. Eclampsia occurs in about 1% of patients with preeclampsia. Virtually all eclampsia is preceded by preeclampsia.

• The **pathophysiology** of eclamptic seizures is unknown but may occur when mean arterial pressure exceeds the capacity of cerebral autoregulation, leading to cerebral edema and increased intracranial pressure.

• Eclampsia can occur antepartum, peripartum, or postpartum and has been reported as late as 3 to 4 weeks postpartum. Patients may have associated hypertension and proteinuria, but a small percentage have neither.

- **Management** of eclampsia is an obstetric emergency that requires immediate treatment, including
  - Appropriate management of ABC's (airway, breathing, and circulation) with measures taken to avoid aspiration.
  - Seizure control with 6 g $MgSO_4$ IV bolus. If the patient has a seizure during or after the loading dose, an additional 2 g IV bolus of $MgSO_4$ can be given.
  - Treatment of seizures refractory to $MgSO_4$ with IV phenytoin, an IV barbiturate (e.g., amobarbitol), or a benzodiazepine (e.g., lorazepam)
  - Treatment of *status epilepticus* with lorazepam 0.1 mg/kg IV at a rate ≤2 mg/min Patients with *status epilepticus* may require intubation to correct hypoxia and acidosis and maintain a secure airway.
  - Prevention of maternal injury with padded bedrails and appropriate positioning.
  - Control of severe hypertension (see medications, above)
  - Delivery after maternal stabilization.
    - During acute eclamptic episodes, fetal bradycardia is common. It usually resolves in 3 to 5 minutes. Allowing the fetus to recover in utero from the maternal seizure, hypoxia, and hypercarbia before delivery is optimal. However, if fetal bradycardia persists beyond 10 minutes, abruptio placentae should be suspected.
    - Emergency cesarean section should always be anticipated in case of rapid maternal or fetal deterioration.
- **Outcomes** depend on the severity of disease. Perinatal mortality in the United States ranges from 5.6% to 11.8%, mainly due to extreme prematurity, placental abruption, and IUGR. The maternal mortality rate is from <1.8% in the developed world to 14% in underresourced countries. Maternal complications include aspiration pneumonitis, hemorrhage, cardiac failure, intracranial hemorrhage, and transient or permanent retinal blindness.
- Long-term neurologic sequelae of eclampsia are rare. Central nervous system (CNS) imaging with computed tomography (CT) or magnetic resonance imaging (MRI) should be performed if seizures are of late onset (longer than 48 hr after delivery) or if neurologic deficits are clinically evident. The signs and symptoms of preeclampsia usually resolve within 1 to 2 weeks postpartum. Approximately 25% of eclamptic patients develop pre-eclampsia in subsequent pregnancies, with recurrence of eclampsia in 2% of cases.

SUGGESTED READINGS

Chronic hypertension in pregnancy. ACOG Practice Bulletin Number 29. American College of Obstetricians and Gynecologists. *Obstet Gynecol* 2001;98:177–185.

Diagnosis and management of preeclampsia and eclampsia. ACOG Practice Bulletin Number 33. American College of Obstetricians and Gynecologists. *Obstet Gynecol* 2002;99:159–167.

Haddad B, Kayem G, Deis S, et al. Are perinatal and maternal outcomes different during expectant management of severe preeclampsia in the presence of IUGR. *Am J Obstet Gynecol* 2007;196:237.e1–237.e5.

National High Blood Pressure Education Program. Working Group Report on high blood pressure in pregnancy. *Am J Obstet Gynecol* 2000;183:51.

Sibai B. Diagnosis, prevention and management of eclampsia. *Obstet Gynecol* 2005;105:402–410.

Sibai B. Expectant management of severe preeclampsia remote from term: patient selection, treatment and delivery indications. *Am J Obstet Gynecol* 2007;196:514.

Cardiopulmonary Disorders of Pregnancy

Meredith Birsner and Ernest M. Graham

CARDIAC DISORDERS

Cardiac diseases complicate 1% to 4% of pregnancies in women without preexisting cardiac abnormalities. Pregnancy is associated with major alterations in circulatory physiology, and cardiovascular disease remains a major cause of nonobstetric maternal morbidity in the United States.

Hemodynamic Changes During Pregnancy

- Profound **hemodynamic alterations** occur during pregnancy, labor and delivery, and the postpartum period. These changes begin during the first 5 to 8 weeks of pregnancy and peak in the late second trimester. Normal pregnancy is associated with fatigue, dyspnea, decreased exercise capacity, peripheral edema, and jugular venous distention. Most pregnant women have audible physiologic systolic murmurs created by augmented blood flow, and a physiologic third heart sound (S3) that reflects the volume-expanded state. The enormous changes in the cardiovascular system during pregnancy carry many implications for the management of pregnant patients with cardiac disease.
  - **Blood volume** increases 40% to 50% during normal pregnancy, in part due to estrogen-mediated activation of the renin-aldosterone axis. The rise in blood volume is greater than the increase in red blood cell mass (20% to 30%), contributing to the fall in hemoglobin concentration causing physiologic anemia in pregnancy.
  - **Cardiac output** increases 30% to 50% above baseline by 20 to 26 weeks' gestation, peaks at the end of the second trimester, then plateaus until delivery. The change in cardiac output is mediated by the following: (a) increased preload due to the rise in blood volume, (b) reduced afterload due to a fall in systemic vascular resistance, and (c) a rise in maternal heart rate of 10 to 15 beats/min. Stroke volume increases during the first and second trimesters but declines in the third trimester due to caval compression by the gravid uterus.
- **Labor and delivery.** During labor and delivery, hemodynamic fluctuations can be profound. Each uterine contraction results in the displacement of 300 to 500 mL of blood into the general circulation. Stroke volume increases, causing a rise in cardiac output of an additional 50% with each contraction. Mean systemic pressure also rises due to maternal pain and anxiety. Blood loss during delivery can further alter the hemodynamic state.
- **Postpartum.** The hemodynamic changes during the postpartum state are mainly due to relief of vena caval compression after delivery. Increased venous return augments cardiac output and prompts brisk diuresis. The hemodynamic changes return to the prepregnant baseline within 3 to 4 weeks postpartum.

Cardiac Disease in Pregnancy

- **Signs and symptoms** of cardiac disease overlap common symptoms and findings in pregnancy including fatigue, shortness of breath, orthopnea, palpitations, edema, systolic flow murmur, and a third heart sound.
- **Evaluation** of cardiac disease includes a thorough history and physical examination. Noninvasive testing includes an electrocardiogram (ECG), chest radiograph, and an echocardiogram. The ECG may reveal a leftward shift of the electrical axis, especially during the third trimester when the diaphragm is pushed upward by the uterus. Routine chest radiographs are used to assess cardiomegaly and pulmonary vascular prominence. Echocardiographic evaluation of ventricular function and structural anomalies is invaluable for diagnosis cardiac disease in pregnancy.

Management of Patients with Known Cardiac Disease

- **Before conception.** Whenever possible, women with preexisting cardiac lesions should receive preconception counseling regarding maternal and fetal risks during pregnancy and long-term maternal morbidity and mortality. The New York Heart Association (NYHA) functional class (Table 15-1) is used as a predictor of outcome. Women with NYHA class III and IV face a mortality rate of 7% and a morbidity of over 30%. These women should be strongly cautioned against pregnancy. A risk index using four risk factors has been shown to predict accurately a woman's chance of having adverse cardiac or neonatal complications: (a) a prior cardiac event, (b) cyanosis or poor functional class, (c) left heart obstruction, and (d) systemic ventricular dysfunction.
- **After conception.** If the patient is already pregnant, she requires cardiac assessment as early as possible. If the pregnancy poses a serious threat to maternal health, she should be counseled about the option of termination of the pregnancy. Patients need close monitoring and follow-up by both a perinatologist and cardiologist, with attention to signs or symptoms of worsening congestive heart failure (CHF) throughout the pregnancy. Each visit should include the following: (a) cardiac

TABLE 15-1	New York Heart Association (NYHA) Functional Classification
NYHA Class	**Symptoms**
I	No symptoms and no limitation in ordinary physical activity such as shortness of breath when walking or climbing stairs.
II	Mild symptoms (mild shortness of breath and/or angina) and slight limitation during ordinary activity.
III	Marked limitation in activity due to symptoms, even during less-than-ordinary activity such as walking short distances (20–100 m). Comfortable only at rest.
IV	Severe limitations. Experiences symptoms even while at rest. Mostly bedbound.

Criteria Committee of the New York Heart Association. *Nomenclature and Criteria for Diagnosis of Diseases of the Heart and Great Vessels*, 8th Ed. Boston, MA: Little Brown, 1979.

examination and cardiac review of systems, (b) documentation of weight, blood pressure, and pulse, and (c) evaluation of peripheral edema.
- **During pregnancy.** If symptoms worsen, hospitalization, bed rest, diuresis, or correction of an underlying arrhythmia may be required. Sometimes, surgical correction during pregnancy becomes necessary. When possible, procedures should be performed during the early second trimester to avoid the period of fetal organogenesis and before more significant hemodynamic changes of pregnancy occur.

Antibiotic Prophylaxis for Endocarditis
- The 2007 American Heart Association (AHA) guidelines for prevention of infective endocarditis (IE) represent a marked change from prior AHA guidelines. Antibiotic prophylaxis is no longer recommended based on increased lifetime risk of IE as IE is more likely to result from frequent random bacteremia with daily activities than from bacteremia caused by specific dental, gastrointestinal (GI), or genitourinary (GU) procedures. Prophylaxis is based now on the risk of adverse outcome with the procedure, and it is not recommended for GU procedures except in high-risk patients with GU infections, to prevent wound infection and sepsis. Antibiotic prophylaxis for IE is not recommended for vaginal delivery or hysterectomy. See Chapter 24.

Specific Cardiac Conditions
Cardiomyopathy
- **Cardiomyopathy**, idiopathic or caused by myocarditis or toxins, manifests during pregnancy with signs and symptoms of CHF including chest pain, dyspnea, paroxysmal nocturnal dyspnea, and cough. Echocardiography demonstrates chamber enlargement and reduced ventricular function. The heart becomes uniformly dilated, filling pressures increase, and cardiac output decreases. Eventually, heart failure develops and is often refractory to treatment. The 5-year survival rate is approximately 50%; therefore, careful preconception counseling is important, even if the patient is asymptomatic.
  - **Hypertrophic cardiomyopathy** with or without left ventricular outflow tract obstruction is an autosomal dominant disorder with a variable phenotype and incidence of 0.1% to 0.5% in pregnancy. Most women with hypertrophic cardiomyopathy do well in pregnancy, and complications are uncommon with prior prepregnancy risk stratification via NYHA functional class and multidisciplinary specialist management. The potential does exist for poor tolerance of the circulatory overload of pregnancy. Major complications include pulmonary edema secondary to diastolic dysfunction, dysrhythmias secondary to myofibrillar disarray, functional class decline, obstetric complications, and poor fetal outcomes.
  - **Peripartum cardiomyopathy** is an idiopathic dilated cardiomyopathy that develops in the last month of pregnancy or within 5 months of delivery and is characterized by left ventricular systolic dysfunction with ejection fraction (LVEF) <45%. Incidence is 1 in 1,300 to 1 in 15,000. Risk factors include advanced maternal age, multiparity, multiple gestations, black race, obesity, malnutrition, gestational hypertension (HTN), preeclampsia, poor antenatal care, breast feeding, cesarean section, low socioeconomic status, family history, and abuse of tobacco, alcohol, or cocaine.
    - Of the patients who survive, approximately 50% recover normal left heart function. The mortality rate is 25% to 50%, half of those die within the first month of presentation and the majority die within three months postpartum. Prognosis is related to left ventricular dysfunction at presentation. Death results from progressive CHF, thromboembolic events, and arrhythmias.

○ Medical management includes fluid and salt restriction, digoxin, diuretics, vasodilators, and anticoagulants; bed rest can predispose to thromboembolism. Cardiac transplantation may be required in advanced unresolving disease. For patients diagnosed antenatally, invasive cardiac monitoring should be considered during labor and until at least 24 hr postpartum. Supplemental oxygen and regional analgesia for pain control should be administered and a passive second stage of labor facilitated by operative vaginal delivery. Cesarean section is reserved for obstetric indications as it carries an increased risk of blood loss and pulmonary embolism. Intensive care unit monitoring should commence immediately postpartum for detection and management of autotransfusion-induced pulmonary edema.

Valvular Disease

- **Mitral valve prolapse (MVP)** is the most common congenital heart defect in women. It rarely has implications for maternal or fetal outcomes. It is the most common cause of mitral regurgitation (MR) in women.
- **MR** is usually well tolerated during pregnancy. Medical management includes diuretics in the rare event of pulmonary congestion or vasodilators for systemic HTN. Acute, severe worsening of MR can result from ruptured chordae and must be repaired surgically. Women with severe MR before pregnancy should undergo operative repair before conception. Patients with advanced disease may require central monitoring during labor.
- **Aortic regurgitation (AR).** AR may be encountered in women with rheumatic heart disease, a congenitally bicuspid or deformed aortic valve, IE, or connective tissue disease. AR is generally well tolerated during pregnancy. Medical management includes diuretics and vasodilators. Ideally, women with severe AR should undergo operative repair before conception; as in MR, surgery during pregnancy should be considered only for control of refractory NYHA functional class III or IV symptoms.
- **Aortic stenosis (AS).** The most common etiology of AS in pregnant women is a congenitally bicuspid valve. Mild AS with normal left ventricular function is usually well tolerated during pregnancy. Asymptomatic severe disease can be managed conservatively with bed rest, oxygen, and beta blockade. Moderate-to-severe AS markedly increases the medical risk of pregnancy; patients are advised to delay conception until correction is performed. Symptoms, such as dyspnea, angina pectoris, or syncope, usually become apparent late in the second trimester or early in the third trimester. Women with bicuspid aortic valves are also at increased risk for aortic dissection and should be followed carefully.
  - Severe symptomatic AS can be managed by percutaneous aortic balloon valvuloplasty prior to labor and delivery, but not without significant risk to both mother and fetus. Spinal and epidural anesthesia are discouraged because of their vasodilatory effects. Because this disorder is characterized by a fixed afterload, adequate end-diastolic volume and therefore adequate filling pressure are necessary to maintain cardiac output. Consequently, great care must be taken to prevent hypotension and tachycardia caused by blood loss, regional anesthesia, or other medications. Patients should be hydrated adequately and placed in the left lateral position to maximize venous return. As with mitral stenosis (MS), hemodynamic monitoring with a pulmonary arterial catheter should be considered during labor and delivery.
- **Pulmonic stenosis (PS)** frequently accompanies other congenital cardiac anomalies, but as an isolated lesion, PS rarely complicates pregnancy. Patients with cyanotic

congenital cardiac disease tolerate pregnancy more poorly than those with acyanotic lesions. Echocardiogram-guided percutaneous valvotomy is a potential treatment option.

- **Mitral stenosis.** MS in women of childbearing age is usually due to rheumatic fever. Mild-to-moderate MS can be managed with judicious diuresis and beta blockade. Aggressive diuresis should be avoided so as to preserve uteroplacental perfusion. Cardioselective beta blockers, such as metoprolol and atenolol, are used to treat or prevent tachycardia to optimize diastolic filling while preventing deleterious effects of epinephrine blockade on myometrial activity.

  - Patients with moderate-to-severe MS often experience hemodynamic deterioration during the third trimester and/or during labor and delivery; these patients should be managed in conjunction with a cardiologist. Increased blood volumes and heart rate lead to an elevation of left atrial pressure, resulting in pulmonary edema. Additional displacement of blood volume into the systemic circulation during contractions makes labor particularly hazardous. Patients with severe MS who develop NYHA functional class III–IV symptoms during pregnancy should undergo percutaneous balloon valvotomy.

  - Atrial fibrillation in pregnant patients with MS may result in rapid decompensation. Digoxin and beta-blockers can reduce heart rate, and diuretics may be used to reduce blood volume and left atrial pressure. With atrial fibrillation and hemodynamic deterioration, electrocardioversion can be performed safely and promptly. Atrial fibrillation also increases the risk of stroke and necessitates anticoagulation.

  - Most patients with MS can undergo vaginal delivery. However, patients with symptoms of CHF or moderate-to-severe MS should undergo hemodynamic monitoring with a Swan-Ganz catheter during labor, delivery, and for several hours postpartum. Epidural anesthesia is usually better tolerated hemodynamically than general anesthesia.

Congenital Heart Disease

- During pregnancy, women with **congenital heart disease** are at increased risk of cardiac events including pulmonary edema and symptomatic sustained arrhythmias (supraventricular tachycardia [SVT] and ventricular tachycardia [VT]). Risk factors include prior history of heart failure, NYHA functional class ≥II, decreased subpulmonary ventricular ejection fraction, severe pulmonary regurgitation, and smoking. These women also face increased risks of adverse neonatal outcomes including preterm delivery, and infants with growth restriction, respiratory distress syndrome, intraventricular hemorrhage, and intrauterine or neonatal death. Additionally, there is an increased incidence of congenital heart disease in children of women with a congenital abnormality ranging from approximately 3% overall to 50% in women carrying single gene defects with autosomal dominant inheritance (e.g., Marfan's syndrome). Because of the great heterogeneity of congenital heart lesions, each patient needs individual assessment for ability to tolerate the hemodynamic changes of pregnancy.

- **Minimal risk lesions** include small ventricular septal defects (VSDs), atrial septal defects (ASDs), and bicuspid aortic valves without stenosis, insufficiency, or aortic enlargement. These patients have near-normal physiology, have only minimal increased risk during pregnancy, and can receive routine care.

- **Moderate risk lesions** include repaired tetralogy of Fallot without significant pulmonary insufficiency or stenosis, complex congenital heart disease with anatomic right ventricle serving as systemic ventricle, and mild left side valve stenosis.

- **High-risk lesions** for which patients should be counseled against pregnancy due to the risk of maternal cardiac decompensation and death include Eisenmenger's syndrome, severe pulmonary HTN, severe AS or left ventricular outflow tract obstruction, Marfan's syndrome with aortic dilation >45 mm, or symptomatic ventricular dysfunction with ejection fraction <40%. Moderate-risk and high-risk patients should be followed at tertiary care centers with perinatologists and cardiologists experienced in managing pregnant patients with congenital heart disease.
  - **Tetralogy of Fallot**, characterized by right ventricular outflow tract obstruction, VSD, right ventricular hypertrophy, and overriding aorta, is associated with right-to-left shunt and cyanosis. If the defect goes uncorrected, the affected patient rarely lives beyond childhood. In developed countries, almost all patients have had surgical correction with good survival rates (85% to 86% at 32 to 36 years) and good quality of life. Pregnancy is generally well tolerated in patients who have had surgical repair, though these women are at increased risk of right-sided heart failure and arrhythmia.
  - **Coarctation of the aorta.** Severe cases of coarctation of the aorta are usually corrected in infancy. Surgical correction during pregnancy is recommended only if dissection occurs. Coarctation of the aorta is associated with other cardiac lesions as well as berry aneurysms. Coarctation of the aorta is characterized by a fixed cardiac output. Therefore, the patient's heart cannot meet the increased cardiac demands of pregnancy by increasing its rate, and extreme care must be taken to prevent hypotension. Two percent of infants of mothers with coarctation of the aorta may also have cardiac lesions.
  - **Septal defects.** Young women with uncomplicated secundum-type ASD or isolated VSD usually tolerate pregnancy well. ASD is the most common congenital heart lesion in adults. ASDs are usually very well tolerated unless they are associated with pulmonary HTN. Complications, such as atrial arrhythmias, pulmonary HTN, and heart failure, usually do not arise until the fifth decade of life and are therefore uncommon in pregnancy. VSDs usually close spontaneously or are closed surgically if the lesion is large. For this reason, significant VSDs are rarely seen in pregnancy. Rarely, uncorrected lesions lead to significant left-to-right shunts with pulmonary HTN, right ventricular failure, and reversal of the shunt. The incidence of VSD in the offspring of affected parents is 4%; however, small VSDs are often difficult to detect antenatally.
  - **Patent ductus arteriosus (PDA).** PDA is usually tolerated well during pregnancy unless pulmonary HTN has developed. PDA is associated with increased volume, left heart failure, and pulmonary HTN, which usually worsen during pregnancy. Therefore, pregnancy is not recommended for patients with large PDA and associated complications. PDA is not associated with additional maternal risk for cardiac complications if the shunt is small to moderate and if pulmonary artery pressures are normal.
  - **Eisenmenger's syndrome** occurs when an initial left-to-right shunt results in pulmonary arterial obliteration and pulmonary HTN, which eventually causes a right-to-left shunt. This serious condition carries a maternal mortality rate of 50% and a fetal mortality rate of more than 50% if cyanosis is present. In addition, 30% of fetuses exhibit intrauterine growth restriction. Because of increased maternal mortality, termination of the pregnancy should be discussed. If the pregnancy is continued, special precautions must be taken during the peripartum period. The patient should be monitored with a Swan-Ganz catheter, and care should be taken to avoid hypovolemia. Postpartum death most often occurs within 1 week

after delivery; however, delayed deaths up to 4 to 6 weeks after delivery have been reported.

- **Marfan's syndrome** is an autosomal dominant disorder of the fibrillin gene characterized by connective tissue fragility. Cardiovascular manifestations include aortic root dilation and dissection, MVP, and aneurysms. Genetic counseling is recommended. If cardiovascular involvement is minor and the aortic root diameter is smaller than 45 mm, the risk in pregnancy is similar to the general population. If cardiovascular involvement is more extensive or the aortic root is larger than 45 mm, complications during pregnancy and aortic dissection are increased significantly. HTN should be avoided and managed with beta-blockers. Beta blockade is recommended for patients with Marfan's syndrome from the second trimester onward, particularly if the aortic root is dilated. Regional anesthesia during labor is considered safe. Women should labor in the left lateral decubitus position with second stage shortened by operative vaginal delivery and cesarean section reserved for obstetric indications. Losartan, shown to prevent aneurysms in mouse models of Marfan's syndrome, is contraindicated in pregnancy.

- **Idiopathic hypertrophic subaortic stenosis** is an autosomal dominant disorder and manifests as left ventricular outflow tract obstruction secondary to a hypertrophic interventricular septum. Genetic counseling is advised for affected patients. Patients' conditions improve when left ventricular end-diastolic volume is maximized. Pregnant patients fare quite well initially because of an increase in circulating blood volume. Later in pregnancy, however, decreased systemic vascular resistance and decreased venous return may worsen the obstruction. This may cause left ventricular failure as well as supraventricular arrhythmias from left atrial distention. The following labor management points should be kept in mind: (a) inotropic agents may exacerbate obstruction, (b) medications that decrease systemic vascular resistance should be avoided or limited, (c) cardiac rhythm should be monitored and tachycardia treated promptly, and (d) the patient should undergo labor in the left lateral decubitus position with the second stage of labor curtailed by operative vaginal delivery.

- **Transposition of the great arteries (TGA)** is characterized by correct atrioventricular connections and inappropriate ventriculoarterial connections; the aorta arises anteriorly from the right ventricle and the pulmonary artery arises posteriorly from the left ventricle. The Senning operation (using atrial and septal tissues) and Mustard operation (using extrinsic material such as pericardium) redirect atrial blood via baffles to deliver oxygenated pulmonary venous blood to the systemic right ventricle and deoxygenated systemic venous blood to the pulmonary left ventricle. Long-term follow-up demonstrates an 80% survival at 28 years with the majority of survivors in NYHA class I. Pregnancy in women after Senning or Mustard repair is associated with arrhythmias (VT, SVT, atrial flutter), heart failure, and NYHA functional class deterioration as well as a high incidence of serious obstetric complications (65%) and offspring mortality (11.7%).

- **Congenital atrioventricular block.** Although affected patients may need a pacemaker, they usually fare well and do not require special treatment during pregnancy.

Arrhythmias

- **Premature atrial and/or ventricular complexes** are not associated with adverse maternal or fetal outcomes and do not require antiarrhythmic therapy. **Atrial fibrillation** and **atrial flutter** are rare during pregnancy. Rate control can be safely achieved with digoxin or beta-blockers. Electrical cardioversion can be performed safely during any stage of pregnancy. Other arrhythmias should be managed with the assistance of a cardiologist. Nonsustained arrhythmias in the absence of organic cardiac disease are best left untreated or managed with lifestyle and dietary modifications (e.g., decreasing smoking, caffeine, and stress). Serious, life-threatening arrhythmias associated with an aberrant re-entrant pathway should be treated before pregnancy by ablation. If medical therapy is necessary during pregnancy, established drugs should be used. Artificial pacing, electrical defibrillation, and cardioversion should have no effect on the fetus.

Ischemic Heart Disease

- **Ischemic heart disease** is an uncommon but potentially devastating event in pregnancy. Risk factors include HTN, thrombophilia, diabetes, smoking, transfusion, postpartum infection, and age >35. Anterior wall myocardial infarcts are most common. Approximately 67% of myocardial ischemia during pregnancy occurs during the third trimester; if it occurs before 24 weeks' gestation, the option of pregnancy termination should be discussed due to the high incidence of maternal mortality. If delivery takes place within 2 weeks of the acute event, the mortality rate reaches 50%; survival is much improved if delivery takes place longer than 2 weeks after the acute event.
- Medical therapy for acute myocardial infarction should be modified in the pregnant patient. Thrombolytic agents increase the risk of maternal hemorrhage to 8% for women who receive thrombolytic therapy shortly after delivery. Low-dose aspirin and nitrates are considered safe. Beta-blockers are safe, although some have been linked to a slight decrease in fetal growth. Short-term heparin administration has not been associated with increased maternal or fetal adverse effects. Angiotensin-converting enzyme (ACE) inhibitors and statins are contraindicated during pregnancy. Hydralazine and nitrates may be used as substitutes for ACE inhibitors.

Cardiovascular Drugs in Pregnancy

- The most commonly used cardiovascular drugs and their potential adverse effects during pregnancy are shown in Table 15-2.
- **Anticoagulation.** Several conditions require the initiation or maintenance of anticoagulation during pregnancy, and the three most common agents considered during pregnancy are unfractionated heparin (UFH), low molecular weight heparin (LMWH), and warfarin. Anticoagulation choice depends on patient and physician preferences after consideration of the maternal and fetal risks.
  - **Warfarin**, a vitamin K antagonist, freely crosses the placenta and can harm the fetus. The incidence of warfarin embryopathy (abnormalities of fetal bone and cartilage formation) has been estimated at 4% to 10%; the risk is highest when warfarin is administered during the 6th through 12th weeks' gestation. Clinically important embryopathy may be lower if the warfarin dose is ≤5 mg/day. Fetal central nervous system (CNS) abnormalities can occur after exposure during any trimester. Warfarin must be discontinued and switched to a heparin compound, several weeks before delivery.
  - **UFH** does not cross the placenta and is safe for the fetus. Its use, however, has been associated with maternal osteoporosis, hemorrhage at the uteroplacental junction, thrombocytopenia (HIT), thrombosis, and a high incidence (12% to 24%) of thromboembolic events with older generation mechanical valves. High doses of UFH are often required to achieve the desired aPTT due to the hypercoagulable

TABLE 15-2 Cardiovascular Drugs in Pregnancy

Drug	Use	Side Effects	Pregnancy Risk Category	Safe During Breast-Feeding
Adenosine	Arrhythmia	None reported	C	No data
Amiodarone	Arrhythmia	IUGR, prematurity, hypothyroidism, neonatal prolonged QT	C/D	Not recommended
ACE inhibitors	HTN	Oligohydramnios, IUGR, PDA, prematurity, renal failure, neonatal hypotension, anemia musculoskeletal abnormalities	C (first trimester), D (second, third)	Not recommended
Beta-blockers (labetolol, metoprolol, propranolol)	HTN, MI, MS, HCM, arrhythmias, hyperthyroidism, Marfan's syndrome	Fetal bradycardia, LBW, hypoglycemia, respiratory depression	C/D	Compatible
Digoxin	Arrhythmia, CHF	LBW, prematurity	C	Compatible
Diltiazem	Myocardial ischemia, tocolysis	Limited data	C	Compatible
Disopyramide	Arrhythmias	Limited data	C	Compatible
Diuretics	HTN, CHF	Uteroplacental hypoperfusion, fetal hypoglycemia, thrombocytopenia, hyponatremia, hypokalemia	C	Compatible
Flecainide	Arrhythmia	Limited data	C	Compatible
Heparin (UFH)	Anticoagulation	Maternal osteoporosis, hemorrhage, thrombocytopenia	C	Compatible

(Continued)

TABLE 15-2 **Cardiovascular Drugs in Pregnancy** *(Continued)*

Drug	Use	Side Effects	Pregnancy Risk Category	Safe During Breast-Feeding
Hydralazine	HTN	None reported	C	Compatible
Lidocaine	Arrhythmia, anesthesia	Neonatal CNS depression	B/C	Compatible
LMWH	Anticoagulation	Hemorrhage	B	Limited data
Nifedipine	HTN, tocolysis	Fetal distress with maternal hypotension	C	Compatible
Nitrates	HTN, MI, pulmonary edema	Limited data	C	No data
Procainamide	Arrhythmia	Limited data	C	Compatible
Propafenone	Arrhythmias	Limited data	C	No data
Quinidine	Arrhythmias	Premature labor, abortion, (minimal oxytocic effect)	C	Compatible
Sodium nitroprusside	HTN, aortic dissection	Fetal thiocyanate toxicity	C	No data
Sotalol	Arrhythmia, HTN	Limited data	B	Compatible
Verapamil	Arrhythmia, HTN, tocolysis	Limited data	C	Compatible
Warfarin	Anticoagulation	Warfarin embryopathy, fetal CNS abnormalities, fetal hemorrhage	X	Compatible

ACE, angiotensin-converting enzyme; CHF, congestive heart failure; CNS, central nervous system; DVT, deep venous thrombosis; HCM, hypertrophic cardiomyopathy; HTN, hypertension; IUGR, intrauterine growth restriction; LBW, low birth weight; LMWH, low molecular weight heparin; MI, myocardial infarction; MS, mitral stenosis; PDA, patent ductus arteriosus; UFH, unfractionated heparin. Adapted from Elkayam U. Pregnancy and cardiovascular disease. In Braunwald E, ed. *Heart Disease. A Textbook of Cardiovascular Medicine*, 6th Ed. Philadelphia, PA: WB Saunders, 2001:2172–2191, with permission.

state associated with pregnancy. Parenteral infusions should be stopped at least 4 hr before cesarean sections. UFH can be reversed with protamine sulfate.

- **LMWH**, in comparison to UFH, produces a more predictable anticoagulant response, is less likely to cause HIT, is easier to administer and monitor, and has lower risk of osteoporosis and bleeding complications. LMWH does not cross the placenta and is safe for the fetus. Antifactor-Xa levels can be checked 4 hr after the morning dose and the dose adjusted to attain antifactor-Xa levels of 0.7 to 1.2 U mL. Although data support the use of LMWH for DVT treatment in pregnant women, there are no data to guide its use in pregnant patients with mechanical valve prostheses.

RESPIRATORY DISORDERS

Pulmonary Changes During Pregnancy

- Pregnancy causes mechanical and biochemical changes that affect maternal respiratory function and gas exchange. The most prominent factors are the mechanical effect of the gravid uterus on the diaphragm and the effect of increased circulating progesterone on ventilation. Progesterone is thought to increase the sensitivity of the respiratory center to carbon dioxide.
- Elevation of the diaphragm in the second half of pregnancy decreases functional residual capacity (FRC), the resting volume of the lungs at the end of a normal expiration. Despite the alteration in resting diaphragm position, excursion is unaffected and therefore vital capacity is maintained. Airway function is normal during pregnancy, as FEV1 (forced expiratory volume in the first second) and FEV1/FVC (forced vital capacity) are normal. Resting minute ventilation increases by 50% due to increased tidal volume of 40%. Both FEV and peak expiratory flow remain unchanged. As a result of increased minute ventilation, arterial PCO_2 decreases, which is offset by renal bicarbonate excretion, and arterial PO_2 levels are slightly increased. Oxygen consumption increases by 15% to 20% throughout pregnancy, which is compensated by the increased cardiac output. Arterial pH rises slightly from the decrease in PCO_2, resulting in a mild maternal respiratory alkalosis.

Specific Respiratory Disorders

Asthma

- **Asthma** is the most common chronic condition in pregnancy and affects 3% to 12% of gestations. Asthma is more likely to deteriorate in women with severe asthma. Exacerbations are most frequent between 24 and 36 weeks' gestation and are most commonly precipitated by viral respiratory infections and noncompliance with inhaled corticosteroid regimens. Low birth weight (LBW) is more common in infants born to mothers reporting daily symptoms of moderate asthma. For women with severe asthma, a pulmonary examination, peak flow measurement, and review of symptoms should be undertaken at each visit. Smoking cessation must be encouraged. In addition, patients may monitor their peak flow at home and begin treatment before they become dangerously symptomatic. Influenza vaccination is recommended for all healthy pregnant patients and pregnant women with high-risk medical conditions.
  - Because asthma exacerbations can be severe, they should be treated aggressively in pregnancy. Pregnant women tend to decrease use of asthma medications because of fear of fetal malformations, but they need reassurance that it is safer to take their

medications in pregnancy than to risk adverse perinatal outcomes from a severe exacerbation. Prostaglandin $F_2\alpha$ for postpartum hemorrhage should be avoided in asthmatics.

- **Inhaled corticosteroids** including beclomethasone, fluticasone, budesonide, flunisolide, and triamcinolone are the cornerstone of treatment for persistent asthma of all severities. They remain active locally with little systemic absorption and effectively prevent exacerbations.
- **Oral steroids** are indicated for acute exacerbations when patients do not respond adequately to other measures. In acute settings, hydrocortisone 100 mg IV every 8 hr or methylprednisolone 125 mg IV every 6 hr may be used, followed by a tapered dose of oral prednisone.
- **Beta-sympathomimetic** drugs help control asthma via bronchial smooth muscle relaxation and can be used for symptomatic relief in conjunction with inhaled corticosteroids. Short-acting preparations are safe in pregnancy. Few data are available on long-acting preparations.
- **Anticholinergics**, such as aerosolized ipratropium bromide or glycopyrrolate, can also be used to treat severe symptoms. Side effects include tachycardia.
- **Cromolyn and leukotriene antagonists** are useful alternatives for mild persistent asthma or additional treatment for more severe exacerbations.
- **Theophylline**, a phosphodiesterase inhibitor, is rarely used in asthma but remains a last treatment option in moderate or severe asthma. Blood levels are required during the third trimester as clearance increases during this period.
- **Acute asthma exacerbations**, that require hospital observation or admission, are treated with 40% humidified oxygen and beta-agonists initially. Chest radiograph should be obtained. Anticholinergics and inhaled or systemic steroids can be added as needed. Intubation should be considered if the PCO_2 is >40 mm Hg or hypoxia develops.
- **Exacerbations during labor** are rare, perhaps because of the increase in endogenous cortisol. Patients who received steroids throughout their pregnancies may require stress-dose steroids during labor and delivery. General endotracheal anesthesia should be avoided, if possible, because of the increased incidence of bronchospasm and atelectasis.

Cystic Fibrosis
- **Cystic fibrosis (CF)** is an autosomal recessive disorder occurring in approximately 1 in 2,500 live births and is characterized by abnormal epithelial cell chloride transport and thickened glandular secretions. Diagnosis is confirmed by elevated sweat chloride concentration with pilocarpine iontophoresis or by mutation analysis of the cystic fibrosis transmembrane conductance regulator (CFTR) gene. Due to improved treatment modalities, women with CF are living longer—the median survival age for women is now 29 years—and they are more frequently reaching childbearing age.
  - Pregnancy does not compromise long-term survival in CF nor does it affect overall severity or maternal survival. Poor prognostic factors include a vital capacity of <50% of predicted value, cor pulmonale, and pulmonary HTN. Affected patients may have pancreatic insufficiency manifested as diabetes, malabsorption, or liver cirrhosis.
  - Genetic counseling and screening should be offered. Pulmonary function tests should be performed monthly throughout pregnancy and pulmonary infection should be managed aggressively. During labor, fluid and electrolytes should be

followed closely. The increased sodium content of sweat in affected patients may make them prone to hypovolemia during labor. Overall, 70% to 80% of pregnant mothers with CF have successful deliveries of healthy infants.

- Breast milk should be evaluated for sodium content before the infant is allowed to breast-feed; in the event of significant sodium elevation, breast-feeding is contraindicated.

Tuberculosis

- **Tuberculosis (TB)** is a worldwide public health issue and highly prevalent in many urban areas.
  - Screening is by subcutaneous injection of purified protein derivative (PPD). Only 80% of results are positive in the setting of reactivation of disease, however, and if a patient previously received the Bacille Calmette-Guérin (BCG) vaccine, the PPD result may remain positive for life. If the PPD test is positive or TB is suspected, chest radiography with abdominal shielding should be performed, preferably after 20 weeks' gestation.
  - A definitive diagnosis of TB can be made with culture of *Mycobacterium tuberculosis* or acid-fast stain. Sputum samples may be induced using aerosolized saline; the first morning sputum should be collected for three consecutive days. If a sputum is positive for acid-fast bacilli, antibiotic therapy should be initiated while final culture and sensitivity results are pending.
  - Standard treatment in pregnancy consists of isoniazid (INH), pyridoxine supplementation, ethambutol, and pyrazinamide. Streptomycin sulfate should be avoided because of the risk of fetal cranial nerve eight damage. Rifampin should also be avoided during pregnancy unless INH and ethambutol cannot be used. INH prophylaxis for 6 to 9 months is recommended for asymptomatic patients under age 35 with positive PPD results and negative findings on chest radiograph.
  - If the patient has converted to positive PPD results within the last 2 years, INH therapy should be initiated during the pregnancy after the first trimester. If the time since conversion is unknown or longer than 2 years, INH is started during the postpartum period. INH prophylaxis is not recommended for patients over age 35 due to its hepatotoxicity. If treated, tuberculosis should not affect the pregnancy, and pregnancy should not alter the course of the disease.

SUGGESTED READINGS

Cunningham FG, Leveno KJ, Bloom SL, et al., eds. Cardiovascular disease (Chapter 44) and Pulmonary disorders (Chapter 46). In *Williams Obstetrics,* 23rd Ed. New York, NY: McGraw-Hill, 2010.

Easterling TR, Stout K. Heart disease (Chapter 34). In Gabbe SG, Niebyl JR, Simpson JL, eds. *Obstetrics: Normal and Problem Pregnancies,* 5th Ed. Philadelphia, PA: Elsevier, 2007.

Whitty JE, Dombrowski MP. Respiratory diseases in pregnancy. In Gabbe SG, Niebyl JR, Simpson JL, eds. *Obstetrics: Normal and Problem Pregnancies,* 5th Ed. Philadelphia, PA: Elsevier, 2007.

Wilson W, Taubert KA, Gewitz M, et al. Prevention of infective endocarditits: guidelines from the American Heart Association. *J Am Dent Assoc* 2007;138:739–760.

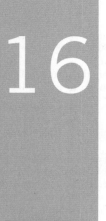

16 Renal Disorders, Gastrointestinal Disorders, and Systemic Lupus Erythematosus in Pregnancy

Hindi Stohl and Teresa Martino

KIDNEY AND URINARY TRACT DISORDERS

Renal Physiology in Pregnancy

- **Structural changes.** During pregnancy, the kidneys increase 1 to 1.5 cm in length and 30% in volume. The collecting system expands more than 80%, with greater dilation on the right side. Mild right-sided hydronephrosis is physiologic as early as 6 weeks' gestation. Renal volume returns to normal within the first week postpartum, but hydronephrosis and hydroureter may not normalize until 3 to 4 months after delivery. Elective pyelography should, therefore, be deferred until at least 12 weeks postpartum.
- **Renal filtration.** Blood volume expansion during pregnancy increases renal plasma flow by 50% to 80%, which in turn results in an increased glomerular filtration rate (GFR). Increased GFR can be seen within one month after conception, peaking at 40% to 50% above prepregnant levels by the end of the first trimester.
  - Elevated GFR increases creatinine clearance, so formulas for GFR based on age, height, and weight do not apply; creatinine clearance is calculated with a 24-hr urine collection in pregnancy.
  - Increased GFR results in lower mean serum blood urea nitrogen (BUN) and serum creatinine during pregnancy (8.5 and 0.46 mg/dL, respectively). A "normal" serum creatinine of 0.9 mg/dL may suggest renal insufficiency in pregnancy.
- **Renal tubular function.** Decreased tubular resorption in pregnancy increases urinary excretion of electrolytes, glucose, amino acids, and protein.
  - Increased calcium clearance is balanced by increased gastrointestinal (GI) tract absorption. Ionized calcium remains stable despite decreased total serum calcium because of the lower serum albumin concentration.
  - Physiologic hyponatremia occurs, with plasma sodium concentration falling by 5 mEq/L during pregnancy. Sodium levels return to baseline by 1 to 2 months postpartum.
  - Urinary excretion of glucose increases 10- to 100-fold, and glucosuria is observed routinely in normal pregnancy. Increased urinary glucose increases the risk of bacteriuria and urinary tract infections (UTIs).

- Renal bicarbonate resorption decreases to compensate for the respiratory alkalosis of pregnancy, lowering serum bicarbonate by about 5 mEq/L in pregnancy.
- **Routine assessment of renal function.** Proteinuria should be assessed at every prenatal visit. A urine dipstick value >1+ should prompt further evaluation by clean-catch urine sample for culture and microscopy. If proteinuria persists with negative culture, a 24-hr urine collection should be obtained. Most gravid patients excrete <260 mg protein/day, and 24-hr total urine protein exceeding 300 mg is abnormal. Serum creatinine persistently >0.9 mg/dL should prompt investigation for intrinsic renal disease. Renal ultrasound, CT pyelogram, or cystoscopy may be appropriate. Renal biopsy is not performed during pregnancy unless the result will change management before delivery.

Urinary Tract Disorders in Pregnancy

Urinary Tract Infection

- **UTIs** are common in pregnancy. Stasis associated with hydroureter and hydronephrosis, bladder trauma with compressed or edematous cystic tissue, vesicoureteral reflux, and increased glucosuria may increase risk. Pregnant women with multiple UTIs or pyelonephritis during pregnancy should receive suppressive therapy.
  - **Asymptomatic bacteriuria (ASB)** is the presence of bacteria within the urinary tract, excluding the distal urethra, without symptoms of infection. ASB is associated with low birth weight and preterm delivery. The prevalence of ASB during pregnancy ranges from 2% to 7%. If left untreated, 20% to 30% of ASB in pregnant women progresses to acute pyelonephritis; treatment reduces this rate to 3%. Screening for bacteriuria is recommended at the first prenatal visit. Women with sickle cell trait have a twofold increased risk of ASB and should be screened every trimester.
    - A clean-catch urine culture with ≥100,000 colonies/mL or catheterized urine culture with ≥100 colonies/mL warrants treatment.
    - *Escherichia coli* accounts for 75% to 90% of infections. *Klebsiella, Proteus, Pseudomonas, Enterobacter* species, and coagulase-negative *Staphylococci* together account for the remainder.
    - Initial therapy is usually empiric, with any of several safe and effective regimens (Table 16-1). Repeat urine culture is obtained 1 to 2 weeks after treatment completion and again each trimester. After a second treatment course, suppressive therapy is prescribed for the remainder of the pregnancy.
  - **Acute cystitis** occurs in approximately 1% to 3% of pregnant women. Symptoms include urinary frequency, urgency, dysuria, hematuria, and suprapubic discomfort. Empiric treatment regimens are the same as for ASB (Table 16-1).
  - **Urethritis** is usually caused by *Chlamydia trachomatis,* and it should be suspected in patients with symptoms of acute cystitis and a negative urine culture. Mucopurulent cervicitis may be present. The treatment of choice is azithromycin 1 g as a single oral dose.

Pyelonephritis

- **Acute pyelonephritis** occurs in approximately 1% to 2% of all pregnancies and is the leading cause of septic shock in pregnancy. Complications include: preterm labor, preterm premature rupture of membranes (PPROM), bacteremia, sepsis, respiratory distress syndrome, and hemolytic anemia. Prompt diagnosis and treatment of pyelonephritis in pregnancy are crucial.
  - Symptoms include high fever, chills, flank pain, nausea, and vomiting. Frequency, urgency, and dysuria are variably present.

TABLE 16-1	Antimicrobial Agents for Treatment of UTI and Asymptomatic Bacteriuria

Single Dose
Amoxicillin, 3 g
Ampicillin, 2 g
Cephalexin, 2 g
Nitrofurantoin, 200 mg
Sulfisoxazole, 2 g
Trimethoprim-sulfamethoxazole, 320/1,600 mg

Short Course (3–7 days)
Amoxicillin, 250–500 mg tid
Ampicillin, 250 mg qid
Cephalexin, 250–500 mg qid
Nitrofurantoin, 100 mg bid
Sulfisoxazole, 1 g then 500 mg qid
Trimethoprim-sulfamethoxazole, 320/1,600 mg bid

Suppression Therapy
Nitrofurantoin, 100 mg qhs
Ampicillin, 250 mg po qd
Trimethoprim-sulfamethoxazole, 160/800 mg qd

- Diagnosis is by clinical findings. Blood and urine cultures, complete blood count (CBC), serum creatinine, and electrolytes should be obtained at admission. Chest x-ray is indicated for dyspnea or tachypnea.
- Treatment includes hospitalization, intravenous (IV) hydration, antipyretics, and broad-spectrum IV antibiotics. Cefazolin, extended-spectrum penicillin, or ampicillin plus gentamicin (clindamycin plus gentamicin for penicillin-allergic patients) are commonly used.
  - Gentamicin is dosed every 8 hr with gentamicin trough monitoring to ensure therapeutic serum levels. Daily dosing is not appropriate due to the pregnancy-related increase in GFR.
  - Transition to an oral regimen after 48 hr afebrile is based on culture sensitivities. Oral therapy is continued to complete a 14-day total antibiotic course. Suppressive therapy (Table 16-1) is then initiated for the remainder of pregnancy due to the recurrence risk of approximately 20%.
  - If there is no response to antibiotic treatment within 72 hr, review dosing and sensitivities and obtain renal ultrasonography to evaluate for anatomic anomalies, nephrolithiasis, and intrarenal or perinephric abscess.

Nephrolithiasis
- **Nephrolithiasis** should be considered in a pregnant patient with suspected UTI and negative urine cultures. The incidence is between 0.3 and 4 per 1,000 pregnancies and is associated with infection and preterm labor.
- Diagnosis is primarily clinical. Classic symptoms include colicky abdominal pain and hematuria. In more than 50% of cases, the stone passes spontaneously after hydration and may be observed directly by filtering the patient's urine. Ultrasonography can assess for obstruction, although detection is hampered by the gravid uterus and

the presence of baseline ureteral dilation during pregnancy. Renal sonogram detects stones in about 60% of cases. Plain abdominal radiography may be helpful since approximately 90% of renal stones are radiopaque. If the patient's clinical symptoms suggest nephrolithiasis despite negative ultrasound and radiographic studies, a limited IV pyelogram, low attenuation CT scan, or ureteroscopy may be diagnostic.
- Initial treatment is with IV hydration and analgesics. Associated infections must be treated aggressively. Indications for surgical intervention include calculus pyelonephritis, impairment of renal function, protracted pain, sepsis, or heavy bleeding. One third of pregnant women with symptomatic stones will require surgical intervention such as stone extraction, ureteral stenting, percutaneous nephrostomy drainage, or surgical exploration. Extracorporeal shock-wave lithotripsy is not recommended in pregnancy.

Glomerulonephritis
- **Glomerulopathies**
  - **Acute glomerulonephritis** is characterized by rapid onset proteinuria, hematuria, and renal insufficiency leading to edema, hypertension, and circulatory congestion. Treatment depends on the etiology, which includes IgA nephropathy, acute poststreptococcal glomerulonephritis, systemic lupus erythematosus (SLE), Henoch-Schonlein purpura, and cryoglobulinemia, to name just a few. Renal biopsy may be necessary for diagnosis. Complications of glomerulonephritis include preterm delivery, intrauterine growth restriction (IUGR), maternal hypertension, and impaired renal function.
  - **Chronic glomerulonephritis** is characterized by progressive worsening of kidney function, with proteinuria and hematuria over years eventually leading to end-stage renal disease.
  - **Rapidly progressive glomerulonephritis** is characterized by rapid progression to end-stage renal failure within weeks to months. Common causes are similar to those for acute glomerulonephritis.
  - **Nephrotic syndrome** is characterized by proteinuria >3 g/day, hypoalbuminemia, hyperlipidemia, and edema. Causes include minimal change disease, membranous glomerulonephritis, focal segmental glomerulosclerosis, amyloidosis, and diabetic nephropathy. Management depends on the etiology. Pregnancies associated with worsening proteinuria, baseline renal insufficiency, or moderate-to-severe hypertension have poorer outcomes. Complications include preterm delivery, preeclampsia/eclampsia, fetal demise, venous and arterial thromboembolism, and disease progression, leading to end-stage renal disease.

Chronic Renal Failure
- **Chronic renal disease** occurs in <0.2% of all pregnancies. The most common causes are diabetes, hypertension, glomerulonephritis, and polycystic kidney disease. The degree of renal impairment is the major determinant of pregnancy outcome and can be categorized as *mild* (serum creatinine <1.5 mg/dL), *moderate* (serum creatinine 1.5 to 3.0 mg/dL), or *severe* (serum creatinine >3.0 mg/dL). In general, patients with mild renal dysfunction experience little disease progression during pregnancy, whereas patients with moderate-to-severe renal insufficiency are at high risk for potentially irreversible loss of renal function. Chronic renal disease with other comorbidity such as hypertension, diabetes, or connective tissue disorder substantially increases both maternal and fetal risks.
  - **Pregnancy complications** with chronic renal disease include perinatal mortality, preeclampsia/eclampsia, preterm birth, and IUGR. Outcome depends on the baseline renal function and presence of comorbidities.

- **Antepartum management** includes the following:
  - Early pregnancy diagnosis and dating. Preconception planning and counseling are encouraged.
  - Baseline laboratory studies including serum creatinine, electrolytes, BUN, 24-hr urine protein and creatinine clearance, urinalysis, and urine culture. Repeat labwork each trimester or when clinically indicated.
  - Antenatal visits every two weeks until 28 to 32 weeks' gestation, then weekly until delivery.
  - Serial ultrasonographic fetal growth examinations every 3 to 4 weeks.
  - Antepartum fetal testing with nonstress test (NST), biophysical profile (BPP), and amniotic fluid index (AFI) starting at 28 weeks for patients with severe disease and as late as 34 weeks for patients with mild disease.

Renal Dialysis

- Pregnancy occurs in 1% to 7% of women on **chronic dialysis**. Up to 50% of these pregnancies result in delivery of a surviving infant. Typically, the infants are born premature, at an average gestational age of 32 weeks. Precipitating factors include polyhydramnios, PPROM, maternal hypertension necessitating premature induction of labor, severe preeclampsia, IUGR, and placental abruption. In some patients, delaying pregnancy until after renal transplantation may be advantageous.
  - Neonatal outcomes are improved with maintenance of the BUN <50 mg/dL on dialysis. Generally, 16 to 20 hr of dialysis a week is necessary. Blood pressure must be controlled, especially during dialysis, to avoid fetoplacental compromise. Electrolytes should be monitored and appropriately corrected for pregnancy. Bicarbonate concentrations, for example, must be managed carefully to avoid dialysis-induced alkalemia. Ultrafiltration goals may be difficult to estimate and should consider fetal and placental growth as well as the plasma volume expansion associated with pregnancy. Continuous fetal monitoring during dialysis after 24 weeks' gestation is recommended to assess fetal tolerance of hemodynamic changes.
  - Anemia is common due to the combined effects of renal failure and pregnancy. Maintain hematocrit above 25% with transfusions and erythropoietin therapy, as needed.

Renal Transplant

- Approximately 1 in 50 women with a **renal transplant** will become pregnant. The incidence of pregnancy after successful renal transplantation is difficult to estimate due to underreporting. The hormonal aberrations associated with end-stage renal disease are usually reversed after kidney transplant, and women often rapidly resume cyclic ovulation and regular menstruation. Pregnancy complications for these patients include increased infections secondary to chronic immunosuppression, preeclampsia, preterm labor, PPROM, IUGR, and low birth weight.
- Management of the transplant patient is a multidisciplinary effort.
  - If the patient requires chronic corticosteroids, she should be screened for gestational diabetes at 20 to 24 weeks and again at 28 to 32 weeks if the initial screen is negative.
  - Antepartum fetal testing should begin by 28 weeks' gestation.
  - Mode of delivery is based on obstetric indications. The pelvic allograft does not obstruct the birth canal in most patients, and vaginal delivery is possible. When cesarean section is indicated, prophylactic antibiotics and careful attention to wound closure are recommended to minimize infectious complications. In addition, knowledge of allograft placement is essential in order to avoid operative

injury, although the transplanted kidney is not usually positioned in an area that is vulnerable, using standard approaches to cesarean section.

LIVER DISORDERS

Hepatic Physiology in Pregnancy

- As the gravid uterus expands into the upper abdomen, the liver is displaced posteriorly and to the right, decreasing its estimated size on physical examination. Treat a palpable liver in pregnancy as abnormal and initiate appropriate workup. Table 16-2 summarizes normal changes in liver function tests during pregnancy.

Hepatic Disorders Unique to Pregnancy

Cholestasis of Pregnancy

- **Intrahepatic cholestasis of pregnancy (ICP)** occurs in about 1 in 1,000 pregnancies in the United States but has significant genetic and geographic variations. Risk factors include a personal or family history of ICP, multiple gestations, and chronic hepatitis C infection. The cause seems to be incomplete bile acid clearance. Complications include preterm labor, meconium ileus, and intrauterine fetal demise. These risks increase progressively with duration, regardless of symptoms. The cause of fetal demise is unknown and rarely happens before term.
  - Initial **diagnosis** is clinical, with confirmation by laboratory testing. The cardinal symptom is pruritis, especially of the palms and soles that worsens at night. Anorexia, malaise, steatorrhea, and dark urine are also common complaints. Jaundice develops in 15% of patients but resolves quickly after delivery. Fever, abdominal pain, hepatosplenomegaly, and stigmata of chronic liver disease are usually absent. Onset is usually late in pregnancy but occasionally occurs in the second trimester.
  - **Differential diagnosis** includes preeclampsia, viral hepatitis, and gallbladder disease.
  - **Laboratory findings** include elevated serum total bile acids, particularly conjugated bile acids and elevated total bilirubin. Serum alkaline phosphatase and transaminase levels are modestly elevated, while serum gamma glutamyl transpeptidase is normal. Serum albumin and prothrombin time are normal.
  - **Treatment** is mainly for symptoms until delivery, which is the definitive therapy. Diphenhydramine, topical emollients, and dexamethasone (12 mg/day for 7 days) can relieve pruritis. Ursodeoxycholic acid (8 to 10 mg/kg/day) or cholestyramine (2 to 4 g 4×/day) is the most effective therapy. They reduce maternal serum bile acids

TABLE 16-2	Liver Function Test Changes During Pregnancy
Alkaline phosphatase	↑
Aminotransferases	↔
Bilirubin	↔
Albumin	↓
Hormone-binding proteins	↑
Lipids	↑
Fibrinogen	↑
PT/aPTT	↔

↑, increased or elevated; ↓, decreased; ↔, unchanged

and decrease pruritus by promoting bile acid excretion. Fat-soluble vitamins (A, D, E, and K) and prothrombin time should be checked periodically for patients taking cholestyramine for extended treatment. If the prothrombin time is elevated, 10 mg/day of oral vitamin K should be administered until the coagulation profile normalizes.

- ICP at term is associated with 3% rate of fetal demise. Antepartum fetal testing is recommended. Delivery should be performed no later than 38 weeks' gestation. When cholestasis is severe, delivery at 36 weeks with or without fetal lung maturity can be considered.
- Recurrence in subsequent pregnancies is approximately 70% and usually more severe. Estrogen-containing oral contraceptives can cause cholestasis in these patients as well.

Acute Fatty Liver of Pregnancy
- **Acute Fatty Liver of Pregnancy (AFLP)** is uncommon, occurring in 1 in 10,000 pregnancies. It typically occurs in primigravid women in the third trimester. It is associated with multiple pregnancies, male fetuses, and with a fetal mitochondrial gene mutation causing long chain 3-hydroxylacyl-CoA-dehydrogenase deficiency. Patients present with nausea, vomiting, epigastric pain, anorexia, jaundice, and malaise. Intra-abdominal bleeding or altered mental status may indicate disease progression to disseminated intravascular coagulation (DIC) or hepatic failure. Laboratory tests may reveal elevated aminotransferases to 1,000 IU/L, leukocytosis, thrombocytopenia, coagulopathy, markedly reduced antithrombin III, hypoglycemia, metabolic acidosis, hyperuricemia, and renal failure. Treatment includes prompt delivery and maternal stabilization with intensive supportive care. Liver function usually normalizes within 1 week postpartum.

Hepatic Disorders Not Directly Related to Pregnancy
Hepatitis
- **Acute and chronic hepatitis**—See Chapter 11.

Cirrhosis
- **Hepatic cirrhosis** leads to metabolic and hormonal derangements that usually induce anovulation, amenorrhea, and infertility. Cirrhosis is associated with 30% to 40% risk of spontaneous abortion, 25% risk of preterm delivery, and up to 18% neonatal mortality. Maternal mortality is estimated at 10% but may be up to 50% in patients with portal hypertension who develop gastrointestinal bleeding during pregnancy. Outcomes are generally poor, but hepatic dysfunction before pregnancy and the presence of portal hypertension correlate with worse maternal/fetal prognosis.
  - Esophageal variceal bleeding is the most common complication, occurring in 18% to 32% of pregnant women with cirrhosis. As in nonpregnant patients, endoscopic variceal ligation is the mainstay of therapy for acute episodes of hemorrhage. Portal decompression shunt placement may also be helpful. Other complications include ascites and bacterial peritonitis, splenic artery aneurysm, portal vein thrombosis, portal vein hypertension, hepatic encephalopathy or coma, postpartum uterine hemorrhage, and death.
  - Vaginal delivery is preferred over cesarean delivery due to the high rate of intraoperative and postoperative complications. In patients with portal hypertension, however, repetitive valsalva in the second stage of labor can increase the risk of significant variceal bleeding. A passive second stage with forceps-assisted delivery may be beneficial.

Budd-Chiari Syndrome

- **Budd-Chiari syndrome** is a veno-occlusive disease of the hepatic vein that increases hepatic sinusoidal pressure and can result in portal hypertension or hepatic necrosis. The disease presents with abdominal pain and the abrupt onset of ascites and hepatomegaly. Cases are often caused by congenital vascular anomalies, myeloproliferative disorders, and thrombophilic disorders. In obstetrics, the disease typically occurs postpartum. Diagnosis is by hepatic Doppler ultrasonography to determine venous occlusion and evaluate the direction and amplitude of blood flow. Acute therapy includes selective thrombolytics and a surgical shunt or transjugular intrahepatic portosystemic shunt (TIPS) for portal hypertension. Chronic Budd-Chiari syndrome is treated with anticoagulation therapy.

Choledochal Cyst

- **Choledochal cysts** are rare, occurring in 1 in 100,000 people. They generally produce abdominal pain, jaundice, and a palpable abdominal mass. Compression by the gravid uterus may lead to cyst rupture, potentially resulting in cholangitis. Surgical management is generally recommended.

GALLBLADDER DISORDERS

Cholelithiasis

- **Cholelithiasis** occurs in up to 10% of pregnancies and is often clinically silent. Biliary stasis from progesterone-induced smooth muscle relaxation and the prolithogenic effect of elevated estrogen levels in pregnancy may predispose to gallstone formation. Symptomatic patients typically complain of vague intermittent right upper quadrant discomfort that occurs with meals. Asymptomatic cholelithiasis requires no treatment during pregnancy.
- **Symptomatic cholelithiasis** and **acute cholecystitis**—See Chapter 19.

OTHER GASTROINTESTINAL DISORDERS

Hyperemesis Gravidarum

- **Hyperemesis gravidarum** is a severe form of nausea and vomiting in pregnancy, characterized by intractable vomiting, dehydration, alkalosis, hypokalemia, and weight loss usually exceeding 5% of prepregnant body weight. It affects 0.3% to 2% of pregnancies and peaks between the 8th and 12th weeks of pregnancy. The etiology may be multifactorial, involving hormonal, neurologic, metabolic, toxic, and psychosocial factors.
  - Nausea (with or without vomiting) occurs in up to 90% of pregnancies at any time of day, despite the general term "morning sickness." Mean onset of symptoms is 5 to 6 weeks' gestation. While symptoms typically abate by 16 to 18 weeks of gestation, they continue into the third trimester in 15% to 20% of pregnant women and until delivery in 5%.
  - With true hyperemesis gravidarum, persistent vomiting leads to plasma volume depletion and elevated hematocrit, and metabolic derangements that include increased BUN, hyponatremia, hypokalemia, hypochloremia, and metabolic alkalosis. A complete workup includes pelvic sonogram for multiple gestation and molar pregnancy and thyroid function tests to evaluate hyperthyroidism. Some patients with hyperemesis gravidarum have transient benign hyperthyroidism, which usually resolves spontaneously as pregnancy continues.

- **Treatment** depends upon the severity of symptoms. Usually, IV hydration and antiemetic therapy are sufficient. Patients may require hospitalization for intractable emesis, electrolyte abnormalities, and severe hypovolemia. In severe cases requiring prolonged IV hydration, parenteral nutrition may be initiated. Thiamine supplementation (100 mg qd intramuscularly or intravenously) is given prior to administration of glucose to prevent Wernicke encephalopathy. Oral feeding with a bland diet should be introduced slowly as tolerated. If symptoms are refractory to medical and supportive care, a psychiatry consultation may be considered.
  - There are no drugs approved specifically for the treatment of nausea and vomiting in pregnancy; however, the following medications have been clinically effective:
    - Pyridoxine (vitamin B_6) 10 to 25 mg PO three times daily.
    - Doxylamine succinate 12.5 mg PO three times daily taken with pyridoxine 10 to 50 mg.
    - Metoclopramide hydrochloride (Reglan) 5 to 10 mg PO or IV three times daily.
    - Promethazine hydrochloride (Phenergan) 12.5 to 25 mg PO four times daily.
    - Prochlorperazine (Compazine) 10 to 50 mg PO, IV, or IM three or four times daily.
    - Ondansetron hydrochloride (Zofran) 4 to 8 mg PO three times daily.
    - Methylprednisolone (Medrol) 16 mg PO or IV every 8 hr for 3 days may be used for refractory cases after 10 weeks' gestation. There is a theoretical risk of cleft lip and palate when administered in the early to mid first trimester.

Acid Reflux

- **Gastroesophageal reflux disease (GERD)** and the resulting symptom of "heartburn" are very common during pregnancy. The incidence is 30% to 50% but may approach 80% in selected populations. Symptoms begin late in the first trimester and become more frequent and severe with increasing gestational age. Risk factors include multiparity and history of GERD before pregnancy.
  - **Treatment** is medical and aimed at neutralizing or decreasing reflux. Lifestyle modification is key in treating mild disease. Elevating the head of the bed at night, avoiding meals within 3 hr of bedtime, and consuming smaller but more frequent meals can help. Dietary modification is recommended, including reduced consumption of fatty foods, chocolate, and caffeine. Cigarette smoking and alcohol consumption can exacerbate GERD and are discouraged in all patients.
    - More persistent symptoms can be treated with over-the-counter antacids (e.g., calcium carbonate) or sucralfate 1 g PO tid. An H_2 blocker, such as cimetidine or ranitidine, may be prescribed. Proton pump inhibitors (e.g., omeprazole) and promotility agents (e.g., metoclopramide) are generally effective and may be used if necessary. Endoscopy is considered if therapeutic measures are unsuccessful and symptoms are very severe.

Peptic Ulcer Disease

- **Peptic ulcer disease (PUD)** is not common in pregnancy, and the hormonal changes of pregnancy usually decrease PUD severity and symptoms.
  - **Treatment** during pregnancy is similar to treatment for GERD and consists of diet modification, avoiding nonsteroidal anti-inflammatory drugs (NSAIDs), and starting H_2 blockers or proton pump inhibitors. Avoid indomethacin for tocolysis of patients with PUD. Diagnosis of *Helicobacter pylori* infection is usually reserved for those with active ulcers; treatment regimens for *H. pylori* without tetracycline are selected.

Inflammatory Bowel Disease

- **Inflammatory Bowel Disease (IBD),** including **ulcerative colitis** and **Crohn's disease,** often presents in reproductive age women. IBD increases the risk for preterm birth, low birth weight, and IUGR. Disease activity at conception seems to correlate with disease activity during pregnancy.
  - **Treatment** is largely pharmacologic, usually with sulfasalazine and corticosteroids. Because sulfasalazine may interfere with the folate absorption, supplemental folate should be prescribed. Corticosteroids are secreted in breast milk, and therefore, breast-feeding should be delayed several hours after taking the medication. Immunosuppressive agents, such as azathioprine, 6-mercaptopurine, cyclosporine, or infliximab, are used for more severe disease. Limited experience shows that all these medications are safe during pregnancy. Methotrexate and mycophenylate are not used in pregnancy. Antibiotics, particularly metronidazole and cephalosporins, are used for perirectal abscesses/fistulae. There is limited data regarding the safety of antidiarrheal medications such as Kaopectate, Lomotil, and Imodium in pregnancy but significant teratogenicity is unlikely. Surgical intervention is indicated only for severe complications of IBD.
  - The **mode of delivery** may be affected by IBD. Vaginal delivery can usually be attempted unless there is severe perineal disease. Crohn's disease may cause perineal scarring, which can make vaginal delivery difficult. Cesarean section should be considered in patients with active perianal disease due to the risk of wound complications and fistulae formation.

Pancreatitis

- **Pancreatitis** is an uncommon cause of abdominal pain in pregnancy, with an incidence of 1 in 1,000 to 1 in 3,800 pregnancies.
  - The **presentation** is usually midepigastric or left upper quadrant pain with radiation to the back, nausea, vomiting, ileus, and low-grade fever. Cholelithiasis is the most common cause of pancreatitis during pregnancy. Ultrasound is of limited use for acute pancreatitis in pregnancy because of the enlarged uterus and overlying bowel gas.
  - **Management** consists of IV hydration, analgesics, and bowel rest. Most cases of gallstone pancreatitis can be managed medically. See Chapter 19 for surgical management.

Appendicitis

- **Appendicitis**—See Chapter 19.

SYSTEMIC LUPUS ERYTHEMATOSUS

SLE is a multisystem autoimmune disease with a complex etiology resulting from interactions between genetic and environmental factors. The incidence of SLE in pregnancy is about 1 in 1,250. African-American women have fivefold higher risk than Caucasians.

- Pregnancy does not appear to alter the long-term prognosis of most SLE patients. Ideally, patients with known SLE should not attempt pregnancy unless their disease has been well controlled for at least 6 months. Only about one third of lupus patients will have worsening disease and a "flare" during pregnancy, but it can be severe. Patients with SLE have increased risk of spontaneous abortion, premature birth, IUGR, fetal death, cesarean delivery, and preeclampsia. The risk of preeclampsia in SLE patients is higher in patients with a history of antiphospholipid antibodies, renal disease, hypertension, or diabetes.

- **Diagnosis** is based on history, physical examination, and laboratory tests. SLE should be considered in any pregnant woman with a photosensitive rash, polyarthritis, undiagnosed proteinuria, false-positive syphilis screening test, or multiple spontaneous abortions. Positive laboratory findings include positive antinuclear antibody (ANA) titer higher than 1:160, elevated anti-SS-A (Ro) and anti-SS-B (La) antibody titers, decreased C3 and C4 complement levels, positive lupus anticoagulant test, and elevated anticardiolipin or anti–double-stranded DNA (dsDNA) antibody titers.
- **Management** of pregnancy with SLE consists of the following:
  - **First trimester.** Initial laboratory studies include CBC, serum creatinine, urinalysis, 24-hr urine collection for protein and creatinine, and a lupus panel (i.e., ANA, anti-Ro and anti-La antibody titers, lupus anticoagulant levels, anticardiolipin antibody, anti-dsDNA antibody titers, CH50, and C3/C4 complement levels). Evaluate for lupus flare at each visit.
  - **Second trimester.** Repeat laboratory studies including CBC, serum creatinine, microscopic urinalysis, and 24-hr urine protein and creatinine. Obstetric ultrasonography should be performed every 4 weeks after 20 weeks' gestation to monitor fetal growth. In women with anti-Ro or anti-La antibodies, M-mode fetal echocardiography should begin at 16 to 18 weeks' gestation, repeated weekly to assess for possible heart block.
  - **Third trimester.** Fetal testing with weekly NST and/or BPP may be initiated as early as 28 weeks depending on the clinical scenario (see Chapter 6). In the presence of IUGR, fetal Doppler ultrasonographic studies should be performed. Betamethasone or dexamethasone should be administered to patients with poor fetal testing results or worsening maternal disease before 34 weeks in case there is early delivery.
  - **Postpartum.** Repeat first trimester labs (above), perform usual obstetric evaluation, and recommend continued follow-up with a rheumatologist.
- Pharmacological treatment is with NSAIDS, immunosuppressants, and antimalarials.
  - Because of the risk of premature closure of the ductus arteriosus and oligohydramnios after 24 weeks, NSAIDS are usually limited to low-dose aspirin (81 mg PO daily).
  - Immunosuppressive agents such as corticosteroids and azathioprine are used for patients with significant end-organ involvement. Mycophenylate and methotrexate are avoided.
  - Antimalarial drugs can control dermatologic disease. Hydroxychloroquine can be safely continued in pregnancy if needed.
  - Antihypertensive agents are used as needed for blood pressure control (see Chapter 14).
- The presence of antiphospholipid antibodies or lupus anticoagulant is associated with fetal death, particularly in the second trimester. Low-dose aspirin and moderate-dose heparin (unfractionated or low molecular weight) improve fetal outcome but with more maternal complications. Anticoagulation for women with thromboembolic events is continued for approximately 3 to 6 months postpartum.

Lupus Flare
- **Lupus flares** are diagnosed clinically. Patients present with fever, malaise, arthritis, rash, or lymphadenopathy. Laboratory findings include low C3 or C4 complement levels, active sediment on urine microscopy (i.e., cellular casts or more than 20 RBCs or WBCs per high-power field), elevated anti-dsDNA antibody titer, hemolytic anemia, thrombocytopenia, and leukopenia.

- Distinguishing a lupus flare from preeclampsia can be challenging. Factors that are *not* helpful include the level of proteinuria, thrombocytopenia, hypertension, or hyperuricemia. Factors that *are* useful include the following: complement levels, which are low in lupus flare and usually normal in preeclampsia; serum transaminase levels, which are generally normal in a lupus flare but may be elevated in preeclampsia; the presence of red blood cell casts on urinalysis implies active lupus; and very gradual onset of proteinuria, which is characteristic of lupus renal flare. If differentiating between preeclampsia and a lupus flare is crucial for further management, renal biopsy may be performed.
- **Treatment** of lupus flare during pregnancy includes corticosteroids. Either prednisone 60 mg PO daily for 2 to 3 weeks then tapered to the lowest maintenance dose, or pulse dose methylprednisolone 1,000 mg IV daily for three days followed by taper are options depending on severity and presentation. Monitor closely for glucose intolerance, hypertension, preeclampsia, and fetal compromise.

Neonatal Lupus

- **Neonatal lupus syndrome** is rare, characterized by skin, hematologic, and other systemic lupus lesions, and sometimes by congenital heart block appearing up to a month after birth. It usually presents only in infants of mothers with anti-Ro (SS-A) or anti-La (SS-B) antibodies. Subsequent pregnancies carry up to 25% recurrence risk. Although no antepartum treatment is proven to reverse fetal heart block, maternal dexamethasone treatment may be beneficial.

SUGGESTED READINGS

Boffa MC, Lachassinne E, Boinot C, et al. European registry of babies born to mothers with antiphospholipid syndrome: a result update. *Lupus* 2009;18(10):900–904.

Clowse ME, Magder LS, Witter F, et al. The impact of increased lupus activity on obstetric outcomes. *Arthritis Rheum* 2005;52(2):514–521.

Cunningham FG, Cox SM, Harstad TW, et al. Chronic renal disease and pregnancy outcome. *Am J Obstet Gynecol* 1990;163:453–459.

Dietrich CS III, Hill CC, Hueman M. Surgical diseases presenting in pregnancy. *Surg Clin North Am* 2008;88(2):403–419; vii–viii.

Goodwin TM. Hyperemesis gravidarum. *Obstet Gynecol Clin North Am* 2008;35(3):401–417; viii, Review.

Hay JE. Liver disease in pregnancy. *Hepatology* 2008;47(3):1067–1076.

Macejko AM, Schaeffer AJ. Asymptomatic bacteriuria and symptomatic urinary tract infections during pregnancy. *Urol Clin North Am* 2007;34(1):35–42.

Petri M. The Hopkins Lupus Pregnancy Center: ten key issues in management. *Rheum Dis Clin North Am* 2007;33(2):227–235; v, Review.

Vidaeff AC, Yeomans ER, Ramin SM. Pregnancy in women with renal disease. Part I: general principles. *Am J Perinatol* 2008;25(7):385–397.

Vidaeff AC, Yeomans ER, Ramin SM. Pregnancy in women with renal disease. Part II: specific underlying renal conditions. *Am J Perinatol* 2008;25(7):399–405.

17 Hematologic Disorders of Pregnancy

Sherrine A. Ibrahim and Linda M. Szymanski

ANEMIA

The Centers for Disease Control and Prevention's **definition of anemia** is hemoglobin (Hgb) or hematocrit (Hct) value less than the fifth percentile in a healthy reference population at the same stage of pregnancy. Typical values include Hgb <11.0 g/dL in the first and third trimesters and <10.5 in the second trimester (Fig. 17-1). Racial differences have been noted, with lower Hgb and Hct levels seen in African-American women compared with white women. The Institute of Medicine suggests lowering the value for Hgb by 0.8 g/dL and hematocrit by 2% in African Americans.

Diagnoses for Anemia
- Anemia is commonly classified by mean red blood cell volume (MCV) as normocytic, microcytic, and macrocytic (Table 17-1).

Physiologic Anemia of Pregnancy
- **Physiologic anemia of pregnancy** occurs because plasma volume increases more during pregnancy (25% to 50%) than red blood cell mass (10% to 25%), causing hemodilution and reduction in hematocrit of 3% to 5%. These changes begin at approximately 6 weeks' gestation and normalize by 6 weeks postpartum.

Iron-deficiency Anemia
- **Iron deficiency anemia** is the most common anemia diagnosed during pregnancy, accounting for nearly 50% to 75% of all cases.
  - **Diagnosis** is based on the slow onset of symptoms, such as weakness and lethargy, and in severe cases, glossitis, stomatitis, koilonychia (in which the outer surfaces of the nails are concave), pica, impaired thermogenesis, and gastritis.
  - **Laboratory findings.** If a microcytic anemia is present, iron studies are indicated (Table 17-2). Measurement of serum ferritin levels has the greatest sensitivity and specificity for the diagnosis of iron deficiency. Serum ferritin levels <10 to 15 ng/mL (or μg/L) generally indicate iron deficiency anemia. A typical diagnostic cutoff is <12 ng/mL.
  - **Treatment.** Although it is important for pregnant women to maintain healthy iron levels, insufficient data exist regarding the benefits of iron supplementation for anemia prophylaxis and treatment during pregnancy. The CDC currently recommends daily elemental iron supplementation (30 mg) for prophylaxis and 60 to 120 mg of daily elemental iron if iron deficiency anemia has been diagnosed. A 325 mg tablet of ferrous sulfate contains 65 mg elemental iron; a 300 mg tablet of ferrous gluconate contains 34 mg elemental iron. ACOG guidelines recommend supplemental iron for women with iron deficiency anemia. For patients who do not respond to or cannot tolerate oral therapy, or for those with severe anemia, intravenous (IV) iron is an alternative. In women with Hgb <6 g/dL, fetal well-being may be compromised secondary to abnormal fetal oxygenation, and maternal transfusion may be indicated.

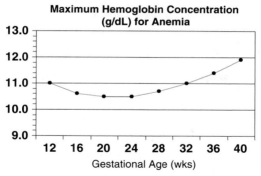

Figure 17-1. Cutoff values for anemia, defined as a hemoglobin level below the fifth percentile based on values from pregnant women with adequate iron supplementation. (Data adapted from Centers for Disease Control and Prevention; *MMWR* 1998; 47 [No. RR-3].)

Hemoglobinopathies

- **Hemoglobinopathies** are genetic abnormalities in the globin portion of the hemoglobin molecule (HbA) that can be either qualitative, resulting in structural abnormalities like sickle cell anemia, or quantitative, resulting in a decreased number of normal globin chains as in the thalassemias. Normal hemoglobin is comprised of 96% to 97% HbA, 2% to 3% HbA2, and <1% HbF.

Sickle Cell Disease

- **Sickle cell disease (SCD)** describes a group of hemoglobinopathies that involve sickle hemoglobin (HbS), including SCD (often called "sickle cell anemia"), sickle cell–hemoglobin C (HbSC), and sickle-thalassemia hemoglobin (HbS-Thal). Homozygosity for HbS (HbSS) is the most common phenotype, occurring primarily among

TABLE 17-1	Classification of Anemia by Mean Corpuscular Volume	
Microcytic (MCV <80 fL)	**Normocytic (MCV 80–100 fL)**	**Macrocytic (MCV >100 fL)**
Iron deficiency	Early iron deficiency	Vitamin B_{12} deficiency
Thalassemias	Acute blood loss	Folic acid deficiency
Anemia of chronic disease (late)	Sickle cell disease	Drug induced (zidovudine)
Sideroblastic anemia	Anemia of chronic disease	Ethanol abuse
Lead poisoning	Infection (osteomyelitis, HIV, mycoplasma, EBV)	Liver disease
Copper deficiency	Bone marrow disease	Myelodysplastic syndromes
	Chronic renal insufficiency	
	Hypothyroidism	
	Autoimmune hemolytic anemia	

MCV, mean corpuscular volume. Adapted from Anemia in Pregnancy. Practice Bulletin Number 95. American College of Obstetricians and Gynecologists. *Obstet Gynecol* 2008;112:201–207.

TABLE 17-2	Laboratory Studies in Various Anemias		
Type of Anemia	Serum Iron	Serum Ferritin	Total Iron Binding Capacity (TIBC)
Iron deficiency anemia	↓	↓	↑
Anemia of chronic disease	↓	↑ ↔	↓ ↔
Sideroblastic anemia	↑	↑	↓
Thalassemia	↔ to ↑	↔ to ↑	↔ to ↑

Adapted from Anemia in Pregnancy. Practice Bulletin Number 95. American College of Obstetricians and Gynecologists. *Obstet Gynecol* 2008;112:201–207.

people from sub-Saharan Africa, South and Central America, Saudi Arabia, India, and Mediterranean countries. Approximately 1 in every 500 to 600 African-American newborns have SCD, an autosomal recessive disorder. Affected patients may experience hemolytic anemia, recurrent pain crises, infection, and infarction of more than one organ system. Hgb S results from a single substitution of valine for glutamic acid at the sixth position of the beta (β)-globin chain. When deoxygenated, HbS is less soluble and tends to polymerize into rigid aggregates and distort into a sickle shape. These cells undergo extravascular hemolysis, leading to a severe chronic anemia, and may become trapped in the microvasculature, causing vascular obstruction, ischemia, and infarction. This cascade results in a vaso-occlusive crisis, which can be associated with severe pain, fever, organ dysfunction, and tissue necrosis. Vaso-occlusive crises may be triggered by infection, hypoxia, acidosis, dehydration, or psychological stress. A serious complication is acute chest syndrome, one of the leading causes of hospitalization and death in patients with SCD. Acute chest syndrome is characterized by a combination of respiratory symptoms, new lung infiltrates, and fever.

- **Diagnosis.** The anemia is normocytic, normochromic with a hemoglobin concentration of 6 to 10 g/dL and hematocrit of 18% to 30%. The reticulocyte count is increased to 3% to 15%. Lactate dehydrogenase is elevated, and haptoglobin is decreased. The peripheral blood smear may show sickle cells, target cells, and Howell-Jolly bodies. Diagnosis is confirmed by hemoglobin electrophoresis, which typically shows 85% to 100% HbS, absent HbA, normal HbA2, and moderately elevated HbF (usually <15%). Jaundice may result from RBC destruction, leading to unconjugated hyperbilirubinemia.
- **Treatment.** Hydroxyurea may be used to reduce intracellular sickling but is not recommended in pregnancy because it is teratogenic in animal studies. Infections are treated aggressively with antibiotics. Severe anemia is treated with blood transfusion. Pain crises are managed with oxygen, hydration, and analgesia. Controversy surrounds prophylactic exchange transfusion and is reserved for the most severe cases. Additionally, the risks involved with transfusions must be taken into account. Advantages of transfusion are an increase in HbA level, which improves oxygen-carrying capacity and a decrease in HbS-carrying erythrocytes. If a transfusion is given, leukocyte-depleted packed red cells, phenotyped for major and minor antigens, should be used.
- **Pregnancy considerations.** Patients with SCD are at increased risk for sickling during pregnancy because of increased metabolic requirements, vascular stasis, and a relative hypercoagulable state. Common complications during pregnancy in

women with SCD include spontaneous abortion, intrauterine growth restriction (IUGR), increased rate of fetal death in utero, low birth weight, preeclampsia, and premature birth. Women with SCD also experience greater risk of urinary tract infection (UTI), bacteriuria, pulmonary infections and infarction, and, possibly, more painful crises. Women with SCD should receive the pneumococcal vaccine before pregnancy and folate supplementation of 1 to 4 mg/day. Iron supplements should be prescribed only if iron is deficient. The intensity of fetal surveillance varies according to the clinical severity of the disease. In advanced cases, twice weekly assessment of fetal well-being should begin at 32 weeks' gestation, and monthly sonography should be performed to evaluate fetal growth. All African-American patients should undergo a hemoglobin electrophoresis to assess carrier status. If both the patient and the father of the baby are found to be hemoglobinopathy carriers, genetic counseling is indicated. Amniocentesis or chorionic villus sampling (CVS) may be offered for prenatal diagnosis. After delivery, patients should practice early ambulation and wear thromboembolic deterrent stockings to prevent thromboembolism.

- No well-controlled studies have evaluated oral contraceptives in SCD; however, low-dose combined contraceptives appear to be a good choice in some women with SCD. Use of intrauterine devices (IUD) is debated due to a potential for increased infection or increased blood loss with the copper IUD; however, benefits generally outweigh the risks. Progestin-only pills, depot medroxyprogesterone, and barrier devices are also recommended for contraception. Medroxyprogesterone acetate (Depo-Provera) injections may decrease the number of pain crises.

Sickle Trait

- **Sickle cell trait (HbAS)** is common in African Americans (1 in 12, or 8%) and is also prevalent in persons of Mediterranean, Middle Eastern, Indian, Caribbean, and Central and South American descents. Women with sickle cell trait have double the frequency of UTI, especially during pregnancy, and should be screened each trimester. No direct fetal compromise exists from maternal sickle cell trait. Partners should be screened because the risk of having a child with SCD becomes one in four if the father is also a carrier.

Thalassemias

- The term **thalassemia** encompasses a group of inherited blood disorders that can cause severe microcytic hypochromic anemia. Alpha (α)-thalassemia and Beta (β)-thalassemia result from absent or decreased production of structurally normal α- and β-globulin chains, respectively, generating an abnormal ratio of α to non-α chains (see Table 17-3). The excess chains form aggregates that lead to ineffective erythropoiesis and/or hemolysis. A broad spectrum of syndromes is possible, ranging from no symptoms to transfusion-dependent anemia and death. Both diseases are transmitted as autosomal recessive traits.
- **Alpha-thalassemia** is associated with Southeast Asian, African, Caribbean, and Mediterranean origin and results from a deletion of one to all α genes, located on chromosome 16. Excess β globins then form β-globin tetramers called Hb H. A fetus would be affected because fetal Hb also requires α chains.
- **Beta-thalassemia** is associated with Mediterranean, Asian, Middle Eastern, Caribbean, and Hispanic origin. More than 200 alterations (mostly point mutations) in β-globin genes, located on chromosome 11, have been reported. The two consequences of these gene defects are the following: β^0, which is the complete absence of the β chain; and β^+, which is decreased synthesis of the β chain.

TABLE 17-3 Findings in Thalassemia

	Genotype[a]	Lab/Clinical Findings	Specifics
Alpha Thalassemias			
Silent carrier	– α/α α	Normal or slight microcytosis.	Asymptomatic. 25%–30% of African Americans.
α-Thalassemia trait	– –/α α (Asian) – α/– α (African)	Mild microcytic, hypochromic. Normal hbg electrophoresis.	Asymptomatic anemia not treatable with iron. Both genotypes identical clinically; position of deleted genes determines severity in offspring (– –/α α at risk of fetus with HbH or hydrops).
HbH disease	– –/– α	Moderate-severe microcytic, hypochromic anemia (Hb 8–10 g/dL). ↑ reticulocytes (5%–10%). HbH= 2%–40%; ↓ HbA2, HbF normal. Normal serum iron. Heinz bodies on peripheral smear. Splenomegaly, bony abnormalities.	Anemia worsens during pregnancy, infection, and with oxidant drugs. Treat with long-term transfusion, splenectomy, and iron chelation. May have cholelithiasis.
Hydrops fetalis "Hb Bart's Disease"	– –/– –	Marked anemia (Hb 3–10), ↑ nucleated erythrocytes, 80%–90% Hb Bart's; 10%–20% HbH. No HbA. Hydrops, heart failure, pulmonary edema, transverse limb reduction defects, hypospadias.	Diagnosis often made in pregnancy by sonogram noting hydropic fetus. Usually results in death. Survival possible with intrauterine transfusion.
Beta Thalassemias			
β-Thalassemia minor	β⁰/β	Asymptomatic or mild microcytic anemia (Hb 8–10 g/dL). ↑ HbA2, ↑HbF, ↓HbA.	Heterozygous. Confers resistance to falciparum malaria. Often misdiagnosed as iron deficient.
"β-Thalassemia trait"	β⁺/β	Mild or no anemia. Basophilic stippling. ↔ ↑ erythrocytes. No splenomegaly, MCV 60 to normal.	
β-Thalassemia intermedia	Varies, 2 β mutations (at least 1 mild)	Mild-moderate anemia. Prominent splenomegaly, bony deformities, growth retardation, iron overload.	Clinical diagnosis. May be asymptomatic to severely symptomatic. Present with symptoms later in life. Chronic transfusions not required.

(Continued)

| TABLE 17-3 | Findings in Thalassemia *(Continued)* | | |

	Genotype[a]	Lab/Clinical Findings	Specifics
Beta Thalassemias *(continued)*			
Thalassemia major "Cooley's anemia"	β^0/β^0	Hb as low as 2–3 g/dL. MCV <67 fL. ↓ reticulocytes. ↑↑ HbF, variable HbA2, no Hb A	Homozygous. Severity depends on amount of globin produced (β^0/β^0 more severe— no globin.) Manifests at age 6–9 months when HbF changes to HbA. With transfusions and chelation, may survive into 3rd–5th decade. Die young from infectious or cardiac complications.
	β^+/β^+	↑ HbF, ↓ HbA, variable HbA2 Splenomegaly; bone changes (increased hematopoiesis), severe iron overload.	

[a]Genotype: β and δ—single gene per chromosome. α gene is duplicated producing two genes per haploid and four per diploid. Adapted from Hemoglobinopathies in pregnancy. ACOG Practice Bulletin Number 78. American College of Obstetricians and Gynecologists. *Obstet Gynecol* 2007;109: 229–237.

- **Diagnosis.** Thalassemia is usually microcytic and hypochromic with a MCV of <80 fL, similar to iron deficiency anemia but with important differences in clinical presentation and laboratory testing.
- **Laboratory findings.** In general, thalassemias, especially the traits, are often misdiagnosed as iron deficiency anemia. However, the anemia is not corrected with iron. A microcytic anemia in the absence of iron deficiency suggests thalassemia and additional testing including electrophoresis and iron studies are warranted. Suspicion for the presence of α-thalassemia is raised by the finding of microcytosis and a normal RDW with minimal or no anemia in the absence of iron deficiency or β-thalassemia. Pedigree studies are often helpful during workup of patients with α-thalassemia. Molecular genetic testing, such as quantitative PCR, is needed for diagnosis. Quantitative hemoglobin electrophoresis is required for the diagnosis of β-thalassemia and should be suspected in cases of elevated HbA2 (>3.5%).
- **Pregnancy and thalassemia.**
  - Women with trait status for either thalassemia require no special care.
  - Women at high risk for or diagnosed with thalassemia should be offered preconception counseling and information about the availability of prenatal diagnosis. First-trimester, DNA-based prenatal testing (CVS) is available if both members of the couple are carriers. Preimplantation genetic diagnosis may also be an option for affected parents.
  - Women with HbH may have successful pregnancies, with maternal outcome related to the severity of her anemia.
  - Pregnancy may exacerbate the anemia, necessitating transfusions, and place women at an increased risk for pre-eclampsia, congestive heart failure, and premature delivery.

- Information on pregnancy in women with β-thalassemia major or intermedia is more limited, although successful pregnancies have been reported. These women require close medical evaluation and follow-up.
- If asplenic, vaccinations need to be up-to-date.
- Thalassemia may confer an increased risk of neural tube defects secondary to folic acid deficiency, so up to 4 mg/day periconceptual folic acid supplementation is recommended. Iron supplements should be prescribed only if iron deficiency is present; otherwise, iron overload can result.
- **Antepartum fetal testing** should be undertaken in anemic thalassemia patients.
  - Periodic fetal sonography to assess fetal growth as well as nonstress testing to evaluate fetal well-being is recommended.
  - Ultrasonography is also useful to detect hydrops fetalis but usually at a later gestational age. Options are also becoming available for affected fetuses. Intrauterine blood transfusions have shown good success in fetuses with hydrops fetalis.

Megaloblastic Anemia

- **Megaloblastic anemia** is the result of impaired DNA synthesis, leading to ineffective erythropoiesis.
  - Megaloblastic anemia is a much greater problem in underdeveloped countries and is primarily the result of dietary folic acid deficiency. Folic acid requirements increase from 50 μg/day in the nonpregnant state to up to 800 μg/day during pregnancy. Phenytoin, nitrofurantoin, trimethoprim, and alcohol decrease absorption of folic acid.
  - A less common cause of megaloblastic anemia is vitamin B_{12} deficiency, often from a long-term vegetarian diet or decreased intestinal absorption due to tropical sprue, regional enteritis, GI resection for bariatric surgery, or chronic giardiasis.
  - Megaloblastic anemia in pregnancy may lead to poor outcomes. Animal studies suggest that it may be related to abruptio placentae, preeclampsia, IUGR, and prematurity. Folic acid deficiency is also linked to open neural tube defects.
- **Diagnosis.** Megaloblastic anemia is often slowly progressive and tends to occur in the third trimester. Weight loss and anorexia may occur in addition to the usual symptoms of anemia, roughness of the skin, and glossitis. It can also manifest as bleeding due to thrombocytopenia or as an infection resulting from leukopenia.
- **Laboratory findings**:
  - Macrocytic, normochromic anemia involving erythrocytes, leukocytes, and platelets.
  - Peripheral blood smear shows hypersegmented neutrophils, oval macrocytes, and Howell-Jolly bodies.
  - To diagnose folate deficiency, consider the erythrocyte folate level as it is a better indicator of whole body stores than the serum level that can vary widely.
- **Treatment.** Determining which deficiency exists is important before treatment.
  - Folate deficiency is generally treated with daily folic acid supplementation of 1 mg/day. Within 7 to 10 days, the white blood cell and platelet counts should return to normal. Hemoglobin gradually increases to normal levels after several weeks of therapy.
  - If the anemia is due to vitamin B_{12} deficiency, folate supplementation may ameliorate the anemia, masking the B_{12} deficiency; it may also precipitate neurologic deficits. Vitamin B_{12} deficiency is treated with intramuscular cobalamin. Affected patients may require monthly (1 mg) injections for life.

THROMBOCYTOPENIA

Thrombocytopenia is defined as a platelet count <150,000/μL, and occurs in about 10% of pregnancies. Clinical signs, such as petechiae, easy bruising, epistaxis, gingival bleeding, and hematuria, are usually not seen until platelets are <50,000/μL. Counts below 50,000/μL may also increase surgical bleeding. The risk of spontaneous bleeding increases only when platelet counts fall below 20,000/μL, and significant bleeding may occur with platelet counts <10,000/μL. Thrombocytopenia, depending on the severity and etiology, may or may not be associated with serious maternal and/or fetal morbidity and mortality. Many conditions can cause thrombocytopenia during pregnancy.

Gestational Thrombocytopenia

- **Gestational thrombocytopenia,** also referred to as incidental thrombocytopenia of pregnancy or essential thrombocytopenia, affects up to 8% of pregnancies and represents the most common diagnosis in over 75% of cases of mild thrombocytopenia during pregnancy. It generally occurs late in gestation and is not associated with fetal thrombocytopenia. The decreased platelet count is likely due to hemodilution and increased physiologic platelet turnover. Platelet counts usually return to normal within 2 to 12 weeks after delivery. Gestational thrombocytopenia can recur in subsequent pregnancies, though the recurrence rate is unknown.
  - **Diagnosis.** Gestational thrombocytopenia is a diagnosis of exclusion; therefore, the first step is to take a careful history to rule out other causes. Platelet counts obtained before pregnancy should be reviewed and any laboratory data available from prior pregnancies.
    - Three criteria should be present: (a) mild thrombocytopenia (70,000 to 150,000/μL), with 2/3 between 130,000 and 150,000/μL; (b) no previous history of thrombocytopenia, except during pregnancy; and (c) no bleeding symptoms.
    - There are no specific diagnostic tests to distinguish gestational thrombocytopenia from mild idiopathic thrombocytopenic purpura (ITP). In fact, many women with gestational thrombocytopenia have platelet-associated IgG and serum antiplatelet IgG, making it difficult to distinguish from ITP using platelet antibody testing.
  - **Management.** In gestational thrombocytopenia, *no intervention is necessary.* Women with gestational thrombocytopenia are not at risk for maternal or fetal hemorrhage or bleeding complications.
    - Monitor platelets closely to detect decreases below 50,000.
    - Document normal neonatal platelet count. Approximately 2% of the offspring of mothers with gestational thrombocytopenia have mild thrombocytopenia (<50,000/μL). However, infants generally do not suffer from severe platelet deficiency.
    - Reevaluate platelet count in the postpartum period to ensure return to normal.

HELLP Syndrome

- **Hemolysis, elevated liver enzymes, and low platelet (HELLP) syndrome** is the most common pathologic cause of maternal thrombocytopenia. It occurs in approximately 10% to 20% of women who have severe preeclampsia and is often an early finding in preeclampsia. Platelets will reach nadir at 24 to 48 hr after delivery. In women who remain severely thrombocytopenic after delivery, plasma exchange and/or corticosteroids may be considered. In addition to improving neonatal outcome before 34 weeks' gestation, corticosteroids may also improve maternal outcomes. When given in the antepartum period, transient improvements are seen in maternal platelet counts. Small placebo-controlled trials have not shown decreased morbidity when steroids are continued post partum. Neonatal complications are typically the result of extreme prematurity.

Idiopathic Thrombocytopenic Purpura (ITP)

- **ITP** is the most common autoimmune disease in pregnancy, occurring in 1 to 2 of 1,000 pregnancies, accounting for 5% of pregnancy-associated thrombocytopenia. ITP is the most common cause of thrombocytopenia in the first trimester. Antiplatelet antibodies directed at platelet surface glycoproteins, leading to increased destruction of platelets by the reticuloendothelial system (primarily the spleen), result in thrombocytopenia. The course of ITP is not typically affected by pregnancy.
- **Diagnosis.** Diagnosis is based on the history, physical exam, complete blood count, and peripheral smear. ITP is a diagnosis of exclusion, and there is no diagnostic test. If thrombocytopenia is mild, it is difficult to distinguish ITP from gestational thrombocytopenia. Detection of platelet-associated antibodies is consistent with, but not diagnostic of, ITP since they may also be present in women with gestational thrombocytopenia and preeclampsia. Platelet antibody testing has a fairly low sensitivity (49% to 66%). However, the absence of platelet-associated IgG makes the diagnosis of ITP less likely. ITP is more likely if the platelet count is <50,000/μL, or in the presence of an underlying autoimmune disease or history of previous thrombocytopenia. In contrast to gestational thrombocytopenia, the thrombocytopenia with ITP typically occurs early in pregnancy. Findings include the following:
  - Persistent thrombocytopenia (platelet count <100,000/μL with or without accompanying megathrombocytes on the peripheral smear).
  - Normal or increased megakaryocytes determined from bone marrow.
  - Secondary causes of maternal thrombocytopenia should be excluded (e.g., preeclampsia, HIV infection, systemic lupus erythematosus, drugs).
  - Absence of splenomegaly.
- **Antenatal management.** Pregnant women with platelet counts over 50,000/μL at any time during the pregnancy and women with counts of 30,000 to 50,000/μL in the first or second trimester do not routinely require treatment. If the platelet count is <10,000/μL or is 10,000 to 30,000/μL in the second or third trimester, or the patient is bleeding, treatment is required. Two treatments are available: glucocorticoids and intravenous gamma globulin (IVIG).
  - Glucocorticoids suppress antibody production, inhibit sequestration of antibody-coated platelets, and interfere with the interaction between platelets and antibodies.
    - Oral prednisone is started at 1 to 2 mg/kg/day and is tapered to the lowest dose supporting an acceptable platelet count (usually over 50,000/μL) and tolerable side effects. Patients usually respond within 3 to 7 days and approximately 75% respond within 3 weeks. One fourth of patients may achieve complete remission.
    - High-dose glucocorticoids, such as methylprednisolone, may be administered at 1 to 1.5 mg/kg IV in divided doses. Very little crosses the placenta. Response is usually seen in 2 to 10 days.
    - Side effects of glucocorticoids include increased gestational hypertension and diabetes.

- High-dose IVIG (400 mg/kg/day for 5 days or 1 g/kg/day for 2 days) is another therapeutic option. The proposed mechanism of action of IVIG is prolongation of the clearance time of IgG-coated platelets by the maternal reticuloendothelial system. Eighty percent of patients treated with IVIG respond within days, and remission lasts 3 weeks. The main drawbacks are cost and inconvenience to the patient.
- Splenectomy is an option in the second trimester in women who fail glucocorticoid and IVIG therapy and are experiencing bleeding and platelet counts <10,000/μL. With splenectomy, remission occurs in 75% of women; however, data in pregnancy are limited. Individuals with splenectomies should be immunized against pneumococcus, *Hemophilus influenzae,* and meningococcus.
- Immunosuppressive therapy is controversial and usually not pursued because, although its efficacy is well established in nonpregnant patients, it is potentially harmful to the developing fetus. The therapeutic regimens have side effects, and the goal of therapy is to raise the platelet count to a safe level (over 20,000 to 30,000/μL), with the least amount of intervention possible, keeping in mind that a safe platelet count is not necessarily a normal platelet count. Pregnant women with ITP should be instructed to avoid nonsteroidal anti-inflammatory agents, salicylates, and trauma.
- **Intrapartum management.** As pregnancy approaches term, more aggressive measures to increase maternal platelet counts may be indicated to allow for adequate hemostasis during delivery and epidural anesthesia. Platelet counts over 50,000/μL are usually adequate for either vaginal or cesarean delivery and are usually also adequate for regional anesthesia, although some recommend a platelet count over 100,000/μL to avoid epidural hematomas. Prophylactic platelet transfusion may be appropriate with a maternal platelet count <10,000 to 20,000/μL before vaginal delivery or <50,000/μL before a cesarean section if bleeding is present. For cesarean section, the transfusion should begin at the time of incision. One "pack" of platelets will increase the platelet count by 5,000 to 10,000/μL. Transfused platelets will have a shorter half-life because of circulating antibodies.

Neonatal Thrombocytopenia
- In mothers with ITP, placental transfer of the IgG platelet antibodies can result in fetal or **neonatal thrombocytopenia**. Approximately, 10% of neonates will have severe thrombocytopenia (<50,000/μL). The general consensus is that no correlation exists between maternal platelet count (or the presence of maternal platelet antibodies) and fetal platelet count. The most reliable indicator of fetal thrombocytopenia is a history of thrombocytopenia in a previous sibling after delivery. Fetal platelet count cannot be predicted accurately, and even fetal scalp sampling or percutaneous umbilical blood sampling does not provide reliable estimates. In ITP, the neonatal platelet count declines after delivery, reaching a nadir at 48 to 72 hr of life. Notification of a pediatrician for close monitoring of the neonatal platelet count is very important in preventing the devastating sequelae of neonatal intracranial hemorrhage (ICH), a rare event. Some recommend obtaining umbilical cord platelet counts at delivery.
  - **Delivery mode.** Because ICH appears to be more of a neonatal than intrapartum event, and due to the limitations in obtaining an accurate fetal platelet count, using the fetal platelet count to determine route of delivery is not recommended. A survey of US perinatologists reported that most prefer not to perform invasive tests to evaluate fetal platelets and support a trial of labor. Unfortunately, no

randomized, controlled studies have compared delivery mode in these neonates. For years, the assumption that a fetus with a platelet count lower than 50,000/μL is at significant risk for ICH, coupled with the belief that cesarean delivery is less traumatic than spontaneous vaginal delivery, led to the recommendation of cesarean delivery for severe fetal thrombocytopenia in ITP patients. However, there is no evidence that cesarean section decreases the risk of ICH. Cesarean section should be reserved for obstetric indications only.

THROMBOEMBOLIC DISEASE

Thromboembolic disease is linked with both adverse maternal and fetal/neonatal outcomes. The term **venous thromboembolism (VTE)** encompasses **deep vein thrombosis (DVT)** and **pulmonary embolism (PE)**.

- Pregnant women are up to five times more likely to experience a VTE than age-matched nonpregnant women.
- Incidence of VTE ranges from 0.76 to 2.0 episodes per 1,000 pregnancies.
- Approximately 80% of VTEs in pregnancy are DVT and 20% are PE.
- Approximately two thirds of all DVTs occur in the antepartum period and appear to be evenly divided among the three trimesters.
- PE occurs more frequently postpartum.
- Cesarean delivery imparts a greater risk than a vaginal delivery (three to five times greater).

Risk Factors for VTE

- Pregnancy is considered a hypercoagulable state. Fibrinogen, coagulation factors, and plasminogen activator inhibitor-1 (PAI-1) levels are increased; free protein S levels are decreased, and fibrinolytic activity is decreased.
- One of the most significant risk factors is a personal history of VTE. Maternal medical conditions including heart disease, SCD, lupus, obesity, diabetes, and hypertension increase risk. Other risk factors include surgery, family history of VTE, bed rest or prolonged immobilization, smoking, age older than 35, multiple gestation, preeclampsia, and postpartum infection.
- **Thrombophilias** may be inherited or acquired.
  - Pregnancy may trigger an event in women with an underlying thrombophilia.
  - Fetal death in utero, severe IUGR, abruption, and severe early-onset preeclampsia may be the result of underlying thrombophilias that affect uteroplacental circulation; however, this is controversial.
  - **Inherited thrombophilias** (Table 17-4)
    ○ Increase the risk of a maternal thromboembolic event approximately eightfold.
    ○ Are present in over half of all maternal thrombotic events.
    ○ Antithrombin deficiency and homozygosity for factor V Leiden mutation are the most potent of the inherited thrombophilias. Double or compound heterozygotes (for both factor V Leiden and prothrombin G20219A) are also at greater risk of VTE.
  - **Acquired thrombophilias**
    ○ Include persistent antiphospholipid antibody syndromes (APS) (lupus anticoagulants or anticardiolipin antibodies). APS is present in 15% to 17% of women with recurrent pregnancy loss.
    ○ Hyperhomocysteinemia can be either acquired or inherited.

| TABLE 17-4 | Inherited Thrombophilias and Risk of VTE in Pregnancy |

Thrombophilia	Odds Ratio
Factor V Leiden homozygosity	34.4
Prothrombin G20210A homozygosity	26.4
Factor V Leiden heterozygous	8.3
Prothrombin G20210A heterozygous	6.8
Protein C deficiency	4.8
Antithrombin deficiency	4.7[a]
Protein S deficiency	3.2
Methylenetetrahydrofolate reductase (MTHFR) C677T homozygote	0.74
Factor V Leiden + Prothrombin G20210A (compound heterozygosity)[b]	88.0
Antiphospholipid antibody syndrome[c]	15.8

[a]Likely an underestimate. Others report 25- to 50-fold increase. Adapted from Robertson L, Greer I. Thromboembolism in Pregnancy. *Curr Opin Obstet Gynecol* 2005;17:113–116; [b]Gebhardt GS, Hall DR. Inherited and acquired thrombophilias and poor pregnancy outcome: should we be treating with heparin? *Curr Opin Obstet Gynecol* 2003;15:501–506; and [c]James AH, Jamison MG, Brancazio LR, et al. Venous thromboembolism during pregnancy and the postpartum period: incidence, risk factors, and mortality. *Am J Obstet Gynecol* 2006;194(5):1311–1315.

- Routine screening for thrombophilias is not recommended in all pregnant women and screening indications are controversial. ACOG no longer recommends thrombophilia testing in women with recurrent fetal loss, placental abruption, IUGR, or preeclampsia. A thrombophilia workup (Table 17-5) should be considered for the following:
  ○ VTE during pregnancy (workup after delivery).
  ○ Personal or family history of VTE (first-degree relative with VTE before age 50 in absence of other risk factors).
  ○ APS screening may be appropriate for women with repeated fetal losses.

Manifestations and Diagnosis of VTE
DVT
- Over 70% of **DVTs** in pregnancy develop in the iliofemoral veins, which are more likely to embolize, and the majority are on the left side. **Diagnosis** of DVT is difficult in pregnancy because expected changes in pregnancy may mimic the symptoms of DVT. Additionally, many patients are asymptomatic. If symptoms exist, the most common include calf or lower extremity swelling, pain or tenderness, warmth, and erythema. Homan's sign (calf pain with passive dorsiflexion of the foot) is present in <15% of cases, and a palpable cord is present in <10% of cases. Symptoms of an iliac DVT include abdominal pain, back pain, and swelling of the entire leg. In pregnant women with clinical suspicion of DVT, diagnosis is confirmed in <10%.
- **Venous duplex imaging,** including compression ultrasound, color, and spectral Doppler sonography, has replaced contrast venography as the gold standard and is the most commonly available noninvasive diagnostic method, with a sensitivity of 97% and specificity of 94% in symptomatic proximal DVT. If the deep venous system is normal, the presence of a clinically significant thrombus is unlikely.

TABLE 17-5	Thrombophilia Testing

Primary Tests Recommended by (ACOG)
Activated protein C resistance screen (95% of positives due to Factor V Leiden) followed by analysis for Factor V Leiden (PCR) if positive
Prothrombin G20210A genotype
Antithrombin functional assay (activity)
Protein C activity
Protein S activity and free and total antigen levels

Other Tests (Not Recommended by ACOG)
Activated Partial Thromboplastin Time (aPTT)
Dilute Russell Viper Venom Time (dRVVT)
Anticardiolipin antibodies (IgG and IgM)
Lupus anticoagulant
4G/4G PAI-1 mutation (if not available, plasma PAI-1 activity)
MTHFR mutation screen and/or fasting plasma homocysteine levels
ANA (if early PEC)

Testing should be remote from thrombotic event, not during pregnancy, and while off anticoagulants, except DNA tests. Adapted from Inherited thrombophilias in pregnancy. ACOG Practice Bulletin Number 113. American College of Obstetricians and Gynecologists. *Obstet Gynecol* 2010;116:212–222.

Limitations include poor sensitivity for asymptomatic disease and difficulty in detecting iliac vein thromboses.

- **Magnetic resonance imaging (MRI).** Studies in nonpregnant patients show a sensitivity of 100% and specificity of 98% to 99% for pelvic and proximal DVTs, while maintaining a high accuracy in detecting below the knee DVTs.
- D-**dimer test** is a sensitive, but nonspecific test for DVT; however, it is not necessarily useful in pregnancy because D-dimer normally increases with gestational age. A normal D-dimer result may be reassuring if clinical suspicion is low. Depending on the assay used, some researchers believe D-dimer may provide important information in combination with other tests in certain circumstances.

PE

- **PE** remains the leading cause of maternal mortality in developed countries, accounting for approximately 20% of deaths. The risk of PE is greatest immediately postpartum, particularly after cesarean delivery, with a fatality rate of nearly 15%. PE most commonly originates from DVT in the lower extremities, occurring in nearly 50% of patients with proximal DVT. Symptoms of sudden shortness of breath, chest pain, and cough or signs of tachypnea and tachycardia, typically associated with PE are all common in pregnancy. Because of the serious consequences of PE and the increased incidence in pregnancy, clinicians must have a low threshold for evaluation. **Diagnosis** starts with a careful history and physical examination and then diagnostic tests to rule out other possible etiologies, such as asthma, pneumonia, or pulmonary edema.
- An arterial blood gas (ABG), electrocardiogram, and chest x-ray should be performed. ABG values are altered in pregnancy and must be interpreted using pregnancy-adjusted normal values. More than half of pregnant women with a documented PE have a normal alveolar-arterial gradient.
- A chest x-ray helps rule out other disease processes and enhances interpretation of the ventilation-perfusion (V/Q) scan. The risks associated with various radiologic

tests indicated for PE workup are minimal compared with the consequences of a missed PE.

- **Pulmonary angiography** is the gold standard for PE diagnosis, but it is expensive and invasive.
- **Computed tomographic (pulmonary) angiography (CTA)** is becoming the recommended imaging test in pregnant women with suspected PE. CTA is easier to perform, more readily available, more cost-effective, and provides a lower dose of radiation to the fetus than a V/Q scan. CTA is also useful in detecting other abnormalities that may be contributing to the patient's symptoms (e.g., pneumonia, aortic dissection). Newer technology, multidetector CT pulmonary angiography, allows visualization of finer pulmonary vascular detail and provides greater diagnostic accuracy.
- Historically, the **V/Q scan** has been the primary diagnostic test for PE. It is interpreted as low, intermediate, or high probability for PE. High-probability scans (i.e., segmental perfusion defect with normal ventilation) confirm PE, with a positive predictive value over 90% when pretest likelihood is high. V/Q scans are limited in their usefulness because of the large proportion of indeterminate results. Most fetal radiation exposure occurs when radioactive tracers are excreted in the maternal bladder. Therefore, exposure can be limited by prompt and frequent voiding after the procedure. If patient is postpartum and breast-feeding, breast milk should not be used for 2 days after a V/Q scan.
- If pregnant women have a nondiagnostic lung scan, **bilateral venous duplex** imaging of the lower extremities is recommended to evaluate for DVT. If DVT is found, PE can be diagnosed. If no DVT is seen, **arteriography** may be performed for further evaluation before a commitment to long-term anticoagulation is made, or a repeat venous duplex imaging in 1 week.
- According to the Centers for Disease Control and Prevention, in all stages of gestation a dose of <5 rads (0.05 Gy) represents no measurable noncancer health effects. After 16 weeks' gestation, congenital effects are unlikely below 50 rads. The risk for childhood cancer from prenatal radiation exposure is 0.3% to 1% for 0 to 5 rads. Any of the proposed modalities for diagnosis of PE are well below the dose levels that increase congenital abnormalities. Radiation exposure from a two-view chest radiograph is <0.001 rad. A higher dose of fetal radiation is provided with V/Q scan (0.064 to 0.08 rad) compared with CTA (0.0003 to 0.0131 rad). Pulmonary angiography provides approximately 0.2 to 0.4 rad with the femoral approach and <0.05 rad with the brachial approach. Maternal radiation dose is higher with CTA than V/Q scan.

Treatment of VTE

- When VTE is suspected, **anticoagulation** with unfractionated heparin (UFH) or low-molecular-weight heparin (LMWH) should be initiated until the diagnosis is excluded. Neither heparin crosses the placenta; thus, there is no risk for teratogenicity or fetal hemorrhage, although bleeding at the uteroplacental junction is possible. Neither drug is secreted into breast milk. Although UFH has been standard treatment for the prevention and treatment of VTE during pregnancy, recent evidence-based clinical practice guidelines now recommend LMWH. Table 17-6 lists dosing regimens. Thromboembolic deterrent stockings and leg elevation should be used for DVT.
- Weight-adjusted **LMWH** should be used for the treatment of VTE (Table 17-6). Advantages of LMWH include fewer bleeding complications, lower risk of heparin-induced thrombocytopenia (HIT) and osteoporosis, longer plasma half-life, and more predictable dose-response relationships. Theoretical concerns have been raised regarding once daily dosing compared to twice daily dosing (i.e., prophylactic or therapeutic) secondary to the increased renal clearance in pregnancy possibly

prolonging trough LMWH levels. However, no comparison data of the two regimens are available. Additionally, recent data suggest daily dosing in the treatment of acute VTE is effective. Monitoring of LMWH levels remains controversial. LMWH cannot be monitored using activated partial thromboplastin time (aPTT), as aPTT probably be normal. Antifactor Xa activity levels may be measured 4 hr after injection, with a therapeutic goal of 0.6 to 1.0 U/mL (slightly higher if once daily dosing is used); however, frequent monitoring is typically not recommended, except at extremes of body weight. If trough levels are evaluated with therapeutic dosing (i.e.,

TABLE 17-6	Thromboprophylaxis Regimens in Pregnancy

Prophylactic
LMWH
    Enoxaparin 40 mg SC q 24 hr
    Enoxaparin 30 mg SC q 12 hr[a]
    Dalteparin 5,000 U SC q 24 hr
    Tinzaparin 4,500 U SC q 24 hr
UFH
    UFH 5,000 U SC q 12 hr
Alternative[b]
    UFH 5,000–7,500 U SC q 12 hr in 1st trimester
    UFH 7,500–10,000 U SC q 12 hr in 2nd trimester
    UFH 10,000 U SC q 12 hr in 3rd trimester (unless aPTT elevated)

Intermediate-Dose
LMWH
    Enoxaparin 40 mg SC q 12 hr
    Dalteparin 5,000 U SC q 12 hr
UFH
    UFH SC q 12 hr; doses adjusted to target peak antifactor Xa levels
      (4 hours after injection) of 0.1 to 0.3 U/mL

Treatment (Weight-Adjusted) Dose
LMWH
    Enoxaparin 1 mg/kg SC q 12 hr (or Enoxaparin 1.5 mg/kg SC q 24 hr[c])
    Dalteparin 200 U/kg SC q 24 hr or 100 U/kg SC q 12 hr
    Tinzaparin 175 U/kg SC q 24 hr
UFH
    UFH SC q 12 hr; doses adjusted to obtain midinterval (6 hr postinjection)
      therapeutic aPTT (often a ratio of 1.5–2.5)

Postpartum Anticoagulation (for 4–6 wk)
Warfarin with a target INR of 2.0–3.0 with initial UFH or LMWH overlap
    until INR ≥2.0 for 2 d
Prophylactic LMWH or UFH

[a]Some experts recommend twice daily dosing of enoxaparin secondary to pharmacokinetic properties of LMWH in pregnancy; however, comparison data are lacking. Additionally, women at the extremes of weight may require different dosing. [b]James AH, Brancazio LR, Ortel TL, et al. Thrombosis, thrombophilia, and thromboprophylaxis in pregnancy. *Clin Adv Hem Oncol* 2005;3:187–197. [c]Chunilal SD, Bates SM. Venous thromboembolism in pregnancy: diagnosis, management and prevention. *Thromb Haemost* 2009;101:428–438. Adapted from Bates SM, Greer IA, Pabinger I, et al. Venous thromboembolism, thrombophilia, antithrombotic therapy, and pregnancy: American College of Chest Physicians Evidence-Based Clinical Practice Guidelines (8th Ed). *Chest* 2008;133:844S–886S.

12 hr after dosing), goal level is 0.2 to 0.4 IU/mL. Current guidelines do not provide definitive monitoring recommendations; however, some researchers advocate checking levels periodically (every 1 to 3 months).

- **UFH** is administered either intravenously or subcutaneously (SC). IV UFH may be a better initial therapy option in unstable patients (e.g., large PE with hypoxia or extensive iliofemoral disease) or patients with significant renal impairment (i.e., creatinine clearance <30 mL/min). The goal of the initial bolus dose (typically 80 U/kg) and subsequent maintenance dosing (typically 18 U/kg/hr) is to achieve a midinterval (6 hr postinjection) therapeutic aPTT (often described as an aPTT ratio of 1.5 to 2.5 times normal). Measuring anti-factor Xa heparin levels may assist in evaluating heparin dosing (target level 0.3 to 0.7 IU/mL). Many facilities have standard protocols for heparin titration. IV treatment should be maintained in the therapeutic range for at least 5 days, and therapy may then be continued with either adjusted-dose SC heparin injections or LMWH. If maintained on UFH, the aPTT should be monitored every 1 to 2 weeks. The aPTT response to heparin in pregnant women is often attenuated secondary to elevated heparin-binding proteins and increased factor VIII and fibrinogen. The therapeutic dose may need to be adjusted. Thus, it may be difficult to achieve target aPTT levels late in pregnancy. The major concerns with UFH use during pregnancy are bleeding, osteopenia, and thrombocytopenia. The risk of major bleeding with UFH is approximately 2%. Bone density reductions have been reported in 30% of patients on heparin for over 1 month. HIT occurs in up to 3% of nonpregnant patients and should be suspected when platelet count decreases to <100,000/μL or <50% of baseline value 5 to 15 days after beginning heparin or sooner with recent heparin exposure. Typical onset is between 5 and 10 days after starting heparin. In 25% to 30% of patients who develop HIT, onset occurs rapidly (within 24 hr) after starting heparin and is related to recent exposure to heparin. After obtaining a starting platelet level, ACOG recommends checking platelets again on day 5 and then periodically for the first 2 weeks of therapy. Others suggest platelets be monitored at 24 hr and then every 2 to 3 days for the first 2 weeks or weekly for the first 3 weeks. If HIT is acquired and ongoing anticoagulant therapy is required, danaparoid sodium is used.
- **Warfarin sodium** crosses the placenta and, therefore, is a potential teratogen and may cause fetal bleeding. Warfarin is likely safe during the first 6 weeks' gestation, but between 6 and 12 weeks' gestation, a risk of skeletal embryopathy exists, consisting of stippled epiphyses and nasal and limb hypoplasia. One third of fetuses exposed to warfarin late in pregnancy develop CNS injuries, hemorrhage, or ophthalmologic abnormalities. Warfarin may be used postpartum and may be given to nursing mothers.
- Temporary **inferior vena cava filters** are indicated in women in whom anticoagulants are contraindicated. They may be inserted within a week of elective induction or cesarean section and removed postpartum.

Prophylaxis for VTE in Pregnancy

Antepartum

- Limited data exist regarding the use of prophylactic anticoagulation for VTE during pregnancy. Women need to be stratified by risk, and clinical judgment applied. Although recommendations vary, women at very high risk for VTE probably benefit from UFH or LMWH throughout pregnancy and postpartum. At a minimum, postpartum prophylaxis is usually recommended in women at elevated risk for VTE. Table 17-7 summarizes recommendations.

TABLE 17-7 Approach to Pregnant Patients at Risk for VTE

Clinical Indication	Antepartum Management	Postpartum Anticoagulation? (if yes, see Table 17-6)
No Thombophilia Present		
History of a single VTE associated with a transient risk factor that is no longer present; no thrombophilia	Clinical surveillance	Yes
History of a prior VTE where transient risk factor was pregnancy or estrogen related	Clinical surveillance *OR* Prophylactic or Intermediate-dose LMWH/UFH	Yes
History of a prior idiopathic VTE, not on long-term anticoagulation; no thrombophilia	Clinical surveillance *OR* Prophylactic or Intermediate-dose LMWH/UFH	Yes
Low Risk Thrombophilia		
Low-risk thrombophilia with single prior VTE, not on long-term anti-coagulation	Clinical surveillance *OR* Prophylactic or Intermediate-dose LMWH/UFH	Yes
Other Thrombophila Present		
Known thrombophilia, but no prior VTE	Clinical surveillance *OR* Prophylactic LMWH / UFH if low-risk; prophylactic LMWH/ UFH if high-risk.	Yes
High-risk thrombophilia with a prior single VTE, not receiving long-term anticoagulation	Prophylactic, Intermedi-ate- *or* adjusted-dose LMWH/UFH	Yes
Other Clinical Situations		
History of multiple (≥2) episodes of VTE, not on long-term anticoagulation	Prophylactic, Intermediate-dose, or Adjusted-dose LMWH/UFH	Yes
Receiving long-term anticoagulation for prior VTE	Adjusted-dose LMWH/ UFH	Resume long-term anticoagulation

Low-risk thrombophilia: heterozygous for factor V Leiden or prothrombin G20210A, protein C or protein S deficiency.

High-risk thrombophilia: antithrombin deficiency, homozygous for factor V Leiden or prothrombin G20210A or compound heterozygous for both, persistent positive antiphospholipid antibodies.

Adapted from Bates SM, Greer IA, Pabinger I, et al. Venous thromboembolism, thrombophilia, anti-thrombotic therapy, and pregnancy: American College of Chest Physicians Evidence-Based Clinical Practice Guidelines (8th Ed.). *Chest* 2008;133:844–886; and Duhl AJ, Paidas MJ, Ural SH, et al. Antithrombotic therapy and pregnancy: consensus report and recommendations for prevention and treatment of venous thromboembolism and adverse pregnancy outcomes. *Am J Obstet Gynecol* 2007;197:457.e1–e21.

At Delivery

- The risk of maternal hemorrhage may be minimized with carefully planned delivery. If possible, induction of labor or scheduled cesarean section should be considered in women on therapeutic anticoagulation dosing regimens, so therapy may be discontinued at an appropriate time. When used in therapeutic doses, LMWH should be discontinued 24 hr before elective induction of labor or cesarean delivery. Epidural or spinal anesthesia should not be administered within 24 hr of the last therapeutic dose of LMWH. A common approach is to transition from LMWH to UFH at 36 to 38 weeks' gestation. If the patient goes into spontaneous labor and is receiving SC UFH, she should be able to receive regional analgesia if the aPTT is normal. If significantly prolonged, protamine sulfate may be administered at 1 mg/100 U of UFH. If the patient is at very high risk for VTE, IV UFH can be started and then discontinued 4 to 6 hr before expected delivery. When receiving LMWH once daily for prophylaxis, regional anesthesia can be administered 12 hr after the last dose. Also, LMWH should be withheld for at least 2 to 4 hr after the removal of an epidural catheter.

Postpartum

- Postpartum anticoagulation may be resumed within 12 hr of cesarean delivery and 4 to 6 hr after vaginal delivery. If at high risk of bleeding postpartum, IV UFH may be chosen initially since its effect dissipates more rapidly and may be reversed with protamine sulfate. Warfarin can be started when adequate hemostasis is assured with initial overlap with UFH or LMWH until INR is ≥2.0 for 2 consecutive days, with a target INR of 2.0 to 3.0. Anticoagulation should be administered for at least 6 weeks postpartum for DVT and 4 to 6 months for PE.

SUGGESTED READINGS

James AH. Thromboembolism in pregnancy: recurrence risks, prevention and management. *Curr Opin Obstet Gynecol* 2008;20:550–556.

Marik PE, Plante LA. Venous thromboembolic disease and pregnancy. *N Engl J Med* 2008;359:2025–2033.

Rogers DT, Molokie R. Sickle cell disease in pregnancy. *Obstet Gynecol Clin North Am* 2010;37(2):223–237.

Rosenberg VA, Lockwood CJ. Thromboembolism in pregnancy. *Obstet Gynecol Clin N Am* 2007;34:481–500.

Sukenik-Halevy R, Ellis MH, Fejgin MD. Management of immune thrombocytopenic purpura in pregnancy. *Obstet Gynecol Surv* 2008;63(3):182–188.

Thrombocytopenia in pregnancy. Practice Bulletin Number 6. American College of Obstetricians and Gynecologists. *Int J Gynaecol Obstet.* 1999;67(2):117–128.

18 Alloimmunization

S.J. Hanson, Anya J. Bailis, and Janyne E. Althaus

Alloimmunization in pregnancy refers to maternal antibody formation against fetal red blood cell (RBC) or platelet antigens. Antibody-coated erythrocytes or platelets are destroyed by the fetal immune system, leading to anemia or thrombocytopenia. Antibodies are formed after uncrossed transfusion or fetomaternal hemorrhage (FMH), when foreign or fetal blood components enter the maternal circulation. Untreated alloimmunization can cause significant fetal and newborn morbidity from hemolytic anemia (*hydrops fetalis*) or neonatal alloimmune thrombocytopenia (NAIT) or death.

RED CELL ALLOIMMUNIZATION

Red cell alloimmunization to all clinically significant antigens occurs in approximately 25 of 10,000 births. The most common targeted red cell antigen is the Rhesus "D" (or Rh D) antigen. Maternal blood type is usually described as ABO+ or ABO–, signifying the presence (+) or absence (–) of the Rh D antigen. Rh alloimmunization usually refers to the development of antibodies to Rh D antigen. Other important red cell antigens include the ABO blood group antigens and more than fifty other minor antigens (e.g., Duffy and Kell). Not all antibodies lead to fetal anemia (e.g., Lewis and "I" antibodies).

Pathophysiology

- Exposing an Rh⁻ woman to Rh D antigen initiates an immune response that produces anti-D immunoglobulin G (IgG), a process termed **Rh sensitization**.
- Fifteen percent of Caucasians and eight percent of African Americans and Hispanic Americans are Rh⁻. The populations with the highest and lowest Rh⁻ prevalence are Spanish Basque (30%) and Native Americans (1%).
- During pregnancy, the RBCs of an Rh⁺ fetus are targeted by maternal IgG.
- Fetal anemia develops as Rh⁺ fetal red cells are sequestered and hemolyzed.
- The fetal response to anemia includes increased erythropoietin production and hematopoiesis. As hemolysis outpaces production, more immature RBCs appear in the fetal circulation (*erythroblastosis fetalis*).
- If left untreated, *hydrops fetalis* develops secondary to fetal portal hypertension, reduced hepatic protein synthesis, increased cardiac output, increased hydrostatic pressure, and increased capillary leakage.
- **FMH** with transplacental passage of Rh⁺ fetal erythrocytes into the maternal circulation is the main cause of Rh sensitization.
  - An immune response is generated with as little as 0.1 mL of blood, an amount that routinely passes into maternal circulation in normal pregnancies.
  - Fetal RBC antigens are present by 38 days of gestation, so even first-trimester events can theoretically cause alloimmunization, including ectopic pregnancy, spontaneous or therapeutic abortion, or (rarely) threatened abortion and molar pregnancy.
  - Invasive procedures such as chorionic villus sampling, amniocentesis, fetal blood sampling, or external cephalic version can also lead to FMH and alloimmunization.

- FMH is most likely to occur at delivery.
- Cesarean delivery, multifetal delivery, abruption, bleeding previa, or manual placental delivery may increase the quantity of FMH.
- Maternal trauma can also result in FMH.

Prevention

- Before the development of anti-D immunoglobulin (commonly called RhoGAM), 17% of all Rh⁻ women developed antibodies during pregnancy and 10% of those were affected by hemolytic disease of the fetus or newborn.
- With preventive measures, only 0.1% of pregnancies in Rh⁻ mothers are complicated by anti-Rh D antibody production (see Table 18-1).
- RhoGAM is pooled sterile human IgG antibodies to the Rh D antigen.
- RhoGAM prevents alloimmunization by clearing Rh D fetal RBCs from maternal circulation, downregulating the maternal B-cell–mediated immune response, and possibly obscuring antigen sites on the fetal RBCs.
- The standard RhoGAM dose is 300 μg IM.
- 10 μg of RhoGAM IgG "neutralizes" 1 mL of fetal blood. The standard dose protects against up to 30 mL of fetal blood entering the maternal system.
  - Quantification of FMH with a Kleihauer-Betke (KB) test guides additional RhoGAM dosing.
  - Perform a postpartum KB test for all Rh⁻ mothers with Rh⁺ infants to ensure adequate immunoglobulin coverage.
- "Mini-dose" RhoGAM (50 μg) IM is sufficient in the first trimester.
- In the United States, RhoGAM is given at 28 weeks, and again postpartum after neonatal Rh⁺ status is confirmed.
- The half-life of Rhogam is 24 days but can be detected on maternal antibody screens for up to 12 weeks.

Management of Rh Unsensitized Patients (Fig. 18-1)

- Rh⁻ pregnant patients should be screened at the **first prenatal visit**.
  - Antibody is detected by **indirect Coombs test**, in which maternal serum is exposed to Rh⁺ red cells. Lack of agglutination signifies the absence of circulating antibody in maternal serum and suggests unsensitized status.

TABLE 18-1	Indications for RhoGAM Administration in Rh⁻, Unsensitized Women with Negative Antibody Screen

First-trimester spontaneous or elective abortion
Ectopic pregnancy
Amniocentesis, fetal blood sampling, or chorionic villi sampling
Molar pregnancy
Second-trimester or third-trimester bleeding (e.g., placenta previa or abruption)
Intrauterine fetal demise
External cephalic version
Abdominal trauma
Threatened abortion[a]
Routine prophylaxis 24–28 wk
Birth of an Rh⁺ infant

[a]Use is recommended in the United States, but evidence is limited. RhoGAM is not given to Rh⁺ or sensitized Rh⁻ women.

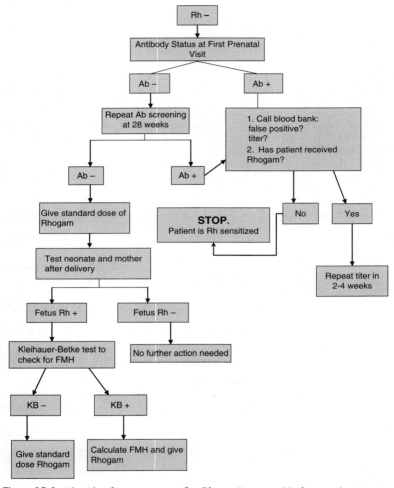

Figure 18-1. Algorithm for management of an Rh-negative, unsensitized woman in pregnancy.

- Repeat antibody screen at **28 weeks' gestation**.
  - If the indirect Coombs test is positive (i.e., agglutination), the laboratory must distinguish between sensitization and RhoGAM administration earlier in pregnancy.
  - If the positive result is from a prior RhoGAM dose, a standard dose RhoGAM injection is given to provide coverage through the remainder of the pregnancy.
  - If the positive result is from sensitization, RhoGAM is not given.
  - If the screen is negative at 28 weeks, the standard dose is administered.
- **After delivery** both the patient and infant are screened.
  - If the neonate is Rh⁻, no Rhogam is necessary.
  - If the neonate is Rh⁺ and the mother is antibody negative, the standard dose of Rhogam is given, and a KB test is performed to evaluate extra RhoGAM dosing, if needed.

- If the neonate is Rh⁺ and the mother is antibody positive with a titer >1:4, no RhoGAM is given and her next pregnancy is managed as Rh-sensitized.
- When in question, Rhogam is given. The risk of giving RhoGAM to a sensitized person is negligible compared with the consequences of permanent sensitization.

Management of the Rh Sensitized Patients (Fig. 18-2)

- An Rh⁻ patient with anti-D titer >1:4 should be considered sensitized, and her fetus is at risk for hemolytic anemia. The following tests further assess the fetus:
- **Sonogram** should be arranged at the first prenatal visit regardless of gestational age.
  ○ Accurate gestational dating is critical to interpret other tests and to time any interventions properly.
  ○ Use serial ultrasounds to monitor development of *hydrops fetalis.*

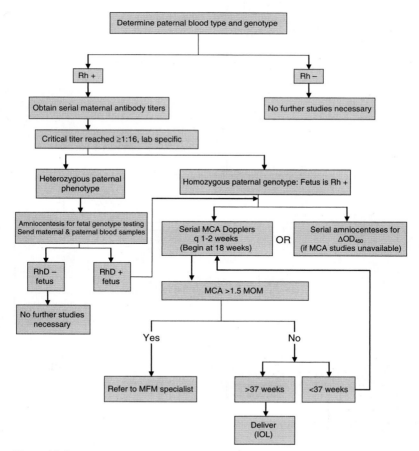

Figure 18-2. Algorithm for management of Rhesus alloimmunized women in pregnancy.

- **Paternal blood typing** is performed to determine whether the fetus can inherit the Rh D antigen. If the father is Rh⁻ and paternity is certain, intervention is unnecessary. All possible paternity candidates must have ABO and Rh status determined.
  - If the father is heterozygous for Rh D, the fetus has a 50% chance of being Rh⁺.
  - If the father is homozygous for Rh D, the fetus will be Rh⁺ and is at risk.
  - If paternity is unknown or testing is not possible, the fetus is assumed to be Rh⁺.
- Follow **serial maternal D antibody titers** monthly until 24 weeks, then every 2 weeks. Most Rh-sensitized patients have a chronic low D antibody titer. The fetus is not at risk until a critical titer is reached.
  - The critical titer is an absolute value of ≥1:16, or an increase of more than one titer dilution (e.g., 1:2 to 1:8). The tests should be performed in the same laboratory. Note that some labs report titers as the denominator only (i.e., titer of 1:2 is reported as "2").
  - Once maternal antibodies exceed the critical titer, the fetus is at risk for the remainder of the pregnancy regardless of titer value. Additional testing is required.
  - In the first affected pregnancy, titers correlate well with fetal status. In subsequent pregnancies, the titer is less predictive, so hydrops assessments should begin at 18 weeks.
- **Fetal blood typing** is determined by amniocentesis if the critical titer is reached and the paternal antigen status is unknown or heterozygous (Fig. 18-3).

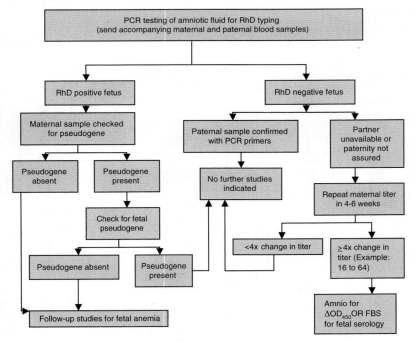

Figure 18-3. Determination of fetal Rh status.

- Fetal blood genotype is determined from amniotic fluid cells by polymerase chain reaction (PCR). The false-negative rate is up to 1.5%.
- Discrepancies between fetal genotype and phenotype can occur, so both maternal and paternal blood samples should be sent along with the amniotic fluid.
- If the fetus is Rh⁺, the maternal sample is checked for the Rh pseudogene, which can cause false-positive results.
- If the fetus is Rh⁻, the paternal sample should be analyzed. Occasionally, spontaneous gene rearrangement results in a fetus mistakenly labeled as Rh⁻, when in fact, it did inherit the paternal D antigen.
- If the fetus is Rh⁻ and a paternal sample is unavailable, the maternal titer is repeated in 4 to 6 weeks. If it remains stable, the clinician can be reasonably certain that the fetus is indeed Rh⁻. A rise in the titer should raise suspicion that the fetus is actually Rh⁺ and managed accordingly.
- Follow **middle cerebral artery (MCA) Dopplers** as a noninvasive alternative to amniocentesis to track fetal anemia. Most centers follow Dopplers every 1 to 2 weeks to detect evolving anemia.
  - The anemic fetus preferentially shunts blood to the brain, called "brain sparing." The combination of increased blood flow and lower blood viscosity (due to the anemia) increases the systolic velocity in the arteries of the head.
  - A peak systolic velocity >1.5 MoM suggests clinically significant anemia.
  - MCA Doppler testing is 87% sensitive. The positive predictive value is 53%, and the negative predictive value is 98%.
  - MCA Dopplers can only be performed in centers with trained, experienced personnel. False-positive and false-negative results can easily derive from technical difficulties.
  - Reliability of MCA Dopplers decreases after 35 weeks and after fetal blood transfusion.
- **Amniocentesis** may also be used to follow fetal anemia. In 1961, Liley demonstrated that amniotic fluid bilirubin levels due to fetal hemolysis are directly proportional to the spectrophotometric absorbance at 450 nm (ΔOD450). This measure correlates well with fetal status. Most centers begin serial amniocentesis at 24 to 26 weeks. ΔOD450 trends are more reliable than a single value, so serial amniocenteses should be plotted.
  - The **Liley curve** has three prognostic zones (Fig. 18-4):
    - Zone 1: The fetus is unaffected or only mildly affected; repeat amniocentesis in 10 to 14 days.
    - Zone 2: The fetus has mild-to-moderate hemolysis. A value in upper Zone 2 (>80%) is an indication for fetal blood sampling. A value in the lower zone (<80%) should prompt repeat testing in 10 to 14 days.
    - Zone 3: The fetus is likely to be anemic. Fetal death is highly probable in 7 to 10 days without intervention. Fetal blood sampling is indicated.
  - Exposing the specimen to light, or administering maternal corticosteroids will falsely lower the ΔOD450.
  - The **Queenan curve** is an extrapolation of the Liley curve, used at earlier gestational ages.
- **Percutaneous umbilical blood sampling (PUBS)** allows direct fetal blood sampling and, if necessary, transfusion. PUBS transfusion is performed between 18 and 35 weeks' gestation. After 35 weeks, delivery is preferred.
  - PUBS carries a risk of fetal death, so it is performed only when MCA Doppler or ΔOD450 values are elevated.

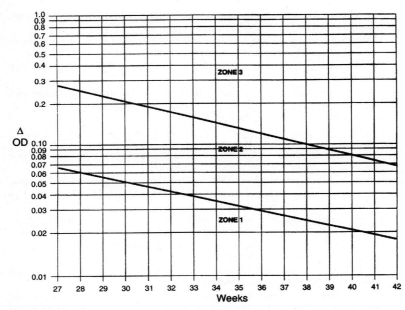

Figure 18-4. Liley curve depicting degrees of Rh sensitization. ΔOD, optical density at 450 nm. (From Liley AW. Liquor amnii analysis in management of pregnancy complicated by rhesus sensitization. *Am J Obstet Gynecol* 1961;82:1359–1370.)

- ○ PUBS should only be performed in a facility with trained personnel and a NICU capable of caring for the preterm neonate if complications occur.
- **Fetal testing** with serial nonstress tests and/or biophysical profiles is performed weekly beginning at 28 to 32 weeks (see Chapter 6).
- **Delivery** is recommended at or after 35 weeks if the fetus has required transfusion or develops abnormal Doppler studies.
  - ○ If the maternal critical titer is not reached, induction of labor between 37 and 39 weeks with or without confirmation of fetal lung maturity is preferred as risks of hemolysis outweigh the risks of immaturity.
  - ○ Route of delivery should be determined by obstetrical indications. Cesarean delivery is not required.
  - ○ Affected neonates may be anemic or jaundiced. Mild cases are treated with phototherapy. Neonatal exchange transfusion may be performed for more severe disease.
- **Subsequent pregnancy management** is guided by titer and outcome.
  - ○ If a patient previously had an affected infant (i.e., *hydrops fetalis* or need for intrauterine transfusion), titers are not helpful in managing future pregnancies.
  - ○ If the father is Rh⁺ heterozygous, amniocentesis at 15 to 18 weeks can determine fetal blood type.
  - ○ If the father is Rh⁺ homozygous, all fetuses will be Rh⁺. No amniocentesis is required.
  - ○ If the fetus is Rh⁺, begin serial amniocentesis or MCA Doppler evaluation every 1 to 2 weeks at 18 weeks' gestation.

Minor RBC Antigens

Other RBC antigens in the erythrocyte Rh complex include the following: **C, c, E, e, Kell, Duffy, and Lewis**.

- Only **anti-c** causes severe disease. Isolated anti-C, anti-E or anti-e generally causes milder disease.
  - If the mother is sensitized to any of these, management is generally the same as for Rh D alloimmunization.
  - Paternal status must be determined by red cell phenotype. Blood and Rh typing are not sufficient.
- The **Kell** group is the most common minor RBC antigen. At least seven different Kell antigens have been identified. The most common is K.
  - Kell alloimmunization usually results from prior maternal transfusion; Kell is not routinely screened for blood transfusions.
  - Unlike the other red cell antigens, anti-Kell antibodies cause both hemolysis and suppression of fetal erythropoietin/erythropoiesis.
  - ΔOD450 and serial titers are not helpful.
  - Serial MCA Dopplers guide clinical management.
- The **Duffy** group also confers risk of fetal hydrops.
- The **Lewis** antigens, Le^a and Le^b, are not innate red cell antigens. They are secreted by other tissues and acquired by red cells. Antibodies to Lewis antigens do not result in fetal hydrops.

PLATELET ALLOIMMUNIZATION

NAIT is also called fetal alloimmune thrombocytopenia (FAIT) or fetomaternal alloimmune thrombocytopenia (FMAIT). The overall incidence of NAIT is 1 to 2:1,000 deliveries, although this varies by ethnicity. Over 15 platelet antigens have been identified to date. HPA-1a causes more than 80% of NAIT cases in HPA-1b homozygous mothers (1% to 2% of Caucasians).

Pathophysiology

- The sensitizing process is similar to RBC alloimmunization but with a specific paternal platelet antigen.
- Antibody-mediated destruction of fetal platelets in the most severe cases can result in fetal intracranial hemorrhage (ICH) or visceral hemorrhage.
- Maternal antibody transfer can occur as early as the first trimester.
- The fetus of the primary sensitizing pregnancy can develop serious NAIT sequelae.
- Ten to twenty percent of fetuses with NAIT have ICH. Twenty-five to fifty percent can be detected in utero by ultrasound.
- Fetal death in utero occurs in approximately 14% of cases.

Diagnosis of NAIT

- **Diagnostic workup** is prompted by clinical suspicion. There is no screening test for NAIT. The differential diagnosis for fetal/neonatal thrombocytopenia includes idiopathic thrombocytopenic purpura (ITP). In ITP, maternal platelets are also affected and mothers are thrombocytopenic.
- NAIT evaluation is initiated for the following:
  - Sonographic detection of in utero fetal hemorrhage,
  - Neonatal thrombocytopenia after delivery,

- Prior pregnancy affected by NAIT or fetal hemorrhage, or
- The mother's sister was diagnosed with NAIT.
- The NAIT workup includes the following:
- Maternal antiplatelet antibody testing.
  - Antiplatelet antibodies are not always present or may be only intermittently present.
  - If antigen-specific antiplatelet antibodies are present in maternal blood, parental platelet genotype discordance should confirm the NAIT diagnosis.
- Maternal and paternal platelet genotyping to assess antigen discordance.
  - If the paternal genotype is heterozygous for a platelet-specific antigen that the maternal genotype lacks, then the fetus has a 50% chance (for each discordant antigen) of being at risk for NAIT. Platelet genotyping from fetal blood, placental tissue, or amniotic fluid should be performed.
  - If the paternal genotype is homozygous for a platelet-specific antigen that the maternal genotype lacks, then all pregnancies are at risk.
  - If the maternal and paternal genotypes are the same, the risk of an affected pregnancy is very low. There is, however, the possibility of as yet unknown discordant platelet antigens.

Management of NAIT

- **Management** of pregnancies at risk for NAIT varies among centers. There is no consensus on optimal treatment.
- Maternal antibody titers are not useful and do not guide treatment.
- **Intravenous gamma immune globulin (IVIG)** with or without corticosteroids is currently the best noninvasive therapy. **Corticosteroids** are usually reserved for persistent fetal thrombocytopenia despite IVIG treatment. At our institution, we initiate weekly IVIG at 13 weeks.
- **Fetal blood sampling** is the only way to determine fetal platelet status in pregnancies at risk for NAIT. We usually perform fetal blood sampling between 24 and 28 weeks, and we transfuse antigen-screened platelets for severe fetal thrombocytopenia.
- Anemia of unknown pathogenesis often accompanies thrombocytopenia, so RBC transfusion is often indicated.
- Weekly transfusions may be required until delivery due to the short half-life of transfused platelets.
- **Vaginal delivery** is recommended. There is no benefit to cesarean delivery except for the usual obstetric indications. The timing is controversial and is related to fetal status. Confirm fetal platelet count before delivery and consider transfusing prior to induction. Document fetal lung maturity for early induction of labor if possible.
- After delivery, neonatal platelet counts reach a nadir within the first few days after birth, and gradually improve over weeks as maternal antiplatelet antibodies resolve.
- Term infants with platelets <30,000/μL and preterm infants with platelets <50,000/μL are transfused with platelets ± IVIG.
- Cranial ultrasound is necessary to rule out ICH if platelets are <50,000/μL at birth.
- The recurrence rate is high in subsequent pregnancies (85% to 90%), and those fetuses tend to be more seriously affected.
- At our institution, we start empiric IVIG therapy early in the second trimester to decrease the risk of ICH if paternity is the same or if platelet incompatibility is known, but this practice is under investigation.

SUGGESTED READINGS

Althaus J, Blakemore KJ. Fetomaternal alloimmune thrombocytopenia: the questions that still remain. *J Mat Fetal and Neonatal Med* 2007;20(9):633–637.

Bussel JB, Zabusky MR, Berkowitz RL, et al. Fetal alloimmune thrombocytopenia. *N Engl J Med* 1997;337:22.

Management of alloimmunization. ACOG Practice Bulletin Number 75. American College of Obstetricians and Gynecologists. *Obset Gynecol* 2006;108(2):457–464.

Mari G, Deter RL, Carpenter RL, et al., for the Collaborative Group for Doppler Assessment of the Blood Velocity in Anemic Fetuses. Noninvasive diagnosis by Doppler ultrasonography of fetal anemia due to maternal red-cell alloimmunization. *N Engl J Med* 2000;342:9–14.

Moise KJ Jr. The usefulness of middle cerebral Doppler assessment in the treatment of the fetus at risk for anemia. *Am J Obstet Gynecol* 2008;198:161.

Prevention of Rh D alloimmunization. ACOG Practice Bulletin Number 4. American College of Obstetricians and Gynecologists. *Int J Gynecol Obstet* 1999;66(1):63–70.

Surgical Disease and Trauma in Pregnancy

Jill Edwardson and Nancy A. Hueppchen

GENERAL CONSIDERATIONS

- One in five-hundred pregnant women will require nonobstetric surgery.
- The goals for diagnosis and management of surgical disease during pregnancy are to provide definitive treatment and to maintain a successful pregnancy.
- Diagnosis in pregnancy can be difficult due to the physiologic changes of pregnancy; presentation and symptoms may not be typical.
- Always consider and discuss the potential harm to the fetus for any intervention.
- Risks of nonobstetric surgery during pregnancy include preterm labor (PTL), preterm delivery, and fetal loss. Overall, there is a 9% risk of preterm delivery with surgery during pregnancy.

Anatomic and Physiologic Changes in Pregnancy

- The gravid uterus displaces abdominal organs cephalad and brings adnexal structures into the abdomen.
- Uterine compression of the inferior vena cava decreases venous return and may cause supine hypotension syndrome. Whenever possible, the pregnant patient should be placed in the left lateral decubitus position for surgery.
- Relative leukocytosis makes evaluation of infection more difficult.
- Increased plasma volume, decreased hematocrit, and generally lower blood pressure make acute blood loss assessment more difficult.
- The hypoalbuminemia of pregnancy predisposes to edema.

Diagnostic Radiology and the Pregnant Patient

- Pregnancy should not impede the use of necessary imaging studies for critical diagnoses.
- High doses of ionizing radiation can harm the developing fetus, causing embryonic demise, congenital anomalies, growth restriction, or severe mental retardation.
- An exposure <5 rad is not associated with increased fetal anomalies or pregnancy loss.
- Chest x-ray gives 0.02 to 0.07 millirad.
- CT of the abdomen/pelvis gives 2.5 to 3.2 rad.
- Ionizing radiation at all gestational ages has been related to a small increase in risk for childhood cancers.
- A single abdominopelvic CT in pregnancy does not cause fetal neurologic deficits; one excess case of cancer is predicted per 500 fetal exposures.
- Iodinated radiographic contrast is rated Category B in pregnancy. It crosses the placenta and poses potential harm to the fetal thyroid. ACOG recommends avoiding

iodinated contrast in pregnancy; in cases where contrast imaging is required, the newborn should have thyroid function testing in the first week of life.
- MRI in pregnancy has no known harmful effects. Gadolinium contrast is associated with intrauterine growth restriction and congenital anomalies in animal testing. Clinical judgment and full discussion of risks and benefits should inform its use in pregnant women.

SURGICAL DISEASES IN PREGNANCY

- The optimal timing for surgery in pregnancy is the second trimester. Surgery during the first trimester carries increased risk of spontaneous abortion from disruption of the corpus luteum. Inadequate operative exposure and risk of PTL complicate third trimester surgery.
- For nonemergent surgery, preoperative assessment of fetal viability, gestational age, and anatomic anomalies provides useful information in the event of a surgical or obstetric complication.
- Preoperative and postoperative fetal heart rate monitoring appropriate for gestational age are recommended.
- Intraoperative considerations include the following: positioning in left lateral decubitus, avoiding uterine manipulation, optimizing maternal oxygenation, and avoiding wide variations of blood pressure. Intraoperative fetal heart rate monitoring is not routinely recommended but should be addressed on an individual basis after viable gestational age.
- Current data do not support routine use of intraoperative tocolytic agents. Tocolysis may be considered, however, for postoperative PTL if there is no evidence of uterine infection.

Acute Appendicitis

- **Acute appendicitis** is the most common surgical complication of pregnancy, occurring in 1/1,000 to 1/5,000 pregnancies. The incidence of appendicitis is not increased in pregnancy, although appendiceal perforation is more common, particularly in the third trimester. Perforation rates are 43% in pregnancy and only 4% to 19% in nonpregnant patients. This may be related to delayed diagnosis or reluctance to operate on pregnant women.
- **Clinical presentation** includes the following: anorexia, nausea, vomiting, fever, abdominal pain, rebound tenderness, and leukocytosis with bandemia.
  - A retrocecal appendix may cause right flank or back pain.
  - Seventy percent of pregnant patients with appendicitis demonstrate rebound, guarding, and referred pain, although these findings are less specific in pregnancy.
  - Some features of appendicitis are similar to normal symptoms of pregnancy, such as leukocytosis and back pain. However, bandemia can be revealing, and careful physical examination can exclude musculoskeletal pain.
- The **differential diagnosis** includes the following: ectopic pregnancy, pyelonephritis, acute cholecystitis, pancreatitis, pulmonary embolism, right lower lobe pneumonia, preeclampsia with liver involvement, pelvic inflammatory disease, PTL, abruptio placentae, degenerating myoma, round ligament pain, adnexal torsion, ovarian cyst, and chorioamnionitis. Pyelonephritis is the most common misdiagnosis.

- **Diagnostic evaluation** with ultrasonography is most accurate in the first and second trimesters. It is useful in excluding other diagnoses throughout pregnancy. MRI or CT may be necessary to visualize and evaluate the appendix. MRI is more than 97% accurate in diagnosing appendicitis.
- **Management**
  - Both maternal and perinatal morbidity and mortality are increased for appendicitis in pregnancy. Surgery should not be postponed until the presentation of generalized peritonitis. Treatment is only delayed if the patient is in active labor.
  - For ruptured appendix with active labor, cesarean section may be appropriate. A stable, nonseptic patient with a ruptured appendix in the later stages of labor may have a vaginal delivery.
  - Perioperative antibiotics with a second-generation cephalosporin, extended spectrum penicillin, or triple antibiotic therapy (ampicillin, gentamicin, clindamycin) are administered in all cases and continued postoperatively until 24 to 48 hr afebrile in cases of peritonitis, perforation, or periappendiceal abscess.
  - Laparoscopy may be useful if the diagnosis is uncertain (e.g., with history of pelvic inflammatory disease) and especially in the first trimester. Open laparoscopy is advisable after 12 to 14 weeks' gestation due to the increased risk of uterine perforation on entering the abdomen.
  - Laparotomy is indicated if suspicion for appendicitis is high, regardless of gestational age. It is also preferred for cases of rupture or generalized peritonitis.
  - The role of preoperative or postoperative tocolysis is not well studied and should be used only for standard obstetric indications.
- **Obstetric complications** of appendicitis include PTL (10% to 15%), spontaneous abortion, and maternal mortality. For uncomplicated appendicitis, the fetal loss rate is about 5%. Perforated appendicitis increases fetal loss to 20% to 25% and carries a maternal mortality risk of up to 4%.

Acute Cholecystitis

- **Acute cholecystitis** is common, affecting about 1 in 1,000 pregnant women. The increased gallbladder volume, delayed emptying, and decreased intestinal motility during pregnancy predispose to cholelithiasis. Preexisting gallstones rarely cause acute cholecystitis, however, due to the progesterone-induced decrease in gallbladder contractions approximately, 3% to 10% of pregnant women have asymptomatic cholelithiasis. Cholelithiasis is the main cause of cholecystitis in pregnancy, accounting for more than 90% of cases.
- **Clinical presentation** includes anorexia, nausea, vomiting, fever, and mild leukocytosis. Symptoms may be localized to the flank, right scapula, or shoulder. Murphy's sign is seen less frequently in pregnancy or may be displaced.
- The **differential diagnosis** includes the following: acute fatty liver of pregnancy, abruptio placentae, pancreatitis, acute appendicitis, HELLP syndrome (hemolysis, elevated liver enzymes, and low platelets), peptic ulcer disease, right lower lobe pneumonia, myocardial infarction, and herpes zoster.
- **Diagnostic evaluation** consists of history and physical examination, laboratory tests (leukocyte count, serum amylase, and total bilirubin), and ultrasonography of the right upper quadrant. MR cholangiogram and endoscopic retrograde cholangiopancreatography (ERCP) may be performed in pregnancy.
- **Management**
  - Conservative initial management includes bowel rest, intravenous hydration, analgesia, and fetal monitoring. A short course of indomethacin may be considered to decrease inflammation and relieve pain.

- Antibiotics are warranted if symptoms persist for 12 to 24 hr or infection develops.
- Coverage for enteric Gram-negative flora is desired. Typical regimens include the following: piperacillin/tazobactram (Zosyn) or ceftriaxone plus metronidazole.
- ERCP with sphincterotomy, or percutaneous cholecystotomy, have been reported for more severe cases.
- Surgical management is required in approximately 25% of cases and is indicated for failure of conservative therapy, recurrence in the same trimester, suspected perforation, sepsis, or peritonitis.
- Early cholecystectomy, even in noncomplicated cases, decreases the length of hospital stay and the rate of preterm delivery; some centers proceed to surgery quickly.
- While laparoscopic cholecystectomy may be performed in all trimesters, consider scheduling cases in the second trimester, if possible.
- Intraoperative cholangiography is safe after organogenesis is complete; it is generally avoided unless gallstone pancreatitis is suspected.
- **Complications** of acute cholecystitis in pregnancy include the following: gangrenous cholecystitis, gallbladder perforation, choledocholithiasis, and cholecystoenteric fistulas. Severe complications such as ascending cholangitis and gallstone pancreatitis are associated with 15% maternal mortality and 60% fetal loss.

Bowel Obstruction

- **Bowel obstruction** during pregnancy is most commonly caused by adhesions (60%) or volvulus (25%).
- Conservative management includes bowel rest, intravenous hydration, and nasogastric suction. Proceed with surgical management if the patient develops an acute abdomen.

Ovarian Torsion and Ruptured Corpus Luteum

- **Torsion** occurs when an adnexal mass twists on its vascular pedicle. A disproportionate share of these cases occur in pregnancy (up to one fourth of all torsion). Causes of adnexal torsion include the following: corpus luteum cysts, dermoids, other neoplasms, and ovulation induction.
- **Clinical presentation** includes the following: acute pain (usually unilateral) with or without diaphoresis, nausea, and vomiting. An adnexal mass may be palpable.
- **Differential diagnosis** includes the following: acute appendicitis, ectopic pregnancy, degenerating uterine myoma, diverticulitis, small bowel obstruction, pelvic inflammatory disease, and pancreatitis.
- **Diagnostic evaluation** is by history and physical examination and ultrasonography with Doppler flow to visualize masses, rule out ectopic pregnancy, and observe blood flow to the ovaries.
- **Conservative management** is indicated for ruptured corpus luteum cysts in hemodynamically stable patients. Corpus luteum cysts usually involute by 16 weeks' gestation.
- **Operative management** is indicated for acute abdomen, torsion, or infarction.
  - Cysts that are persistent, larger than 6 cm, or contain solid elements may require surgery. A laparoscopic approach is often used in the management of adnexal masses in pregnancy.
  - If the ovarian corpus luteum is disrupted, progestins can be used postoperatively to prevent miscarriage up to 10 weeks of pregnancy.
- **Complications** of torsion include adnexal infarction, chemical peritonitis, and PTL.

Breast Mass During Pregnancy

- About 1 in 3,000 pregnant women in the United States is affected by **breast cancer**. Pregnant patients tend to be diagnosed late. The average delay between symptoms and diagnosis is 5 months.
- **Diagnostic evaluation** is similar to that of nonpregnant patients (see Chapter 2).
  - Mammography, with abdominal shielding, is safe in pregnancy; however, there is a 50% false-negative rate.
  - Breast ultrasonography may differentiate solid and cystic masses without radiation exposure but may also give false-negative results.
  - A clinically suspicious breast mass, even with negative imaging, should be biopsied, regardless of pregnancy. Fine needle aspiration and core biopsy are safe in pregnancy.
- **Management** of pregnant patients should avoid external beam radiation and hormonal treatments.
  - Chemotherapy may be used after the first trimester, but the patient should be counseled about risks to the fetus.
  - Methotrexate, tamoxifen, and anthracycline should be avoided during pregnancy.
  - Pregnancy termination should be discussed. However, no survival benefit is shown for first-trimester termination.

Pregnancy After Bariatric Surgery

- Bariatric surgery is increasingly common among reproductive-age women.
- Conception should be delayed for 12 to 18 months after bariatric surgery, during the period of most rapid weight loss.
- Limited data on pregnancy after bariatric surgery suggest that there is no increase in adverse fetal outcomes. Complications such as gestational diabetes, preeclampsia, and fetal macrosomia may be less common in patients following bariatric surgery than in their obese counterparts but may still occur with greater frequency than the general population.
- Patients who have had gastric banding may need band adjustment during pregnancy.
- Bariatric surgery patients should be appropriately counseled about nutritional goals and risks. Vitamin and mineral deficiencies, including B_{12}, folate, iron, and calcium, should be monitored.

TRAUMA IN PREGNANCY

Ten to twenty percent of pregnant women experience physical injury. **Trauma** is the leading cause of death for women of childbearing age and is the number one cause of maternal death during pregnancy, accounting for 40% to 50% of maternal deaths. The leading causes of trauma in pregnancy include motor vehicle accidents (50%), falls (20% to 30%), physical abuse (10% to 20%), gun violence (4%), sexual assault (2%), and thermal injury/burns (1%).

- During the first trimester, the uterus is mostly protected by the bony pelvis.
- Complications from trauma include PTL and delivery, premature rupture of membranes (PROM), placental abruption, fetal-maternal hemorrhage with risk of alloimmunization, direct fetal injury, fetal demise, and maternal bladder rupture.
  - Placental abruption is identified in 6% of trauma cases.
  - Fetal injury can include skull fractures and intracerebral hemorrhage from blunt pelvic trauma or direct injury from a penetrating wound.

- Fetomaternal hemorrhage occurs in 9% to 30% of trauma cases. Signs include fetal anemia, fetal tachycardia, and fetal demise.
- Due to the risk of fetomaternal hemorrhage, all Rh-negative pregnant women should receive Rhogam, if appropriate, after trauma.

Trauma Assessment in Pregnancy

- **Assessment of the pregnant trauma patient** is the same as for nonpregnant patients. The mother should be stabilized first, a primary survey conducted, oxygen administered to maintain saturation >95%, and IV access obtained. Intubation should be performed early, if necessary, to maintain fetal oxygenation and reduce the risk of maternal aspiration.
- **Primary assessment**
  - If the gestational age is >20 weeks, place the patient in the left lateral decubitus position or supine with a wedge under the right hip in order to displace the gravid uterus off the inferior vena cava.
  - Two large-bore intravenous catheters should be placed and crystalloid administered in a volume three times the estimated blood loss (i.e., 3:1 ratio).
  - Initiate blood transfusion for estimated blood loss (EBL) >1 L. Patients may lose up to 1,500 mL of blood before becoming unstable due to the increased blood volume in pregnancy.
  - Avoid vasopressors, if possible, as they depress uteroplacental perfusion. Do not withhold them if they are needed, as for cardiogenic or neurogenic shock. See Chapter 3.
- **Secondary assessment** is performed after initial stabilization.
  - Examine the patient's entire body, particularly the abdomen and uterus.
  - Assess fetal well-being and estimate gestational age with ultrasound.
  - Assess fetal heart rate by doptones or continuous monitoring, depending on gestational age, and place a tocodynamometer for uterine contractions.
    - ○ Greater than four contractions per hour during the first 4 hr of monitoring and/or a positive Kleihauer-Betke (KB) test are concerns for abruption. Fewer than four contractions per hour over 4 hr of fetal monitoring and a negative KB are not associated with increased adverse outcomes.
  - Perform a pelvic examination to evaluate for bleeding, ruptured membranes, and cervical change.
- **Diagnostic evaluation**
  - CT scan should be performed if indicated and the patient is stable. It should not be delayed due to pregnancy.
  - Ultrasonography may be used to screen for abdominal injury and to evaluate fetal age and viability. Ultrasound in trauma is 61% to 83% sensitive and 94% to 100% specific in detecting intra-abdominal injury during pregnancy.
  - Diagnostic peritoneal lavage (DPL) is riskier in pregnant patients than in nonpregnant patients but still has a morbidity rate of <1%. Typically, CT and ultrasound are sufficient and DPL is not needed.
  - Laboratory studies include blood type and antibody screen, cross-match for anticipated needs, CBC, KB test, coagulation profile, and toxicology screen including blood alcohol level.
  - Cesarean delivery for fetal distress, abruptio placentae, uterine rupture, or unstable pelvic or lumbosacral fracture in labor may be considered if the mother is stable, depending on gestational age, fetal status, and uterine injury.

- Tocolysis in trauma cases is controversial but not contraindicated. Standard tocolytic agents produce symptoms that can complicate assessments, however, such as tachycardia (betamimetics), hypotension (calcium channel blockers), and altered sensorium (magnesium sulfate).
- Fetal monitoring protocols after trauma vary among institutions and have not been evaluated rigorously. We typically monitor patients for 2 to 4 hr after any trauma. If >4 to 6 contractions per hour are detected, continuous monitoring is extended to 24 hr; injuries that are more serious, significant pain, vaginal bleeding, or nonreassuring fetal monitoring warrant extended observations as well.

Specific Traumatic Injuries

Blunt Trauma

- Motor vehicle collision is the most common cause of blunt trauma. Pregnant women should wear seat belts with the lap belt secured over the bony pelvis and not across the fundus. The shoulder strap should be placed across the woman's chest.
- Physical examination includes careful assessment for vaginal bleeding and PROM.
- Laboratory testing includes: CBC, type and screen, and KB test.
- Perform radiographic studies as indicated.
- Complications include retroperitoneal hemorrhage (more common in the pregnancy from the marked engorgement of pelvic vessels), abruptio placentae, preterm labor, and uterine rupture.
  - Abruptio placentae occurs in up to 38% of major and 3% of minor blunt trauma cases.
  - Uterine rupture occurs in <1% of trauma cases, usually from direct high-energy abdominal impact. It often results in fetal death.
  - Complications are more likely in the presence of pelvic fractures. Pelvic fracture with retroperitoneal hemorrhage in a pregnant woman causes significantly increased blood loss compared to nonpregnant patients.
  - Splenic rupture is the most common cause of intraperitoneal hemorrhage.
  - Bowel injuries are less common during pregnancy.
- Fetal death is most commonly caused by maternal death and correlates with severity of injury, expulsion from the vehicle, and maternal head injury.

Penetrating Trauma

- Gunshot and stab wounds are the most common causes of penetrating trauma.
- The health of the mother is of primary concern and takes precedence over the fetus, unless vital signs cannot be maintained in the mother, in which case perimortem cesarean section should be considered.
- Gunshot wounds to the abdomen carry a fetal mortality rate of 41% to 71%. Evaluation includes thorough examination of all entrance and exit wounds with radiographs or CT to help localize the bullet.
- Stab wounds carry a more favorable prognosis than gunshot wounds. CT may help assess the extent of injuries.
- Exploratory laparotomy is performed for any penetrating trauma to the abdomen.
  - Laparotomy for maternal indications is not considered a reason to perform a cesarean section, unless a fetal indication for delivery is present or if the gravid uterus prevents appropriate intra-abdominal exploration.

Thermal Injuries/Burns
- Both maternal and fetal outcomes after burn injury are related to the extent of burn area, maternal age and health at baseline, and the gestational age of the fetus. As the burn surface area approaches 50%, mortality exceeds 60% to 70%. In general, mortality parallels burn area for term or near-term pregnant patients with extensive thermal injury.

CARDIOPULMONARY RESUSCITATION (CPR) IN PREGNANCY

- Fetal survival is improved by restoring maternal circulation.
- Causes of cardiac arrest in pregnant patients include: trauma/hemorrhage, pulmonary embolism, amniotic fluid embolism, stroke, maternal cardiac disease, anesthetic complications, and flash pulmonary edema.
- Standard Advanced Cardiac Life Support (ACLS) protocols are obeyed without modification for pregnancy.
  - Leftward uterine displacement should be used during compressions.
  - Administer drugs per protocol. Pressors should not be withheld as fetal outcome depends on successful maternal resuscitation.
  - Intubate early to reduce aspiration risk.
- **Perimortem or emergency cesarean section** is rarely required except in patients with a viable fetus who do not respond to resuscitation.
  - Perimortem delivery improves maternal resuscitation by increasing venous return and cardiac output.
- **The decision to proceed with postmortem cesarean section** should be made within 4 minutes of cardiac arrest with delivery by 5 minutes for the best outcome. If delivery is delayed more than 10 to 15 minutes, fetal death is likely.
  - Infant survival has been reported up to 35 minutes after maternal arrest. Attempt delivery if any signs of fetal life are detected.
  - Delivery does not need to be emergent for maternal brain death unless fetal compromise is present.
- **Perimortem cesarean** should be performed immediately at the bedside. A sterile field is unnecessary. Generally, a midline vertical skin incision is made with a scalpel and carried down to the uterus. The hysterotomy is also performed by midline vertical incision. After delivery of the fetus and placenta, the uterus is closed using running locked sutures. Continue CPR throughout the procedure. If maternal survival is possible, start broad-spectrum antibiotics. Careful documentation of the circumstances and indications for this procedure is essential.

SUGGESTED READINGS

Chames MC, Pearlman MD. Trauma during pregnancy: outcomes and clinical management. *Clin Obstet Gynecol* 2008;51(2):398–408.

Dietrich CS, Hill CC, Hueman M. Surgical diseases presenting in pregnancy. *Surg Clin N Am* 2008;88:403–419.

Guidelines for diagnostic imaging during pregnancy. ACOG Committee Opinion Number 299. American College of Obstetricians and Gynecologists. *Obstet Gynecol* 2004 (reaffirmed 2009);104:647–651.

Nonobstetric surgery in pregnancy. ACOG Committee Opinion Number 284. American College of Obstetricians and Gynecologists. *Obstet Gynecol* 2003;102:431.

Obstetric aspects of trauma management. ACOG Educational Bulletin Number 251, September 1998, reaffirmed 2006. American College of Obstetricians and Gynecologists. *Int J Gynaecol Obstet* 1999;64:87–94.

Parangi S, Levine D, Henry A, et al. Surgical gastrointestinal disorders during pregnancy. *Am J Surg* 2007;193(2):223–232.

Patel SH, Reede DL, Katz DS, et al. Imaging the pregnant patient for nonobstetric conditions: Algorithms and radiation dose considerations. *Radiographics* 2007;27:1705–1722.

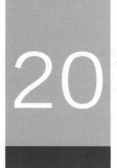

20 Postpartum Care and Breast-feeding

Jacqueline Baselice and Shari Lawson

POSTPARTUM CARE

Immediate postpartum care includes monitoring vital signs, managing/relieving pain, and observing for complications. Patients who have had a cesarean section should receive special attention, recognizing that they are postsurgical patients. As the risk of postpartum complications decreases, attention should be turned to education. Important issues to cover include maternal self-care, appropriate sexual and physical activity, breast-feeding, and infant care and nutrition.

Common postpartum complications

- **Postpartum hemorrhage** has various definitions: (a) estimated blood loss >500 mL for a vaginal delivery and >1,000 mL for a cesarean delivery; (b) a 10% change in hematocrit between admission and the postpartum period; or (c) excessive bleeding that produces symptoms requiring erythrocyte transfusion. Excessive blood loss that occurs within 24 hr of delivery is termed *primary* or *acute* postpartum hemorrhage, while more than 24 hr after delivery (up to 6 weeks) is termed *secondary* or *late* postpartum hemorrhage. The incidence of postpartum hemorrhage is approximately 4% with vaginal delivery and 6% with cesarean delivery.
- **Postpartum febrile morbidity** is defined as a temperature higher than 38.0°C on at least two occasions at least 4 hr apart, after the first 24 hr postpartum. The differential diagnosis includes breast engorgement, atelectasis, urinary tract infection, and endomyometritis. All maternal fevers should be reported to the newborn nursery.
  - **Urinary tract infection** is common in pregnancy and after catheterization; culture should be considered based on clinical examination.
  - **Endomyometritis** complicates 1% to 3% of vaginal deliveries and is up to ten times more common after cesarean delivery. It presents as fever, uterine fundal tenderness, malaise, or foul-smelling lochia and is usually a polymicrobial infection of Gram-positive aerobes (groups A and B streptococci, enterococci), Gram-negative aerobes (*Escherichia coli*), and anaerobes (*Peptostreptococcus, Peptococcus, Bacteroides*) from the genital tract. Bacteremia may be present in 10% to 20% of cases.
    - Endomyometritis should be treated with intravenous antibiotics until the patient is clinically improved and afebrile for 24 to 48 hr. ACOG recommends treatment with gentamicin (1.5 mg/kg every 8 hr) and clindamycin (900 mg every 8 hr), with the addition of ampicillin (2 g every 4 to 6 hr) if fever persists after initial treatment. Some practitioners simply begin initial therapy with the triple antibiotic regimen. Further treatment with oral antibiotic therapy is unnecessary once the patient has been afebrile for at least 24 hr and her symptoms have improved. Response to antibiotic treatment is usually prompt. Persistent fever after 48 to 72 hr of antibiotic treatment necessitates further evaluation.

- Other causes of postpartum fever include: **breast engorgement, pneumonia** (particularly if the patient received general anesthesia), **retained products of conception** (especially if bleeding is heavier than normal), **pelvic abscess, wound infection, infected hematoma, ovarian vein thrombosis**, and **septic pelvic thrombophlebitis (SPT)**.
- **SPT** is rare but more frequent after cesarean section. It is characterized by high spiking fevers despite appropriate antibiotics. Patients tend to feel well between fevers and have no complaint of pain. Imaging is frequently obtained to look for an abscess, but the pelvic clots with SPT are not always seen on CT or MRI, so the diagnosis is made based on clinical examination and exclusion of other causes. Continued antibiotics and the potential addition of heparin anticoagulation are suggested, though debatable, treatments.
- **Hypertension** is defined as blood pressure (BP) of 140/90 or higher, taken with the patient in a seated position on two or more occasions at least 6 hr apart. Preeclampsia or eclampsia can present postpartum, even in the absence of antenatal complications. Any pressure reading of 140/90 or higher should be evaluated by repeating BP measurement, dipping urine for protein, and evaluating for other signs and symptoms of preeclampsia. In those women who had antenatal pre-eclampsia, postpartum diuresis and normalization of BP are generally expected. Hypertension from preeclampsia can persist for up to 6 weeks, however, and may require temporary treatment.

Postpartum Immunizations

- **Immunizations/injections** that may be offered postpartum include hepatitis A and B, rubella, rubeola, pertussis, and varicella, all as indicated. See Chapter 1.
  - **Rh D immunoglobulin.** An unsensitized Rh-negative woman who delivers an Rh-positive infant should receive 300 μg of Rh D immunoglobulin within 72 hr of delivery even if Rh immunoglobulin was given antepartum. If there is laboratory evidence of excessive maternal-fetal hemorrhage, additional doses may be required. The blood bank should perform a rosette test or Kleihauer-Betke test to assess the amount of maternal-fetal blood mixing and to calculate the additional amount of Rh D immunoglobulin to administer.
  - **Rubella vaccine.** Mothers who are rubella nonimmune should receive the measles-mumps-rubella (MMR) vaccine prior to discharge after delivery. Use of monovalent rubella vaccine (i.e., Rubivax) is generally not appropriate because MMR is more cost-effective and because many women without immunity to rubella also lack immunity to rubeola (measles). Breast-feeding is neither a contraindication to MMR vaccination nor should breast-feeding be discouraged after MMR injection.

Discharge from Hospital

- When no complications occur, mothers may be discharged 24 to 48 hr after vaginal delivery and 24 to 96 hr after cesarean delivery. The following criteria should be met:
  - Vital signs are stable and within normal limits.
  - Uterine fundus is firm and decreasing in size (within 24 hr postpartum a uterus without fibroids should decrease to 20-week size).
  - The amount and color of lochia are appropriate—red, less than a heavy period, and decreasing.
  - Urine output is adequate.

- Perineal pain is adequately controlled with sitz baths, ice packs, and analgesics.
- Any surgical incisions or vaginal repair sites are healing well without signs of infection.
- The mother is able to eat, drink, ambulate, and void without difficulty.
- No medical or psychosocial issues are identified that preclude discharge.
- The mother has demonstrated knowledge of appropriate self-care and care of her infant.
- The issue of contraception has been addressed.
- Appropriate immunizations and Rh immunoglobulin, if appropriate, have been administered.
- Follow-up care has been arranged for mother and infant.
- Infant nutritional needs have been addressed.

Outpatient Postpartum Visit

- **The postpartum visit** can be scheduled for 4 to 6 weeks postpartum unless a problem that requires closer follow-up is identified. For example, women with hypertensive complications should have a BP check and brief assessment within 1 week of discharge. Immunization status should be reviewed and vaccines that were not given immediately postpartum may be offered. The following are other important elements of routine postpartum visits:

Physical Exam
- BP, breast, abdomen, and pelvic examination (including vaginal repair assessment).
- At 2 weeks postpartum, the nonmyomatous uterus is usually not palpable abdominally.
- By 6 weeks postpartum, the uterus should return to 1.5 to 2.0 times its nonpregnant size.
- By 6 weeks postpartum, lochia should be essentially absent.
- If lochia is persistent, it should be reevaluated at 10 to 12 weeks. If still bleeding, evaluation is warranted, including measurement of serum human chorionic gonadotropin.

Sexual Activity and Contraception
- See below in breast-feeding section and Chapter 29 for contraception topics.
- When the perineum is healed and bleeding decreased, sexual activity may be safely resumed.
- Any significant dyspareunia should be evaluated.

Depression Screening
- Assess psychosocial well-being; consider depression screening surveys.
- If there is evidence of depression, antidepressant medication should be considered, and the patient should be referred for mental health care.
- Thyroid-stimulating hormone level may be determined to evaluate postpartum hypothyroidism.

Antenatal Complications
- Patients with preeclampsia should be followed to rule out chronic hypertension or nephrotic syndrome.
- Women with gestational diabetes should be screened for diabetes (see Chapter 13).

BREAST-FEEDING

Recommendations

- The American Academy of Pediatrics advises exclusive breast-feeding for the first 6 months of life and partial breast-feeding (plus complementary foods) for at least 12 months. See Table 20-1.
- The World Health Organization recommends continued partial breast-feeding for 2 or more years.
- Breast-feeding should be encouraged as soon as possible after delivery. Infants and mothers who initiate breast-feeding within the first hour after delivery have a higher success rate than those who delay.

TABLE 20-1	Benefits of Breast-feeding

For Newborns	For Mothers
<ul><li>Excellent nutrition matched to needs.</li><li>Milk content changes with developmental needs (i.e., more protein/minerals after delivery and increased water, fat, and lactose later).</li><li>Secretory IgA at high levels in colostrum. Passive immunity passed to infant.</li><li>Boosts cellular immunity by promoting phagocytosis by macrophages and leukocytes.</li><li>Bifidus factor in milk promotes *Lactobacillus bifidus* proliferation, protecting from diarrheal pathogen proliferation.</li><li>Decreases the rate and/or severity of bacterial meningitis, bacteremia, diarrhea, respiratory tract infection, necrotizing enterocolitis, otitis media, urinary tract infections, and late-onset sepsis in preterm infants.</li><li>21% reduced infant mortality in breast-fed infants in the United States.</li><li>Breast milk proteins are human specific, thus delaying or reducing some environmental allergies.</li><li>May decrease the incidence and severity of eczema.</li></ul>	<ul><li>Supports early bonding between mother and infant.</li><li>Oxytocin release during milk let-down increases uterine contractions, thereby decreasing postpartum blood loss and facilitating uterine involution.</li><li>Decreased lifetime risk of ovarian and premenopausal breast cancer proportional to duration of breast-feeding.</li><li>Decreased incidence of osteoporosis and postmenopausal hip fracture.</li><li>Lower cost compared with formula feeding.</li><li>Faciliates pregnancy-spacing due to lactational amenorrhea.</li></ul>

- Newborns should be fed every 2 to 3 hr until satiety. Feeding for at least 5 minutes at each breast at each feeding on postpartum day 1 and gradually increasing feeding time over the next few days will allow optimal milk let-down with less nipple soreness.
- Arouse nondemanding infants every 4 hr for feeding. Frequent breast-feeding establishes maternal milk supply, prevents excessive engorgement, and minimizes neonatal jaundice.
- Breast-feeding may be associated with initial minor discomfort. Painful breasts should be assessed and positioning reevaluated. Nursing on the less sore breast first, rotating stress points on nipples, and breaking suction before removing the infant may help. Nipple tenderness can be treated with lanolin cream.
- Breast-feeding increases maternal caloric requirements by 500 to 1,000 kcal/day and increases the risk of deficiencies in magnesium, vitamin B_6, folate, calcium, and zinc. Thus, women should be encouraged to continue taking their prenatal multi-vitamin supplement. Human milk may not provide adequate iron for premature newborns or for infants older than 6 months. These infants, and babies of mothers with iron-deficiency, should receive iron supplements.
- Women who are not breast-feeding will experience breast engorgement about 3 days postpartum, which is often uncomfortable. Breast binding, ice packs, and avoiding nipple stimulation are recommended.
- Healthy People 2010 goals are 75% of all mothers breast-feeding immediately postpartum, 50% at 6 months, and 25% at 12 months.

Contraindications to Breast-feeding

- Some structural problems make breast-feeding difficult and sometimes impossible. These include tubular breasts, hypoplastic breast tissue, true inverted nipples (rare), and surgical alterations that sever the milk ducts.
- Contraindications to breast-feeding include the following:
  - Mother actively using drugs of abuse, including excessive alcohol.
  - Infant with galactosemia.
  - Maternal human immunodeficiency virus (HIV) infection in a developed country. In developing countries, the benefits of breast-feeding may outweigh the small risk of HIV transmission.
  - Maternal active, untreated tuberculosis or women with human T-cell lymphotropic virus type I or II. Women can give their infant expressed breast milk and can breast-feed once their treatment regimen is well established.
  - Active untreated maternal varicella. Once the infant has been given varicella zoster immunoglobulin, expressed milk is allowed if there are no lesions on the breast. Within 5 days of the appearance of the rash, maternal antibodies are produced, making breast milk beneficial for passive immunity.
  - Active herpes lesions on the breast.
  - Mothers who are receiving diagnostic or therapeutic radioactive isotopes or have had recent exposure to radioactive materials.
  - Mothers receiving antimetabolites or chemotherapeutic agents.

Noncontraindications

- Healthy term infants with acquired or congenital cytomegalovirus should breast-feed for the benefit of maternal antibodies.
- Babies of mothers with hepatitis A or B may breast-feed as soon as the infant receives appropriate immunoglobulin and hepatitis vaccination. Special attention to avoid broken skin on or around the nipples of mothers with hepatitis B should be advised.

- Mothers with hepatitis C may breast-feed. There is no evidence for hepatitis C transmission via breast milk. Again, advise no feeding on bleeding or broken skin.

Breast-feeding and Maternal Medications

- Nearly all antineoplastic, thyrotoxic, and immunosuppressive medications are contraindicated during breast-feeding (Table 20-2). In general, breast-feeding can continue during maternal antibiotic therapy. Although all major anticonvulsants are secreted in breast milk, they need not be discontinued unless the infant exhibits excessive sedation. The Web site of the American Academy of Pediatrics (www.pediatrics.org) contains updated information on medication use in breast-feeding.

Breast-feeding and Contraception

- **Contraception during lactation.** In the nonbreast-feeding woman, the average time to first ovulation is 45 days (range 25 to 72 days). The mean time to ovulation is 190 days in women who are breast-feeding exclusively (Fig. 20-1).
- The **lactational amenorrhea method** is 95% to 99% protective in the first 6 months postpartum if strict criteria are followed. Feedings must be every 4 hr during the day and every 6 hr at night, and supplemental feedings should not exceed 5% to 10%.
- **Nonhormonal methods** (e.g., condom, intrauterine device, sterilization) are preferred contraception in lactating women.
- **Progestin-only contraceptives** (e.g., mini-pill, progestin injectables, progestin implants) do not affect the quality of and may increase the volume of breast milk. These are the preferred methods of hormonal contraception. The progestin is detectable in breast milk, but no evidence suggests adverse effects on the infant. The levonorgestrel intrauterine device (Mirena) is a progesterone-only option with greater efficacy; it may be inserted at the 6-week postpartum visit, and some studies suggest immediate postpartum insertion is feasible.

TABLE 20-2	Medications Contraindicated During Breast-feeding
Medication	**Reason for Discontinuation**
Bromocriptine mesylate	Lactation suppression
Cocaine	Cocaine intoxication of the newborn
Ergotamine tartrate	Vomiting, diarrhea, convulsions in the newborn
Lithium	One third to one half of maternal drug levels found in the newborn
Phencyclidine	Potent hallucinogen
Radioactive elements	Enter newborn bloodstream
Cyclophosphamide	Possible neutropenia and immune suppression in the newborn; unknown effect on growth or association with carcinogenesis
Cyclosporine	Same as for cyclophosphamide
Doxorubicin hydrochloride	Same as for cyclophosphamide
Methotrexate sodium	Same as for cyclophosphamide

Adapted from the American Academy of Pediatrics, Committee on Medications, 1994.

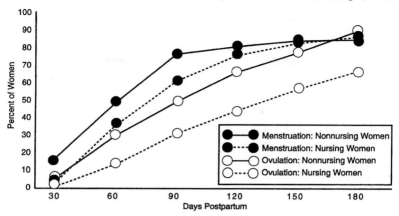

Figure 20-1. Postpartum return of menstruation and ovulation.

- The estrogen in **combination estrogen-progestin oral contraceptive pills (OCPs)** can reduce the quantity and duration of breast milk. WHO recommends waiting at least 6 months before initiating combination OCPs. The U.S. Food and Drug Administration labeling committee recommends not using combination OCPs until the child is completely weaned. ACOG recommends that if combination OCPs are preferred, they should not be started before 6 weeks postpartum, and should only be started after lactation is well established and the infant's nutritional status is good. As with progestin-only contraceptives, some providers may initiate OCPs earlier if lactation is well established, the patient declines other forms of contraception, or the risk of repeat pregnancy is significant.

Mastitis

- **Mastitis** is a breast infection that occurs in 1% to 2% of breast-feeding women, usually between the 1st and 5th weeks postpartum. It is characterized by a localized sore, reddened, indurated area on the breast, and is often accompanied by fever, chills, and malaise.
- Forty percent of mastitis is due to *Staphylococcus aureus* infection. Other common organisms include B-hemolytic streptococci, *E. coli*, and *Haemophilus influenzae*.
- **Treatment** includes continued nursing, nonsteroidal anti-inflammatory pain medication, and antibiotics. Initial antibiotic therapy is often started with dicloxacillin, 500 mg PO four times daily for 10 days. Women should continue to express milk, starting on the affected side, to encourage complete emptying. If there is no improvement in 48 hr, antibiotic coverage should be changed to cephalexin or ampicillin with clavulanate (Augmentin). Continued mastitis, particularly if there is evidence of abscess formation, demands evaluation for the possibility of methacillin-resistant *S. aureus* (MRSA) infection.
- The **differential diagnosis** for mastitis (Table 20-3) includes the following:
  - **Clogged milk ducts:** a tender lump in the breast not accompanied by systemic symptoms that resolves after application of warm compresses and massage. Unrelieved, clogged ducts can lead to galactoceles, cysts filled initially with milk that can become a thick cheesy substance that is difficult to drain. Galactoceles may require ultrasound treatment or needle aspiration if conservative methods fail.

TABLE 20-3	Diagnosis of Postpartum Breast Tenderness		
Finding	Engorgement	Mastitis	Plugged Duct
Onset	Gradual	Sudden	Gradual
Location	Bilateral	Unilateral	Unilateral
Swelling	Generalized	Localized	Localized
Pain	Generalized	Intense, localized	Localized
Systemic symptoms	Feels well	Feels ill	Feels well
Fever	No	Yes	No

From Beckmann CRB, Ling FW, Barzansky BM, et al. *Obstetrics and Gynecology*, 4th Ed. Baltimore, MD: Lippincott Williams & Wilkins, 2002:158, with permission.

- **Breast engorgement:** bilateral, generalized tenderness of breasts, often occurring 2 to 4 days postpartum and associated with low-grade fevers. May be treated with application of warm compresses followed by hand or pump expression of milk and continued breast-feeding.
- **Inflammatory breast cancer:** a rare disease that presents with breast tenderness and breast skin changes.
- **Breast abscess:** a firm, tender, usually well-circumscribed mass. Breast sonography may be required for diagnosis, and incision and drainage may be necessary for treatment.

Decreased Milk Supply

- The normal volume of milk produced at the end of the first postpartum week is 550 mL/day. By 2 to 3 weeks, milk production is increased to approximately 800 mL/day. Production peaks at 1.5 to 2.0 L/day. Exclusively breast-fed newborns can be expected to lose 5% to 7% of birth weight in the first week. If the loss is >7% or very rapid, the adequacy of feeding should be assessed. Glycogen stores in full-term infants generally provide sufficient initial nutrition. Therefore, supplemental feeding should be avoided unless medically indicated. Frequent breast-feeding and good maternal nutrition help maintain milk stores. Sheehan's syndrome (postpartum pituitary necrosis) can also result in lack of milk production from low prolactin levels. It is characterized by postpartum lethargy, anorexia, weight loss, as well as inability to lactate. See Chapter 13.

SUGGESTED READINGS

American Academy of Pediatrics, American College of Obstetricians and Gynecologists. *Breastfeeding Handbook for Physicians*. Elk Grove Village (IL): AAP; Washington, DC: ACOG, 2006.

Breastfeeding: maternal and infant aspects. ACOG Committee Opinion Number 361. American College of Obstetricians and Gynecologists. *Obstet Gynecol* 2007;109:279–280.

French L, Smaill FM. Antibiotic regimens for endometritis after delivery. *Cochrane Database Syst Rev* 2007;1:CD001067.

Postpartum hemorrhage. ACOG Practice Bulletin Number 76. American College of Obstetricians and Gynecologists. *Obstet Gynecol* 2006;108:1039–1047.

Truitt ST, Fraser AB, Grimes DA, et al. Combined hormonal versus nonhormonal versus progestin-only contraception in lactation. *Cochrane Database Syst Rev* 2003;2:CD003988.

21 HIV in Pregnancy

Catherine Eppes and Jean Anderson

The Centers for Disease Control and Prevention (CDC) first reported unusual opportunistic infections in previously healthy gay men in 1981. By 1982, the CDC reported the first case of **Acquired Immunodeficiency Syndrome (AIDS)** transmitted from mother to infant. Today, approximately 33 million people are living with **human immunodeficiency virus (HIV)** infection/AIDS worldwide. One half of the infected are women. About two thirds of infected persons live in sub-Saharan Africa. In 2006, there were 56,300 new HIV infections in the United States with an incidence of 22.8 per 100,000 people. The number of new HIV diagnoses in women is growing fastest among women of childbearing age. In 2004, the CDC reported AIDS as the leading cause of death in African-American women from 25 to 34 years of age. Women account for approximately 27% of new HIV infections in the United States annually, and over three quarters are of reproductive age.

- With the wide use of highly active antiretroviral therapy (HAART) in the developed world, people infected with HIV live longer and lead healthier lives. Improved treatment has reduced morbidity, increased survival, and markedly decreased perinatal transmission. Recent data reported a 150% increase in births to HIV-positive women since widespread use of HAART in pregnancy. This chapter summarizes recommendations regarding the care of HIV-infected women during pregnancy; readers are advised that this is a rapidly evolving field and the most current guidelines should be consulted.

PATHOPHYSIOLOGY OF HIV/AIDS

- HIV is an RNA virus that belongs to the retrovirus (Retroviridae) family and lentivirus subfamily.
- The most common cause of HIV disease in the United States is HIV-1.
- HIV-2, a related strain, is endemic to Western Africa. It is less virulent than HIV-1 and less transmissible. It has a longer incubation period, is associated with lower viral loads, and progresses to AIDS less often than HIV-1. HIV-2 is primarily seen in the United States in immigrants from West Africa.
- Currently, it is estimated that two thirds to three fourths of new cases of HIV in women in the United States result from heterosexual transmission.
- Without any intervention, maternal-to-child transmission (MTCT) of HIV occurs in 14% to 42% of live births, depending on the setting.
- HIV infection results in progressive depletion of helper T cells.
- The subset of T-lymphocytes affected is defined phenotypically by the presence of the CD4 receptor, which is the primary docking protein for HIV.
- Fusion and entry of the virus into the cell are facilitated by coreceptors, including CXCR4 and CCR5.
- Infection results in functional impairment and gradual depletion of CD4 cells, leading to immunodeficiency and subsequent opportunistic infection.

- HIV-RNA level (viral load) reflects active viral replication, and this can be used to track disease progression and therapeutic response. Higher viral loads predict more rapid disease progression.

COUNSELING AND TESTING

- The American College of Obstetricians and Gynecologists (ACOG) and CDC recommend offering **HIV testing** to all pregnant women:
  - as a routine part of antenatal care, unless the woman declines (opt-out approach).
  - with repeat testing in the third trimester to those in areas with high HIV prevalence, to those known to be at risk, and to those who declined earlier testing.
  - as a rapid screen on presentation for any pregnant woman of unknown HIV status.
- It is important to know your state law concerning HIV testing in pregnancy, as rules vary widely.
- Studies have shown that the rate of acceptance of HIV testing varies with the approach:
  - When extensive pretest counseling is required and patients must specifically consent to testing (the opt-in approach), testing occurs less frequently. The opt-out approach includes counseling for basic information about HIV, the rationale for testing, the availability of therapeutic and preventive interventions, and recognition of ability to refuse testing.
- Most patients test positive within 1 month of primary infection. However, seroconversion may take up to 6 months.
- The most commonly used HIV screening test is a laboratory serum **enzyme-linked immunosorbent assay (ELISA)**. A positive or indeterminate test is followed by a **Western blot** for confirmation.
- Rapid HIV immunosorbent assays are available, requiring about 20 minutes to obtain a result. Many of the simple bedside or office rapid tests are clinical laboratory improvement amendments (CLIA) waived. The sensitivity and specificity of these tests are comparable to the ELISA HIV test. Since the positive predictive value declines with decreasing seroprevalence, a positive result with a rapid HIV test must be confirmed by the Western blot test.
- Appropriate posttest counseling is required. Important issues include:
  - the role of safe sex practices in preventing HIV transmission and limiting other sexually transmitted disease (STD) infections, including superinfection with resistant strains of HIV-1.
  - HIV screening of older children who may have been perinatally infected.
  - encouraging substance abuse rehabilitation, if appropriate.
  - encouraging disclosure to sexual partners and health care providers; offer assistance with disclosure and consider issues related to possible domestic violence.

MANAGEMENT OF HIV INFECTION IN PREGNANCY

Preconception

- In pregnancies complicated by HIV disease, the major goals are to optimize maternal health and to reduce the risk of perinatal transmission. Ideally, a treatment plan will be made during preconception counseling. HIV status should be assessed by viral load and CD4 count. Appropriate vaccinations to be administered (ideally

before conception) include: influenza, pneumococcus, hepatitis A, hepatitis B, and tetanus. Rubella vaccine is given prepregnancy, if the CD4 count is >200.
- Women who should be on HAART for maternal viral status should be started on medication prior to pregnancy. Women who do not yet meet HAART criteria are generally not started until after the first trimester.
- Prevention of unintended pregnancy is paramount. Current data suggest that over 50% of pregnancies in HIV-positive women are unintended. In HIV-positive adolescents, the rate of unintended pregnancy is as high as 83%.

Antepartum

- In the United States, approximately 19% of HIV/AIDS cases are due to injection drug use. Noninjection drug use (e.g., crack cocaine) also contributes to HIV transmission, and illicit drug use has been associated with higher vertical transmission rates. Rehabilitation resources should be provided.
- Screening for domestic violence is important. Approximately two thirds of HIV-positive women have a lifetime or recent history of violence.
- Addressing mental health concerns is paramount. Up to 50% of HIV-positive women experience depression—more than twice as often as HIV-positive men or the general population. HIV-positive women should be screened for depression in pregnancy and managed appropriately. Mental health status can affect medication adherence.
- Variables associated with **increased vertical transmission** include the following:
  - High plasma or genital tract HIV viral load
  - Primary HIV infection or advanced AIDS
  - Low CD4 count
  - Sexually transmitted/genital tract coinfection
  - Placental disruption/abruption, chorioamnionitis
  - Active substance abuse
  - Invasive fetal monitoring or assessment (e.g., fetal scalp sampling, chorionic villus sampling, amniocentesis)
  - Prolonged rupture of membranes
  - Preterm delivery
  - Episiotomy
  - Instrumental delivery
  - Breast-feeding

Antiretroviral Therapy During Pregnancy

- Although antiretroviral therapy among asymptomatic HIV-infected nonpregnant adults and adolescents is generally delayed until the CD4 count drops below 350 cells/μL, **all pregnant women should be offered treatment** regardless of CD4$^+$ T cell count or viral load to reduce MTCT (see Table 21-1).
- For women who are not on antiretroviral therapy at the beginning of pregnancy, it may be delayed until after the first trimester.
- Women with opportunistic infections should receive appropriate prophylaxis, as outlined in Table 21-2.
- Decisions regarding an appropriate regimen should consider:
  - Previous antiretroviral treatment and viral resistance.
  - Safety and toxicity profiles for specific drugs during pregnancy (considering both mother and fetus).
  - Medical comorbidities that may contraindicate certain medications.
  - Patient compliance/adherence to treatment.

TABLE 21-1	Antiretroviral Therapy and Rates of Perinatal HIV Transmission

Treatment Category	Vertical Transmission Rate (%)
Untreated	20–30
Zidovudine monotherapy	10
Dual therapy	4
HAART	1–2

HAART, highly active antiretroviral therapy

- Specific drug regimens should be selected in consultation with an HIV specialist.
- To optimally suppress viral replication, minimize the risk of vertical transmission, and minimize the risk of new resistance mutations, strict adherence to the treatment regimen is crucial.
- The use of Zidovudine (AZT) alone in the antenatal period is now generally discouraged except in select circumstances including high CD4 count with very low

TABLE 21-2	Opportunistic Infection Primary Prophylaxis	

Opportunistic Infection	Indication	Recommendation
Pneumocystis jeroveci (formerly called *Pneumocystis carinii*) pneumonia	CD4 <200	Bactrim DS daily (preferred); dapsone 50 mg bid or 100 mg daily is alternative Aerosol pentamidine 300 mg dose every 4 wk (may be considered in first trimester; may not achieve adequate distribution in lung in later pregnancy)
Toxoplasma gondii encephalitis	CD4 <100	Bactrim DS daily (preferred) OR pyrimethamine 50 mg weekly + dapsone 50 mg daily + leucovorin 25 mg weekly OR dapsone 200 mg + pyrimethamine 75 mg + leucovorin 25 mg all weekly
Disseminated *Mycobacterium avium* complex	CD4 <50	Azithromycin 1,200 mg weekly OR Rifabutin 300 mg by mouth daily (be aware of drug interactions with antiretroviral therapy; rule out active TB)

Prophylaxis against opportunistic pathogens is indicated at specific CD4 counts, and this treatment should be initiated or maintained in pregnancy. Consult an HIV expert when treatment or secondary prophylaxis/chronic maintenance therapy is needed. Adapted from Centers for Disease Control and Prevention, National Institutes of Health, HIV Medicine Association/Infectious Diseases Society of America. Treating opportunistic infections among HIV-infected adults and adolescents. *MMWR Recomm Rep* 2004;53(RR15);1–112.

VL (<1,000), patient refusal of HAART, or patient nonadherence to HAART. Combination therapy should be considered for all pregnant women, regardless of CD4 or HIV viral load.

- Patients who do not meet the criteria for antiretroviral therapy outside of pregnancy should have all antiretrovirals discontinued in the immediate postpartum period, after the umbilical cord is clamped.
- Current **antiretroviral medications** can be divided into five classes:
  - nucleoside/nucleotide reverse transcriptase inhibitor (NRTI)
  - nonnucleoside reverse transcriptase inhibitor (NNRTI)
  - protease inhibitor (PI)
  - entry inhibitor
  - integrase inhibitor

HAART During Pregnancy (see Tables 21-3 and 21-4)

- HAART is the combination of three or four drugs from at least two different classes. It can dramatically reduce the risk of vertical transmission. Regimens typically include two NRTIs plus a booster PI or a NNRTI

Nucleoside/Nucleotide Reverse Transcriptase Inhibitors (NRTIs)

- Most extensively studied HIV medication in pregnancy.
- Pregnancy does not alter the pharmokinetic profile.
- Maternal/fetal safety considerations:
  - Lactic acidosis/hepatic steatosis. Life-threatening complication related to mitochondrial toxicity. Associated with long-term use of NRTIs, particularly in combination of didanosine/stavudine
    - Clinical manifestations include malaise, weakness, nausea/vomiting, abdominal pain, liver function abnormalities. Can proceed to multiorgan failure. May be confused with pregnancy complications such as HELLP syndrome or acute fatty liver of pregnancy.
    - Monitor LFTs and electrolytes monthly in last trimester. Evaluate new symptoms thoroughly. Check lactic acid levels with concerning clinical picture, not routinely.
  - Mitochondrial toxicity in NRTI-exposed infant can be associated rarely with neurologic defects.
  - Anemia is most associated with zidovudine. Monitor Hgb/Hct and supplement iron and folate.
    - The increased MCV typical of zidovudine use does not indicate folate or B_{12} deficiency.

Protease Inhibitors (PIs)

- Minimal transplacental passage.
- Most PIs are now used with low-dose ritonavir "boost" to achieve a better pharmacokinetic profile.
- Drug-drug interactions are common. Consult drug-interaction tables for patients on any other medications.
- Pharmacokinetic studies suggest lower blood levels of some PIs in pregnancy with standard dosing.
- Maternal/fetal safety considerations:
  - Hyperglycemia/diabetes. Increased risk in general population taking PIs, but no significant increase in gestational diabetes. Standard glucose screening

TABLE 21-3 Preclinical and Clinical Data on Antiretrovirals in Pregnancy

Antiretroviral Drug	FDA Pregnancy Category	Placenta Passage	Long-Term Animal Carcinogenicity Studies	Animal Teratogenicity Studies
Nucleoside and Nucleotide Analogue Reverse Transcriptase Inhibitors				
Abacavir (Ziagen, ABC)	C	Yes (rats)	Positive (malignant and nonmalignant tumors of the liver, thyroid, preputial and clitoral glands)	Positive (fetal anasarca and skeletal malformations)
Didanosine (Videx, ddI)	B	Yes (human)	Negative	Negative
Emtricitabine (Emtriva, FTC)	B	Yes (mice and rabbits)	Negative	Negative
Lamivudine (Epivir, 3TC)	C	Yes (human)	Negative	Negative
Stavudine (Zerit, d4T)	C	Yes (rhesus monkey)	Positive (liver and bladder tumors)	Negative
Tenofovir (Viread)	B	Yes (human)	Positive (hepatic adenomas)	Negative
Zalcitabine (HIVID, ddC)	C	Yes (rhesus monkey)	Positive (thymic lymphoma)	Positive (hydrocephalus)
Zidovudine (AZT)	C	Yes (human)	Positive (noninvasive vaginal epithelial tumors)	Positive (and fetal resorption)
Nonnucleoside Reverse Transcriptase Inhibitors				
Delavirdine (Rescriptor)	C	Unknown	Positive (hepatocellular adenomas, carcinomas)	Positive (VSD)

Efavirenz (Sustiva)	D	Yes (monkey, rat, rabbit)	Positive (hepatocellular adenomas, carcinomas, pulmonary alveolar/bronchiolar adenomas in females)	Positive (anencephaly, anophthalmia, microophthalmia)
Nevirapine (Viramune)	B	Yes (human)	Positive (hepatocellular adenomas and carcinomas)	Negative
Protease Inhibitors				
Amprenavir (Agenerase)	C	Minimal/variable (human)	Positive (hepatocellular adenomas and carcinomas)	Negative (but deficient ossification and thymic elongation)
Atazanavir	B	Minimal/variable (human)	Positive (hepatocellular adenomas)	Negative
Darunavir (Prezista)	B	Unknown	Not completed	Negative
Fosamprenavir (Lexiva)	C	Unknown	Positive (benign and malignant liver tumors)	Negative (deficient ossification with amprenavir)
Indinavir (Crixivan)	C	Minimal (human)	Positive (thyroid adenomas and carcinomas)	Negative (but extra ribs)
Lopinavir/ritonavir (Kaletra)	C	Yes (human)	Minimal/Variable (human)	Positive (hepatocellular adenomas and carcinomas)

(Continued)

TABLE 21-3 Preclinical and Clinical Data on Antiretrovirals in Pregnancy *(Continued)*

Antiretroviral Drug	FDA Pregnancy Category	Placenta Passage	Long-Term Animal Carcinogenicity Studies	Animal Teratogenicity Studies
Nelfavir (Viracept)	B	Minimal/variable (human)	Positive (thyroid follicular adenomas and carcinomas)	Negative
Ritonavir (Norvir)	B	Minimal (human)	Positive (liver adenomas and carcinomas)	Negative (but cryptorchidism)
Saquinavir (Fortovase)	B	Minimal (human)	Negative	Negative
Tipranavir (Aptivus)	C	Unknown	In progress	Negative (decreased ossification and weights)
Entry Inhibitor				
Enfuvirtide (Fuzeon)	B	Unknown	Not done	Negative
Maraviroc (Selzentry)	B	Unknown	In progress	Negative
Integrase Inhibitors				
Raltegravir (Isentress)	C	Yes (rats)	In progress	Negative (extranumerary ribs)

Adapted from Centers for Disease Control and Prevention, National Institutes of Health, HIV Medicine Association/Infectious Diseases Society of America. Treating opportunistic infections among HIV-infected adults and adolescents. *MMWR Recomm Rep* 2004;53(RR15);1–112.

TABLE 21-4 Pharmacokinetics and Toxicity of Antiretroviral Drugs and Recommendations for Use in Pregnancy

Antiretroviral Drug	Pharmacokinetics in Pregnancy	Concerns in Pregnancy	Rationale for Use in Pregnancy
NRTI-Recommended Agents			
Zidovudine	Not significantly altered in pregnancy, no change in dose indicated	No evidence for human teratogenicity. Well-tolerated short-term safety demonstrated	Preferred NRTI for use in combination therapy
Lamivudine	Not significantly altered in pregnancy, no change in dose indicated	No evidence for human teratogenicity. Well-tolerated short-term safety demonstrated	Because of extensive experience with lamivudine in pregnancy in combination with zidovudine, lamivudine plus zidovudine is the recommended dual NRTI backbone
Alternative agents	Didanosine, Emtricitabine, Stavudine, Abacavir		
Insufficient data to recommend	Tenofovir		
Not recommended	Zalcitabine		
NNRTIs			
Nevirapine	Not significantly altered in pregnancy, no change in dose indicated	No evidence for human teratogenicity. Increased risk of symptomatic liver toxicity (often rash-associated and potentially fatal) among women with CD4 counts >250/μL when first starting treatment	Nevirapine should be initiated in pregnant women with CD4 <250/μL only if benefits outweigh risks
Not recommended	Efavirenz, Delavirdine		

(Continued)

TABLE 21-4 Pharmacokinetics and Toxicity of Antiretroviral drugs and Recommendations for Use in Pregnancy *(Continued)*

Antiretroviral Drug	Pharmacokinetics in Pregnancy	Concerns in Pregnancy	Rationale for Use in Pregnancy
Protease Inhibitors			
Lopinavir/Ritonavir	Consider increasing dose from two tablets twice daily to three tablets twice daily during the third trimester, with return to standard dosing postpartum. Data from older capsule formulation suggest lower blood levels with standard dosing in third trimester	No evidence for human teratogenicity. Well-tolerated short-term safety demonstrated	Pharmacokinetic studies of new tablet formation are underway, but insufficient data to make a definitive recommendation regarding dosing in pregnancy.
Alternative agents	Indinavir, Nelfinavir, Ritonavir, Saquinavir		
Insufficient data to recommend	Amprenavir, Atazanavir, Darunavir, Fosamprenavir, Tipranavir		

Insufficient Data to Recommend Entry Inhibitors and Integrase Inhibitors

Adapted from Centers for Disease Control and Prevention, National Institutes of Health, HIV Medicine Association/Infectious Diseases Society of America. Treating opportunistic infections among HIV-infected adults and adolescents. *MMWR Recomm Rep* 2004;53(RR15);1–112.

recommended at 24 to 28 weeks. Consider earlier screening in women with PI-based antiretroviral therapy started before pregnancy or with other risk factors for glucose intolerance.
- Preterm delivery. There is conflicting data on the risk of preterm birth with combination antiretroviral therapy, particularly PIs. Recent meta-analysis of 14 clinical studies in the United States and Europe found no increase in preterm delivery in treated recipients compared to no therapy.

Nonnucleoside Reverse Transcriptase Inhibitors (NNRTIs)
- Nevirapine (NVP) and efavirenz (EFV), the commonly used NNRTIs, have long half-lives.
  - If a combination regimen NNRTI is stopped, there will be a period of functional monotherapy as the other drugs are metabolized and excreted while NNRTI levels persist. Significant NVP levels have been found up to 3 weeks after a single dose of NVP. This increases risk for NNRTI resistance.
  - If an NNRTI regimen is used during pregnancy with a plan to discontinue after delivery, an NRTI "tail" should be prescribed for approximately 7 days after the final NNRTI dose to reduce resistance risk. Another option is to switch the NNRTI to a PI 3 to 4 weeks before delivery, though this is less studied.
- Maternal/fetal safety considerations:
  - NVP (nevirapine, Viramune) is associated with 12-fold increased risk of symptomatic hepatotoxicity when started in women with CD4 counts >250/μL. Death from fulminant hepatic failure has been reported.
    o Most cases occur within the first 18 weeks of therapy; onset can be abrupt. Women who become pregnant while on nevirapine-containing regimens and have immune reconstitution with higher CD4 counts are at lower risk. Nevirapine naive women with CD4 counts >250/μL should not be started on NVP as part of combination therapy unless benefit clearly outweighs risk.
    o When NVP multidrug therapy is initiated, close clinical and laboratory monitoring is advised.
    o Hepatotoxicity has not been reported with single-dose NVP for peripartum prophylaxis.
  - NVP carries risk for drug rash as high as 17%. Severe hypersensitivity and Stevens-Johnson Syndrome have been reported. Two-week introduction dosing of 200 mg NVP daily, increasing to 200 mg twice daily may be helpful.
- EFV (Efavirenz, Sustiva) is pregnancy category D.
  - Serious teratogenic effects in primates and neural tube defects in humans with early in utero exposure are reported.
  - EFV should be avoided in sexually active HIV-positive women who are not using effective consistent contraception.
  - EFV should also be avoided in pregnancy, particularly in the first trimester.

Entry Inhibitors, Integrase Inhibitors
- There is little data on the use of these newer drugs in pregnancy.

Intrapartum

- **IV zidovudine** should be administered, regardless of antepartum regimen or history of zidovudine resistance. When C-section is planned, IV zidovudine should be administered for at least 3 hr prior to C-section to ensure therapeutic blood levels.

- HAART should be continued throughout labor.
- Single dose NVP has not been shown to decrease transmission further in women on combination antiretroviral therapy.

Postpartum

- Discontinue HAART if not indicated by AIDS status or CD4 count.
- Infants receive zidovudine for 6 weeks postpartum.

Perinatal HIV Transmission: Mode of Delivery

- In general, the recommendation for women with a VL >1,000 copies/mL at 36 weeks is **elective cesarean delivery** at 38 weeks or prior to labor or rupture of membranes with 3 hr of zidovudine administered preoperatively. Before the widespread availability of HIV RNA testing and the use of combination antiretroviral therapy during pregnancy, several studies clearly established that cesarean section, if performed before labor or rupture of membranes, significantly reduces perinatal HIV transmission compared to vaginal delivery.
- In 1999, the International Perinatal HIV Group published a meta-analysis of 15 prospective cohort studies addressing the impact of scheduled cesarean section versus vaginal delivery on MTCT. Scheduled cesarean section decreased the risk of mother-to-child HIV transmission by approximately 50%. HIV infection occurred in 8.4% of infants delivered by scheduled cesarean section versus 16.7% for all other modes of delivery. In those who received prenatal, intrapartum, and neonatal antiretroviral therapy, neonatal HIV transmission occurred in 2% of the 196 women with scheduled cesarean-section delivery compared with 7.3% of the 1,255 who had other modes of delivery.
- **Evidence does NOT support cesarean delivery for patients on combination therapy with VL <1,000 copies/mL.**
- Evidence is mixed regarding C-section in patients who are not on HAART, who present in labor or with ruptured membranes, or who have VL >1,000 copies/mL. Mode of delivery should be selected based on duration of rupture, labor progress, HIV viral load, current antiretroviral therapy, and other clinical factors. Augmentation to shorten the time to vaginal delivery may be considered for some patients.
- HIV-infected women have higher **complication rates** (mostly infectious) from scheduled cesarean deliveries than from vaginal deliveries but less than those associated with urgent or emergent C-sections. They also have more complications than uninfected women after cesarean delivery, particularly with lower CD4 counts. The complications with cesarean section are not of sufficient frequency or severity to outweigh the potential benefit for women with increased risk of vertical transmission.
- More studies are needed to determine the optimal management of PPROM with HIV infection and for patients with newly diagnosed HIV in labor (see Table 21-5).
- Transmission risk increases with low maternal CD4 counts and ROM for longer than 4 hr; there is no clear increased risk with ROM for women with higher CD4 levels. The influence of antiviral therapy on transmission with prolonged ROM is unclear.
- **In general, AROM, invasive monitoring, and instrumental delivery should be avoided.**
- During cases of uterine atony, many antiretroviral drugs interact with methergine, and therefore, this drug should be avoided.

TABLE 21-5 Treatment Recommendations Based on Clinical Scenario in the United States

Clinical Scenario	Testing	Treatment
HIV-infected woman on HAART becomes pregnant	If detectible viremia, resistance testing	• Continue current regimen if successfully suppressing viremia (except EFV) • IV zidovudine intrapartum and continue HAART during labor • Zidovudine for 6 wk postpartum for infant • Continue HAART after delivery
HAART naive HIV-infected pregnant woman with indication for antiretroviral treatment	Resistance testing prior to therapy and once on therapy if suboptimal viral suppression	• Initiate HAART (avoid EFV in first trimester) • Use zidovudine in regimen if feasible • IV zidovudine intrapartum and continue HAART during labor • Zidovudine for 6 wk postpartum for infant • Continue HAART after delivery
HAART naive HIV-infected pregnant woman WITHOUT indications for antiretroviral treatment	Resistance testing before initiation and after treatment begins if suboptimal viral suppression	• Delay HAART until after first trimester • Use zidovudine in regimen if feasible • Do not use NVP in regimen, (increased hepatotoxicity with CD4 >250/μL) • Using zidovudine alone is controversial; only for select situations. • IV zidovudine intrapartum and continue HAART during labor • Zidovudine 6 wk postpartum for infant • Discontinue HAART for mother postpartum

(Continued)

TABLE 21-5 Treatment Recommendations Based on Clinical Scenario in the United States *(Continued)*

Clinical Scenario	Testing	Treatment
HIV-infected pregnant women who has received antiretroviral drugs in the past but not currently	Full antiretroviral history, resistance testing prior to initiating and if suboptimal response on treatment	• Initiate HAART based on resistance testing and history • IV zidovudine intrapartum and continue HAART during labor • Zidovudine 6 wk postpartum for infant • Discontinue HAART for mother postpartum, unless meets criteria for ongoing treatment

HIV-infected women who received no antiretroviral therapy prior to labor	Evaluate need for ongoing maternal therapy postpartum	• IV zidovudine intrapartum and 6 wk postpartum for infant-or-
		• Women: IV zidovudine in labor plus single dose-NVP at onset of labor. May give 3TC during labor and zidovudine/ 3TC for 7 d postpartum to reduce NVP resistance
		  Infant: single dose-NVP plus Zidovudine for 6 wk-or-
		• Women: IV Zidovudine in labor
		  Infant: Zidovudine in combination with additional drugs in consultation with pediatric HIV specialist

HIV-exposed infant born to HIV-infected women who has received no antiretroviral treatment prior to or during labor	Evaluate mother for postpartum treatment indications (CD4 count, viral load, presence of opportunistic infections)	• Zidovudine 6 wk postpartum for infant-or- • Zidovudine in combination with additional drugs. Consult pediatric-HIV specialist

HAART, highly active antiretroviral therapy; EFV, efavirenz; NVP, nevirapine; 3TC, lamivudine. Adapted from Centers for Disease Control and Prevention, National Institutes of Health, HIV Medicine Association/Infectious Diseases Society of America. Treating opportunistic infections among HIV-infected adults and adolescents. *MMWR Recomm Rep* 2004;53(RR15);1–112.

Management in Resource Limited Areas

- Management of HIV-positive pregnancies in resource poor countries can be very different from the recommendations presented here. With limited medications, poor health infrastructure, reduced bottle feeding options, and less laboratory testing availability, these recommendations cannot always apply.

COINFECTION WITH VIRAL HEPATITIS

Some women with HIV will be coinfected with hepatitis B (HBV) or hepatitis C (HCV) virus. Antepartum screening is recommended.

Hepatitis B/HIV Coinfection

- Treatment with interferon alpha or pegylated interferon alpha is not recommended during pregnancy.
- Women with chronic hepatitis B who require HAART or HBV treatment should receive a three drug regimen including a dual NRTI backbone of tenofovir plus lamivudine or emtricitabine. These drugs show activity against HBV. Triple therapy is indicated to prevent HBV drug resistance.
- For women who do not require treatment for either disease and will be receiving antiretroviral drugs for prophylaxis of perinatal transmission only (with discontinuation postpartum), consultation with an expert is recommended.
- An elevation of hepatic enzymes may occur following antiretroviral therapy initiation due to an immune-mediated flare in HBV disease from immune reconstitution syndrome, particularly in women with a low CD4 cell count.
- Hepatitis B may increase the hepatotoxicity of certain agents, specifically PIs and NVP. Women with HIV/HBV coinfection should be counseled about signs and symptoms of liver toxicity.
  - Liver function tests should be obtained 2 weeks after starting treatment and then monthly.
- Infants should receive HBIG and the HBV three dose vaccination series after birth.

Hepatitis C/HIV Coinfection

- The seroprevalence of HCV in HIV positive women is 17% to 54%.
- Pegylated interferon-alpha is not recommended, and ribavirin is contraindicated during pregnancy.
- Coinfection significantly increases perinatal HCV transmission. Maternal HCV/HIV coinfection may also increase risk for perinatal HIV transmission.
- Effective combination therapy with three drugs should be considered for all HCV/HIV-infected women regardless of CD4 count and viral load.
- These women can also experience a transient worsening in symptoms due to immune-mediated flare in HCV disease.
- Hepatitis C may increase the hepatotoxicity of certain agents, specifically PIs and NVP. See recommendations for HBV for testing protocol (above).
- Intrapartum management of HIV/HCV coinfected women is no different from management of HIV infection alone. Decisions concerning mode of delivery in HCV/HIV-coinfected pregnant women should be based on HIV considerations alone.
- Infants should receive HCV RNA testing between 2 and 6 months and HCV antibody after 15 months.

SUGGESTED READINGS

Apetrei C, Marx PA, Smith SM. The evolution of HIV and its consequences. *Infect Dis Clin North Am* 2004;18(2):369–394.

Centers for Disease Control and Prevention. Fact sheet. HIV/AIDS among women. CDC-NCHSTP. Divisions of HIV/AIDS Prevention. Available at http://www.cdc.gov/hiv/topics/women/resources/factsheets/women.htm

Cooper ER, Charuat M, Mofenson L, et al. Combination antiretroviral strategies for the treatment of pregnant HIV-1-infected women and prevention of perinatal HIV-1 transmission. *J Acquir Immune Defic Syndr* 2002;29(5):484–494.

Dao H, Mofenson LM, Ekpini R, et al. International recommendations on antiretroviral rugs for treatment of HIV-infected women and prevention of mother-to-child HIV transmission in resource limited settings: 2006 update. *Am J Obstet Gynecol* 2007;197 (3 Suppl):S42–S55.

Hammer SM. Clinical practice. Management of newly diagnosed HIV infection. *N Engl J Med* 2005;353(16):1702–1710.

Holtgrave DR. Causes of the decline in AIDS deaths, United States, 1995–2002: Prevention, treatment or both? *Int J STD AIDS* 2005;16(12):777–781.

Perinatal HIV Guidelines Working Group. Public Health Service Task Force recommendations for use of antiretroviral drugs in pregnant HIV-infected women for maternal health and interventions to reduce perinatal HIV transmission in the United States. April 29, 2009; pp 1–90. Available at http://aidsinfo.nih.gov/ContentFiles/PerinatalGL.pdf

Scheduled cesarean delivery and the prevention of vertical transmission of HIV infection. ACOG Committee Opinion Number 234, May 2000 (replaces number 219, August 1999). American College of Obstetricians and Gynecologists. *Int J Gynecol Obstet* 2001;73: 279–281.

Obstetric Anesthesia

Natalia A. Colón Guzmán and Jamie Murphy

Labor and delivery is a time of intense pain, often influenced by the psychological, emotional, social, cultural, and physical state of the parturient. Multiple techniques and procedures for pain relief during the birthing process are available. With appropriate counseling of risks and benefits, patients can choose their preferred analgesic treatments.

PAIN PATHWAYS

- In the first stage of labor (cervical dilation) the pain is visceral, produced by the distention of the lower uterus and cervix and ischemia of the uterine and cervical tissues. Visceral pain signals traverse T10-L1 white *rami communicantes* and enter the spinal cord.
- The second stage involves both visceral and somatic pain. The parturient experiences more somatic pain in the late first stage of labor (7 to 10 cm cervical dilation), entering into the second stage from distention of the vagina, perineum, and pelvic floor. Somatic pain signals traverse the pudendal nerve (S2-4) and enter into the anterior spinal cord. The parturient also experiences rectal pressure. See Chapter 27 for more on biologic basis of pain perception.

OVERVIEW OF OBSTETRIC ANALGESIA/ANESTHESIA

- Local, regional, and systemic methods of analgesia and anesthesia are used in obstetrics. Local and regional methods include local injection, peripheral nerve block, and regional block. Systemic methods can be administered intramuscularly, intravenously, or by inhalation. General anesthesia is often used in cases where total motor and sensory loss is necessary (Table 22-1).
- During the first stage of labor, visceral pain is mollified by the preferred use of regional anesthesia, such as an epidural, spinal, or a combination of both.
- In **vaginal deliveries**, the goal is to block nociceptive pathways while preserving motor function so that the parturient is comfortable but can participate actively with second stage expulsive effort. Local anesthesia or peripheral nerve block with pudendal injection, or more systemic analgesia with intravenous (IV) pain medication or spinal/epidural block is used during the second stage of labor.
- In **cesarean sections**, anesthetic selection is often determined by the condition of the mother and fetus, the urgency of the procedure, and physician preference. Operative anesthesia requires a denser and higher block than that used for a vaginal delivery because the pain from surgery is more intense. Regional anesthesia is often used because it is safe, effective, and allows the mother to interact with the newborn soon after delivery. Spinal anesthesia is now widely used due to the pencil-point needles that minimize dural puncture size and reduce the risk of spinal headache. General anesthesia renders the patient unconscious and unable to experience the moment of

TABLE 22-1		Use of Anesthesia in Obstetric Situations				
Situation	Local	Peripheral Nerve Blocks	Regional	Systemic	General	Oral Analgesics
Labor—first stage		X (Paracervical)	X	X		
Vaginal delivery	X	X (Pudendal)	X	X		
Cesarean section	X		X		X	
Urgent	X		X		X	
Postpartum pain			X	X		X
Postoperative pain		X	X	X		X

X marks usual options for obstetric anesthesia. For more information on practice patterns for obstetric anesthesia, see: Bucklin BA, Hawkins JL, Anderson JR, et al. Obstetric Anesthesia Workforce Survey. *Anesthesiology* 2005;103:645–653.

birth and is used in urgent situations or for medical indications. Supplemental local anesthesia can be used by the obstetrician on the operative field as well.

TYPES OF OBSTETRIC ANALGESIA/ANESTHESIA

Local Injection (Field Block)

Indications
- Used before cutting or repairing episiotomies or lacerations during and after the delivery
- Common agents include **lidocaine** (1% to 2%) or **2-chloroprocaine** (1% to 3%), which provide anesthesia for 20 to 40 minutes. The maximum allowed dose of injected lidocaine is 4.5 mg/kg.

Advantages
- Can provide pain relief without special equipment or personnel.
- Local block can relieve most of the pain of simple laceration repair.
- Minimal systemic effect if administered correctly.

Limitations
- May not cover entire field well or may not entirely block pain perception.

Risks/Complications
- Inadvertent IV injection can lead to serious systemic complications.
- Hypotension, arrhythmias, and seizures are rare complications.

Peripheral Nerve Block (Pudendal, Paracervical)

Indications
- **Paracervical block** is used for the first stage of labor in patients for whom an epidural or spinal is contraindicated, unavailable, or undesired.
- **Pudendal block** may be used as supplemental analgesia during the second stage of labor or before operative deliveries if an epidural has not provided adequate relief.

Technique
- Paracervical: Five to ten mL of local anesthetic (e.g., 2% chloroprocaine) is injected in the lateral vaginal fornices at the 4 and 8 o'clock positions to a depth of 3 to 4 mm.
- Pudendal: Ten mL of local anesthetic (e.g., 1% lidocaine) is injected transvaginally about 1 cm medial and posterior to the ischial spine along the sacrospinous ligament at a depth of about 1 cm. Care must be taken to avoid injecting directly into the pudendal vessels.

Advantages
- Peripheral nerve block is highly effective. Paracervical block, for example, may offer relief in 75% of patients.

Limitations
- Total anesthetic injection limits apply, as above.
- In some cases, relief may be inadequate. Twenty to thirty minutes are required before full effect. Pudendal block may be ineffective in up to 50% of patients and is frequently unilateral.

Risks/Complications
- Intravascular injection can result in systemic effects, hematoma formation, and pelvic infection; these are recognized complications.
- Fetal bradycardia is a known side effect of paracervical block, occurring in approximately 15% of cases. Direct fetal injection is also a risk with paracervical block, resulting in fetal cardiac toxicity. Except in select cases in which other analgesia is not available, paracervical block is usually avoided.

Regional Anesthesia (Epidural, Spinal)
- **Epidural and spinal anesthesia** are the preferred methods for obstetric pain control in the United States. They may be administered separately or as a combined spinal-epidural (CSE). Analgesia occurs below the T8-10 levels, with varying degrees of motor blockade.

Indications
- May be used when there is anticipated difficulty with intubation, a history of malignant hyperthermia, cardiovascular or respiratory disorders, or a need to prevent autonomic hyperreflexia in women with high spinal cord lesions.
- Regional anesthesia is preferred in women with preeclampsia because it may increase intravillous blood flow and reduce the need for general anesthesia if cesarean delivery is indicated.
- Maternal request alone is sufficient reason to give regional anesthesia.

Technique
- Table 22-2 lists agents commonly used for obstetric regional anesthesia.
- **Epidural** (Fig. 22-1): A catheter is introduced into the lumbar epidural space through an epidural needle. The catheter is secured to the patient's back with adhesive tape. Medication is administered preferably via continuous infusion pump, rather than intermittent bolus, to provide more consistent pain relief. Local anesthetic, neuraxial opioid, or a combination of both is used. A test dose (typically 3 mL of 1.5% lidocaine with 1:200,000 epinephrine in bolus) should be given to determine catheter placement and avoid complications. Patient-controlled epidural anesthesia allows the patient to self-administer small bolus doses by pressing a

TABLE 22-2	Epidural/Spinal Anesthetics	
Class	**Action**	**Examples**
Local anesthetics	Block conductance through sodium channels in axons. Reversible effect	Amides: lidocaine, bupivacaine, ropivacaine Ester: chloroprocaine
Opioids	Act on opioid receptors in dorsal horn of spinal cord	Morphine, fentanyl, sufentanil, alfentanil, meperidine
Adrenergic agonists	Bind to alpha-2 receptors in the spinal cord	Epinephrine, clonidine, dexmedetomidine
Cholinergic agonists	Increase cholinergic effect via muscarinic receptors in the dorsal horn of spinal cord	Neostigmine

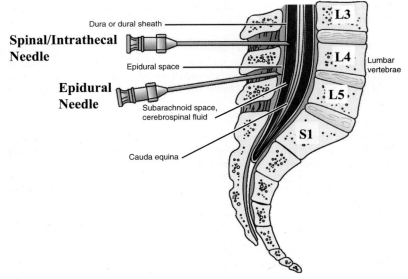

Figure 22-1. Placement of spinal and epidural anesthesia. The spinal cord ends at the conus medullaris near lumbar vertebral bodies L1/L2 in adults, with the cauda equina nerves extending below. Spinal anesthesia is injected directly into the cerebrospinal fluid of the subarachnoid space, while epidural anesthesia is deposited in the epidural space (near L3/L4). Combined spinal-epidural analgesia can be administered with a single needle that allows intrathecal injection followed by epidural catheter placement. L, lumbar; S, sacral. (Adapted from Taylor C, Lillis CA, LeMone P. *Fundamentals of Nursing*, 2nd Ed. Philadelphia, PA: JB Lippincott, 1993, with permission.)

dose-demand button. Pain relief may be further improved by a combination of continuous plus patient-controlled dosing. Breakthrough pain is addressed by increasing the continuous infusion rate or giving a second bolus dose.

- **Spinal:** An opioid, often in combination with local anesthetic, is injected in the subarachnoid space. The onset of action is rapid. Continuous spinal anesthesia can be given by transdural catheter, although there is a significant risk for spinal headache.
- **CSE:** This is the needle-through-needle approach in which a smaller bore spinal needle (i.e., −24 to 27 G) is placed inside the epidural needle. The spinal medication is injected, then the small needle is withdrawn and an epidural catheter threaded into the epidural space as above. A single spinal bolus of opioid, sometimes with local anesthetic, is injected into the subarachnoid space. This method combines the rapid onset of spinal anesthesia with the longer lasting relief of an epidural.

Advantages
- Regional analgesia generally provides excellent pain control but allows the patient to participate actively in the labor and delivery process.

Limitations
- Regional anesthesia cannot be placed in every case due to time, anatomic considerations, comorbidities, or contraindications.
- Twenty to thirty minutes are required for full effect of an epidural.
- Spinal anesthesia lasts only 30 to 250 minutes depending on the drug injected.
- CSE is associated with a higher incidence of fetal bradycardia, with emergency cesarean delivery occurring in 1% to 2% of cases.
- Failure of the spinal component may occur in 4% of cases in which CSE is used.

Contraindications
- Patient refusal.
- Untreated coagulopathy or use of once daily dose of low-molecular weight heparin within 12 hours.
- Thrombocytopenia.
- Infection at injection site.
- Untreated maternal bacteremia.
- Refractory hypotension.
- Increased intracranial pressure caused by a mass lesion.
- History of extensive spinal surgery.

Risks/Complications
- **Infection:** meningitis, epidural abscess, reactivation of latent herpes simplex virus (HSV), and maternal fever.
- **Neurologic complications:** epidural hematoma, neural injury, spinal headache, catheter and needle-related complications, back pain, and nerve palsies.
  - **Spinal headache.** If the subarachnoid space is entered by the epidural needle, a spinal headache may result in up to 70% of patients. Management includes analgesics, supine positioning, hydration, caffeine, and abdominal binding. A **blood patch** can be offered if conservative management fails and the patient desires it.
  - **Back pain.** There is no evidence implicating epidural anesthesia as a cause of chronic back pain.
  - **Nerve palsies.** Injuries to the lumbosacral trunk, lateral femoral cutaneous, femoral, and common peroneal nerves have been reported.

- **Adverse drug reactions.** Local anesthetic toxicity, high spinal block/respiratory distress, allergic reaction, and transient neurologic impairment are possible complications.
  - **Local anesthetic toxicity.** Symptoms include tinnitus, disorientation, and seizures; cardiovascular symptoms include hypotension, dysrhythmias, and cardiac arrest.
  - **High spinal.** Respiratory compromise may result if the block progresses more cephalad than planned.
  - **Motor block.** Motor impairment can reduce maternal expulsive efforts and alter the birthing process and parturient experience.
  - Intrathecal opioids can cause **maternal respiratory depression** and hypoxemia.
- **Hypotension.** Low blood pressure can result with regional anesthesia from sympathetic blockade–induced vasodilation or position-dependent decreased venous return. Hypotension is significant when symptoms develop, such as maternal lightheadedness or fetal bradycardia. Episodes can be treated with bolus IV fluids or low-dose ephedrine (5 mg) or phenylephrine (100 μg). Adequate IV hydration must occur before epidural or spinal access is placed.
- **Fetal complications.**
  - **Nonreassuring fetal monitoring.** Bradycardia and transient heart rate decelerations may occur. Hydration is usually adequate treatment, though pressor support (as above) may be indicated. Repositioning should also be attempted.
  - **Instrumentation.** There is mixed evidence for increased rates of forceps or vacuum delivery with regional anesthesia.
- When compared to IV systemic opioid analgesia, early neuraxial anesthesia does not increase the risk of cesarean delivery.

Systemic Analgesia

Opioids (morphine, fentanyl, meperidine) or mixed opioid agonist-antagonists (butorphanol, nalbuphine) are used for systemic pain relief (see Table 22-3). They can be administered by intramuscular (IM) or intravenous (IV) injection depending on the onset and duration of relief desired.

Indications
- Maternal request

Advantages
- Rapid onset and ease of administration.
- Can be administered via IV patient-controlled anesthesia.

Limitations
- Randomized controlled trials demonstrated higher pain scores during labor for parenteral compared with regional anesthesia.
- It is difficult to obtain adequate pain control throughout labor with only narcotic analgesia.

Risks/Complications
- Maternal respiratory depression requires close monitoring.
- Sedative effects may increase aspiration risk.
- All of the opiates cross the placenta, affecting both fetal and newborn status. Fetal tracings may show decreased variability with maternal narcotic analgesia. Newborns may require extra assistance after delivery including supplemental oxygen and ventilatory support.

TABLE 22-3	Parenteral Agents for Labor Pain				
Agent	**Class**	**Usual Dose**	**Frequency**	**Onset**	**Duration**
Meperidine (Demerol)	Opioid	25–50 mg IV 50–100 mg IM	q1–2 hr q2–4 hr	5 min IV 30–45 min IM	2–3 hr
Fentanyl	Opioid	50–100 µg IV 100 µg IM	q1 hr	1–3 min IV 7–10 min IM	3–4 hr
Morphine	Opioid	2–5 mg IV 5–10 mg IM	q4 hr	3–5 min IV 20–40 min IM	3–4 hr
Nalbuphine (Nubain)	Mixed opioid agonist/antagonist	5–10 mg IV or IM	q3 hr	2–3 min IV 10–15 min IM	3–6 hr
Butorphanol (Stadol)	Mixed opioid agonist/antagonist	1–2 mg IV or IM	q4 hr	5–10 min IV 10–30 min IM	3–4 hr

Adapted from Althaus J, Wax J. Analgesia and Anesthesia in Labor. *Obstet Gynecol Clin N Am* 2005;32:231–244.

General Anesthesia

Indications
- General anesthesia is useful in urgent situations in which epidural/spinal is not available, in cases where regional anesthesia is contraindicated, and in parturients with medical problems that require general anesthesia.

Technique
- Before intubation, the patient receives a nonparticulate antacid, such as sodium citrate, to neutralize gastric pH and decrease aspiration risk. One hundred percent oxygen is administered for 3 to 5 minutes before induction and intubation, to fortify oxygen reserve.
- IV agents are used in a rapid sequence induction to minimize aspiration from the abdominal distention/pressure of the gravid uterus.
- The trachea is intubated quickly with a cuffed endotracheal tube as cricoid pressure is applied to reduce aspiration risk.

Advantages
- Intubation can be performed rapidly in emergent cases.
- Inhaled fluorinated anesthetics cause rapid uterine relaxation which may be used to correct uterine inversion or to facilitate internal/external version or release fetal head entrapment.
- The patient remains still throughout the procedure and does not remember an extensive or prolonged procedure.

Limitations
- The parturient is unable to witness the birth of her child.
- All inhalational agents cross the placenta and can affect the fetus, leading to brief neonatal respiratory depression after delivery; the time from intubation to delivery should be as brief as feasible and safe.

Risks/Complications
- Given the decreased functional residual capacity and increased oxygen requirements of pregnancy, there is **increased maternal morbidity** with general anesthesia/intubation.
- **Aspiration** and hypoxemia can lead to postoperative medical complications.
- **Neonatal respiratory depression.**
- Uterine relaxation can increase surgical **blood loss**. Pitocin, methergine, and misoprostol should all be on hand at the time of obstetric general anesthesia.

SUGGESTED READINGS

Gaiser R, Chapter 2 (Physiologic Changes of Pregnancy); Wong CA, Nathan N, Brown DL, Chapter 12 (Spinal, Epidural, and Caudal Anesthesia); Santos AC, Bucklin BA, Chapter 13 (Local Anesthetics and Opioids). In: Chestnut DH, Polley LS, Tsen LC, et al., eds. *Chestnut's Obstetric Anesthesia: Principles and Practice*, 4th Ed. Philadelphia, PA: Mosby Elsevier, 2009.

Kopp SL, Horlocker TT. Anticoagulation in pregnancy and neuraxial blocks. *Anesthesiol Clin* 2008;26:1–22.

Obstetric analgesia and anesthesia. ACOG Practice Bulletin Number 36. American College of Obstetricians and Gynecologists. *Obstet Gynecol* 2002;100:177–191.

III Gynecology

23 Anatomy of the Female Pelvis

Cara L. Grimes and Chi Chiung Grace Chen

ABDOMINAL WALL

The **anterior abdominal wall** lies ventrally and is outlined superiorly by the lower edge of the rib cage; caudally by the iliac crests, inguinal ligaments, and pubic bone; and dorsolaterally by the lumbar spine and adjacent muscles.

Layers of the Anterior Abdominal Wall

- **Skin**
- **Subcutaneous layer.** This consists of fat globules in a meshwork of fibrous septa. **Camper's fascia** is the more superficial aspect of the subcutaneous layer. **Scarpa's fascia** is the deeper portion and has a more organized consistency than Camper's fascia secondary to more fibrous tissue.
- **Musculoaponeurotic layer.** Located immediately below the subcutaneum, the musculoaponeurotic layer consists of layers of fibrous tissue and muscles that hold the abdominal viscera in place.
  - **Rectus sheath.** The aponeuroses of the external oblique, internal oblique, and transversus abdominis muscles comprise the rectus sheath.
  - The anterior rectus sheath is anatomically different above and below the **arcuate line.** The arcuate line (linea semicircularis, semilunar fold of Douglas) is located midway between the umbilicus and symphysis pubis. It marks the lower edge of the posterior rectus sheath.
    - **Below the arcuate line**, the anterior rectus sheath is composed of the aponeuroses of all the muscles previously mentioned (Fig. 23-1).
    - **Above the arcuate line**, the anterior rectus sheath is composed of the aponeuroses of the external oblique and ventral half of the internal oblique muscles. The posterior rectus sheath is composed of the aponeuroses of the dorsal half of the internal oblique and transversus abdominis muscles (Fig. 23-2).
    - The **linea alba** is the midline ridge of the rectus abdominis muscles. Above the arcuate line, the linea alba marks the fusion of the anterior and posterior rectus sheaths.

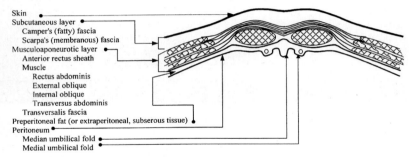

Figure 23-1. Layers of the anterior abdominal wall caudal to the arcuate line.

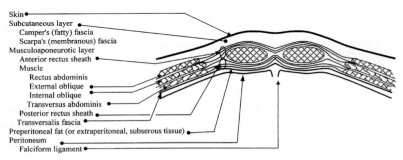

Figure 23-2. Layers of the anterior abdominal wall cephalad to the arcuate line.

- **Abdominal wall muscles**
  - **Oblique flank muscles** lie lateral to the rectus abdominis muscles.
    - ◦ The **external oblique muscle** originates from the lower eight ribs and iliac crest and runs obliquely anteriorly and inferiorly.
    - ◦ The **internal oblique muscle** originates from the anterior two thirds of the iliac crest, the lateral part of the inguinal ligament, and the thoracolumbar fascia in the lower posterior flank. It runs obliquely, anteriorly, and superiorly.
    - ◦ The **transversus abdominis muscle** runs transversely, originating from the lower six costal cartilages, the thoracolumbar fascia, the anterior three fourths of the iliac crest, and the lateral inguinal ligament. The nerves and vasculature of the flank are found between the internal oblique and transverses abdominis muscles and, therefore, are susceptible to injury in transverse incisions.
  - **Longitudinal muscles**
    - ◦ The **rectus abdominis muscle** is a paired muscle, found on either side of the midline, originating from the sternum and cartilage of ribs 5 through 7 and inserting into the anterior surface of the pubic bone.
    - ◦ The **pyramidalis muscle** is a vestigial muscle with a variable presence among individuals. It arises from the pubic bone and inserts into the linea alba several centimeters cephalad to the symphysis ventral to the rectus abdominis muscle.
  - The **transversalis fascia** is a layer of fibrous tissue, located underneath the abdominal wall muscles and outside the peritoneum. The transversalis is separated from the peritoneum by a variable layer of adipose tissue.

- **Peritoneum.** A single layer of serosa lines the posterior aspect of the anterior abdominal wall. Five vertical folds converge toward the umbilicus.
  - The **median umbilical fold** is a single fold created by the **median umbilical ligament** or **obliterated urachus.**
    - The apex of the bladder blends into the median umbilical ligament and is highest in the midline. This relationship should be considered when entering the peritoneal cavity.
  - The **medial umbilical folds** are paired folds lateral to the median umbilical fold, remnants of the obliterated umbilical arteries; they converge at the umbilicus.
  - The **lateral umbilical folds** are paired folds caused by the inferior epigastric vessels. They are less prominent but should be identified before laparoscopic trocar insertion.

Vasculature of the Abdominal Wall

- **Subcutaneous vascular supply (Fig. 23-3)**
  - The **superficial epigastric artery** branches from the femoral artery after it descends through the femoral canal. It runs superomedially approximately 5 cm lateral to the midline.

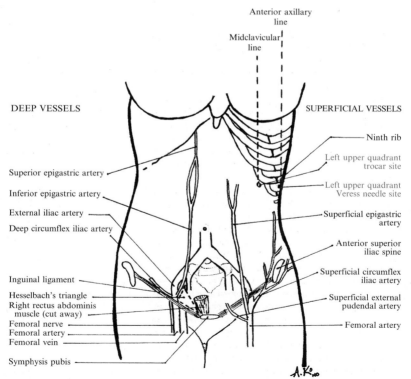

Figure 23-3. Vasculature and laparoscopic landmarks of the anterior abdominal wall. (Original drawing by Alice W. Ko, from *The Johns Hopkins Manual of Gynecology and Obstetrics*, 2nd Ed. Philadelphia, PA: Lippincott Williams and Wilkins, 2002.)

- The **superficial external pudendal artery** branches from the femoral artery and runs medially toward the mons pubis.
- The **superficial circumflex iliac artery** branches from the femoral artery and runs laterally toward the flank.
- **Musculofascial blood supply** parallels the subcutaneous supply (see Fig. 23-3).
  - The **inferior epigastric artery** branches from the external iliac artery, proximal to the inguinal ligament. It runs cephalad, deep to the transversalis fascia and lateral to the rectus muscle. Midway between the pubis and umbilicus, the vessels intersect the lateral border of the rectus muscle and course between the dorsal aspect of the rectus and the posterior rectus sheath. These vessels run between 4 and 8 cm lateral to the midline. After entering the posterior rectus sheath, numerous branches supply all layers of the abdominal wall and anastomose with the superior epigastric vessels.
  - **Hesselbach's triangle** is a space defined laterally by the inferior epigastric artery, medially by the rectus abdominis muscle, and inferiorly by the inguinal ligament.
  - The **superior epigastric artery** branches from the internal thoracic artery and runs caudally to form anastomoses with the inferior epigastric artery.
  - The **deep circumflex iliac artery** also branches from the external iliac artery and runs laterally between the internal oblique and transverses abdominis muscles.

Abdominal Wall Incisions

- **Vertical.** A midline or paramedian incision provides optimal exposure to the abdomen. The incision is made from the symphysis to below the umbilicus, depending on how much space is needed. The incision can always be extended more cephalad and then circumferentially around the umbilicus to the left to avoid the ligamentum teres. The anterior rectus sheath is incised longitudinally. The peritoneum is entered taking care to avoid the superior aspect of the bladder.
- **Pfannenstiel's incision.** This is one of the most common incisions in obstetrics and gynecology. A transverse incision is made approximately two fingerbreadths (3 to 4 cm) above the pubic symphysis. Transverse incisions are generally less painful and more cosmetic than longitudinal incisions as they run along Langer's lines. The incision is continued through the rectus sheath, and then the rectus muscles are dissected cephalad and caudad off the posterior aspect of the rectus sheath. Then, the rectus muscles are separated in the midline to gain entry to the peritoneum through a midline longitudinal incision. The degree of separation of the rectus fascia from the underlying rectus muscles determines the amount of exposure provided by the Pfannenstiel's incision. If more space is needed, the rectus fascia can be separated from the rectus muscle up to the umbilicus. Further exposure is not facilitated by extending the lateral skin incision, and greater risk of injury is present to the ilioinguinal and iliohypogastric nerves either by direct incision or more often by entrapment during fascial closure.
- **Cherney incision.** A modification of the Pfannenstiel incision, the Cherney incision provides better exposure to the pelvis than the Pfannenstiel incision by releasing the inferior attachments of the rectus muscles. After the rectus muscle is dissected off the fascia, as in a Pfannenstiel, the tendinous insertion of the rectus muscle is cut approximately 0.5 cm above the insertion site at the posterior aspect of the pubic bones. The rectus bellies are then moved cephalad, providing excellent exposure to the pelvis. Note the importance of leaving enough tendon on the pubic bone so that the caudal aspect of the rectus muscles can be reapproximated to the tendon with a 2 to 0 delayed absorbable suture in a horizontal mattress fashion during closure.

- **Maylard incision.** The Maylard incision provides the best pelvic exposure of all the incision types. This incision is transverse, like the Pfannenstiel, with two main differences. The Maylard incision is made slightly more cephalad (at the level of the anterior superior iliac spine), and the rectus muscles are not dissected off the fascia. Rather, they are left attached to the rectus sheath and the muscles are transected. The inferior epigastric vessels are identified and ligated before the rectus muscles are transected completely. This helps to prevent blood loss from inadvertent inferior epigastric injury and also serves to preserve blood supply by leaving the vessels attached to the fascia. This type of incision has the potential for greater blood loss but also for better pelvic exposure.

Abdominal Landmarks for Laparoscopy

- **Laparoscopic trocars** are most commonly placed at the umbilicus, suprapubically and laterally (Fig. 23-3).
  - **Umbilical trocar.** The umbilical trocar should be placed at a 45-degree angle in thin women in order to avoid hitting the aorta or common iliacs. In an obese patient, the trocar can be placed at a more perpendicular angle due to the amount of adipose tissue that must be traversed.
  - **Suprapubic trocar.** The suprapubic trocar is placed two fingerbreadths above the pubic symphysis. It is placed under direct visualization and after Foley insertion in order to assure that the bladder is not in line of the trocar path.
  - **Lateral trocars.** The lateral trocars are placed at least 5 cm cephalad to the pubic symphysis and 8 cm lateral to the midline in order to avoid the inferior epigastric vessels. The trocar is placed under direct visualization lateral to the lateral umbilical folds.

PELVIC VISCERA

Vagina

- The **vagina** is shaped like a flattened tube, starting at the distal hymenal ring and ending at the fornices surrounding the proximal cervix. Its average length is 8 cm; this varies greatly with age, parity, and surgical history.
- The vaginal epithelium is nonkeratinized, stratified squamous epithelium lacking mucous glands and hair follicles. Mesonephric duct remnants in the lateral vaginal wall can result in Gartner's duct cysts.
- Deep to the epithelium is the vaginal muscularis, or endopelvic fascia. The term *fascia* is misleading because this is actually fibromuscular tissue that includes fibroblasts, smooth muscle cells, and elastin, in addition to type I and III collagen, all loosely arrayed to create an elastic supportive layer. At the vaginal apex, this fibromuscular layer coalesces to create the cardinal and uterosacral ligaments. The fan-shaped cardinal ligament creates a sheath that envelops the uterine artery and vein, fusing medially with the paracervical ring. The uterosacral portion inserts into the posterior and lateral aspect of the paracervical ring and then curves laterally along the pelvic sidewall to attach to the presacral fascia that overlies the second, third, and fourth sacral vertebrae. Together the cardinal and uterosacral ligaments pull the vagina proximally toward the sacrum, suspending it over the muscular levator plate.
- The endopelvic fascia of the anterior and posterior vaginal wall are known as the **pubocervical fascia** and **rectovaginal fascia**, respectively. Again, these layers are not true fasciae but composed of fibromuscular sheets. Superiorly, the pubocervical fascia attaches to the cervix and the cardinal/uterosacral support of the vaginal apex. Laterally, it coalesces with the fascia of the obturator internus muscle to create

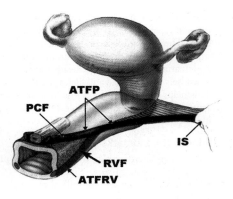

Figure 23-4. Illustration of attachment of rectovaginal fascia (RVF) and arcus tendineus fascia pelvis (ATFP) to the pelvic sidewall. RVF represents the ideal line of suture placement during lateral defect repair. PCF, pubocervical fascia; ATFRV, arcus tendineus fascia rectovaginalis; IS, ischial spine. (From Leffler KS, Thompson JR, Cundiff GW, et al. Attachment of the rectovaginal septum to the pelvic sidewall. *Am J Obstet Gynecol* 2001;185:43, with permission.)

the **arcus tendineus fascia pelvis (ATFP)** or "white line." Inferiorly, it attaches to the pubic symphysis. The rectovaginal fascia in the upper vagina coalesces with the lateral support of the anterior vaginal wall and fuses with the ATFP. The lower half of the rectovaginal fascia fuses with the aponeurosis of the levator ani muscles along a line referred to as the **arcus tendineus fascia rectovaginalis**. At its most inferior point, the rectovaginal septum fuses with the perineal body (Fig. 23-4).

Levels of Pelvic Support
- The pelvic muscles and connective tissue are the primary support for the pelvic organs. The pelvic muscles consist of the **levator ani plate** (i.e., puborectalis, pubococcygeus, and ileococcygeus) and the coccygeus muscle. The **connective tissue attachments** (uterosacral/cardinal ligament complex and the endopelvic fascia) stabilize the pelvic organs in the correct position to receive support from the pelvic muscles. With pelvic muscle weakness or damage secondary to obstetric injury, the endolpevic fascia becomes the primary mechanism of support. This stress can attenuate, stretch, or break the endopelvic fascia resulting in failure of support of the pelvic organs and pelvic organ prolapse.
- There are three levels of support, as described by DeLancey (Fig 23-5).
  - **Level I** is the upper vertical axis or uterosacral/cardinal ligament complex. The uterosacral/cardinal ligament complex supports the cervix and upper vagina to maintain vaginal length and to keep the upper vaginal axis nearly horizontal so that it rests on the rectum and can be supported by the levator plate.
  - **Level II** is the horizontal axis or paravaginal supports. The pubocervical fascia and rectovaginal fascia spread over the vagina and condense into the ATFP to support the midvagina and create the anterior lateral vaginal sulci.
  - **Level III** is the lower vertical axis or perineal body, perineal membrane, and the superficial muscles (bulbocavernosus, ischiocavernosus, superficial and deep transverse perineal muscles). This supports and maintains the normal position of the distal one third of the vagina and introitus, which is nearly vertical in a standing female.
  - Levels I, II, and III are connected through continuation of the endopelvic fascia.

Uterus
- The **uterus** is a fibromuscular organ comprised of the corpus and the cervix.
- **Corpus.** The **endometrium** is the innermost lining of the uterus made up of columnar epithelium and specialized stroma. The superficial layer of the

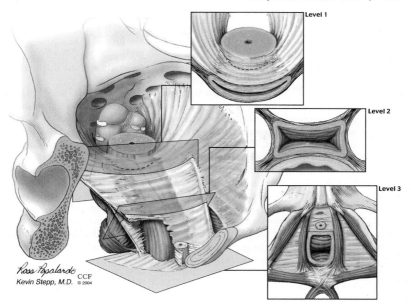

Figure 23-5. DeLancey's levels of pelvic support. (Reprinted from Cleveland Clinic Center for Medical Art & Photography © 2004, with permission. All Rights Reserved.)

endometrium contains hormonally sensitive spiral arterioles, which shed with each cycle. The deeper basal layer is preserved with each cycle and has its own arterial supply. The **myometrium** contains interlacing smooth muscle fibers, and the **serosal** surface of the uterus is formed by peritoneal mesothelium. The **fundus** is the portion of the uterus cephalad to the endometrial cavity. The **cornua** are located where the fallopian tubes insert into the uterine cavity, lateral to the fundus.

- **Cervix.** The cervix is generally 2 to 4 cm in length and has two parts: the **portio vaginalis** (protruding into the vagina) and the **portio supravaginalis** (lying above the vagina). The cervix is made up of dense fibrous connective tissue and is surrounded in a circular fashion by a small amount of smooth muscle into which the cardinal and uterosacral ligaments and pubocervical and rectovaginal fascia insert. The cervix contains a central longitudinal canal connecting the endometrial cavity with the vagina, called the **endocervical canal.** The **internal os** of the cervix is at the junction of the endocervical canal and the endometrial cavity. The **external os** is the distal opening of the cervical canal. The **squamocolumnar junction** is located at the external os. It marks the transition from the squamous epithelium of the ectocervix to the columnar epithelium of the endocervical canal at the external os. The **ectocervix** is the outer portion of the cervix, which is lined with squamous epithelium.

Ligaments of the Uterus
- These ligaments are formed by thickening of the endopelvic fascia or folds of peritoneum.

- The **round ligament** courses from the anterolateral aspect of the uterine corpus through the inguinal canal to insert into the labia majora. It has a fibromuscular element and can give rise to leiomyomas. It contains the **artery of Sampson.** The round ligament provides no support for the uterus.
- The **utero-ovarian ligament** contains the anastomotic vasculature of the uterine and ovarian vessels. It connects the uterus and ovaries.
- The **cardinal ligaments (Mackenrodt's ligaments)** extend from the lateral pelvic walls and insert into the lateral portion of the vagina, uterine cervix, and isthmus. These play an important role in support of the pelvic organs.
- The **infundibulopelvic ligament (IP ligament, suspensory ligament of the ovary)** contains the ovarian vessels. The ovarian arteries branch directly off the aorta. The right ovarian vein feeds into the inferior vena cava while the left vein drains into the left renal vein. The peritoneal layer below the ovarian vessels is called the **avascular space of Graves.** This space is entered during a salpingo-oophorectomy.
- The **uterosacral ligaments** extend from the sacral fascia and insert into the posterior portion of the uterine isthmus and endopelvic fascia. They are composed of connective tissue and smooth muscle and contain the autonomic sympathetic and parasympathetic nerves of the pelvic organs. The cardinal and uterosacral ligaments both play an important role in pelvic organ support. Together they form the parametrium, which is the suspensory tissue that extends from the uterus and provides support for the vaginal apex and uterus.
- The **broad ligament** is the peritoneum that covers the uterus and fallopian tubes. It forms a mesentery around the uterine structures:
- **Mesoteres** contains the round ligament.
- **Mesosalpinx** contains the fallopian tube.
- **Mesovarium** contains the utero-ovarian ligament.

Adnexae

- The **fallopian tubes** are bilateral tubular structures that connect the endometrial cavity to the peritoneal cavity. They are, on average, 10 cm in length. Distally, the tubes have a fimbriated end that is near the ovary and receives each egg after ovulation. The lumen is lined by ciliated columnar epithelium, which helps move the egg or embryo toward the uterine cavity. The fallopian tube has four regions (from proximal to distal): interstitial, isthmic, ampullary, and infundibular.
- The **ovaries** are bilateral, white, flattened oval structures that store ova. The ovary is suspended laterally from the pelvic sidewall by the IP ligament and medially from the uterus by the utero-ovarian ligament. Each ovary rests in the ovarian fossa **(fossa of Waldeyer)**, which is bordered dorsomedially by the hypogastric artery and ventrolaterally by the external iliac artery. The ureter runs at the base of this fossa. The ovary has a fibromuscular and vascular medulla and an outer cortex that contains specialized stroma with follicles, corpora lutea, and corpora albicantia. The ovary is covered by cuboidal epithelium.

Ureter

- The **ureter** courses from the kidneys retroperitoneally, crosses the pelvic brim at the level of the bifurcation of the common iliac artery, and continues in the medial leaf of the broad ligament. It enters the tunnel of Wertheim and passes under the uterine artery 1.5 cm lateral to the cervix at the level of the internal cervical os and enters the trigone of the bladder. The three most common areas of ureteral injury during gynecologic surgery are at the pelvic brim during clamping of the IP ligaments, during clamping of the uterine artery at time of hysterectomy, and near the trigone when mobilizing the bladder off the lower uterine segment.

SURGICAL SPACES OF THE PELVIS

The reproductive, urinary, and gastrointestinal organs found in the pelvis have the ability to change their size and shape independently of each other, which is made possible by their loose attachments via connective tissue planes composed of fat and areolar tissue. These planes are potential spaces that can be entered with surgical dissection. The neurolymphovascular supply to the organs remains in the connective tissue septae, permitting blunt and bloodless dissection of the surgical spaces. Eight avascular spaces are described: prevesical, vesicovaginal, paravesical (2), pararectal (2), rectovaginal, and retrorectal (see Fig. 23-6).

- The **prevesical space**, also known as the **space of Retzius** or **retropubic space**, is separated ventrally from the rectus abdominis by the transversalis fascia. Laterally, the muscles of the pelvic wall, cardinal ligament, and attachment of the pubocervical fascia to the ATFP border the prevesical space. Important structures within the space of Retzius include the dorsal clitoral vessels, obturator nerves and vessels, nerves of the lower urinary tract, iliopectineal line, ATFP, and the arcus tendineus levator ani. Burch urethropexies are performed in this space.
- The **vesicovaginal spaces (also called vesicocervical)** are separated by a thin supravaginal septum. The spaces are bound caudally by the fusion of the junction of the proximal one third and distal two thirds of the urethra with the vagina, ventrally by the urethra and bladder, cephalad by the peritoneum, forming the vesicocervical reflection. This is the space entered when developing a "bladder flap" during cesarean delivery or hysterectomy.

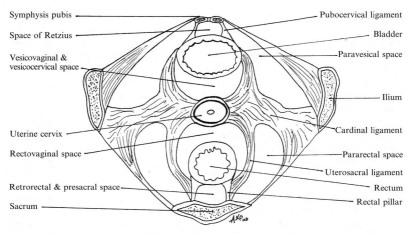

Figure 23-6. Surgical spaces of the pelvis. (Original drawing by Alice W. Ko, from *The Johns Hopkins Manual of Gynecology and Obstetrics*, 2nd Ed. Philadelphia, PA: Lippincott Williams and Wilkins, 2002.)

- The **paravesical spaces** are paired spaces adjacent to the bladder. They are bordered medially by the bladder and obliterated umbilical artery, laterally by the obturator internus, dorsally by the cardinal ligament, ventrally by the pubic symphysis, and caudally by the levator ani. The ureter can be found in the tissue between the paravesical and vesicovaginal spaces. Parametrial tissue obtained in a radical hysterectomy is located between the paravesical and pararectal spaces.

- The **pararectal spaces** are paired spaces adjacent to the rectum. The space is bordered medially by the ureter, uterosacral ligament, and rectum, laterally by the hypogastric vessels and pelvic wall, ventrolaterally by the cardinal ligament, and dorsally by the sacrum. The coccygeus forms the floor of this space. Bleeding can be encountered from the lateral sacral and hemorrhoidal vessels if dissection is carried to the pelvic floor. These spaces allow access to the sacrospinous ligaments.

- The **rectovaginal space** is bordered caudally by the apex of the perineal body; laterally by the uterosacral ligament, ureter, and rectal pillars; ventrally by the vagina; and dorsally by the rectum. The **pouch of Douglas** or **posterior cul-de-sac** is the space between the uterus and rectum bounded inferiorly by the peritoneum. The rectovaginal space is below this peritoneum and cul-de-sac and is developed by incising the peritoneal fold between the uterus and rectum.

- The **retrorectal space** is caudal to the presacral space and bordered ventrally by the rectum, posteriorly by the sacrum, and laterally by the uterosacral ligaments. The **presacral space** is bordered laterally by the internal iliac arteries, cephalad by the bifurcation of the aorta, dorsally by the sacrum, and ventrally by the colon. It contains the presacral nerve (superior hypogastric plexus), the middle sacral artery and vein (originating from the dorsal aspect of the aorta and vena cava), and the lateral sacral vessels.

VASCULATURE OF THE ABDOMEN AND PELVIS

- **Aorta.** From cephalad to caudad, the arteries that stem from the aorta below the diaphragm are: inferior phrenic, celiac trunk, suprarenal, superior mesenteric, renal, ovarian, inferior mesenteric, and middle sacral. The aorta then bifurcates into the common iliac arteries at the level of the fourth lumbar vertebra.

- **Celiac trunk.** The celiac trunk has three main branches: the **left gastric,** the **splenic**, and the **common hepatic** arteries. The **left gastric artery** divides into the esophageal branches and branches that supply the lesser curvature of the stomach. The **splenic artery** divides into pancreatic branches, the **short gastric artery,** which supplies the fundus of the stomach, and the **left gastroepiploic artery,** which supplies the greater omentum and the greater curvature of the stomach. The left gastroepiploic artery anastomoses with the right gastroepiploic, which is a terminal branch of the common hepatic. The **common hepatic artery** has two main divisions: the **proper hepatic artery** and the **gastroduodenal artery**. The proper hepatic artery divides into the **right gastric artery** and enters the lesser omentum to anastomose with the **left gastric artery** and terminates into the **right and left hepatic arteries**. The **cystic artery** often branches from the right hepatic artery and supplies the gallbladder. The **gastroduodenal artery** branches into the **supraduodenal artery**, the **right gastroepiploic artery**, and the **superior pancreatoduodenal artery**. The **right gastroepiploic artery** enters the greater omentum and anastomoses with the left gastroepiploic artery along the greater curvature of the stomach. The **superior pancreatoduodenal artery** supplies the second part of the duodenum and the head of the pancreas.

- The **superior mesenteric artery** branches into the **jejunal** and **ileal artery** branches, the **ileocolic artery**, the **right colic artery**, and the **middle colic artery**.
- The **inferior mesenteric artery** branches into the **left colic artery**, the **sigmoid branches**, and the **superior rectal artery**.
- **Ovarian vessels.** The ovarian arteries originate from the anterior aspect of the aorta and course toward the pelvis, crossing laterally over the **ureters** at the level of the pelvic brim, and passing branches to the ureters and fallopian tubes. They then cross medially over the proximal external iliac vessels and run medially in the infundibulopelvic ligaments. The left ovarian vein drains into the left renal vein, whereas the right ovarian vein drains directly into the inferior vena cava.
- The aorta bifurcates into the **common iliac arteries** at the level of the fourth lumbar vertebra. The common iliac then bifurcates into the **external and internal** (hypogastric) **arteries**. The hypogastric artery divides into an anterior and posterior division 3 to 4 cm after the branching off of the common iliac artery. The **ureter** courses anteriorly to the division of the hypogastric and external iliac arteries.
  - **Anterior division of the hypogastric artery.** Some variance exists in the branching pattern. The branches include the obturator, uterine, vaginal, inferior, and superior vesicals, middle rectal, internal pudendal, and inferior gluteal arteries. The **ureter** passes laterally under the **uterine artery** at the level of the internal cervical os. During hypogastric artery ligation, the anterior division of the hypogastric artery should be doubly ligated with 1-0 silk (do not divide) 2.5 to 3.0 cm distal to the bifurcation of the common iliac to preserve the posterior division of the hypogastric artery, thereby avoiding compromising blood supply to the gluteal muscles. The dissection is done laterally to medially to avoid damaging the hypogastric vein.
  - **Posterior division of the hypogastric artery.** The branches include the iliolumbar, lateral sacral, and superior gluteal arteries, all of which have anastomosing channels in the pelvis.
- **External iliac artery.** The deep epigastric and deep circumflex iliac arteries branch from the external iliac artery before it travels under the inguinal ligament and into the femoral canal, where it becomes the femoral artery.
- **Anastomoses.** The **superior rectal artery** branches off the inferior mesenteric artery, the **middle rectal artery** branches off the anterior division of the hypogastric artery, and the **inferior rectal artery branches** off the pudendal artery (a branch of the hypogastric). This allows for redundant blood flow to the pelvis.

VULVA AND PERINEUM

External Anatomy

- The bony pelvic outlet is bordered anteriorly by the ischiopubic rami and posteriorly by the coccyx and sacrotuberous ligaments. The outlet can be divided into anterior and posterior triangles sharing a common base along a line between the ischial tuberosities.
- **Skin and subcutaneous layer** (Fig. 23-7). The subcutaneous tissue has two nondiscrete layers: Camper's fascia and Colles' fascia.
  - **Camper's fascia** includes the continuation of this layer from the anterior abdominal wall.

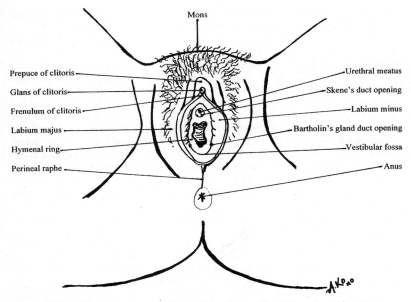

Figure 23-7. Vulva and perineum. (Original drawing by Alice W. Ko, from *The Johns Hopkins Manual of Gynecology and Obstetrics*, 2nd Ed. Philadelphia, PA: Lippincott Williams and Wilkins, 2002.)

- **Colles' fascia** is similar to Scarpa's fascia of the anterior abdominal wall. It fuses posteriorly with the perineal membrane and laterally with the ischiopubic rami.
- The **mons (mons pubis, mons veneris)** is hair-bearing skin overlying adipose tissue that lies on the pubic bones.
- The **labia majora** extend posteriorly from the mons and contain similar hair-bearing skin. The labia majora contain the insertion of the round ligaments.
- The **labia minora** are hairless skin folds that split anteriorly to form the prepuce and frenulum of the clitoris. They overlie loosely organized connective tissue rather than adipose tissue.
- **Gland duct openings**
  - The **greater vestibular (Bartholin) gland** duct opening is seen on the posterolateral aspect of the vestibule 3 to 4 mm lateral to the hymenal ring.
  - The **minor vestibular gland** duct opening is seen in a line above the greater vestibular gland duct opening toward the urethra.
  - The **Skene's ducts** are located inferolateral to the urethral meatus at approximately 5 and 7 o'clock.
- **Specialized glands**
  - **Holocrine sebaceous glands** are located in the labia majora and are associated with hair shafts.
  - **Apocrine sweat glands** are located lateral to the introitus and anus. **Hidradenitis suppurativa** can occur if these glands become chronically infected. **Hidradenomas** are neoplastic enlargements of these glands.

- **Eccrine sweat glands** are also located laterally to the introitus and anus. They can enlarge and form a **syringoma.**

Superficial Compartment of the Vulva

- This compartment lies between the subcutaneous layer and the perineal membrane (Fig. 23-8).
- The **clitoris** consists of the glans, a shaft that is attached to the pubis by a subcutaneous suspensory ligament, and paired crura that stem from the shaft and attach to the inferior aspect of the pubic rami.
- **Ischiocavernosus muscles** overlie the crura of the clitoris. They originate at the ischial tuberosities and free surfaces of the crura and insert into the upper crura and clitoral shaft.
- **Bulbocavernosus muscles** originate in the perineal body and insert into the clitoral shaft. They overlie the centrolateral aspects of the vestibular bulbs and Bartholin's gland.
- **Superficial transverse perineal muscles** originate from the ischial tuberosities and insert into the perineal body.
- The **perineal body (central tendon of the perineum)** is connected anterolaterally with the bulbocavernosus muscle and anteriorly with the perineal membrane, which attaches the perineal body to the inferior pubic rami. The perineal body is attached laterally to the superficial transverse perineal muscles, posteriorly to the external anal sphincter, and superiorly to the distal rectovaginal fascia.
- The **vestibular bulbs** are paired erectile tissues that lie immediately under the skin of the vestibule and under the bulbocavernosus muscles.

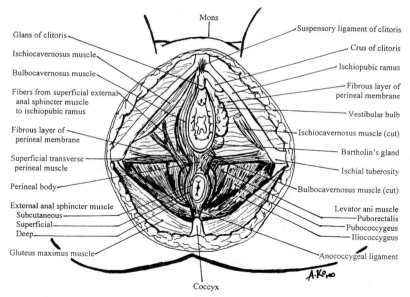

Figure 23-8. Superficial compartment of the vulva. (Original drawing by Alice W. Ko, from *The Johns Hopkins Manual of Gynecology and Obstetrics*, 2nd Ed. Philadelphia, PA: Lippincott Williams and Wilkins, 2002.)

- **Bartholin's glands** lie between the bulbocavernosus muscles and the perineal membrane at the tail end of the vestibular bulb. Their ducts empty into the vestibular mucosa.

Pelvic Floor

- The **pelvic floor** comprises the perineal membrane and the muscles of the pelvic diaphragm. It helps support the pelvic contents above the pelvic outlet.
- The **perineal membrane** is a triangular sheet of dense fibromuscular tissue that spans the anterior triangle. It provides support by attaching the urethra, vagina, and perineal body to the ischiopubic rami. The perineal membrane contains the dorsal and deep nerves and vessels to the clitoris.
- The **muscles of the pelvic diaphragm** comprise the levator ani and coccygeal muscles. These are covered by the superior and inferior fascias (Fig. 23-9).
  - **Levator ani muscles**
    - The **puborectalis** arises from the inner surface of the pubic bones and inserts into the rectum. Some fibers form a sling around the posterior aspect of the rectum.
    - The **pubococcygeus** arises from the pubic bones and inserts into the anococcygeal raphe and superior aspect of the coccyx.
    - The **iliococcygeus** arises from the **arcus tendineus levator ani** and inserts into the anococcygeal raphe and coccyx.
  - The **coccygeus muscle** arises from the ischial spine and inserts into the coccyx and lowest area of the sacrum. It lies cephalad to the sacrospinous ligament.

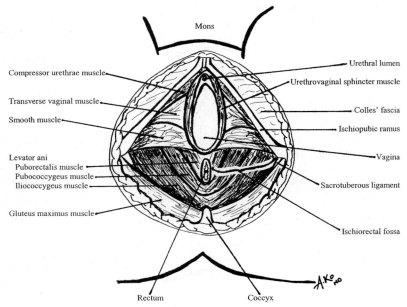

Figure 23-9. Skeletal muscle layer of the perineal membrane. (Original drawing by Alice W. Ko, from *The Johns Hopkins Manual of Gynecology and Obstetrics*, 2nd Ed. Philadelphia, PA: Lippincott Williams and Wilkins, 2002.)

Posterior Triangle
- This area is bounded bilaterally by the ischial tuberosities and posteriorly by the coccyx.
- **External anal sphincter**
  - The superficial portion is attached anteriorly to the perineal body and posteriorly to the coccyx.
  - The deep portion encircles the rectum and blends in with the puborectalis muscle.
- **Internal anal sphincter.** This sphincter is a smooth muscle that is separated from the external sphincter by the intersphincteric groove as well as fibers from the longitudinal layer of the bowel.
- The **ischiorectal fossa** contains the pudendal neurovascular trunk; it is bordered medially by the levator ani muscles and laterally by the obturator internus muscles. It has an anterior recess that lies above the perineal membrane and a posterior portion that lies above the gluteus maximus. This space allows for physiologic expansion of the rectum.

NERVES OF THE PELVIS AND PERINEUM

Pelvic Diaphragm
- The **pudendal nerve** supplies the external anal sphincter and the urethral sphincter.
- The **anterior branch of the ventral ramus of S3 and S4** innervates the levator ani and coccygeal muscles.

Perineum
- The **pudendal nerve** is the sensory and motor nerve of the perineum.
  - The pudendal nerve originates from the sacral plexus (S2-4), exits the pelvis through the greater sciatic notch, hooks around the ischial spine and sacrospinous ligament, and enters the pudendal canal (**canal of Alcock**) in the lesser sciatic notch. It has several terminal branches:
    - The **clitoral nerve** runs along the superficial aspect of the perineal membrane to supply the clitoris.
    - The **perineal nerve** runs along the deep aspect of the perineal membrane. Its branches supply the muscles of the superficial compartment, subcutaneum, and skin of the vestibule, labia minora, and medial aspect of the labia majora.
    - The **inferior hemorrhoidal nerve (inferior rectal)** innervates the external anal sphincter and the perianal skin.

Nerve Injuries in Gynecologic Surgery
- Nerve injuries are encountered from positioning, incisions, use of retractors, and dissection (Table 23-1).

LYMPHATIC DRAINAGE OF THE PELVIS

- The vulva and lower vagina drain to the **inguinofemoral lymph nodes** and then to the **external iliac nodes**. See Chapter 41.
- The cervix drains through the cardinal ligaments to the **pelvic nodes (hypogastric, obturator, and external iliac)** and then to the **common iliac and para-aortic lymph nodes**.

| TABLE 23-1 | Nerve Injuries in Gynecologic Surgery | | |

Nerve	Injury	Motor Loss	Sensory Loss
Femoral L2-4	Deep retraction on psoas muscle, excessive hip flexion	Hip flexion, knee extension, knee DTR, leg adduction	Anteromedial thigh, anteromedial leg and foot
Lateral femoral cutaneous L2-3	Deep retraction on psoas muscle, excessive hip flexion	None	Anterolateral and posterolateral thigh
Genitofemoral branch L1-2	Pelvic sidewall dissection	None	Mons, labia majora, anterior superior thigh
Obturator L2-4	Retroperitoneal surgery, lymph node dissection, paravaginal defect repair	Leg abduction	Anteromedial thigh
Sciatic L4-S3	Extensive endopelvic resection	Hip extension, knee flexion	Lateral calf, dorsomedial foot
Common peroneal L4-S2	Compression from stirrups on lateral calf	Foot dorsiflexion and eversion	Lateral calf, dorsomedial foot
Tibial L4-S3	Compression from stirrups on lateral calf	Foot plantar flexion and inversion	Toes, plantar foot
Iliohypogastric T12	Transverse abdominal incision	None	Mons, labia, inner thigh
Ilioinguinal L1	Transverse abdominal incision	None	Groin, symphysis pubis

DTR, deep tendon reflex. Adapted from Irvin W, Anderson W, Rice L. Minimizing the risk of nerve injury in gynecologic surgery. *Obstet Gynecol* 2004;103:374–382.

- The **uterus** drains through the broad ligament and intraperitoneal ligament to the **pelvic and para-aortic lymph nodes.**
- The **ovaries** drain to the **pelvic and para-aortic lymph nodes.**

SUGGESTED READINGS

Ashton-Miller JA, DeLancey JO. Functional anatomy of the female pelvic floor. *Ann NY Acad Sci* 2007;1101:266–296.

DeLancey JO. Anatomic aspects of vaginal eversion after hysterectomy. *Am J Obstet Gynecol* 1992;166:1717–1728.

DeLancey JO. Structural anatomy of the posterior pelvic compartment as it relates to rectocele. *Am J Obstet Gynecol* 1999;180:815–823.

Law YM, Fielding JR. MRI of pelvic floor dysfunction: review. *Am J Roentgenol* 2008;191: S45–S53.

Weber AM, Walters MD. Anterior vaginal prolapsed: review of anatomy and techniques of surgical repair. *Obstet Gynecol* 1997;89:311–318.

24 Perioperative Care and Complications of Gynecologic Surgery

Jessica B. Russell and Isabel C. Green

PREOPERATIVE CARE

The main objectives of the **preoperative assessment** are completion of a thorough history and physical examination, selection of the ideal surgery, identification of potential limitations, and optimization of the patient's medical condition. The goal is to decrease perioperative morbidity and complications and to optimize outcomes.

Informed Consent

- **Informed consent** should include the rationale and explanation of the procedure as well as alternatives such as expectant management, nonsurgical interventions, and other surgical options. An interactive process should exist between physician and patient. When more than one option is available, the surgeon should provide education and guidance without coercion. Ultimately, the patient must determine which of the options is appropriate.
- Risk discussion should address the specific procedure as well as general surgical risks and should be accompanied by a discussion of interventions intended to minimize those risks. These risks include, but are not limited to bleeding and possible blood transfusion (Table 24-1), organ injury (bladder, ureter, bowel, vessel, or nerve), unanticipated organ removal, need for additional surgery, myocardial infarction, congestive heart failure, thromboembolic complications, infection, and perioperative death. Injury and failure rates should be cited based on personal data and current literature when available. Discussion of interventions such as perioperative antibiotics, deep vein thrombosis (DVT) prophylaxis, and postoperative incentive spirometry should be included. Possible changes in plans due to intraoperative surgical findings should be included in the consent document, as well as the possibility of a change in mode of access (e.g., laparoscopic to open procedure, vaginal to abdominal procedure). Documentation of the preoperative discussions and the patient's response and acceptance of risk, including informed refusal, is crucial.

Medical Evaluation and Optimization

Preoperative Evaluation

- **Preoperative evaluation.** History and physical examination are essential for evaluating surgical eligibility and the need for further testing or consultation. Identifying occult disease and optimizing preexisting conditions are of utmost importance. Abnormal findings and comorbid conditions need to be evaluated appropriately. It may be beneficial for patients with complex preexisting conditions to be comanaged

TABLE 24-1	Risks of Blood Transfusion
Bacterial contamination of platelet components	1:12,000
Bacterial contamination from packed red cells	1:5 million
Hepatitis C virus	1:1.6 million
Hepatitis B virus	1:180,000
Human immunodeficiency virus	1:1.9 million
Fatal red cell hemolytic reaction	1:250,000–1.1 million
Delayed red cell hemolysis	1:1,000–1,500
Transfusion-related acute lung injury (TRALI)	1:5,000
Febrile red cell nonhemolytic reaction	1:100
Allergic urticarial reaction	1:100
Anaphylactic reaction	1:150,000

From Jones HW, Rock WA. Control of pelvic hemorrhage. In: Rock JA, Jones HW, eds. *Te Linde's Operative Gynecology,* 9th Ed. Philadelphia, PA: Lippincott Williams & Wilkins; 2003, with permission.

with a medical specialist. Preoperative consultation with an anesthesiologist is important for the medically complicated patient, those with known difficult airways, and those with a history of anesthesia complications.

- **Preoperative testing and imaging.** Preoperative testing should be based on risk factors for abnormal physiology, including comorbid conditions, tobacco use, exercise intolerance, and irregular examination findings. Mild and even asymptomatic conditions that may be exacerbated by medical and surgical interventions should be anticipated. Guidelines are available from the American Society of Anesthesiologists (ASA) and American Heart Association (AHA)/American College of Cardiology (ACC).
  - Gynecologic patients are strongly advised to have current Pap smear and mammography results. Red blood cell type and screen should be performed on most patients, with exceptions made for very minor outpatient procedures. A pregnancy test will be required on all reproductive age women (<50), and endometrial biopsy is recommended by ACOG for women with abnormal uterine bleeding over the age of 35. Imaging should be individualized, but computed tomography (CT), magnetic resonance imaging (MRI), and pelvic ultrasound are helpful for illustrating anatomy and extent of disease, thereby limiting intraoperative surprises.
- **Preoperative cardiac evaluation.** The preoperative cardiac evaluation should be directed toward the detection of symptoms using directed questioning looking for conditions such as angina, heart failure, and arrhythmias. For women over the age of 45 years, general preoperative workup includes detailed history and physical examination, as well as electrocardiogram (ECG). Additional cardiac workup depends on the planned surgery and the patient's functional status.
  - In low-risk procedures (ambulatory), no additional workup or treatment is needed, and most patients can proceed directly to surgery.
  - A major intraperitoneal surgery is considered an intermediate procedure with a reported cardiac risk of 1% to 5%. These patients need to be assessed by their functional status, which is based on their ability to perform 4 METs of activity or greater without chest pain, dyspnea, or fatigue.

○ A MET is a unit equal to the metabolic equivalent of oxygen uptake while quietly seated; 4 METs is equal to walking on a flat surface or climbing a flight of stairs. If the patient can perform 4 METs of activity without dyspnea or fatigue, she is considered to have a normal functional status and may proceed to intermediate risk surgery without further cardiac testing. If her functional status is <4 METs, additional evaluation may be indicated based on clinical risk factors that include history of ischemic heart disease, history of compensated or prior heart failure, history of cerebrovascular disease (stroke), diabetes mellitus, and chronic kidney disease (defined as a creatinine >2 mg/dL).

- For gynecologic surgeries that are considered higher risk (prolonged surgeries that involve large fluid shifts), patients with a functional capability <4 METs and one to three risk factors warrant further cardiac testing.

Preoperative Management

- **Thromboembolic prophylaxis.** The approximate risk of DVT in hospitalized patients after major gynecology procedures is 10% to 40%. It is the standard of care to offer DVT prophylaxis (Table 24-2).
- **Antibiotic prophylaxis.** See Table 24-3 for preoperative antibiotic prophylaxis. Evidence supports the use of antibiotics in cases of hysterectomy, with data on abdominal and vaginal routes generalized to laparoscopic hysterectomy. Single-dose prophylaxis appears to be as effective as multiple doses, with less risk of adverse events and microbial resistance. To reduce surgical site infections (SSI), first-generation or second-generation cephalosporins are preferred for most patients, with metronidazole or clindamycin reserved for those with severe penicillin allergy.
  - Antibiotic levels should be therapeutic prior to incision. Antibiotics should be redosed according to half-life and blood loss (e.g., cefazolin is redosed every 3 to 4 hr or if >1,500 mL of blood loss).
  - Postoperative antibiotic prophylaxis has not been shown to be effective.
  - Preoperative treatment of bacterial vaginosis (BV) is recommended. BV is a known risk factor for SSI, and treatment with metronidazole 4 days prior to surgery has been demonstrated to decrease the risk of cuff cellulitis.
- **Antibiotic prophylaxis for subacute bacterial endocarditis.** Prophylaxis for bacterial endocarditis is no longer recommended by the AHA for routine GU or GI tract procedures. One exception is in patients undergoing a GU or GI procedure in the setting of active infection.
  - For patients with a prosthetic cardiac valve, previous history of endocarditis, unrepaired cyanotic congenital heart defect including palliative shunts and conduits, completely repaired congenital heart defect with prosthetic material or device during the first 6 months after the procedure, repaired congenital heart defect with residual defect at the site or adjacent to the site of a prosthetic patch or device, cardiac transplant, or cardiac valvulopathy, it may be reasonable to use an antibiotic regimen that covers organisms known to cause endocarditis, particularly *enterococci*. Preferred agents include penicillin, ampicillin, piperacillin, or vancomycin.
- **Bowel preparation.** Bowel preparation with polyethylene glycol nonosmotic electrolyte solution (e.g., Golytely) and a clear liquid diet for 24 hr on the day before surgery is common.
  - Alternative regimens include sodium phosphate (e.g., Fleet Phospho-Soda) or magnesium citrate, with or without enemas.

TABLE 24-2	Thromboprophylaxis for Gynecologic Procedures	
Procedure	Risks	Recommended Thrombophylaxis
Minor procedures	No additional risk factors	Early and frequent ambulation
Entirely laparoscopic	No additional risk factors	Early and frequent ambulation
Entirely laparoscopic	VTE risk factors are present	One or more of LMWH, LDUH, IPC, or GCS
Major gynecologic surgery	No additional risk factors	LMWH, LDUH, or IPC started just before surgery and used continuously while the patient is not ambulating
Major gynecologic surgery	VTE risk factors are present	LMWH or LDUH three times daily, or IPC started just before surgery and used continuously while the patient is not ambulating. Alternatives include combined LMWH or LDUH plus mechanical thromboprophylaxis with GCS or IPC, or fondaparinux
Extensive surgery for malignancy		Same as above for major surgery with VTE risks.

For major gynecologic procedures, recommend that thromboprophylaxis continue until discharge from hospital. For selected high-risk gynecology patients, including some of those who have undergone major cancer surgery or have previously had venous thromboembolism (VTE), consider continuing thromboprophylaxis after hospital discharge with LMWH for up to 28 days. LMWH, low molecular weight heparin; LDUH, low dose unfractionated heparin; GCS, graduated compression sockings; IPC, intermittent pneumatic compression. Adapted from Geerts WH, Bergqvist D, Pineo GF, et al. Prevention of venous thromboembolism: American College of Chest Physicians Evidence-Based Clinical Practice Guidelines (8th Ed.). *Chest* 2008;133 (6 Suppl):381S–453S.

- No conclusive evidence documents that mechanical bowel preparation reduces wound complications, infection, or anastomotic leakage after elective colorectal surgery involving bowel resection. On the contrary, data suggest an increased risk of anastomotic leakage and wound complications that may be explained by incomplete bowel preparations. A bowel prep or enema prior to surgery can be helpful to reduce the bulk in the recto-sigmoid colon and improve visualization in the pelvis.
- **Medications.** Antihypertensive medications, cardiac medications, reflux medications, psychiatric drugs, asthma medications, and antiseizure medications should be taken on the morning of surgery, with a sip of water.
  - Diabetic patients should take one third of the long-acting insulin, and those with an insulin pump should be on their basal rate. No oral hypoglycemics are taken

TABLE 24-3	Antibiotic Prophylaxis for Gynecologic Procedures	
Procedure	Antibiotic	Dose
Vaginal/abdominal hysterectomy	Cefazolin	1 or 2 g IV
	Cefoxitin	2 g IV
	Metronidazole	1 g IV
	Tinidazole	2 g PO (4–12 hrs before surgery)
Hysterosalpingogram (if dilated tubes)	Doxycycline	100 mg twice daily PO × 5 d
Induced abortion/D&C	Doxycycline or	100 mg PO 1 hr before and 200 mg orally after procedure
	Metronidazole	500 mg twice daily PO × 5 d
Laparoscopy	None	None
Laparotomy	None	None
Hysteroscopy	None	None
IUD insertion	None	None
Endometrial biopsy	None	None
Urodynamics	None	None

Adapted from Antibiotic prophylaxis for gynecologic procedures. ACOG Practice Bulletin Number 74. American College of Obstetricians and Gynecologists. *Obstet Gynecol* 2006;108(1):225–234, with permission.

on the day of surgery. Metformin should be stopped 2 days before surgery and not restarted for at least 48 hr after surgery.

- Aspirin and Plavix should be discontinued 7 days before surgery; other NSAIDs should be stopped 3 days before surgery. Patients on an anticoagulant will require a detailed plan of management. Coumadin therapy should be discontinued 4 to 5 days prior to surgery and converted to subcutaneous low molecular weight heparin (LMWH). On the day of surgery, the morning dose of heparin is held and coagulation studies are drawn immediately before surgery.
- Patients who were treated with steroids on a long-term basis (e.g., prednisone >5 mg/day for >3 weeks) usually receive intraoperative stress doses of steroids. Two options are hydrocortisone 50 or 100 mg IV or methylprednisolone 100 mg IV at the time of surgery. The steroids are continued for 24 hr postsurgery.
- Herbal supplements are discontinued 1 to 2 weeks prior to surgery as many have anticoagulant effects.
- These medication adjustments should be arranged in coordination with the patient's primary care physician. Postoperative instructions should address resumption of any discontinued medications.
- **Perioperative β-blockade** had previously been recommended to prevent cardiac events associated with surgery. Newer recommendations support the use of β-blockers in perioperative period in patients already on them. In patients undergoing

intermediate risk surgery with more than one cardiac risk factor, there may be benefit from β-blockade. The benefit of β-blockers in patients with only one cardiac risk factor remains uncertain. Consider the following when using β-blockade in the perioperative period:

- Start β-blockade weeks before surgery.
- Titrate dose to a resting heart rate of 60.
- Continue β-blockade during the intraoperative period.
- Continue β-blockers in the postoperative period for at least a month.
- Longer-acting β-1 selective β-blockers (e.g., atenolol or metoprolol) appear superior to shorter-acting β-blockers (e.g., propranolol).

INTRAOPERATIVE COMPLICATIONS

Hemorrhage

- Incidence of **pelvic hemorrhage** in major gynecologic surgery is reported as 1% to 2% in abdominal hysterectomy and 0.7% to 2.5% for vaginal hysterectomy. Other procedures associated with higher rates of hemorrhage are Burch colposuspension, abdominal sacrocolpopexy, and oncologic lymph node dissection. Previous surgery, large malignant or benign masses, history of pelvic inflammatory disease, and endometriosis can cause anatomic distortion predisposing a patient to injury and pelvic hemorrhage.
  - Control of pelvic bleeding starts with **preventive measures**, such as proper patient positioning, choosing an appropriate incision to ensure adequate exposure, meticulous surgical technique, and limited blunt dissection. Once hemorrhage is encountered, communication with anesthesia and operating room staff is essential.
  - Hemorrhage management is centered on four basic actions: (a) assess vital signs, (b) obtain adequate intravenous access, (c) resuscitate with judicious use of fluid or blood components, and (d) achieve hemostasis.
    - **Direct pressure** should be applied to sites of bleeding, allowing time for proper identification and control with electrocautery, ligation, or surgical clips. Difficult bleeding in the presacral area can also be managed with **bone wax** or **sterile tacks**.
    - **Hypogastric artery ligation** may be used for uncontrolled venous bleeding as it lowers pulse pressure.
    - Topical hemostatic agents, such as fibrin glue, Gelfoam, and Surgicel, can be applied to small venous bleeding sites.
    - **Pelvic packing**, using moist laparotomy pads, may be used temporarily for continued hemorrhage or left intra-abdominally with postoperative ICU monitoring. The patient is usually returned to the OR in 48 to 72 hr to remove the packs, irrigate, and close.
  - See also Chapter 3.
- **Postoperative bleeding** may be detected through changes in vital signs consistent with hypovolemia, patient restlessness, disproportionate pain relative to surgery or analgesics, abdominal ecchymosis, and abdominal distention. A larger than anticipated reduction in postoperative hematocrit should raise suspicion. These findings should prompt further evaluation to determine whether active bleeding is present. Orthostatic blood pressures, serial blood counts, and imaging studies (i.e., ultrasound or CT) should be performed as indicated. A stable hematoma can often be managed conservatively. Active bleeding requires blood replacement, and re-exploration is often necessary. With the availability of interventional radiology,

pelvic artery embolization has clinical success rates of 90% for postsurgical and posttraumatic hemorrhage and avoids the additional morbidity of reoperation.

Ureteral Injury

- **Ureteral injury** rates have been reported from 0.4% to 2.5% during benign pelvic surgery, and only one third are recognized intraoperatively. Most commonly reported rates of injury are 0.1% to 1.7% during abdominal hysterectomy and 0% to 0.1% for vaginal hysterectomy. The highest rates are seen in laparoscopic surgery, with an odds ratio of 2.6 when compared to the abdominal route. During vaginal hysterectomy, the ureter can be traumatized at its entry point at the trigone. Laparoscopic procedures, especially ablation of endometriosis, carry an increased risk of ureteral injury near the uterosacral ligament.

- **Prevention and detection.** Steps taken to avoid ureteral injury during hysterectomy include development of the vesicouterine space, skeletonization of the uterine arteries, and cephalad traction on the uterus, all of which deflect the ureters laterally and downward. These measures are equally important in laparoscopic and abdominal surgery. The ureter can be visualized in the pararectal space on the medial leaf of the broad ligament. The pelvic ureter approaches within 1 cm of the infundibulopelvic ligament, lies 1.5 cm lateral to the internal cervical os, and approaches within 0.9 cm of the upper third of the vagina. These distances are important during dissection, clamp placement, and in the consideration of thermal injury with the use of cautery. Preoperative intravenous pyelograms (IVP) and ureteral stenting have a questionable role in decreasing ureter injury risk.

- **Intraoperative cystoscopy** with indigo carmine is an excellent test for assessing ureteral integrity and allows immediate corrective surgery to be undertaken if an injury is detected. This technique is recommended for all urogynecologic surgery and major gynecologic surgery to identify and prevent sequelae of intraoperative urinary tract injury, as well as decrease liability from an undetected injury.

- **Management.** In cases of crush injury without transection, stenting the ureter for an extended period and placing a drain at the site of injury may be sufficient therapy. Complete transection above the pelvic brim or partial transection is repaired by suturing the defect end-to-end (**uretero-ureterostomy**). Reimplantation into the bladder (**uretero-neocystostomy**) is performed if the injury is within 6 cm of the ureterovesical junction. Mobilization of the bladder along the external iliac vessels with attachment to the psoas tendon (**psoas hitch**) can be used to bridge the gap and decrease tension at the anastomotic site when necessary. In cases of insufficient residual ureteral length, a Boari flap or ileal interposition can be performed. **Transuretero-ureterostomy** for injuries high in the pelvis is no longer recommended. Drains should be placed near the anastomosis to prevent urinoma formation and detect leakage. Delayed diagnosis of a ureteral injury may require retrograde pyelography with cystoscopy and stent placement or percutaneous nephrostomy with antegrade stent placement. The recovery potential of the kidney depends on the duration of the obstruction, the degree of obstruction, the degree of backflow, the presence or absence of infection, and the extent to which each kidney was functional before the injury.

Bladder Injury

- The rate of **bladder injury** in benign gynecologic surgery is 0.5% to 1%. The rate during abdominal hysterectomy is 0.2% to 2.3%, which is increased compared to the vaginal hysterectomy rate of 0.3% to 1.5%. Major lacerations may require mobilization of the bladder for tension-free repair. Multiple cystotomies may be joined into one defect. A one-layer or two-layer closure with 2-0 or 3-0 synthetic absorbable suture in two layers is required, and the security should be assessed by placing sterile milk or methylene blue retrograde into the bladder. A Foley or suprapubic catheter is left in place for 7 to 14 days. A small cystotomy that occurs with a trocar during placement of a midurethral sling requires catheterized decompression for only 24 to 48 hr.

- A missed bladder or ureteral injury usually results in postoperative urinary ascites or urinoma, abdominal or flank pain, and distention with fever, chills, oliguria, nausea, and vomiting. These patients may have elevated blood urea nitrogen and creatinine levels and may respond to aggressive hydration and bladder rest. Unrecognized surgical injuries are the most common cause of genitourinary fistulas in the developed world.

Bowel Injury

- Inadvertent **bowel injury** occurs most often in gynecologic surgeries from an abdominal approach and is reported in 0.1% to 1% of abdominal hysterectomies and 0.1% to 0.8% of vaginal hysterectomies.
- A systematic evaluation of the bowel should be performed at the end of a procedure. Serosal injuries can be closed with permanent or delayed absorbable 3-0 suture. Gastrostomies, enterotomies, or colostomies may be closed in two layers, using a continuous mucosal repair with 3-0 absorbable suture and an imbricating seromuscular interrupted permanent 3-0 suture.
  - Suture lines should be perpendicular to the longitudinal axis of the lumen to avoid luminal constriction. In cases of multiple enterotomies, the bowel may be resected and reanastomosed. A nasogastric tube can be used for decompression in stomach and small bowel injuries. Distal colonic injury does not warrant colostomy except in cases of previous radiation or infection.

Nerve Injury

- Malpositioning or retractor placement is the usual cause of **nerve injury** in gynecologic surgery. However, hematoma formation, a foreign body, or transection can also be complicating factors. See Chapter 23.
  - **Common peroneal nerve** injury is most often caused by compression at the lateral epicondyle from the stirrups and may result in a transient, postoperative foot drop.
  - **Lateral femoral cutaneous nerve** injury can result from placement of self-retaining retractors or hyperflexion of the hips in lithotomy position and results in anterior lateral thigh paresthesia and pain. One should be aware of the location, depth, and the exact pressure exerted by the lateral sidewall retractors on the iliopsoas muscle.
  - **Femoral nerve** injury can result in motor or sensory injury, or both, and may occur when the deep retractors rest on the psoas muscle or when the thighs are severely flexed on the abdomen in the lithotomy position. Passing below the relatively firm inguinal ligament, the femoral nerve is vulnerable to compression at that point. Postoperatively, the patient may experience weakness in the quadriceps muscle and difficulty walking.
  - The **sciatic nerve** can be injured when the surgical assistant rests on the dorsal aspect of the thigh during vaginal surgery or when the hip is flexed and the knee is suddenly straightened. This tends to happen more commonly with free hanging

("candy cane") stirrups. As with common peroneal nerve injury, this injury typically leads to foot drop.

- The **obturator nerve** may be injured during dissection, or with leg positioning. Excessive external rotation at the hip may result in a stretch injury. Patients may complain of difficulty walking and will have weakness of the internal compartment muscles, and demonstrate deficiency in adduction.
- The **iliohypogastric and ilioinguinal nerves** are at risk for injury or entrapment when a Pfannenstiel incision extends beyond the lateral margin of the inferior rectus abdominis muscle, or during trocar placement and port site closure. Typically, patients report a sharp or burning pain radiating from the incision to the suprapubic area or paresthesias in this area.
- Most compression and stretch injuries resolve completely over several weeks to months. Physical therapy is required in cases with motor deficits. In cases of ilioinguinal or iliohypogastric injury, infiltration of local anesthesia in this area can help in diagnosis of this type of nerve injury and provide temporary relief of the symptoms. Neurectomy is usually indicated if a local nerve block is found to be effective. The key to treatment is prevention: proper patient positioning, periodic reassessment during long surgeries, proper retractor placement, and careful dissection.

Complications Specific to Laparoscopy

- One analysis of 70,000 cases in Finland reported complication rates (per 1,000) as follows: overall, 3.6; major complications, 1.4; intestinal injury, 0.6; ureteral injury, 0.3; bladder injury, 0.3; and vascular injuries, 0.1.
- **Port placement.** The majority of injuries during laparoscopy occur during access. A recent Cochrane review finds no clear advantage of one entry technique over another. However, open entry may be prudent in patients with a history of multiple lower abdominal surgeries or inflammatory bowel disease. The left upper quadrant or "Palmers point" is an alternate site for insertion of the Veress needle for creation of a pneumoperitoneum and primary trocar insertion when significant periumbilical adhesions are suspected (see Chapter 23). The gastric contents must be aspirated with a nasogastric or oral gastric tube prior to using this method. The skin incision is made between the left midclavicular and anterior axillary lines approximately 2 fingerbreadths below the left costal margin to avoid the superior epigastric vessels. The Veress needle is inserted perpendicularly and shallowly into the peritoneal cavity to allow insufflation; then, a 5-mm trocar can be inserted. This approach offers two advantages: (a) short distance between layers of the anterior abdominal wall and (b) less chance of adhesions in the left upper quadrant in patients with a history of prior surgery. During primary port placement, the small bowel, iliac artery, and colon are the most commonly injured structures. With secondary ports, abdominal wall vessels, iliac arteries, and aorta are at most risk for injury. A systematic review of the field should be performed in every case after gaining primary access prior to Trendelenburg, and all secondary ports should be inserted under direct visualization.
- **Extraperitoneal insufflation of CO_2.** Misplacement of a Veress needle in the preperitoneal space causes this complication and can impair visualization due to peritoneal tenting. In most cases, CO_2 can be allowed to escape and needle placement attempted again. If this is not successful, open laparoscopy is performed. Mediastinal emphysema is an uncommon complication that requires observation for respiratory compromise and, in severe cases, may require ventilation.
- **Vessel injury.** The Veress needle or trocar may traumatize omental, mesenteric, major abdominal, or pelvic vessels. Trendelenburg position should never be

obtained prior to trocar placement; the table should be flat. The sacral promontory should be palpated as a landmark of the aortic bifurcation. In thin patients, the Veress needle is directed at 45 degrees and in obese patients at 90 degrees. Confirmation of peritoneal access is obtained as follows. A 5-mL syringe filled with saline is attached to the Veress needle and aspiration is performed to ensure neither blood nor bowel contents are returned. Some saline is then instilled through the Veress without resistance, and the syringe is removed. The remaining saline in the tip of the Veress should easily fall into the abdominal cavity with elevation of anterior abdominal wall. If bright red blood is aspirated through the Veress needle, leave it in place and proceed to laparotomy; this will aid in identifying the injury site.

- The *superficial epigastric* vessels may be identified by transillumination, especially in thinner patients; however, the deeper *inferior epigastric* vessels should be identified intra-abdominally prior to accessory trocar placement. The landmarks for the inferior epigastric vessels are the medial umbilical ligaments and the entry point of the round ligament into the inguinal canal. The inferior epigastric vessels begin their cephalad course between these structures. The secondary trocars are inserted perpendicularly lateral to the edge of the rectus muscles. Upon penetration of the fascia, the trocar is directed toward the vesicouterine pouch in order to decrease the risk of vessel laceration. Maintaining the perpendicular insertion until the peritoneal cavity is entered is essential to prevent damage to the inferior epigastric vessels.

- Management of inferior epigastric vessel injury includes balloon tamponade with a foley or suture ligature using a Carter Thompson or Endoclose device. Consider enlarging the incision at the trocar site or proceeding to laparotomy to improve visualization. Damage to major retroperitoneal vessels generally requires emergent laparotomy and consultation with a vascular surgeon.

- **Bowel injury.** Intestinal injuries have been reported at a rate of <0.5%. Approximately half of these injuries occur on entry and half occur as a result of electrocautery, either direct thermal injury or due to coupling. Most bowel injuries are not recognized at the time of surgery. If bowel perforation with the Veress needle is suspected, the needle should be withdrawn and insufflation attempted at another site. If the laparoscope enters the bowel lumen, it should be left in place to limit contamination and to facilitate identification of the injured site. Generally, puncture sites from the pneumoperitoneum needle can be managed conservatively. Repair may be accomplished by routine laparoscopic or open techniques. A thermal injury is often treated by oversewing of the bowel, or resection in cases of significant injury. Monopolar energy has been shown to have a thermal spread up to several centimeters away; therefore, extreme caution should be used when using monopolar cautery on strands of tissues attached to bowel. Symptoms of bowel injury can range from increased pain at the trocar site to abdominal distention and diarrhea to sepsis. CT scan is the best imaging study to confirm the diagnosis. Access injuries or traumatic injuries often present early, in the first hours or days postoperatively. Thermal injury may present late (3 to 7 days after surgery) due to a delay in the perforation after necrosis at the site of injury. Unrecognized bowel injury is one of the most common causes of postoperative death from laparoscopy.

- **Bladder injury.** Prevention is best achieved by decompression of the bladder with a foley, avoiding low suprapubic ports (<5 cm above pubic symphysis), and direct visualization during trocar placement. Bladder injury is not restricted to port placement, and also occurs during dissection of the vesicouterine space. Low anterior fibroids and history of prior cesarean section increase that risk. Injury may be detected by the presence of air or blood in the drainage bag of an indwelling Foley catheter. The size of the injury dictates treatment. Needle perforations can be managed expectantly. Lacerations <10 mm long will heal spontaneously if the bladder is drained continuously with a Foley catheter for 3 to 4 postoperative days. Larger injuries require suturing, as described earlier. This can be performed laparoscopically by surgeons experienced in laparoscopic suturing technique.

- **Ureteral injury.** Laparoscopical-assisted vaginal hysterectomy is the leading gynecologic procedure in which ureteral injury occurs. Electrocautery instruments are also associated with injuries during laparoscopic surgery. Careful exposure and identification of anatomy is the best way to reduce risk of injury to the ureter. If ureteral injury is suspected, indigo carmine administration and cystoscopy should be performed intraoperatively.

- **Dehiscence and hernia.** The overall incidence of incisional dehiscence and hernia is approximately 0.02% and is greater with trocar-cannula systems ≥10 cm in diameter. Richter's hernias, which typically have a delayed diagnosis, contain a portion of the intestinal wall in a peritoneal defect. General recommendations for fascial closure are to close all defects ≥10 mm and defects >5 mm that are lateral to the rectus sheath or after significant tissue extraction or peritoneal stretch. Both fascia and peritoneum should be closed.

Complications Specific to Hysteroscopy

- **Fluid overload.** Fluids are delivered into the uterine cavity with sufficiently high pressure to allow intravasation of the distention media into the vascular system. Serious complications can occur if intravasation is excessive. The risks and allowable fluid deficits vary according to type of distention media used.
  - Electrolyte-containing media (normal saline and lactated ringers) are relatively safe, but fluid overload is still possible. These media can be used with bipolar but not monopolar instruments. Alternative fluid media carry increased risks with overload.
  - Hyskon, a high viscosity 32% solution of dextran 70, provides a clear field because it does not mix with blood. In the bloodstream, it acts as a volume expander, potentially leading to acute noncardiogenic pulmonary edema. Dextran molecules can trigger disseminated intravascular coagulation and anaphylaxis. In an acute setting, dextran molecules must be removed from the circulation with plasmapheresis.
  - Three percent sorbitol and 1.5% glycine are low-viscosity, hypotonic, electrolyte-free solutions. When absorbed into the bloodstream, they cause hyponatremia, arrhythmias, cerebral edema, coma, and death.
  - Mannitol 5% is an iso-osmolar media that can also cause hyponatremia. Absorption is increased as a function of increasing flow pressure, uterine size, and operative time. Automated fluid-monitoring systems have made the exact measurements of input and output of the distending medium much easier. The surgeon should be aware of the deficit at all times and should be updated frequently by operating room staff (Table 24-4).

- **Uterine perforation** may be managed conservatively, particularly with a blunt instrument, with close monitoring, or overnight hospitalization. In cases of active bleeding or perforation with electrosurgical instruments, conversion to laparoscopy or laparotomy is required.

TABLE 24-4	Guidelines for Fluid Management During Hysteroscopy

- Fluid input and output should be monitored preoperatively and intraoperatively by an individual assigned to this task. Results should be reported to the surgical team at regular intervals.

- Low-viscosity, electrolyte-poor fluids: A fluid deficit of 750 mL implies excessive intravasation of fluid. Surgeon should consider termination of procedure in patients with high cardiovascular risk or comorbid conditions.

- Nonelectrolyte solutions: A fluid deficit of 1,000–1,500 mL implies excessive intravasation of fluid but depends on patient weight and other factors. The infusion should be stopped, procedure concluded, and electrolyte and fluid status assessed. Diuretics and other interventions should be initiated as needed.

- Electrolyte solutions: A fluid deficit of 2,000 mL implies excessive intravasation of fluid. Management is same as previous.

- Discontinuing the infusion at lower thresholds should be considered in outpatient settings, with limited acute care and laboratory services.

- Automated fluid monitoring systems facilitate early recognition of fluid imbalance.

Adapted from Loffer FD, Bradley LD, Brill AI, et al. Hysteroscopic fluid monitoring guidelines. The ad hoc committee on hysteroscopic training guidelines of the American Association of Gynecologic Laparoscopists. *J Am Assoc Gynecol Laparosc* 2000;7:167–168, with permission; and American College of Obstetricians and Gynecologists (ACOG). Technology Assessment in Obstetrics and Gynecology, Hysteroscopy. *Obstet Gynecol* 2005;106(2)439–442, with permission.

POSTOPERATIVE COMPLICATIONS

Postoperative Fever

- A common definition of **fever** requires a temperature at or above 38°C (100.4°F) on two occasions at least 4 hr apart. Febrile morbidity within the first 48 hr of surgery has been estimated to occur in up to 50% of gynecologic surgery patients. Atelectasis has not been shown to be causal for fever during this period. Noninfectious etiologies, such as medications, malignant hyperthermia, thrombotic or embolic events, ureteral injuries, cardiovascular events, endocrine abnormalities, and transfusion reactions, should be included in the differential diagnosis and workup for postoperative fever.
- **Evaluation.** Evaluation should include a review of the patient's history and a thorough examination, with specific attention to sites as follows: pulmonary examination, palpation of the suprapubic region, costovertebral angles, evaluation of incision, catheter and line sites, extremities, and pelvic examination to evaluate the vaginal cuff for cellulitis, hematoma, or abscess.
- **Testing.** Initial laboratory and radiologic assessment should be tailored to the individual patient. Complete blood count with differential, urinalysis, and urine culture should be performed. Urinalysis will be of limited value in patients with bladder catheters. Blood cultures seldom yield positive results except in patients with high

fever or risk factors for endocarditis and are most sensitive when drawn at the time of the fever. Imaging studies may include chest and abdominal radiographs, IVP, ultrasonography of the pelvis and kidneys, contrast bowel studies, and CT scan. Chest CT, or ventilation perfusion (V/Q) scan should also be considered to rule out pulmonary embolism (PE).

Postoperative Infection

- **Urinary tract infection.** The bladder is a common site of infection in surgical patients, largely due to contamination with indwelling Foley catheters. Pyelonephritis is a rare complication. The treatment is hydration and antibiotic therapy tailored to the pathogen.
- **Respiratory infection.** Preventive measures are early ambulation and intensive respiratory therapy (i.e., incentive spirometry, chest physical therapy) for reversal of hypoventilation and atelectasis. Patient education prior to surgery has an important role in compliance with postoperative incentive spirometry. Patients at risk of postoperative pneumonia include those with an ASA status of 3 or higher, preoperative hospital stay of 2 days or longer, surgery lasting 3 hr or longer, surgery in the upper abdomen or thorax, nasogastric suction, postoperative intubation, or a history of smoking or obstructive lung disease. Smoking cessation should be encouraged preoperatively, not only for respiratory complications but also for wound healing.

Wound Infection

- **Prevention.** Risk factors for SSI include age, nutritional status, diabetes, smoking, obesity, coexistent infections at a remote body site, colonization with microorganisms, altered immune response, and length of preoperative stay.
- **Surgical closure.** Studies in cesarean-section patients have shown closure of the subcutaneous fat compared with nonclosure reduces wound complications (defined as hematoma, seroma, wound infection, wound separation). In women with fat thickness ≥2 cm, suture closure of subcutaneous fat decreases the risk of wound disruption. Further trials are justified to investigate suturing materials and techniques. Whether these findings can be extrapolated to gynecologic surgery is unclear. Recent meta-analyses have failed to show that the routine use of closed suction drains prevents surgical infections.
- **Wound care.** Wound care has recently shifted away from an aggressive cleaning approach to one that emphasizes a clean but moist environment and minimizes the mechanical irritation caused by frequent dressing changes. Hydrogel applications play an important role, and vacuum systems can aid in wound drainage and facilitation of blood flow to the wound, resulting in more rapid closure.

Incisional or Vaginal Cuff Cellulitis

- Fever, leukocytosis, and pain localizing to the pelvis may accompany a severe cellulitis in which adjacent pelvic tissues are involved. Broad-spectrum antibiotic therapy should be initiated. If an abscess is suspected at the cuff or incision, drainage is indicated in the operating room or under ultrasound guidance. Intra-abdominal abscesses are characterized by persistent fever and leukocytosis. Radiologic confirmation with ultrasonography or CT scan is usually needed for diagnosis.
- Treatment involves parenteral antibiotics, with possible drainage in cases of large collections or failure to improve on antibiotics alone. Sonographic or CT scan–guided drain placement has obviated the need for surgical exploration in many

circumstances. Re-exploration in cases of active infection or abscess is approached with reservation due to associated high morbidity.

Necrotizing Fasciitis

- Group A Streptococcus can cause a progressive, inflammatory infection of the deep fascia, with necrosis of the subcutaneous tissues. Surgeons must be acutely aware of this potentially life-threatening complication in any patient with a wound infection. Clinically, the infection results in extensive soft-tissue destruction, including necrosis of skin, subcutaneous tissue, and muscle. Erythema and induration around the wound should be marked and followed closely. Extensive and aggressive surgical debridement and broad-spectrum antibiotic therapy are warranted at first suspicion. Treatment delay and obesity increase an already high mortality rate.

Venous Thromboembolism (VTE)

- **Deep vein thrombosis.** DVT involves unilateral lower-extremity swelling, pain, and erythema. A palpable cord may be detected. Duplex doppler ultrasonographic imaging has replaced venography as the gold standard for diagnosing DVT.
- **Pulmonary embolism.** The signs and symptoms of PE include anxiety, shortness of breath, tachypnea, chest pain, hypoxia, tachycardia, and mental status changes. Even when a PE is suspected, evaluation should be prompt and thorough; chest radiograph, electrocardiogram (ECG), and arterial blood gas assessment are the first-line tests. The chest radiograph helps distinguish between pneumonia and embolism. ECG findings are usually nonspecific except for tachycardia, but they help rule out an ischemic cardiac event. Laboratory evaluation with arterial blood gas test may show hypoxemia, hypocapnia, respiratory alkalosis, and an increased arterial-alveolar gradient.

Imaging

- Radionucleotide imaging (V/Q scan) and contrast-enhanced CT arteriography are the current studies available for the evaluation of a suspected PE. V/Q scans have a high sensitivity but a low specificity. Contrast-enhanced CT arteriography is rapid, easily accessible in most large hospitals, and less prone to interference from other underlying pulmonary disease. Its sensitivity is greatest for detecting emboli in the main, lobar, or segmental pulmonary arteries. In most institutions, the CT arteriography has replaced the V/Q scan as the first-line diagnostic imaging study.

Therapy

- Intravenous unfractionated heparin (UFH) has been the traditional treatment for DVT and PE. Recent studies have established that LMWH and the pentasaccharide fondaparinux are equivalent to UFH. The half-life of LMWH is longer, the dose response is more predictable, and less bleeding may occur while producing an equivalent antithrombotic effect. When using UFH, oral therapy with Coumadin is started as early as possible, and the patient is discharged when a therapeutic international normalized ratio value is reached. Placement of a vena caval filter may be necessary in patients with acute thromboembolism and active bleeding or a high potential for bleeding, patients who are on medical therapy with a history of multiple venous thrombi, and patients with a history of heparin-induced thrombocytopenia. Bleeding that occurs after the use of heparin-related compounds can be reversed with protamine sulfate; Coumadin-related bleeding can be reversed with vitamin K or with plasma or factor IX concentrates. The most effective treatment is prevention. See also Chapter 17.

Ileus and Bowel Obstruction

- **Diagnosis.** Infection, peritonitis, electrolyte disturbances, extensive manipulation of the GI tract, and prolonged procedures may cause postoperative ileus. Postoperative adhesions occur in 60% to 90% of patients who undergo major gynecologic surgery and represent one of the most common causes of intestinal obstruction. The prevalence of ileus or small bowel obstruction following hysterectomy is 0.2% to 2.2%. Nausea, vomiting, and distention may be present with both. Absent and hypoactive bowel sounds are more likely to occur with ileus, whereas borborygmi, rushes, and high-pitched tinkles are more characteristic of postoperative obstruction. Abdominal radiographs show distended loops of large and small bowel, with gas present in the rectum in the setting of ileus. Single or multiple loops of distended bowel with air-fluid levels are seen in postoperative obstruction. These findings may be difficult to distinguish in the early postoperative period. In prolonged cases, it may be helpful to obtain a study with oral contrast to identify a transition point.
- **Treatment.** Ileus is treated with bowel rest, intravenous fluids, electrolyte repletion, and nasogastric suction in cases of persistent vomiting. Most cases of partial obstruction will respond to conservative management with bowel rest and nasogastric decompression. Increasing abdominal pain, progressive distention, fever, leukocytosis, or acidosis should increase the suspicion for complete bowel obstruction, which may require re-exploration. In cases with delayed improvement, a CT scan may help identify bowel perforation or abscess. Parenteral nutrition should also be considered in patients with prolonged GI compromise.

Diarrhea

- **Diarrhea** is not uncommon after abdominal and pelvic surgery. Prolonged or multiple episodes, however, may represent a pathologic process, such as impending small bowel obstruction, colonic obstruction, or pseudomembranous colitis. *Clostridium difficile*–associated colitis may result from exposure to any antibiotics; stool testing can confirm clinical suspicions. Extended oral metronidazole therapy and hydration are needed for adequate treatment, and oral vancomycin may be necessary in refractory cases.

Genitourinary Fistulae

- In the United States, most **genitourinary fistulae** are the result of pelvic surgery, usually after an abdominal hysterectomy for benign conditions. In the developing world, most fistulas are due to obstetric trauma secondary to absent or poor obstetric care. Patients may present with persistent vaginal discharge or recurrent urinary tract infections.
- The simplest initial test for a genitourinary fistula is the tampon test. A tampon or cotton ball is inserted into the vagina. The bladder is then filled with methylene blue through a Foley catheter. The appearance of dye at the urethral end of the tampon suggests urethral urinary loss. Dye at the vaginal apex suggests a vesicovaginal fistula. A wet but undyed tampon is suggestive of a ureteral-vaginal fistula. Fluid pooling in the vagina can also be sent for a creatinine level. Further workup may include IVP, cystoscopy, voiding cystourethrogram, retrograde ureteral studies, and MRI. Simple fistulas often resolve with drainage by either foley catheter or percutaneous nephrostomy tube placement to allow healing and decreased inflammation. Surgical repair is necessary if this is unsuccessful.

ROUTINE POSTOPERATIVE CARE

• See Chapter 3.

SUGGESTED READINGS

Antibiotic prophylaxis for gynecologic procedures. ACOG Practice Bulletin Number 104. American College of Obstetricians and Gynecologists. *Obstet Gynecol* 2009;113:1180–1189.

Douketis JD, Berger PB, Dunn AS, et al. The perioperative management of antithrombotic therapy: American College of Chest Physicians Evidence-Based Clinical Practice Guidelines (8th Ed.). *Chest* 2008;133(6 Suppl):299S–339S.

Jones HW, Rock WA. Control of pelvic hemorrhage. In Rock JA, Jones HW, eds. *Te Linde's Operative Gynecology*, 9th Ed. Philadelphia, PA: Lippincott Williams & Wilkins, 2003.

Tapson VF. Acute pulmonary embolism. *N Engl J Med* 2008;358(10):1037–1052.

Wilson W, Taubert KA, Gewitz M, et al. Prevention of infective endocarditis: guidelines from the American Heart Association. *Circulation* 2007;116(15):1736–1754. Epub 2007 Apr 19.

Infections of the Genital Tract

Matthew W. Guile and Jean Keller

INFECTIONS OF THE LOWER GENITAL TRACT

Symptoms caused by **infections of the lower genital tract** are among the most common presenting complaints of gynecologic patients. This chapter reviews the following: vulvar infections, parasitic infections, ulcerative lesions, vaginitis, cervicitis, and pelvic inflammatory disease. Urinary tract infections are covered in Chapter 16.

Vulvar Infections

Human Papillomavirus (HPV)

- HPV infection is the most common sexually transmitted disease (STD) in the United States, with an estimated 80% of sexually active women having acquired genital HPV by the age of 50. Most HPV infection is asymptomatic or subclinical, with the majority of patients clearing the infection within 2 years.
- There are over 100 types of HPV, of which approximately 30 are mucosal and can infect the lower genital tract in women. HPV types 6 and 11 cause ***condyloma acuminata*** or genital warts. HPV can be classified as low-, intermediate-, and high-risk for the development of **squamous cell carcinoma**, with the majority of cervical cancer caused by four types, 16, 18, 31, and 45 (see Chapter 42).
- Peak **incidence** is highest among 15- to 25-year-olds, soon after the onset of sexual activity. Pregnant, immunosuppressed, and diabetic patients are at increased risk.
- **Signs and symptoms** of genital warts include soft, sessile, and/or verrucous lesions on any mucosal or dermal surface that range in size and formation. Lesions are usually multifocal and asymptomatic, although itching, burning, bleeding, and pain can occur.
- **Diagnosis.** Genital warts are usually diagnosed by gross inspection, and colposcopic examination may aid in the identification of cervical or vaginal lesions. HPV testing is not warranted for the diagnosis of genital warts. Biopsy is recommended if there is no response to standard therapy or if there are hyperpigmented, flat, ulcerated, bleeding or atypical lesions, or in immunocompromised patients. Condyloma acuminatum must be differentiated from the lesion of secondary syphilis, condyloma lata.
- **Treatment.** There are multiple modalities for the treatment of genital warts, including surgical excision, application of topical cytotoxic or keratolytic agents, cytodestructive techniques, and immune modulators. Therapy should be based on the location, size, and number of lesions and the preference of the patient. Lesions may spontaneously regress and recur. A combination of approaches may be required, although no therapy can ensure complete eradication of the virus (Table 25-1).

TABLE 25-1 Treatment Options for Genital Warts

Therapy	Application	Clearance Rate (%)	Recurrence Rate (%)	Use in Pregnancy
Patient applied				
Imiquimod 5% cream	Apply three times a week at bedtime for up to 16 wk. Wash the area 6–10 hr after application.	40–77	13	Contraindicated
Podofilox 0.5% solution or gel	Apply bid for 3 d, no treatment for 4 d, repeat the cycle for up to four times.	68–88	16–34	Contraindicated
Provider administered				
Podophyllin resin at 10%–25% in benzoin	Can be repeated weekly, as needed	38–79	21–65	Contraindicated
Surgical excision	—	89–93	19–22	Only if obstructing vaginal delivery
Cryotherapy	Can be repeated every 1–2 wk	70–96	25–39	Permitted
Topical trichloroacetic acid or bichloroacetic acid (80%–90% solution)	Apply small amount q1–2wk until the wart sloughs off. Typical course is six treatments.	81	36	Permitted
Alternative regimens				
CO_2 laser excision	—	72–97	6–49	Not recommended
Interferons	Inject at the edge of and beneath the wart with a 26- to 32-gauge needle.	36–53	21–25	Not recommended

From Centers for Disease Control and Prevention. Sexually transmitted diseases treatment guidelines, 2006. *MMWR* 2006;55(No. RR-11), with permission.

- **Prevention.** In June 2006, an HPV vaccine was licensed by the US Food and Drug Administration for use in women aged from 9 to 26 years old that protects against the four types of HPV (types 16, 18 and types 6, 11). Types 16 and 18 account for 70% of all cervical cancer and 6 and 11 for 90% of all genital warts. See also Chapters 42 and 43.

Molluscum Contagiosum

- **Molluscum** is a benign poxvirus infection of the skin found worldwide, but is most common in the developing world. It is spread by skin contact (sexual or nonsexual), autoinoculation, and fomites. The incubation period ranges from several weeks to months.
- **Signs and symptoms** include the appearance of dome-shaped papules with central umbilication ranging from 2 to 5 mm in diameter. Multiple lesions may arise but generally are fewer than 20. The lesions are usually asymptomatic but occasionally pruritic and may become inflammed and swollen. They are usually self-limited, lasting for 6 to 12 months, but may take as long as 4 years to resolve.
- **Diagnosis.** The characteristic appearance of molluscum contagiosum lends itself to clinical diagnosis by gross inspection. When in doubt, a crush preparation (i.e., microscopic examination of white, waxy material expressed from a nodule) can be performed. Intracytoplasmic molluscum bodies confirm the diagnosis. Immuno-compromised patients with HIV/AIDS or other conditions can develop giant lesions (>15 mm in diameter) and large numbers of lesions that may be resistant to standard therapy.
- **Treatment.** Molluscum contagiosum is usually self-limited. Multiple regimens have been evaluated in clinical trials, with none being convincingly efficacious. Many practitioners employ watchful waiting. Lesion visibility and patient preference may prompt therapy, which consists of evacuation of the core material with cryofreezing, curettage, or laser ablation.

Parasites

Pediculosis Pubis

- **Pubic lice** infect approximately three million people a year in the United States. This is the most common STD but can also be transmitted through infected bedding and clothing. The ectoparasite *Phthirus pubis* is usually restricted to the pubic, perineal, and perianal areas but may infect the eyelids and other body parts. The parasite deposits eggs at the base of the hair follicle. The incubation period is 1 week and the crab louse lives for about 6 weeks but dies within 24 hr without blood.
- **Symptoms** of infection include intense pruritus in the affected area, sometimes accompanied by maculopapular lesions. Occurrence of a large number of bites over a short period may lead to systemic manifestations, such as mild fever, malaise, or irritability.
- **Diagnosis** is made by gross visualization of lice, larvae, or nits in the pubic hair or microscopic identification of crablike lice under oil.

Scabies

- **Scabies** is caused by the mite *Sarcoptes scabiei* var. *hominis*. It is transmitted via prolonged close contact (sexual or nonsexual) and may infect any part of the body, especially flexural surfaces of the elbows, wrists, finger webs, axilla, genitals, and buttocks. Fomite transmission is considered possible through clothing, bedding, or towels. The adult female burrows beneath the skin, lays eggs, and travels quickly across the skin. Crusted or Norwegian scabies is highly infectious and is an aggressive infestation in immunodeficient, debilitated, or malnourished persons, and is associated with increased treatment failure.

- **Symptoms** include the insidious onset of severe intermittent pruritus approximately 3 to 6 weeks after the initial exposure. Subsequent infections can become symptomatic within 24 hr of reinfection. The intense pruritus may worsen at night and include most of the body. The characteristic lesion is the burrow, a 1- to 10-mm curving track that serves to house the mite. Other lesions include papules and vesicles.
- **Diagnosis** can often be made clinically based on history and gross appearance of the burrows. Skin scrapings can be obtained for microscopic examination under oil.
- **Treatment** (Table 25-2) for pediculosis pubis and scabies requires an agent that kills both adult organisms and eggs. Treat pruritus with antihistamines.
  - Toxic effects of lindane include seizures and aplastic anemia. This agent is not recommended for use in pregnant or lactating women, children younger than age 2, or patients with extensive dermatitis.

TABLE 25-2	Treatment Options for Parasites	
	Pediculosis Pubis	**Scabies**
Permethrin (Nix) cream—*Safe in pregnancy*	Apply 1% cream rinse to the affected areas, wash off after 10 min, and comb the infested areas with a fine-toothed comb.	Apply 5% cream to all areas of the body from the neck down and wash off after 8–14 hr.
Lindane 1% (Kwell) lotion, cream, or shampoo—*Not for use in pregnancy*	Not first-line due to toxicity.	Apply 1 oz. of lotion or 30 g of cream in a thin layer to all areas of the body from the neck down and thoroughly wash off after 8 hr.
Pyrethrins with piperonyl butoxide—*Safe in pregnancy*	Apply to the affected area and wash off after 10 min.	Treat pruritus with antihistamines.

Clothes and linens should be laundered in hot water and heat dried or removed from body contact for at least 72 hr. Sexual partners should be treated. From Centers for Disease Control and Prevention. Sexually transmitted diseases treatment guidelines 2006. *MMWR* 2006;55(No. RR-11), with permission.

Genital Ulcers

- The most common infectious causes of genital ulcers in young, sexually active women are herpes simplex virus (HSV), *Treponema pallidum* (syphilis), and *Haemophilus ducreyi* (chancroid). Genital herpes is the most prevalent of the three. All these lesions are associated with increased risk of HIV acquisition.

Genital Herpes

- Fifty million people in the United States have **genital herpes**, a chronic sexually transmitted infection caused by HSV. Multiple types of herpes virus have been identified. Historically, HSV-2 accounts for the majority of genital infections; however, HSV-1 now accounts for up to 50% of first-episode cases. HSV-1 genital infections are less likely to recur and less commonly result in asymptomatic viral shedding. The majority of persons infected with HSV-2 have not been diagnosed with genital herpes, and intermittent viral shedding accounts for most HSV transmission.
- **Clinical diagnosis** of genital herpes is both insensitive and nonspecific. The classic presentation of multiple, painful, vesicular or ulcerative lesions is absent in many patients.
- Herpetic outbreaks can last as long as 2 to 6 weeks in a first-episode primary infection and up to 7 days in recurrent outbreaks. Classically, lesions are preceded by vulvar paresthesias or pruritus, followed by the formation of multiple vesicles that coalesce into ulcerations which may be painful. Outbreaks are self-limiting, and lesions heal without scar formation. The prodrome of itching or burning in the affected area is important for counseling patients on when to start antiviral therapy since systemic symptoms are usually absent. The majority of patients with HSV-2 will experience recurrent outbreaks in the first year with declining frequency over time. Patients should be counseled that asymptomatic shedding of virus with possible transmission to sexual partners can occur in the absence of outbreaks.
- **Complications** include herpes encephalitis (rare but potentially life threatening) and urinary tract infection (which can cause urinary retention or severe pain).
- **Diagnosis.** Clinical suspicion is based on history and the appearance of lesions. Obtain laboratory confirmation with type-specific virologic and serologic testing. Documentation of HSV-1 or HSV-2 is useful for prognosis and counseling.
  - **Virology.** Isolation of the virus in culture is the gold standard; however, sensitivity is low. Viral culture isolates should be typed to determine HSV-1 or HSV-2. Lack of detection does not prove absent infection.
  - **Serology** can confirm clinical suspicion in the absence of a positive culture; antibodies develop within weeks of infection. Assays that differentiate glycoprotein 1 (HSV-1) from glycoprotein 2 (HSV-2) are recommended.
- **Treatment.** See Table 25-3.
  - Systemic antiviral therapy for HSV may reduce symptoms and complications of infection.
  - Suppressive therapy can reduce recurrence in up to 80% of patients. Daily suppressive therapy with valacyclovir 500 mg a day has been shown to decrease transmission in discordant couples.
  - Recurrences will decrease over time regardless of suppressive therapy, so providers should address continued suppressive therapy yearly.
  - Topical antiviral therapy has not shown any benefit and is not recommended.

TABLE 25-3	Treatment for Genital Herpes	
Stage	**Treatment**	**Duration**
Primary outbreak— outpatient	Acyclovir, 400 mg PO tid	7–10 d
	Acyclovir, 200 mg PO 5×/d	
	Famciclovir, 250 mg PO tid	
	Valacyclovir, 1 g PO bid	
Episodic recurrences (begin treatment with prodrome or within 1 d of lesion outbreak)	Acyclovir, 400 mg PO tid	5 d
	Acyclovir, 800 mg PO tid	2 d
	Acyclovir, 800 mg PO bid	5 d
	Famciclovir, 125 mg PO bid	5 d
	Famciclovir, 1 g PO bid	1 d
	Valacyclovir, 1 g PO qd	5 d
	Valacyclovir, 500 mg PO bid	3 d
Daily suppression therapy	Acyclovir, 400 mg PO bid	As needed
	Famciclovir, 250 mg PO bid	
	Valacyclovir 500 mg PO qd	
	Valacyclovir, 1 g PO qd	

From Centers for Disease Control and Prevention. Sexually transmitted diseases treatment guidelines 2006. *MMWR* 2006;55(No. RR-11), with permission.

- The virus cannot be completely eradicated and remains latent in the cell bodies of sacral nerves S2, S3, and S4.
- An effective HSV vaccine is not yet available.
- **Counseling.** Patients should be advised to remain abstinent from the onset of prodromal symptoms until complete re-epithelialization of lesions. Couples should discuss the role of suppressive therapy in decreasing transmission risk. Counseling should be appropriate to the HSV type.
- **During pregnancy**, women with primary HSV should be treated with antiviral therapy. Perinatal transmission is possible, and therefore, cesarean delivery is recommended for women with active lesions or prodromal symptoms of genital HSV at delivery. Many providers prescribe suppressive therapy for pregnant women with a history of genital herpes beginning at 36 weeks' gestation. Also see Chapter 11.

Syphilis
- The spirochete *T. pallidum* is the etiologic agent of the systemic disease syphilis. The disease is contagious only when mucocutaneous lesions are present. This occurs through contact with a chancre, condyloma lata, or mucosal lesion. The organism can penetrate skin or mucous membranes, incubating over a period of 10 days to 3 months. Syphilis has a complex course characterized by the immunologic response to the spirochete.
- Primary, secondary, and tertiary syphilis stages occur over years to decades, with periods of inactive or latent disease.
  - **Primary syphilis** usually presents as a hard, painless, solitary chancre appearing on the vulva, vagina, or cervix, although extragenital lesions may occur. Lesions

that occur on the cervix or in the vagina often go unrecognized. Nontender inguinal lymphadenopathy is frequently present. The primary chancre resolves spontaneously within 2 to 6 weeks.

- **Secondary syphilis** occurs after hematogenous spread of the spirochete and is characterized by protean manifestations including generalized nonpruritic papulosquamous rash typically on the palms and soles, irregular rash, mucous patches, patchy alopecia, condyloma lata, and generalized lymphadenopathy. Systemic symptoms such as fever, headache, and malaise also occur.
- **Latent syphilis** is defined by seropositivity without evidence of clinical manifestations. Latent syphilis documented as acquired during the previous year is referred to as early latent. All other latent syphilis is either late latent or latent syphilis of unknown duration. The late latent phase (>1 year) is not infectious by sexual transmission, but the spirochete may transplacentally infect the fetus.
- **Tertiary syphilis** develops in up to one third of the untreated or inadequately treated patients and refers to gummas, locally destructive lesions of the bone, skin, or other organs. Cardiovascular involvement in tertiary syphilis includes aortic aneurysm and aortic valvular insufficiency.
- **Neurosyphilis** can occur during any stage of syphilis, and all patients with clinical evidence of CNS involvement should have examination of the cerebrospinal fluid (CSF) performed. It is not synonymous with tertiary syphilis. CSF should be tested for fluorescent treponemal antibody absorption (FTA-ABS) reactivity.
- **Diagnosis.** *T. pallidum* cannot be cultured in vitro. The diagnosis is made definitively by identifying the spirochete through dark-field microscopy or by direct fluorescent antibody tests of lesion exudate or tissue. The majority of syphilis infection is diagnosed presumptively with nonspecific serologic tests, such as the Venereal Disease Research Laboratory (VDRL) or rapid plasma reagin (RPR). A positive VDRL or RPR requires confirmation with specific serologic tests. These are FTA-ABS or microhemagglutination assay for antibody to *T. pallidum*. False-positive nontreponemal tests are associated with pregnancy, autoimmune disorders, chronic active hepatitis, intravenous drug use, febrile illness, and immunization. Serologic tests become positive 4 to 6 weeks after exposure, usually 1 to 2 weeks after the appearance of the primary chancres. The specific FTA-ABS test remains positive indefinitely. The diagnosis of neurosyphilis cannot be made with a single test, but requires a combination of reactive serologic tests, CSF analysis, and reactive VDRL-CSF with or without clinical symptoms.
- **Pregnancy.** All women should be screened for syphilis in early pregnancy, and this is mandated in most states. In high-risk patients or in high prevalence areas, syphilis testing should be repeated twice in the third trimester (i.e., at 28 to 32 weeks' gestation and again at delivery).
- **Treatment** options are listed in Table 25-4. Individuals with an allergy to penicillin may be desensitized and treated with benzathine penicillin.
- **Follow-up.** Definitive criteria for treatment cure or failure have not been established. Clinical follow-up and serologic VDRL or RPR titers should be obtained (preferably at same lab) every 6 months for 1 year or at 3, 6, 9, 12, and 24 months if HIV-positive. If signs or symptoms persist, or there is a fourfold increase in titer, then treatment has failed or the patient has been reinfected. If titers remain stable or do not decrease fourfold (e.g., 1:16 to 1:4) in 6 months, treatment failure may have occurred. These patients should undergo HIV testing, lumbar puncture for CSF evaluation, and retreatment.

TABLE 25-4   Recommended Treatment for Syphilis

Phase	Medication	Dosage	Duration
Primary and secondary syphilis and early latent syphilis (<1 yr)	Benzathine penicillin G	2.4 million U IM	1 dose
Penicillin allergy (nonpregnant)	Doxycycline *or* tetracycline	100 mg PO qid 500 mg PO bid	2 wk 2 wk
Late latent syphilis (>1 yr) and secondary syphilis without neurosyphilis	Benzathine penicillin G	2.4 million U IM (7.2 million U total)	q wk × 3 wk
Penicillin allergy (nonpregnant)	Doxycycline *or* tetracycline	100 mg PO qid 500 mg PO bid	4 wk 4 wk
Neurosyphilis	Aqueous crystalline penicillin G	3–4 million U IV q4h (18–24 million U per day)	10–14 d
Alternate regimen (if compliance assured)	Procaine penicillin PLUS Probenecid	2.4 million U IM qd 500 mg PO qid	10–14 d 10–14 d
Syphilis during pregnancy	Penicillin Desensitize if allergic	Parenteral regimen appropriate for the stage of syphilis	—
Primary or secondary syphilis in HIV positive patients	Benzathine penicillin G Desensitize if allergic	2.4 million U IM	1 dose
Latent syphilis in HIV positive patients	Benzathine penicillin G Desensitize if allergic	2.4 million U IM (7.2 million U total)	q wk 3 wk

From Centers for Disease Control and Prevention. Sexually transmitted diseases treatment guidelines 2006. *MMWR* 2006;55(No. RR-11), with permission.

Other Ulcerative Lesions
- **Granuloma inguinale, lymphogranuloma venereum**, and **chancroid** are other infections that cause genital ulcers. They are rare in the United States, but should be considered in any patient with ulcers that are not diagnosed as syphilis or HSV.

Vaginitis
- **Vaginitis** is characterized by pruritus, discharge, odor, dyspareunia, and dysuria. The vagina is normally colonized by several organisms, including *Lactobacillus acidophilus*, diphtheroids, *Candida*, and other flora. Its physiologic pH is approximately 4.0, with peroxide-producing *L. acidophilus* inhibiting overgrowth of pathogenic bacteria. Vaginal fluid is typically white, odorless, and seen in dependent areas of the vagina.
- **Diagnosis** of vaginitis usually requires microscopic examination of the vaginal discharge. The three major types of vaginitis and their distinguishing characteristics are described in Table 25-5.

Bacterial Vaginosis
- **Bacterial vaginosis (BV)** is the most common cause of vaginitis. No single infectious agent is responsible, rather there is a shift in the composition of vaginal flora, with up to tenfold increase in anaerobic bacteria such as *Prevotella*, *Gardnerella vaginalis*, and *Mobiluncus* species, and a decrease in the concentration of *Lactobacillius* species. BV is not sexually transmitted. It has been implicated as a risk factor for preterm premature rupture of membranes and preterm delivery. BV has been associated with endometritis, salpingitis, and vaginal cuff cellulitis after invasive procedures including endometrial biopsy, hysterectomy, therapeutic abortion, intrauterine device (IUD) insertion, cesarean section, and uterine curettage.
- **Diagnosis.** BV is diagnosed by the presence of at least three of the Amsel criteria: (a) homogenous thin white discharge coating the vaginal walls, (b) vaginal pH >4.5, (c) clue cells on microscopic examination, and (d) fishy odor before or after the addition of 10% potassium hydroxide (KOH) to the sample (whiff test). Commercially available point-of-care card tests to detect elevated pH and trimethylamine are now available and may be useful when a microscope is not available.

TABLE 25-5	Distinguishing Characteristics of Vaginitis		
	Bacterial Vaginosis	***Trichomonas* Vaginitis**	**Candidal Vaginitis**
Vaginal pH	≥4.5	5.0–7.0	—
Type of discharge	Thin, white, adherent; amine (fishy) odor with potassium hydroxide (KOH)	Thin, frothy, white, gray, yellow; copious	Thick, white, curdlike
Wet smear	Clue cells, no WBCs	Trichomonads, WBCs	Hyphae and buds, WBCs

WBCs, white blood cells. From Amsel R, Totten PA, Spiegel CA, et al. Nonspecific vaginitis. Diagnostic criteria and microbial and epidemiologic associations. *Am J Med* 1983;74(1):14–22.

TABLE 25-6	Treatment for Bacterial Vaginosis		
Medication	**Dosage**	**Duration**	**Use in Pregnancy**
Metronidazole (Flagyl)	500 mg PO bid	7 d	Recommended
Clindamycin phosphate cream 2%	1 full applicator (5 g) intravaginally qhs	7 d	Not recommended
Metronidazole (MetroGel) gel 0.75%	1 full applicator (5 g) intravaginally qhs	5 d	Not recommended
Alternative regimens[a]			
Clindamycin ovules	100 g intravaginally qhs	3 d	Not recommended
Clindamycin hydrochloride	300 mg PO bid	7 d	Second and third trimesters (preferred)

[a]Extended-release metronidazole (750 mg) and single-dose clindamycin intravaginal cream are also available. Metronidazole 250 mg PO tid for 7 days is also recommended in pregnancy. From Centers for Disease Control and Prevention. Sexually transmitted diseases treatment guidelines 2006. *MMWR* 2006;55(No. RR-11), with permission.

- **Treatment.** Treatment regimens are shown in Table 25-6. The data is insufficient to support the prophylactic treatment of BV before other invasive treatments.
- **Follow-up.** Recurrence of BV is not unusual. A different regimen should be used to treat recurrences. Follow-up in 1 month for asymptomatic pregnant women at high risk for preterm delivery should be considered.

Trichomoniasis
- **Trichomoniasis** is a sexually transmitted infection by the unicellular protozoan *Trichomonas vaginalis*. *Trichomonas* can survive on wet towels and other surfaces and thus can be nonsexually transmitted. Its incubation period ranges from 4 to 28 days.
- **Diagnosis.** Vaginal exam may reveal a frothy, malodorous yellow-green discharge with vulvar irritation. The cervix may appear erythematous and friable. Some women have minimal or no symptoms. A wet smear preparation that is promptly reviewed may reveal the flagellated, mobile protozoon with a sensitivity of approximately 70%. Point-of-care tests are available and have higher sensitivity than vaginal examination, but false-positives can occur. Culture should be obtained in women who have clinical suspicion for trichomonas when microscopic evaluation is negative.
- **Treatment** consists of one 2-g dose of either metronidazole or tinidazole by mouth. Alternatively, metronidazole 500 mg PO bid for 7 days can be used. Metronidazole gel has an efficacy of <50% and is not recommended. The patient's sexual partners should be treated as well. While trichomoniasis has been associated with premature rupture of membranes and premature birth, treatment of the infection has not been found to reduce these risks and may in fact increase the risk of premature birth.
- **Follow-up** is unnecessary for women who become asymptomatic after treatment. Most organisms are susceptible to metronidazole but low-level resistance has been documented for 2% to 5% of vaginal trichomonas. If treatment failure occurs, 2 g of either tinidazole or metronidazole once a day for 5 days is recommended. Sexual partners must be treated and the patients should be instructed to avoid intercourse until the treatment is completed and symptoms have resolved.

Candida Vaginitis

- Candida vaginitis is not a sexually transmitted infection. *Candida* spp. are a normal vaginal inhabitant in up to 25% of women. *Candida albicans* accounts for 80% to 92% of the cases of vulvovaginal candidiasis (VVC). Lifetime incidence of VVC is 75%, with 40% to 45% of women having repeated infections, and the majority of women with uncomplicated VVC have no identifiable precipitating factors. Complicated or recurrent VVC occurs in 5% of women. These are often non-albicans species and are most often found in immunocompromised women, uncontrolled diabetics, or pregnant women.
- **Diagnosis.** The signs and symptoms include pruritus, vulvar fissures, or excoriations, vaginal irritation, external dysuria, erythema, and edema. The diagnosis of uncomplicated VVC is often made clinically on the basis of history and physical exam and can usually be confirmed by the presence of hyphae and spores on saline or 10% KOH wet preparation. Culture should be performed in women not responding to treatment, in cases where a non-albicans species is suspected, or with recurrent VVC to establish species and sensitivity.
- **Treatment.** Symptomatic patients, including pregnant women, should be treated. See Table 25-7. Only topical therapies are recommended in pregnancy. For severe VVC, extended treatment with topical azoles up to 14 days or fluconazole 150 mg in two doses 72 hr apart is recommended. Maintenance therapy with 150 mg of fluconazole or clotrimazole 200 mg twice a week or 500 mg once a week is recommended. Maintenance therapy is effective in reducing recurrence in up to 50% of women.
- **Follow-up.** If symptoms persist or recur, patients should return for follow-up.
- **Treatment of male partners** is not indicated unless the partner has symptoms of yeast balanitis or in cases of recurrent VVC.

TABLE 25-7	Treatment for Uncomplicated Yeast Infections

Intravaginal agents
Butoconazole 2% cream 5 g intravaginally for 3 d[a]
Butoconazole 2% cream 5 g (sustained release), single application
Clotrimazole 1% cream 5 g intravaginally for 7–14 d[a]
Clotrimazole 100 mg vaginal tablet for 7 d
Clotrimazole 100 mg vaginal tablet, two tablets for 3 d
Clotrimazole 500 mg vaginal tablet, one tablet in a single application
Miconazole 2% cream 5 g intravaginally for 7 d[a]
Miconazole 100 mg vaginal suppository, one suppository for 7 d[a]
Miconazole 200 mg vaginal suppository, one suppository for 3 d[a]
Miconazole 1200 mg vaginal suppository, 1 suppository for 1 d
Nystatin 100,000-unit vaginal tablet, one tablet for 14 d
Tioconazole 6.5% ointment 5 g intravaginally in a single application[a]
Terconazole 0.4% cream 5 g intravaginally for 7 d
Terconazole 0.8% cream 5 g intravaginally for 3 d
Terconazole 80 mg vaginal suppository, one suppository for 3 d

Oral agent
Fluconazole 150 mg oral tablet, one tablet in single dose

[a]Over-the-counter (OTC) preparations. From Centers for Disease Control and Prevention. Sexually transmitted diseases treatment guidelines 2006. *MMWR* 2006;55(No. RR-11), with permission.

Cervicitis

- **Cervicitis** is characterized by two major diagnostic signs: a purulent cervical exudate and sustained cervical bleeding in response to manipulation by an examining swab. The primary pathogens of mucopurulent cervicitis are the two sexually transmitted organisms *Chlamydia trachomatis* and *Neisseria gonorrhoeae*. In the majority of cases, no etiologic agent is identified; limited data has implicated BV, *Mycoplasma genitalium*, and frequent douching as other causes of cervicitis.

Chlamydia

- **Chlamydia trachomatis** is the most frequently reported sexually transmitted bacterial disease in the United States. Risk factors include age <25, low socioeconomic status, multiple sex partners, and unmarried status.
- **Microbiology.** *C. trachomatis* is an obligate intracellular organism that preferentially infects the squamocolumnar cells in the transition zone of the cervix.
- **Signs and symptoms.** Chlamydia cervicitis is asymptomatic in about 75% of cases. Patients with Chlamydia may complain of abnormal vaginal discharge, burning with urination, spotting, or postcoital bleeding. A yellow mucopurulent discharge may be present.
- **Diagnosis.** Nucleic acid amplification testing (NAAT) using polymerase chain reaction is the preferred method of diagnosis for chlamydia and gonorrhea cervicitis and can be performed on either cervical or urine samples. Screening is important as up to 75% of patients are asymptomatic. Cell culture for chlamydia infection has a high false negative rate, and is not widely available. Women with cervicitis should be evaluated for trichomonas and BV (Table 25-8).
- **Treatment.** Presumptive therapy can be initiated based upon clinical findings and STD risk assessment (see Table 25-9). Treatment for coinfection with gonorrhea is recommended if local prevalence is >5%. Concomitant treatment for BV or trichomonas should be given if detected. Sexual partners should be referred to a clinic for treatment.
  - A test of cure is necessary only in pregnant patients or if symptoms persist.

TABLE 25-8   Testing for Gonorrhea and Chlamydia Infection

	N. gonorrhoeae		C. trachomatis	
	Sensitivity	Specificity	Sensitivity	Specificity
Endocervical culture	70–85	100	60–70	100
Immunoassay	>80	97–100	Not reliable	
Nucleic acid probe	77–97	96–100	92	99.7
PCR/LCR	95	100	96.7	99.7

Values are in percentages. PCR, polymerase chain reaction; LCR, ligase chain reaction. Adapted from Black CM. Current methods of laboratory diagnosis of *Chlamydia trachomatis* infections. *Clin Microbiol Rev* 1997;10(1):160–184; Van Dyck E, Ieven M, Patten S, et al. Detection of *Chlamydia trachomatis* and *Neisseria gonorrhoeae* by enzyme immunoassay, culture, and three nucleic acid amplification tests. *J Clin Microbiol* 2001;39(5):1751–1756; and Koumans EH, Johnson RE, Knapp JS, St. Louis ME. Laboratory testing for *Neisseria gonorrhoeae* by recently introduced non-culture tests: a performance review with clinical and public health considerations. *Clin Infect Dis* 1998;27:1171–1180.

TABLE 25-9	Treatment for *Chlamydia Trachomatis*		
Medication	Dosage	Duration	Use in Pregnancy
Recommended			
Azithromycin	1 g PO	1 dose	Recommended
Doxycycline	100 mg PO bid	7 d	Contraindicated
Amoxicillin (in pregnant women)	500 mg PO tid	7 d	Acceptable
Alternative			
Erythromycin base	500 mg PO qid	7 d	Recommended
Erythromycin ethylsuccinate	800 mg PO qid	7 d	Alternative
Ofloxacin	300 mg PO bid	7 d	Contraindicated
Levofloxacin	500 mg PO qd	7 d	Contraindicated

From Centers for Disease Control and Prevention. Sexually transmitted diseases treatment guide-lines 2006. *MMWR* 2006;55(No. RR-11), with permission.

Gonorrhea
- Risk factors for **gonorrhea** are essentially the same as those for *Chlamydia* cervicitis.
- **Microbiology.** *N. gonorrhoeae* is a Gram-negative diplococcus that infects columnar or pseudostratified epithelium. Genital, pharyngeal, and disseminated infections may occur. The incubation period is 3 to 5 days.
- **Signs and symptoms.** Similar to chlamydial infections, 50% of patients with *gonococcal cervicitis* are asymptomatic. When present, symptoms include vaginal discharge, dysuria, or abnormal uterine bleeding. The most commonly infected site is the endocervix.
- **Diagnosis.** Culture and NAAT are available for the diagnosis of *N. gonorrhea*. NAAT is recommended for the diagnosis of cervical gonorrhea. Culture is the most widely available option for detection in the nongenital sites and is used when antibiotic sensitivity testing is indicated (see Table 25-8).
- **Treatment** options are listed in Table 25-10. Due to increasing resistance, fluoroquinolones are no longer recommended for the treatment of *N. gonorrhea*. Because coinfection with *Chlamydia* is common, treatment of both is recommended unless the NAAT is negative. Sexual partners should be referred for treatment. Although azithromycin 2 g PO is effective against uncomplicated gonorrhea, it is not recommended secondary to expense and GI upset.

INFECTIONS OF THE UPPER GENITAL TRACT

Pelvic Inflammatory Disease (PID)
- **PID** is an infection of any combination of the endometrium, fallopian tubes, ovaries, myometrium, parametrium, and pelvic peritoneum.
- **Pathophysiology and microbiology.** PID is caused by the spread of infection via the cervix. Although PID is often associated with sexually transmitted infections of the lower tract, the process is polymicrobial. *N. gonorrhoeae* and *C. trachomatis* are implicated in many cases, but numerous exogenous and endogenous microorganisms

TABLE 25-10 Treatment for *Neisseria Gonorrhoeae*

Uncomplicated gonococcal infections of the cervix, urethra, and rectum[a]
Recommended regimens
Ceftriaxone 125 mg intramuscular (IM) in a single dose
OR

Cefixime 400 mg orally once or 400 mg by suspension (200 mg/5 mL)
PLUS
Treatment for chlamydia unless ruled out

Alternative regimens
Single-dose cephalosporin treatments include ceftizoxime 500 mg IM; or cefoxitin 2 g IM with probenicid 1 g orally; or cefotaxime 500 mg IM.

Uncomplicated gonococcal infections of the pharynx[a]
Recommended regimens
Ceftriaxone 125 mg IM in a single dose
PLUS
Treatment for chlamydia unless ruled out

Disseminated gonococcal infection (DGI)
Recommended regimen
Ceftriaxone 1 g IM or IV every 24 hr until 24–48 hr after clinical improvement then switch to oral medicines to complete 1 wk of therapy.

Alternative regimens
Cefotaxime 1 g IV every 8 hr
OR

Ceftizoxime 1 g IV every 8 hr

Oral followup regimen
Cefixime 400 mg orally twice daily
OR

Cefixime 400 mg suspension (200 mg/5 mL) twice daily
OR

Cefpodoxime 400 mg orally twice daily

A cephalosporin-based intravenous regimen is recommended for the initial treatment of DGI. This is particularly important when gonorrhea is detected at mucosal sites by nonculture tests. Fluoroquinolones may be an alternative treatment option if antimicrobial susceptibility can be documented by culture.

[a]These regimens are recommended for all adult and adolescent patients, regardless of travel history or sexual behavior. From Centers for Disease Control and Prevention. Sexually transmitted diseases treatment guidelines 2006. *MMWR* 2006;55(No. RR-11); from Updated recommended treatment regimens for gonococcal infections and associated conditions – United States, April 2007 at http://www.cdc.gov/std/treatment/2006/updated-regimens.htm, with permission.

may be involved, including anaerobes, *G. vaginalis, Haemophilus influenza,* Gram-negative rods, *Streptococcus agalactia,* and enteric species. Other organisms include *Mycoplasma* spp. and *Ureaplasma* spp. Diagnosis of PID should include testing for *N. gonorrhea* and *C. trachomatis* and screening for HIV.

- **Prevention.** There are no signs and symptoms pathognomic for PID, and the clinical picture does not accurately predict the extent of tubal involvement. A high degree of suspicion for PID and treatment based on minimal or subtle signs may help reduce the incidence of long-term sequelae. One in four women with PID will experience tubal infertility, an ectopic pregnancy, or chronic pelvic pain. Treatment of sexual partners and education is important in reducing the rate of recurrent infections.
- **Risk factors** include a previous history of PID, multiple sex partners, adolescence, BV, and current infection by a sexually transmitted organism.
- **Signs and symptoms.** The most common presenting symptom is abdominopelvic pain. Other complaints are variable, including vaginal discharge, dyspareunia, abnormal bleeding, right upper quadrant pain, fever and chills, nausea, and dysuria.
- **Diagnosis** of PID is difficult because the presenting signs and symptoms vary widely. Because of the sequelae of PID, especially infertility, ectopic pregnancy, and chronic pelvic pain, health care providers should maintain a low threshold for the diagnosis of PID based on minimal criteria.
  - **Minimal criteria.** Empiric treatment should be initiated in sexually active young women and other women at risk for STDs if they are experiencing pelvic or lower abdominal pain, if no other cause can be identified, and if one or more of the following are present on pelvic examination:
    ○ Cervical motion tenderness
    ○ Uterine tenderness
    ○ Adnexal tenderness
  - **Additional criteria for diagnosis, which increase specificity**
    ○ Oral temperature >101 °F (>38.3 °C)
    ○ Abnormal cervical or vaginal mucopurulent discharge
    ○ Presence of white blood cells in the vaginal secretions, on saline microscopy
    ○ Elevated erythrocyte sedimentation rate
    ○ Elevated C-reactive protein
    ○ Laboratory documentation of cervical infection with *N. gonorrhoeae* or *C. trachomatis*
  - **Criteria that are specific for PID**
    ○ Endometrial biopsy with histopathologic evidence of endometritis
    ○ Transvaginal sonography or magnetic resonance imaging techniques showing thickened, fluid-filled tubes with or without free pelvic fluid or tubo-ovarian complex
    ○ Laparoscopic abnormalities consistent with PID
- **Treatment** for PID should have as its goals the prevention of tubal damage that leads to infertility and ectopic pregnancy and prevention of chronic infection. Many patients can be successfully treated as outpatients, and early ambulatory treatment should be the initial therapeutic approach. Antibiotic choice should target the major etiologic organisms (*N. gonorrhoeae* and *C. trachomatis*) but should also address the polymicrobial nature of the disease (Table 25-11).
- **Criteria for hospitalization**
  - Surgical emergencies (e.g., appendicitis) cannot be excluded
  - The patient is pregnant
  - The patient does not respond clinically to oral antimicrobial therapy

- The patient is unable to follow or tolerate an outpatient oral regimen
- The patient has severe illness, nausea and vomiting, or high fever
- The patient has a tuboovarian abscess
- **Sequelae.** Approximately 25% of PID patients experience long-term sequelae. Infertility due to tubal occlusion affects anywhere from 6% to 60% of women following an episode of PID, depending on severity, whereas the risk of ectopic pregnancy is approximately six to ten times the normal. Chronic pelvic pain and dyspareunia have also been reported and are associated with the presence of adhesive disease and the number of episodes. Fitz-Hugh-Curtis syndrome is the development of fibrous perihepatic adhesions resulting from the inflammatory process of PID that may result in acute right upper quadrant pain and tenderness.

Endometritis (Nonpuerperal)

- **Pathophysiology.** Endometritis is caused by the ascension of pathogens from the cervix to the endometrium. Pathogens include *C. trachomatis, N. gonorrhoeae, Ureaplasma urealyticum,* and *M. genitalium.* Chronic endometritis is often linked to common bacteria such as *streptococci, staphylococci,* and *Escherichia coli.* Organisms that produce BV may also produce histologic endometritis, even in women without symptoms. Endometritis is also an important component of PID and may be an intermediate stage in the spread of infection to the fallopian tubes.
- **Signs and symptoms**
  - **Chronic endometritis.** Many women are asymptomatic. The classic symptom of chronic endometritis is intermenstrual vaginal bleeding. Postcoital bleeding, menorrhagia, and a dull, constant lower abdominal pain are other complaints.
  - **Acute endometritis.** Uterine tenderness is common.

TABLE 25-11   **Treatment for Pelvic Inflammatory Disease (PID)**

Parenteral treatment for severe PID
Transition to oral therapy, which usually can be initiated within 24 hr of clinical improvement, should be guided by clinical experience.

Recommended parenteral regimen A
Cefotetan 2 g IV every 12 hr
   OR
Cefoxitin 2 g IV every 6 hr
   PLUS
Doxycycline 100 mg orally or IV every 12 hr

Recommended parenteral regimen B
Clindamycin 900 mg IV every 8 hr
   PLUS
Gentamicin loading dose IV or IM (2 mg/kg body weight) followed by maintenance dose (1.5 mg/kg) every 8 hr. Single daily dosing may be substituted.

   Alternative parenteral regimen
   Ampicillin/sulbactam 3 g IV every 6 hr
     PLUS
   Doxycycline 100 mg orally or IV every 12 hr

(Continued)

TABLE 25-11	Treatment for Pelvic Inflammatory Disease (PID) *(Continued)*

Oral treatment for mild to moderate PID
Parenteral and oral therapies have similar efficacy in treatment of women with mild to moderate PID. Women who do not respond to oral therapy within 72 hr should be reevaluated to confirm the diagnosis and should be administered parenteral therapy on either an outpatient or in-patient basis.

Recommended oral regimen
Ceftriaxone 250 mg IM in a single dose
   PLUS
Doxycycline 100 mg orally twice a day for 14 d
   WITH OR WITHOUT
Metronidazole 500 mg orally twice a day for 14 d
   OR
Cefoxitin, 2 g IM in a single dose, and
Probenecid, 1 g orally administered concurrently in a single dose
   PLUS
Doxycycline 100 mg orally twice a day for 14 d
   WITH OR WITHOUT
Metronidazole 500 mg orally twice a day for 14 d
   OR
Other parenteral **third-generation cephalosporin** (e.g., **ceftizoxime** or **cefotaxime**)
   PLUS
Doxycycline 100 mg orally twice a day for 14 d
   WITH OR WITHOUT
Metronidazole 500 mg orally twice a day for 14 d

For full details and alternative oral treatment regimens, see updated Centers for Disease Control guidelines. Adapted from Centers for Disease Control and Prevention. Sexually transmitted diseases treatment guidelines 2006. MMWR 2006;55(No. RR-11); Updated recommended treatment regimens for gonococcal infections and associated conditions – United States, April 2007 at http://www.cdc.gov/std/treatment/2006/updated-regimens.htm, with permission.

- **Diagnosis.** The diagnosis of chronic endometritis is established by endometrial biopsy and culture. The classic histologic findings of chronic endometritis are an inflammatory reaction of monocytes and plasma cells in the endometrial stroma (five plasma cells per high-power field). A diffuse pattern of inflammatory infiltrates of lymphocytes and plasma cells throughout the endometrial stroma or even stromal necrosis is associated with severe cases of endometritis.
- **Treatment.** The treatment of choice for chronic endometritis is doxycycline, 100 mg PO bid for 10 days. Broader coverage of anaerobic organisms may also be considered, especially in the presence of BV. When endometritis is associated with acute PID, the treatment should focus on the major etiologic organisms, including *N. gonorrhoeae* and *C. trachomatis*, and should also include broader polymicrobial coverage.
- See Chapter 20 for puerperal **endomyometritis**.

SUGGESTED READINGS

Biggs WS, Williams RM. Common Gynecologic Infections. *Prim Care Clin Office Pract* 2009;36:33–51.

Gynecologic herpes simplex virus infections. ACOG Practice Bulletin Number 57, reaffirmed 2006. American College of Obstetricians and Gynecologists. *Obstet Gynecol* 2004;104:1111–1117.

Mers D, Wolff T, Gregory K, et al. for the US Preventive Services Task Force. USPSTF Recommendations for STI Screening. *Am Fam Physician* 2008;77(6):819–824.

Soper DE. Pelvic inflammatory disease. *Obstet Gynecol* 2010;116:419-428.

Vaginitis. ACOG Practice Bulletin Number 72, reaffirmed 2008. American College of Obstetricians and Gynecologists. *Obstet Gynecol* 2006;107:1195–1206.

van der Wouden JC, van der Sande R, van Suijlekom-Smit LWA, et al. Interventions for cutaneous molluscum contagiosum. *Cochrane Database of Systematic Reviews* 2009;4: CD004767.

Wiley D, Masongsong E. Human papillomavirus: The burden of infection. *Obstet Gynecol Surv* 2006;61(6):S3–S14.

26 Ectopic Pregnancy

Jacqueline Baselice and Melissa Yates

An **ectopic pregnancy (EP)** is one that implants outside of the uterine cavity.

EPIDEMIOLOGY OF EP

- Two percent of all pregnancies are ectopic.
- EP is the leading cause of death in the first trimester.
- EP is responsible for 6% of all pregnancy-related deaths.
- At least one third of pregnancies that occur after failure of tubal sterilization procedures are EPs.
- In assisted reproductive technology (ART), the incidence of EP is approximately 3% to 5%. These pregnancies tend to be recognized at an earlier stage due to the close monitoring in these patients.
- Ninety-seven percent of ectopic pregnancies are implanted within the fallopian tube, although implantation can occur within the abdomen, cervix, ovary, or uterine cornua. The most common etiology for ectopic pregnancy is tubal pathology.
- **Risk factors for EP** include previous EP (even if previous EP was treated by salpingectomy), pelvic inflammatory disease, previous tubal surgery, infertility, current or previous use of an intrauterine device (IUD), two or more pregnancy termination procedures, diethylstilbestrol exposure, age >40, smoking, greater than three previous spontaneous abortions, and assisted reproduction.
- **Risk factors for recurrent EP** include previous spontaneous miscarriage, with likelihood increasing with each miscarriage, and a history of pelvic surgery. No significant increase exists with a history of pelvic infections when these patients are compared to those with a primary presentation of EP.
- Forty percent of EPs have an unknown etiology.

DIAGNOSIS OF EP

Presentation

- **Classic triad** (present in <50% of patients) is history of amenorrhea followed by abnormal vaginal bleeding, abdominal or pelvic pain, and a tender adnexal mass.
- **Pain** (95% of patients with rupturing EPs). Usually located in the lower quadrants but can be anywhere within the abdomen. Cervical motion tenderness (CMT) is present in 75% of patients with ruptured EP.
- **Vaginal spotting** (60% to 80% of patients). Scant, dark brown bleeding, either intermittent or continuous.
- EP may present as a surgical emergency, and therefore, timely diagnosis is essential (Fig. 26-1).

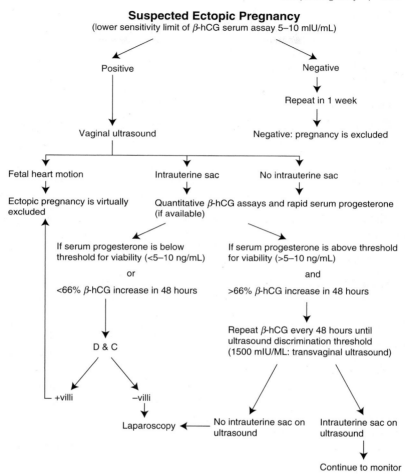

Figure 26-1. Evaluation of the stable patient with suspected EP. Hormonal parameters can vary depending on the assay technique and reference standard used. The discriminatory threshold for sonographic detection of an intrauterine gestational sac must be established by each institution. (Reused with permission from Damario MA, Rock JA. Ectopic pregnancy. In Rock JA, Jones HW III, eds. *TeLinde's Operative Gynecology*, 9th Ed. Philadelphia, PA: Lippincott Williams & Wilkins, 2003:516.)

Differential Diagnosis

- The differential diagnosis includes conditions unrelated to pregnancy, in addition to pregnancy-related problems. See Chapter 27.

- **Salpingitis** presents with similar symptoms and examination findings but negative pregnancy test results, an elevated WBC, and temperature elevation.
- **Threatened abortion.** In this condition, bleeding is usually heavier, pain is localized to the lower mid abdomen, and CMT is generally absent.
- **Appendicitis.** Amenorrhea or abnormal vaginal bleeding is usually absent. Persistent right lower quadrant pain, with fever and GI symptoms, suggests appendicitis. CMT, if present, is usually less severe than with EP. Pregnancy test results are negative.
- **Ovarian torsion.** Pain is initially intermittent and later becomes constant as vascular supply is compromised. Findings may include an elevated WBC and a palpable adnexal mass, but pregnancy test results are negative.
- **Other conditions.** Normal intrauterine pregnancy, heterotopic pregnancy (especially in the case of ART), ruptured ovarian cyst, bleeding corpus luteum, endometriosis, diverticulitis, and dysfunctional uterine bleeding. Gastroenteritis, urinary tract infection, or renal calculus early in pregnancy may also mimic an EP.

Physical Examination

- **Ruptured unstable EP.** If unstable, may have signs of hypovolemic shock, including tachycardia, hypotension, and confusion. Abdominal exam may have signs consistent with peritonitis, including guarding, rigidity, or rebound tenderness. Up to 15% of women may complain of shoulder pain, secondary to diaphragmatic irritation from hemoperitoneum. This is a surgical emergency.
- **Stable EP.** Tenderness in patients with EP may be generalized (45%), located bilaterally in the lower quadrants (25%), or located unilaterally in a lower quadrant (30%). Rebound tenderness may or may not be present. CMT, resulting from peritoneal irritation, is usually present but is not specific for EP. A palpable adnexal mass or mass in the cul-de-sac is reported in approximately 40% of cases; absence of a palpable mass does not rule out EP.

Laboratory Evaluation

- If EP is diagnosed before rupture, a laboratory diagnosis may be made and conservative treatment offered.

Quantitative Gonadotropin Levels

- **Quantitative beta human chorionic gonadotropin (β-hCG).** The titer climbs in a linear fashion from 2 to 4 weeks after ovulation in normal pregnancy, doubling every 48 to 72 hr until it reaches 10,000 mIU/mL.
  - β-hCG that increases <50% in 48 hr is almost always associated with an abnormal pregnancy.
  - Levels of β-hCG are more likely to plateau (<15% change) with an EP than with a spontaneous abortion.
  - A β-hCG level of <1,500 mIU/mL accompanied by pain and vaginal bleeding increases the likelihood of an EP by 2.5 times.
  - Patients with a single β-hCG of 2,000 mIU/mL and no identifiable gestational sac on transvaginal ultrasound (TVUS) should have a repeat β-hCG in 12 to 24 hr. A rapidly falling β-hCG can indicate a completed spontaneous abortion.
  - Seventeen percent of patients with EP will have normal β-hCG doubling times (>66% rise in 48 hr).

Hemoglobin and Hematocrit

- Baseline blood counts should be obtained. Serial measurements are useful if the diagnosis of ruptured EP is uncertain. An acute drop in **hemoglobin or hematocrit** over the first few hours of observation is more revealing than the initial reading. After acute hemorrhage, initial readings may be at first unchanged or only slightly decreased; a subsequent decline represents restoration of depleted blood volume by hemodilution.

Metabolic Panel
- Baseline creatinine and liver transaminases should be obtained in preparation for methotrexate (MTX) treatment for EP. Any signs of renal, hepatic, or hematologic dysfunction are a contraindication to MTX treatment.

Progesterone
- A normal intrauterine pregnancy should be associated with a serum progesterone value of 25 ng/mL or greater. A value of <5 ng/mL indicates a nonviable pregnancy.
- Of limited utility, as many patients will have serum progesterone levels between 10 and 20 ng/mL. A progesterone level may be used to predict viability of a pregnancy of unknown location but is insufficient for EP diagnosis.

Diagnosis by Imaging: Transvaginal Ultrasound
- **Most common sites of EP.** Ampullary (70%), isthmic (12%), fimbrial (11.1%), ovarian (3.2%), interstitial and cornual (2.4%), abdominal (1.3%), and cervical (0.15%).
- **The discriminatory zone** (β-hCG 1,500 to 2,000). Depending on the institution, TVUS should detect evidence of an intrauterine pregnancy (IUP) when the β-hCG level is >1,500 to 2,000 mIU/mL.
  - When the β-hCG level is below 2,000, ultrasound diagnosis of EP should be based upon visualization of an adnexal mass rather than absence of intrauterine gestational sac.
- Combined intrauterine and extrauterine pregnancy (i.e., heterotopic pregnancy) is rare, except among women conceiving through IVF. Serial hCG concentrations are not interpretable in the presence of both a viable intrauterine pregnancy and EP. On ultrasound examination, the diagnosis is suggested by visualization of both an ectopic and an intrauterine pregnancy or the presence of echogenic fluid in the cul-de-sac in the presence of an intrauterine pregnancy. Surgery (e.g., salpingostomy or salpingectomy) is the standard treatment of heterotopic pregnancy with a tubal component since the intrauterine pregnancy is a contraindication to medical therapy.
- **Radiologic signs of EP** include an empty uterus, cystic or solid adnexal masses, dilated and thick-walled fallopian tubes, free echogenic fluid in pelvis, hematosalpinx, and extrauterine gestational sac that contains a yolk sac, with or without an embryo.
- **Doppler technology** can be used to demonstrate increased blood flow to the adnexa that contains an EP. In one study, patients with EP had a 20% increase in blood flow to the affected adnexa versus only 3% flow discrepancy in patients without an EP. Caution is advised with interpreting this method because a normal corpus luteum may also demonstrate increased blood flow. In most cases, two separate structures will be visualized: the ovary and the affected fallopian tube.
- **Pseudosac.** Ten percent of ectopic pregnancies have a pseudosac in the uterus that lacks the "double decidual" sign of an intrauterine pregnancy. A pseudosac tends to be oval in shape with irregular margins versus the smooth margins of an IUP. It also tends to appear centrally in the intrauterine cavity.
- An EP >2 cm in size can be visualized with TVUS.
- Adnexal cardiac activity may be seen if the β-hCG titer is >15,000 mIU/mL.

Diagnosis by Pathology: Dilation and Curettage (D&C)

- When β-hCG concentration is above 1,500 to 2,000 mIU/mL and TVUS fails to confirm an IUP, D&C should be considered to distinguish between an abnormal IUP and an EP.
- In a recent study of patients with a β-hCG level above 2,000 mIU/mL and no visible IUP on ultrasound, 45.7% had an EP as compared with 54.3% who had a spontaneous abortion. Of the patients with a β-hCG level below 2,000 mIU/mL with similar findings, 68.8% had an EP, whereas 31.2% had a spontaneous abortion.
- Women with abnormally rising or plateauing β-hCG <2,000 should undergo curettage before initiation of MTX to ensure that a patient with a spontaneous abortion is not treated unnecessarily.
- Absence of chorionic villi in a curettage specimen suggests the presence of EP; however, the sensitivity is only 70% as it may represent a completed spontaneous abortion. β-hCG values should continue to be followed.
- If the β-hCG level is rising or has reached a plateau after D&C, MTX treatment should be initiated.

TREATMENT FOR EP

Initial management is based on the patient's stability. Patients in shock or with a surgical abdomen should be resuscitated with intravenous fluids, using two large-bore intravenous cannulas, have an indwelling catheter placed to monitor urine output, and be taken to the operating room as soon as possible (see Chapter 3). Blood should be obtained for a type and cross match, CBC, prothrombin time, partial thromboplastin time, and complete metabolic panel (especially if MTX treatment is being considered). For the stable patient with an EP, various medical or surgical therapeutic options may be considered.

Medical Management: Methotrexate

- **Mechanism of action.** As a folic acid antagonist, MTX inactivates dihydrofolate reductase, causing depletion of tetrahydrofolate, which is necessary for DNA and RNA synthesis. The result is inhibition of growth of the rapidly dividing trophoblast cells of an EP
- **Criteria for MTX therapy** are listed in Table 26-1.
- **Absolute and relative contraindications to MTX therapy** are listed in Table 26-2.
- **Prior to administration of MTX**
  - Determine patient's blood type and give Rhogam, if necessary.
  - Obtain a CBC and metabolic panel including liver and renal function studies.
- **Drug side effects** of MTX include nausea, vomiting, stomatitis, diarrhea, gastric distress, dizziness, elevated liver transaminases, pneumonitis, neutropenia (rare), and reversible alopecia (rare).
  - In one meta-analysis, 36.2% of patients experienced side effects that correlated with effectiveness of treatment in both single dose and multidose protocols.
  - The most common side effects are elevated transaminases, mild stomatitis, and GI upset.
- **Treatment side effects**
  - Perhaps the most significant side effect is abdominal pain that arises 2 to 3 days after treatment, presumably from the cytotoxic effect of the drug causing tubal

TABLE 26-1   Criteria for Methotrexate Therapy

Stovall and Ling, 1993[a]
Hemodynamic stability
Increase in β-hCG titers after curettage
Transvaginal sonogram showing an unruptured EP of <3.5 cm in greatest
    diameter
Desire for future fertility

American College of Obstetricians and Gynecologists, 1990[b]
Gestational sac size of ≤3 cm
Desire for future fertility
Stable or rising β-hCG levels with peak values of <15,000 mIU/mL
Intact tubal serosa
No active bleeding
EP fully visible at laparoscopy
Cervical and cornual pregnancy (in selected cases)

β-hCG, beta human chorionic gonadotropin. [a]Adapted from Stovall TG, Ling FW. Single-dose methotrexate: an expanded clinical trial. *Am J Obstet Gynecol* 1993;168:1759–1762. [b]From Ectopic pregnancy. ACOG Technical Bulletin Number 150. American College of Obstetricians and Gynecologists. *Int J Gynaecol Obstet* 1992;37(3):213–219.

TABLE 26-2   Contraindications to Methotrexate Therapy

Stovall and Ling, 1993[a]
Hepatic dysfunction: aspartate aminotransferase level >2 times normal
Renal disease: serum creatinine level >130 mmol/L (1.5 mg/dL)
Active peptic ulcer disease
Blood dyscrasia: leukocyte count <3,000 cells/μL or platelet count 100,000/μL

American College of Obstetricians and Gynecologists, 2008[b]
Absolute contraindications
Breastfeeding
Overt or laboratory evidence of immunodeficiency
Alcoholism, alcoholic liver disease, or other chronic liver disease
Preexisting blood dyscrasia, such as bone marrow hypoplasia, leukopenia,
    thrombocytopenia, or significant anemia
Peptic ulcer disease
Hepatic, renal, or hematologic dysfunction

Relative contraindications
Gestational sac larger than 3.5 cm
Embryonic cardiac motion

[a]Adapted from Stovall TG, Ling FW. Single-dose methotrexate: an expanded clinical trial. *Am J Obstet Gynecol* 1993;168:1759–1762. [b]From Medical Management of Ectopic Pregnancy. ACOG Practice Bulletin Number 94. American College of Obstetricians and Gynecologists. *Obstet Gynecol* 2008;111: 1479–1485.

abortion. This pain may complicate the diagnosis of ruptured ectopic and require hospital admission for close observation. NSAIDS should be avoided for analgesia due to risk of interaction with MTX.

- Increase in β-hCG levels during first 1 to 3 days of treatment
- Vaginal bleeding or spotting
- 10% risk of tubal rupture
- **MTX dosing regimens**
  - **Single dose versus multidose treatment.** Treatment protocols that involve single or multiple injections of MTX have been developed (Table 26-3). Benefits of a

TABLE 26-3	Methotrexate Treatment Protocols for Ectopic Pregnancy		
	Single-Dose Regimen[a]	Two-Dose Regimen[b]	Fixed Multidose Regimen[c]
Schedule	Day 1, repeat if necessary	Days 0 and 4	Days 1, 3, 5, 7
Medication			
Methotrexate	50 mg/m² IM	50 mg/m² IM	1 mg/kg IM
Leucovorin	None	None	0.1 mg/kg IM (days 2, 4, 6, 8)
Surveillance	Measure hCG on days 4 and 7, checking for 15% decrease from days 4–7.	Measure hCG on days 4 and 7, checking for 15% decrease from days 4–7.	Measure hCG on MTX dose days and continue until 15% decrease between values.
	If <15% decrease, repeat dosing (50 mg/m²) on day 7 and measure hCG on days 11 and 14. If >15 % decrease, measure hCG levels weekly until reaching nonpregnant level.	If <15% decrease, repeat dosing (50 mg/m²) on days 7 and 11, measuring hCG levels.	If <15% decrease or increase, consider repeating MTX regimen.

[a]Stovall TG, Ling FW. Single-dose methotrexate: an expanded clinical trial. *Am J Obstet Gynecol* 1993;168:1759–1762. [b]Barnhart K, Hummel AC, Sammel MD, et al. Use of "2-dose" regimen to treat ectopic pregnancy. *Fertil Steril* 2007;87:250. [c]Rodi IA, Sauer MV, Gorril MJ, et al. The medical treatment of unruptured ectopic pregnancy with methotrexate and citrovorum rescue: preliminary experience. *Fertil Steril* 1986;46:811–813. Adapted from Medical Management of Ectopic Pregnancy. ACOG Practice Bulletin Number 94. American College of Obstetricians and Gynecologists. *Obstet Gynecol* 2008;111:1479–1485.

single dose include decreased cost, better side-effect profile, improved patient compliance, and no need for leucovorin rescue treatment. The benefit of the multidose regimen is a lower failure rate. A systematic review reported a failure rate of 14.3% or higher with single-dose MTX when pretreatment β-hCG levels are higher than 5,000 mIU/mL, compared with a 3.7% failure rate for hCG levels <5,000 mIU/mL. If hCG levels are higher than 5,000 mIU/mL, the two-dose regimen may be appropriate while still avoiding the need for leucovorin rescue and improved patient compliance.

- The overall success rate for MTX is 89%.
- The success rate of single dose treatment is reported to be 88.1% versus 92.7% for the multidose regimen (p = 0.035).
- Patients with previous EPs are four times more likely to fail MTX treatment.
- **Special indications for MTX treatment** include known EP in difficult locations, such as cervical, ovarian, or cornual pregnancies in which the risk of surgical management outweighs the risk of attempted medical management.
- **Treatment monitoring.** Concentration of β-hCG often rises after the initial MTX injection. The level of β-hCG should drop by at least 15% from day 4 to day 7 following administration. TVUS is not an appropriate modality for determining treatment failure. Enlargement of the ectopic mass and/or free fluid in the pelvis are common findings after MTX injection and may prompt unnecessary interventions.
- **Treatment failure** is generally defined as a need for subsequent surgical intervention, although some studies use the term to describe the failure of a single MTX injection to lower β-hCG concentration by at least 15%.

Surgical Management

- Surgical management is the appropriate course of treatment in hemodynamically unstable patients or patients who have failed MTX therapy. Surgical management is also indicated in patients who have had a previous ectopic in the same fallopian tube.
- The surgical techniques should be tailored to the specific findings and situation, and they include salpingostomy, salpingectomy, partial salpingectomy, segmental resection, cornual resection, and possible hysterectomy for interstitial pregnancy.
  - **Salpingostomy.** A linear incision is made on the antimesenteric border over the pregnancy, which usually extrudes from the incision and is removed. Bleeding points are cauterized with laser or needlepoint cautery, and the incision is left to heal by secondary intention. EPs located in the ampulla are ideal candidates.
  - **Salpingectomy.** Involves the removal of the entire tube on the affected side. Consideration must be given to tubal damage at the time of surgery, especially in the case of a second EP in the same tube. Candidates for salpingectomy include women who have completed childbearing and patients with uncontrolled bleeding.
  - EP after tubal ligation is most often located in the fimbriated end of the tube. In this case, both fimbria should be surgically removed and the proximal segments of the tube cauterized to prevent recurrent ectopics.

Laparoscopy

- Minimally invasive laparoscopy is the preferred surgical approach in the hemodynamically stable patient. It usually provides a definitive diagnosis, although early EPs are missed 4% to 8% of the time. Not all patients are ideal candidates (e.g., patients with large body habitus or previous abdominal surgeries). Surgical approaches include linear salpingostomy and salpingectomy.

- **Contraindications to laparoscopy** may include pelvic adhesions, hemoperitoneum, pregnancy >4 cm, and hemodynamic instability.
- Linear salpingostomy requires postoperative MTX in 15% of cases. Serial β-hCG levels must be followed weekly.
- Tubal rupture is not an absolute indication for salpingectomy, especially if the rupture site is linear and small. The rupture site can be used to evacuate the pregnancy and preserve the tube.
- Salpingectomy is indicated when the tube continues to bleed after linear salpingostomy, when an EP occurs in a tube with previous damage, or when an EP occurs in a tube with a previously identified hydrosalpinx in a patient who is currently undergoing IVF.
- Copious irrigation of the pelvis is indicated to prevent adhesions and trophoblastic implants.

Laparotomy
- Laparotomy is indicated for a patient with obvious hemorrhage and hemodynamic compromise. After hemostasis is obtained, the treatment of choice is complete or partial salpingectomy. With a ruptured interstitial or cornual pregnancy, cornual resection may be required. Laparotomy is also indicated when adhesive disease precludes adequate visualization through the laparoscope.

Complications of Surgical Management
- Persistent trophoblastic tissue and persistent EP are considered surgical failures. Levels of β-hCG should be followed weekly after salpingostomy, until nonpregnant levels are reached. Surgically managed EPs can be given a dose of MTX for eradication of persistent trophoblastic tissue if β-hCG levels are found to plateau, in lieu of reoperation.

FOLLOW-UP AND PROGNOSIS

- After one EP, approximately 60% of patients conceive spontaneously.
- The recurrence risk ranges from 10% to 27%, which is 5 to 10 times greater than the risk for EP in the general population. The risk of recurrence increases in patients who have had two or more EPs. Only one out of three will conceive, and 20% to 57% of these will have EPs.
- Subsequent tubal patency rates are similar (80% to 85%) for patients treated medically or with salpingostomy.
- Patients with badly damaged fallopian tubes and those whose tubes have been removed can conceive through in vitro fertilization.
- Patients should be advised to use reliable contraceptive methods until initial inflammation resolves (6 to 12 weeks). Contraception will avoid confusion between rising β-hCG levels from a new pregnancy and those from a persistent EP, if conception occurs in the immediate postoperative period.
- Patients should undergo extensive counseling regarding their risk for recurrent EP and the necessity for early medical attention for subsequent pregnancies. The latter includes serial determinations of β-hCG levels until an early ultrasound examination can document an IUP or EP.
- Postoperative RhoGAM must be given to an Rh-negative woman to prevent Rh alloimmunization in a future pregnancy. See Chapter 18.

SUGGESTED READINGS

Barnhart KT, Gosman G, Ashby R, et al. The medical management of EP: a meta-analysis comparing "single-dose" and "multidose" regimens. *Obstet Gynecol* 2003;101:778–784.

Bouyer J, Coste J, Shojaei T, et al. Risk factors for EP: a comprehensive analysis based on a large case-control, population-based study in France. *Am J Epidemiol* 2003;157:185–194.

Gerton GL, Fan XJ, Barnhart K, et al. Presumed diagnosis of EP. *Obstet Gynecol* 2002;100: 505–510.

Lipscomb GH, McCord ML, Stovall TG, et al. Predictors of success of methotrexate treatment in women with tubal ectopic pregnancies. *N Engl J Med* 1999;341:1974–1978.

Lipscomb GH, Stovall TG, Ling FW. Nonsurgical treatment of EP. *N Engl J Med* 2000;343:1325–1329.

27 Chronic Pelvic Pain

K. Joseph Hurt and Richard P. Marvel

Chronic pelvic pain (CPP) is a common and often difficult problem, with direct medical costs estimated at $1 to $2 billion per year in the United States. CPP affects quality of life, increases work absenteeism, decreases overall productivity, and limits normal physical, social, emotional, and sexual function. The differential diagnosis is extensive, and the cause is often multisystem and multifactorial. CPP is the diagnosis for 10% to 20% of gynecology office referrals.

TYPES OF PELVIC PAIN

There are no standard diagnostic criteria, but a reasonable **definition of CPP** is cyclic or noncyclic pain in the lower abdomen, pelvis, lower back, or buttocks of at least 6 months duration that causes functional disability and motivates the patient to seek medical help. Because of varied definitions, the epidemiology and natural history of CPP are not well described. **Acute pelvic pain** can be defined with the same criteria but lasts <30 days.

- CPP is most common in younger adult women. Four to fifteen percent of reproductive-aged women are affected, similar to other common disorders such as asthma, migraine headache, and lower back pain.
  - **Dysmenorrhea** (pain associated with menstrual cycles) occurs in up to 90% of women. Risk factors include age <30 years, BMI <20, tobacco use, early menarche, menometrorrhagia, and history of pelvic inflammatory disease (PID), tubal ligation, and physical/sexual assault.
  - **Dyspareunia** (pain during sexual activity) occurs in 1% to 40% of women. Risk factors include female circumcision, history of PID, anxiety, depression, sexual assault, and postmenopausal status.
  - **Noncyclic pelvic pain** (with no relation to menses) occurs in 4% to 40% of women. Risk factors include anxiety, depression, prior cesarean section, pelvic adhesions, endometriosis, menorrhagia, and history of miscarriage or physical/sexual abuse.
- Up to 90% of patients with CPP will undergo one or more *unsuccessful*, and often unneccessary, gynecologic procedures. At least 40% of gynecologic laparoscopies are performed for CPP, but only 30% to 60% of those surgeries reveal a cause. Ten to twenty percent of hysterectomies are performed with the primary indication of CPP, but relief is not universal.

BIOLOGY AND CLASSIFICATION OF PAIN PERCEPTION

Acute **pain perception** is an evolutionary protective mechanism causing reflexive withdrawal from noxious stimuli. Individuals with congenitally impaired pain sensation have shorter lifespans.

- **Pain receptors** respond to intense mechanical stress or local inflammatory/pain mediators (e.g., histamine, bradykinin, substance P). That stimulus is transduced to an electrical impulse that is transmitted via A-delta (fast myelinated) and C-fiber (slow unmyelinated) dorsal root ganglion neurons to synapse in the dorsal horn of the spinal cord. Second order pain neurons then cross the anterior commissure and travel via the lateral spinothalamic tract to the thalamus where they synapse again. Third order pain neurons project from the thalamus to the insular cortex (emotional content), the anterior cingulate cortex (planning/motivational function), and the primary sensory cortex (primary pain perception).

- **Pain afferent pathways** can be modulated in the brain and spinal cord by descending pathways that can augment or diminish pain sensation. The possible interactions between acute pain perception, chronic pain pathway activation, and higher level/emotional modulation of pain circuitry underlie the complex pathophysiology of CPP. Normal descending inhibition of dorsal horn synaptic activity, for example, is decreased in chronic pain syndromes such as irritable bowel syndrome (IBS). Emotional factors such as depression and anxiety also decrease the pain threshold.
- **Nociceptive somatic pain** (e.g., postoperative pain, trauma, inflammation) is produced by heat, cold, mechanical, and chemical stimuli. Deep somatic pain is detected within muscles, ligaments, and bone. Deep visceral pain from internal organs is poorly localized and has some overlap with somatic sensory tracts in the spinal cord, causing "referred pain." The T10-L1 afferent visceral pain fibers that innervate the uterus, adnexa, and cervix also supply the lower ileum, sigmoid colon, and rectum. Pelvic pain sensations can originate in any of those closely related structures.
- **Neuropathic pain** (e.g., postherpetic neuralgia, diabetic neuropathy, nerve entrapment, taxol chemotherapy neuropathy) is due to peripheral or central nerve damage causing a malfunction in pain detection. It is commonly perceived as a chronic burning or tingling pain and produced from both local and systemic processes.
- Current **pain theory** incorporates the Descartean concept of sensory specificity (i.e., a single stimulus is conducted along a dedicated pain pathway) and more recent ideas regarding the modulating influence of emotional, cognitive, cultural, attentive, and suggestive factors on both initial transmission and ultimate perception.
- **Psychogenic pain** (e.g., somatization) is another possible etiology in a complete biopsychosocial model, representing the physical manifestation of unresolved emotional or psychologic conflict.
- It is not merely academic to keep these concepts in mind when treating CPP, since it can be difficult to determine whether a patient has a symptom of nociceptive stimulation or an ongoing malfunction of pain perception, or both. Acutely painful processes, PID for example, may eventually resolve but leave permanently remodeled pelvic structures (e.g., adhesions) that can cause chronic pain. An extended inflammatory stimulus (e.g., inflammatory bowel disease) can lead to higher order pain sensitization and hyperesthesia. Pain associated with intense emotional content (e.g., childhood sexual abuse) can alter neurocognitive development, leading to hypervigilence and heightened pain sensation.
- Though gynecologists often think of CPP as originating from either gynecologic or nongynecologic sources, it may be more helpful to take a broader view. Anatomic localization (e.g., abdominal wall, bowel, bladder, perineum), affected organ system (e.g., gastrointestinal, genitourinary, musculoskeletal, psychiatric), and type of pain (e.g., somatic, visceral, neuropathic, psychogenic) are possible diagnostic paradigms.

EVALUATION OF CPP

The **evaluation of CPP** starts with a complete medical history and the goal of establishing an enduring therapeutic physician-patient relationship.

History and Physical Exam

- **Prior records** (including past history, test results, operative notes, and pathology reports) should be reviewed to avoid redundant tests or procedures and to gauge the effectiveness of prior interventions and progress over time.
- **Pain inventory questionnaires** can be helpful in recording subjective and objective data and may increase the efficiency of initial data gathering. Useful resources are available from the International Pelvic Pain Society (IPPS) at www.pelvicpain.org. Pain questionnaires are helpful in allowing the patient to develop a coherent and relevant narrative before appearing at the office and allow rapid review of symptoms, permitting the interview to focus on pain issues. A personal body pain map is extremely helpful in focusing the differential and examination.
- Adequate time should be allotted for a **complete medical and psychosocial history**, without rushing the patient. A detailed review of systems including genitourinary, gastrointestinal, musculoskeletal, and psychoneurologic questions is important.
  - Establish a detailed understanding of the intensity, location, character, and duration of the pain and any association with intercourse, menstruation, defecation, recent or distant surgery, radiation treatments, or abdominopelvic infections. Precipitating and relieving factors should be reviewed.
  - Screening for physical or sexual abuse, domestic violence, and other psychosocial stressors (e.g., death of loved one, divorce) should be completed. Twenty to sixty percent of patients with CPP report a history of sexual or childhood abuse. A complete mental health history and depression screening are helpful; mood and personality disorders are frequently comorbid with CPP.
  - Current, usual, and worst pain can be recorded using a pain scale (e.g., visual analogue scale). Associated symptoms such as weight loss, hematochezia, and perimenopausal/postmenopausal bleeding should prompt a thorough investigation for malignancy.
- The **physical exam** begins with a general and neurologic assessment. Fully explain the plan and exam techniques, to relieve anxiety and promote patient cooperation and comfort. The IPPS physical exam form or similar tools may be useful for recording the complete assessment. The exam should help narrow the differential, rule out systemic disease or neoplasm, and suggest additional testing.
  - Evaluate the **general appearance**, including dress, nutrition, posture, apparent age, gait, and pain behaviors. Evaluate **posture (both seated and standing) and gait** (for any hip height and leg length discrepancy).
  - Ask the patient to **indicate the precise location** of her pain. If she is able to use a single finger, a discrete source is more likely than if she uses a broad sweeping motion of the entire hand.
  - Note the presence of **scars or hernias** on abdominal exam. Gently attempt to elicit pain with palpation of the skin, fascia, or muscle. Especially note any reproducible tenderness. Appropriate **trigger point mapping** should be performed if fibromyalgia is in the differential.
  - Look for **Carnett's sign** (i.e., increased abdominal tenderness when the patient lifts her head and shoulders in the supine position) suggesting abdominal wall rather than intra-abdominal pathology. Pain with the **Betty maneuver** (i.e., thigh abduction against resistance) may suggest piriformis syndrome. The **obturator sign** (i.e., pain with flexion and internal rotation of the hip while lying supine) and the **psoas sign** (i.e., pain with hip flexion against resistance) can indicate inflammation or dysfunction within those muscles. The **straight leg raise test** evaluates radiculopathy

or intervertebral disc disease. The **FAbER test** (i.e., pain with Flexion/Abduction/External Rotation of the hip) assesses hip and sacroiliac joint pathology.

- A thorough **neurologic examination**, including sensation, muscle strength, and reflexes, may be required. Examine the spine for scoliosis while the patient is sitting, standing, walking, and bending at the waist.
- The **gynecologic exam** starts with external observation and then palpation with cotton swabs to define hyperesthetic areas (even if the skin appears normal). Colposcopic examination of the vulva and vestibule may be helpful. Light touch and pinprick sensation testing of the vulva is required.
  - Start the internal examination with a single-digit vaginal exam. Assess the vestibule, vaginal walls, rectum, urethra, bladder trigone, pubic arch, pelvic floor muscles, cervix, and vaginal fornices. Initial assessment of the uterus and adnexa are performed with a single digit as well.
  - Visual inspection of the vaginal vault can begin with a single speculum blade. Assess the vaginal cuff or cervix, cervical os, paracervix, and vaginal muscosa.
  - Finally, perform a bimanual exam of the uterus, adnexa, and other pelvic contents followed by rectovaginal exam. Fecal occult blood testing may be indicated. The bimanual exam, being the most invasive part of the evaluation, should be performed last. Some patients will be unable to tolerate any additional evaluation following the bimanual exam.

Imaging and Laboratory Testing

- **Imaging and diagnostic testing** are tailored to the differential.
  - Pelvic ultrasonography is of little benefit unless uterine or adnexal pathology is suspected. Transvaginal imaging may better assess the pelvic structures than the transabdominal approach.
  - MRI can be helpful in selected cases, especially if adenomyosis is suspected.
  - Plain x-ray of the chest, spine, abdomen, or joints, or CT scan is rarely indicated.
  - Colonoscopy can assess colorectal cancer, inflammatory bowel disease, diverticulosis, and invasive endometriosis. It is indicated in cases with persistent diarrhea or hematochezia.
- **Laboratory testing** is guided by the history and physical and may include urine pregnancy test, vaginal pH and wet mount, gonorrhea and chlamydia PCR, CBC, ESR, TSH, RPR, hepatitis B surface antigen, HIV test, urinalysis/microscopy, and urine culture. There is no standard laboratory panel for CPP. Serum CA-125 testing is not useful unless a cancer workup is initiated. Endocrine testing for FSH, estradiol, and GnRH stimulation test may be indicated for suspected ovarian remnant syndrome.

Laparoscopy and Consults

- Although **pelviscopy** is performed for more than 40% of CPP cases, it should be employed only when noninvasive evaluation is completed and for cases in which a diagnosis can be reasonably anticipated. Laparoscopy is not a substitute for a complete history and physical or for diagnoses that can be made without a procedure. Most causes of CPP are *not* detectable by laparoscopy. It is performed when endometriosis is suspected.
- Selected evaluation by neurology, gastroenterology, anesthesiology, urology, psychiatry, or physical therapy **consultants** can provide important multidisciplinary perspective and assist in forming a complete treatment plan. Often, patients have

been through a long, tedious, and piecemeal evaluation by multiple providers followed by redundant diagnostic and treatment failures. Performing a complete and multidisciplinary assessment from the start may reach a successful outcome more efficiently and reassure a demoralized and anxious patient. In addition, some tests are only appropriately obtained via consultation, such as nerve conduction studies or electromyography, if they are necessary. Cystoscopy and evaluation for interstitial cystitis (IC) are frequently indicated early in the workup.

DIFFERENTIAL DIAGNOSIS OF PELVIC PAIN

The **differential diagnosis** of pelvic pain is extensive, and many cases deserve multiple diagnoses.

- Selected **causes of acute pelvic pain** are listed in Table 27.1. Some of these may be the initiating event leading to a chronic pain state.
- Selected **causes of chronic pelvic pain** are listed in Table 27.2. Previously undiagnosed medical illness should also be considered, such as neoplasia, sickle cell disease, hyperparathyroidism, urolithiasis, lead/mercury intoxication, lactose intolerance, chronic constipation, chronic appendicitis, and chronic fatigue syndrome.
- The clinical satisfaction of applying Occam's razor and assigning only one unifying diagnosis after a thorough workup for CPP is not likely; management of multiple disease processes is often required. The following disorders, in addition to being primary etiologies, are frequently comorbid with CPP and deserve special consideration.
  - **Dysmenorrhea** is reported in up to 80% of women with CPP. It is characterized by cramping pelvic or suprapubic pain that radiates to the lower back or thighs, often with mood or behavioral changes. Nausea/vomiting, diarrhea, irritability, and fatigue may be present. The pathophysiology is inflammatory prostaglandin release upon progesterone withdrawal at the end of the menstrual cycle. Patients with hyperalgesia may experience significantly longer and more intense menstrual pain. Managing "normal menstrual pain" can be an important consideration for patients with CPP.
  - **Endometriosis** is diagnosed in up to 70% of pelvic pain patients, though biopsy-proven disease is present in perhaps only 30%. See Chapter 35. Up to 80% of patients treated with laparoscopic excision of endometriosis have short-term pain relief, but less than half of those continue to report improved pain scores at 1 year.
  - **Irritable bowel syndrome (IBS)** is a primary or secondary diagnosis in 40% to 60% of patients with CPP. See Table 27.3. Associated symptoms of IBS include abdominal distention, bloating, fatigue, and headache; symptoms are sometimes worse before menses. When other causes *have been ruled out*, this may be the primary diagnosis.
  - **Pelvic adhesions** are eventually diagnosed in about 25% of women with CPP, but a causal relationship is debatable. Pain localization, but not intensity, correlates with the presence of isolated adhesions detected during pelviscopy. Adhesiolysis is not proven to provide dramatic relief.
  - **Interstitial cystitis (IC)** is a chronic inflammatory disorder with aspects of a chronic visceral pain syndrome that frequently coexists with other causes of CPP. Diagnosis is made by cystoscopy and hydrodistention under anesthesia, with findings of glomerulations or Hunner's ulcers (see Chapter 28). Treatment is with

TABLE 27-1   Differential Diagnosis of Acute Pelvic Pain

Etiology	Mechanism	Testing/Diagnosis[a]	Treatment
Ectopic pregnancy	Fallopian tube stretch; generalized peritoneal irritation; hemoperitoneum	hCG, ultrasound	Medical or surgical treatment (Chapter 26)
Adnexal torsion	Twisting of ovary/tube on vascular pedicle causes venous occlusion leading to ischemia/necrosis	Ultrasound	Surgical correction or removal (Chapter 19)
Hemorrhagic corpus luteum cyst or hemorrhagic follicular cyst	Rapid expansion of an ovarian cyst with blood causes ovarian capsule stretch; hemoperitoneum	Ultrasound	Conservative management with fluids/pain meds; laparoscopy/laparotomy for severe persistent bleeding
Endometritis	Polymicrobial ascending intrauterine infection can lead to PID/TOA. Acute = neutrophils and microabscesses in glands; Chronic = plasma cells in stroma	Ultrasound, CBC, ESR, gonorrhea/Chlamydia testing, endometrial biopsy	Intravenous antibiotic treatment (Chapters 7 and 25)
Pelvic inflammatory disease/tubo-ovarian abscess	Polymicrobial pelvic peritoneal inflammation from ascending infection	See endometritis, above	In- or out-patient management with antibiotics depending on severity; rarely surgical washout (Chapter 25)
Septic pelvic thrombophlebitis/ovarian vein thrombosis	Typically with puerperal infection or septic abortion. Other sources must be ruled out	Blood cultures, CBC, ESR, lower extremity Dopplers, CT or MRI	Broad-spectrum antibiotics ± heparin or enoxaparin (Chapter 7)
Uterine fibroid degeneration/torsion	Rapid growth, especially in pregnancy outstrips blood supply leading to infarction; pedunculated fibroid twisting on pedicle leads to ischemia/necrosis. Fibroids can also cause chronic pressure/pain	Ultrasound	Pain medications, laparoscopic excision, uterine artery embolization, hysterectomy (Chapter 34)
Mittelschmerz	Midcycle ovulatory pain with follicular rupture and prostaglandin leakage	H&P	NSAIDs if necessary; hormonal ovulation suppression

[a]A thorough history and physical exam are the initial diagnostic process for all the disorders discussed in this chapter. Additional or specific testing is listed as appropriate.

TABLE 27-2 Differential Diagnosis of Chronic Pelvic Pain

Category	Etiology	Mechanism	Testing/Diagnosis	Treatment
Cyclic/recurrent gynecologic	**Endometriosis**	• Ectopic endometrial tissue infiltration and inflammation. Can progress from cyclic to noncyclic pain as adhesions develop	• H&P, ±imaging, laparoscopy with biopsy	• Ovulation suppression, surgical ablation, excision of endometriomas (Chapter 35)
	Endosalpingiosis Adenomyosis	• Ectopic fallopian tube epithelium • Endometrial stroma and glands deeper than 2 mm within the myometrium → menorrhagia and dysmenorrhea by uncertain mechanism	• Biopsy, pelvic washings • MRI	• Ablation, GnRH agonists • NSAIDs, OCPs, GnRH agonists, progesterone IUD, hysterectomy
	Primary/secondary dysmenorrhea	• Primary = uterine menstrual pain. Secondary = menstrual pain due to structural pathology	• H&P, rule out other causes	• NSAIDs, OCPs, GnRH agonists, LUNA procedure, Transcutaneous electrical nerve stimulation, treatment of secondary causes
	Ovarian remnant syndrome	• FSH stimulation of inadequately excised ovarian tissue at time of oophorectomy. Similar mechanism if ovaries are purposefully conserved at hysterectomy	• Surgical history, serum FSH, and estrogen in premenopausal range	• Adhesiolysis and removal of all ovarian tissue may cure >90%.
	Cervical stenosis	• Blocked cervical os → hematometra, retrograde menstruation	• Pelvic exam, ultrasound	• Dilation of cervical os in the office or under sedation in operating room
Noncyclic gynecologic	**Abdominopelvic adhesions**	• Scar tissue from infection, trauma, endometriosis. Left-sided sigmoid adhesions are a frequent finding.	• H&P, laparoscopy	• Laparoscopy/laparotomy and adhesiolysis
	Uterine retroversion	• Rare cause of deep dyspareunia and dysmenorrhea. Very rare cause of uterine pelvic incarceration in early pregnancy	• Pelvic exam, ultrasound, pessary test for symptom relief	• Hodge pessary or laparoscopic uterine suspension

Condition	Description	Workup	Treatment
Chronic endometritis/ chronic PID	Pelvic tuberculosis, tuboovarian abscess, chronic chlamydial endometritis → inflammation. More frequent in populations with high rates of STDs	Cervical Chlamydia PCR, endometrial biopsy, ultrasound, laparoscopy	Antibiotic therapy; erythromycin or doxycycline × 2–4 wk (Chapter 25)
Chronic vulvovaginitis	Recurrent or chronic yeast, trichomonas, or fungal infections	H&P, wet prep, culture	Antibiotics, boric acid vaginal suppositories (Chapter 25)
Vaginal cuff pain	Posthysterectomy chronic low-grade cuff cellulitis, seroma, neuroma, or nerve entrapment	H&P, pelvic exam, anesthetic blocks	Cuff resection/revision, cuff anesthesia injection, chemical neurolysis
Contact vulvitis	Contact irritant from lotion, soaps, clothing, etc.	H&P	Eliminate offending agents, ±apply topical steroids
Vulvodynia	Vulvar hyperalgesia due to neuropathic and pelvic floor pain	Exam, ±biopsy	Vaginal physical therapy, biofeedback, TCA (Chapter 39)
Vulvar vestibulitis	Subset of vulvodynia. Nonspecific vestibular inflammation → severe entry dyspareunia	H&P, ± vulvar skin biopsy	Vestibulectomy/perineoplasty if conservative management fails (Chapter 41)
Pudendal neuralgia	Pudendal nerve injury or entrapment	H&P, nerve block	Avoid sitting. Pain medications, nerve block, or surgical decompression for severe cases
Pelvic congestion syndrome	Pelvic vein insufficiency from pelvic varicosities, vascular stasis with tissue edema. Pain with increased intra-abdominal pressure, prolonged standing. Increased risk with collagen vascular disease (e.g., Ehlers-Danlos)	History of postcoital aching pain + ovarian point tenderness; pelvic venography (transuterine contrast injection with real-time radiography)	Medroxyprogesterone acetate, endovascular embolization, hysterectomy
Pelvic organ prolapse	Trauma or intrinsic laxity of vaginal or uterine supporting tissues causing discomfort or pain	Exam, POP-Q measurements	See Chapter 28

(Continued)

TABLE 27-2 Differential Diagnosis of Chronic Pelvic Pain *(Continued)*

Category	Etiology	Mechanism	Testing/Diagnosis	Treatment
Gastrointestinal	Irritable bowel syndrome	• Functional bowel disorder	• H&P, rule out other causes, see Table 27.3	• Increase dietary fiber, loperamide, stool softeners, dicyclomine
	Inflammatory bowel disease (ulcerative colitis and Crohn's disease)	• Chronic bowel inflammation.	• Cramping lower abdominal pain and bloody diarrhea, stool studies, colonoscopy, biopsies	• Anti-inflammatory drugs, steroids. Refer to gastroenterology.
	Diverticular disease	• Colonic outpouchings of mucosa/submucosa due to muscularis weakness at sites of higher pressure present in >10% of women over age 40. Can become infected/inflamed	• AXR, Barium enema, colonoscopy	• Antibiotics for infection, increased dietary fiber and hydration
	Intermittent bowel obstruction	• Mechanical partial obstruction, usually secondary to adhesions	• AXR (upper GI with small bowel follow through study), CT scan, biopsy of any mass	• Bowel decompression and conservative management or surgical adhesiolysis
Urologic	Interstitial cystitis (IC)	• Chronic noninfectious cystitis and hyperesthesia	• H&P, potassium sensitivity testing, cystoscopy, hydrodistension	• Hydrodistension, intravesicle DMSO, oral pentosan polysulfate, low-dose TCA, antihistamines (Chapter 28)
	Chronic/recurrent urinary tract infection	• Bacterial or fungal infection, often due to anatomic abnormalities, causes irritative voiding symptoms. Increases with age and PMP status	• Urinalysis, urine culture, test of cure	• Antibiotics, ±prophylactic suppression

Urethral syndrome	Chronic urethral inflammation, infection, or obstruction, similar to IC	History of dysuria, frequency, urgency, and slow painful urine stream; exam, cystoscopy, urine culture, Chlamydia PCR	Hormone replacement therapy in PMP women, biofeedback, DMSO, NSAIDs, muscle relaxants, and alpha antagonists may be useful.
Urethral diverticulum	Herniation of the urethral lining; pocket may become infected/inflamed. It is a rare cause of chronic pain.	History of dysuria, dyspareunia, and postvoid dribbling. Urinalysis, urine culture, ±cytology, voiding cystourethrography, double-balloon positive pressure urethrography, ultrasound, MRI, urethroscopy	Antibiotics for infection, surgical excision
Detrusor-sphincter dyssynergia	Urethral sphincter relaxation does not occur in coordination with detrusor activity causing increased bladder pressure and urine retention. Often from CNS injury or multiple sclerosis	Urodynamics, EMG study	Urethral stent, transurethral sphincterotomy, botulinum toxin injection, and catheterization are possible treatments.
Musculoskeletal **Levator ani syndrome**	Pelvic floor muscle spasm → chronic or recurrent rectal or vaginal pain or dyspareunia	Pain reproduction or trigger point detection on vaginal or rectal exam	Heat packs, muscle relaxants, massage, physical therapy, relaxation techniques
Osteoarthritis	Referred pelvic pain from chronic degenerative loss of cartilage especially at the hip, knee, sacroiliac, and vertebral joints	Musculoskeletal exam, joint x-rays	Weight loss, lifestyle modification, NSAIDs, physical therapy, joint replacement surgery
Thoracolumbar syndrome	Hypermobility of thoracolumbar junction in patients with lumbar fusion → referred anterior abdominal and lateral hip pain	Musculoskeletal exam, spinal/hip x-rays	Physical therapy, NSAIDs, orthopedic referral may be appropriate.

(Continued)

TABLE 27-2 Differential Diagnosis of Chronic Pelvic Pain *(Continued)*

Category	Etiology	Mechanism	Testing/Diagnosis	Treatment
Musculoskeletal (continued)	**Myofascial pain syndrome Fibromyalgia**	• Irritability, spasm, pain of pelvic floor or abdominal muscles • Global myofascial pain syndrome due to abnormal pain processing/signaling	• H&P, pelvic exam, EMG testing • 11 of 18 painful diagnostic trigger points	• Physical therapy, trigger point injection, muscle relaxant • Exercise, physical therapy, warm packs, massage, NSAIDs, biofeedback, relaxation techniques, low-dose SSRIs, muscle relaxants, trigger point injections
	Coccydynia	• Trauma to the coccyx can cause S1-S4 nerve pain referred to pelvic floor.	• Dynamic spine/coccygeal x-rays, MRI, diagnostic local anesthetic injection	• Local anesthetic or steroid injections, NSAIDs, TCAs, physical therapy, rarely coccygectomy
	Hernia	• Inguinal, obturator, spigelian, umbilical, etc.	• Exam, CT scan	• Manual reduction, binders, avoiding increased intra-abdominal pressure, surgical correction
	Lumbar vertebral compression fracture	• Osteoporosis, trauma, malignancy → lumbar spine fractures	• Spinal x-ray, CT or MRI, DEXA scan	• Referral for treatment, physical therapy, rehabilitation, lumbar orthotic brace, occupational therapy, pain medication; surgery for neurologic impairment
	Piriformis syndrome	• Sciatic nerve impingement by piriformis muscle spasm or overuse syndrome → buttock, thigh, leg pain. Running and biking can exacerbate.	• Rule out lumbar disk herniation (i.e., sciatic root impingement), complete neurologic exam, spinal imaging	• NSAIDs, muscle relaxants, physical therapy, local steroid/anesthetic/botulinum toxin injection

Neurologic	Nerve entrapment	Surgical injury of ilioinguinal or iliohypogastric nerve can cause neuroma formation. Obturator internus can press on obturator nerve. Mechanical nerve impingement or stretch can lead to neuropathy.	History, anatomic correlation, and diagnostic nerve block	Transcutaneous neurolysis, myofascial release procedure, local anesthetic injection, or surgical neurectomy if medical therapy fails
	Peripheral neuropathy/neuritis/neuralgia	Numerous local and systemic processes that damage peripheral nerves → persistent numbness, burning, tingling pain	H&P, evaluate for systemic disease and infectious causes (e.g., zoster)	TCAs, gabapentin, pregabalin, valproate, transcutaneous electrical nerve stimulation
	Abdominal migraine	Neuronal hyperexcitation → paroxysmal abdominal pain ± nausea/vomiting/flushing. Usually in children, rare in adults	H&P, family history, rule out other causes, consider neuroimaging	Sleep, antiemetics, TCAs, refer to neurology
Psychiatric[a]	Posttraumatic disorders	Sexual or physical abuse, especially in childhood	History, psychiatric assessment, rule out organic pathology	Psychotherapy, treat depression, SSRI antidepressants
	Somatization disorder	Internal psychological conflict and hypersensitivity to pain stimuli	Four different sites of pain plus two GI, one sexual, and one pseudoneurologic symptom (per diagnostic criteria). Rule out organic pathology	Psychiatry referral, cognitive-behavioral therapy, antidepressants

This list is not exhaustive but represents the multiple systems and variety of diagnoses in the workup of CPP. General treatments are listed only to indicate *possible* therapies used for each condition. [a]Also include a broader psychiatric differential such as bipolar disorders, personality disorders, depression, and substance abuse. AXR, abdominal x-ray; DMSO, dimethyl sulfoxide; DEXA, dual energy x-ray absorptiometry; EMG, electromyography; LUNA, laparoscopic uterosacral nerve ablation; OCP, hormonal oral contraceptive pills; PCR, polymerase chain reaction; PID, pelvic inflammatory disease; PMP, postmenopausal; SSRI, selective serotonin reuptake inhibitors; STD, sexually transmitted disease; TCA, tricyclic antidepressants.

TABLE 27-3	Rome III Diagnostic Criteria for IBS

Recurrent abdominal pain/discomfort:
- Of at least 3 days/month for the preceding 3 months
- With symptoms first appearing at least 6 months before diagnosis

And at least two of the following characteristics:
- Symptoms improved/relieved with defecation
- Onset associated with a change in the frequency of defecation
- Onset associated with a change in the appearance/form of stool

Adapted from Longstreth, et al. Functional Bowel Disorders. *Gastroenterology* 2006;130: 1480–1491, and see: www.romecriteria.org

oral pentosan sulfate (Elmiron), antihistamines, and low-dose tricyclic antidepressants (e.g., amitriptyline). Bladder installation of an anesthetic cocktail of lidocaine, heparin, steroids, and sodium bicarbonate can provide significant pain relief on an intermittent or continuous basis.

- **Pelvic congestion syndrome** (symptomatic varicose veins of the pelvis) can be objectively diagnosed by transcervical pelvic venogram. Randomized trials show correlation between venogram scores and pain, with improvement after treatment.
- **Myofascial pain** is comorbid with 10% to 20% of CPP. Physical therapy is the mainstay of treatment. Selective serotonin reuptake inhibitors (SSRIs) and muscle relaxants may be useful adjuncts.
- **Dyspareunia** can be a primary or secondary symptom in CPP. Additionally, the psychological effect of CPP on relationships and sexual function should be addressed in the evaluation and treatment plan.
- **Low back pain** is often a separate treatable problem that can exacerbate CPP.
- The incidence of **depression, anxiety,** and **drug abuse** is increased in patients with CPP and should be investigated in the initial workup. It may not be clear whether these problems are a cause or result of pain. Increased depression scores, however, correlate with increased pain scores, so simultaneous treatment is most effective.

MANAGEMENT OF CPP

Management of CPP depends upon the etiology and comorbidities (Table 27.2). The best outcomes may come from a rehabilitation approach with a consistent provider, personalized multidisciplinary treatment, extensive patient education and counseling, and regular office visits. The physician must be open-minded and supportive but offer realistic and explicit goals for therapy. The patient, desperate for a diagnosis and possibly with exaggerated or nonanatomic pain or nonphysiologic sensations, should always be taken seriously. Tailor treatments to the patient and address the underlying etiology, associated pain syndrome, psychological needs, and physical therapy concerns. Develop an accurate problem list and plan of management for each pain component. There is no strong evidence to support medical versus surgical management. At 1 year, about half of surgical patients report improved pain while the rest report no change or worsening symptoms; similar proportions have been reported with medical treatment.

Medical Therapy

- **Medical therapies** are selected to correct or arrest underlying pathology and to relieve pain symptoms. Analgesics should be dosed on noncontingent schedules with additional breakthrough pain treatment as needed.
  - **Nonsteroidal anti-inflammatory drugs (NSAIDs)** (e.g., acetaminophen, ibuprofen, aspirin, naproxen) are a mainstay of pain treatment, especially if inflammation is present. Contraindications to NSAID treatment (e.g., liver disease for acetaminophen, renal failure or peptic ulcer disease for NSAIDs) must be excluded. Prescribe medications with adequate dosing and frequency. Higher than usual doses may be required.
  - **Opioid analgesia** with oral tramadol, codeine, oxycodone, and hydrocodone may be indicated. IV medications are rarely indicated for CPP. Combination long- and short-acting opioids can be beneficial. See Chapter 48 for a stepwise approach to pain management.
  - **Hormonal treatment** is frequently used for endometriosis and dysmenorrhea.
    - Continuous oral contraceptive pills and GnRH agonists (e.g., goserelin, depot lupron) prevent ovulation and may help pain associated with menses, including endometriosis.
    - There is good evidence that **medroxyprogesterone** 50 mg orally each day helps control endometriosis and pelvic congestion syndrome symptoms. Depot medroxyprogesterone acetate 150 mg IM every 3 months is another option.
  - **Thiamine (Vitamin B$_1$)** 100 mg PO daily, **vitamin E** supplementation, and oral **magnesium** supplementation are possible nutritional approaches to dysmenorrhea, though effectiveness data are limited.
  - **SSRI antidepressants** (e.g., fluoxetine, sertraline) have not been shown to work well for pain, but they are useful for treatment of comorbid depression or anxiety disorders that can increase pain perception. **SSNRI medications** (i.e., duloxetine, venlafaxine, milnacipran) are effective for depression, anxiety, and neuropathic pain.
  - **Tricyclic antidepressants** (e.g., amitryptiline, nortryptiline) are the most effective neuropathic pain medications; they may act by lowering the pain threshold (see Table 27.2). **Antiseizure medications** (e.g., gabapentin, pregabalin, carbamezapine) are useful for neuropathic pain.
  - **Muscle relaxants** (e.g., cyclobenzaprine, baclofen) are sometimes useful for muscule spasm, but they should be used as adjuncts or second-line agents with nonsteroidal drugs, until a course of physical therapy can be completed.

Surgical Treatment

- **Surgical therapies** are indicated for specific diagnoses or for patients who do not improve with medical treatments.
  - Surgical treatment of severe endometriosis or suspected intervisceral adhesions (i.e., **adhesiolysis**) can be curative in some cases. Patients should understand that there is a strong possibility that additional therapies or medication may be required and that the surgical procedure can lead to unforeseen complications.
  - **Laparoscopic uterosacral nerve ablation** (LUNA) has been used for dysmenorrhea in patients with endometriosis who desire to maintain fertility, but several controlled clinical trials show that it is ineffective.
  - The superior hypogastric plexus is excised with **presacral neurectomy**. There is some evidence showing modest pain reduction for patients with midline pelvic pain due to dysmenorrhea/endometriosis. The procedure can lead to complications

such as ureteral injury and uncontrolled bleeding and should be performed by experienced surgeons only.

* **Pudendal nerve release** from Alcock's canal by transgluteal or transperineal approach is performed for some patients with pudendal nerve entrapment, though there are only limited data by which to judge the procedure.
* **Hysterectomy** can be performed for patients with evidence of uterine pain (e.g., adneomyosis, some cases of endometriosis) who have completed their childbearing and have not responded well to medical management. Sixty to eighty percent of appropriately selected patients report pain improvement.

Other Treatment Options

* Neurologic/pain anesthesia therapies are useful for CPP that can be discretely localized or is due to a specific peripheral nerve injury. Local anesthetic (e.g., lidocaine) can be injected for **cutaneous nerve or trigger point block**. Longer acting **peripheral nerve blocks** can benefit some patients. **Botulinum toxin** injection can improve unresponsive spasmodic muscular disorders. Referral to an anesthesia pain specialist may be warranted.
* **Physical therapy** by a provider with expertise in pelvic floor disorders can be helpful in both evaluation and treatment of CPP. Stretching, strengthening, hot/cold applications, pelvic floor training, transcutaneous electrical nerve stimulation, and biofeedback can be used.
* **Psychotherapy** is almost always beneficial for a patient with chronic pain. Psychological disorders can be diagnosed and managed, and cognitive behavioral therapy, psychotherapy, or counseling can benefit almost all CPP patients. If abuse is reported, the patient should be referred for psychological counseling regardless of the degree to which that history contributes to her pain. In some cases, referral for family or relationship counseling may be indicated as well.
* **Alternative/holistic therapies** such as massage, relaxation techniques, and acupuncture may be appropriate adjunctive interventions for many patients and enhance the effectiveness of traditional medical or surgical therapy. These should be discussed with the patient and integrated in her treatment plan early on.

SUGGESTED READINGS

Bettendorf B, Shay S, Tu F. Dysmenorrhea: contemporary perspectives. *Obstet Gynecol Surv* 2008;63(9):597–603.

Bhutta HY, Walsh SR, Tang TY, et al. Ovarian vein syndrome: a review. *Int J Surg* 2009;7:516–520.

Chronic pelvic pain. ACOG Practice Bulletin Number 51. American College of Obstetricians and Gynecologists. *Obstet Gynecol* 2004, reaffirmed 2008;103:589–605.

Hillis SD, Marchbanks PA, Peterson HB. The effectiveness of hysterectomy for chronic pelvic pain. *Obstet Gynecol* 1995;86(6):941–945.

Howard FM. Chronic pelvic pain. Clinical gynecologic series: an expert's view. *Obstet Gynecol* 2003;101:594–611.

Lamvu G, Williams R, Zolnoun D, et al. Long-term outcomes after surgical and nonsurgical management of chronic pelvic pain: one year after evaluation in a pelvic pain specialty clinic. *Am J Obstet Gynecol* 2006;195:591–600.

Latthe P, Mignini L, Gray R, et al. Factors predisposing women to chronic pelvic pain: systematic review. *Br Med J* 2006; 332(7544):749–755.

28 Urogynecology and Reconstructive Pelvic Surgery

Cara L. Grimes and Stuart Shippey

Urogynecology is the subspecialty of obstetrics and gynecology that addresses all aspects of pelvic floor dysfunction in women.

NORMAL BLADDER FUNCTION

- **Anatomy.** The bladder is both an elastic-muscular reservoir and a pump for urination. The urethra serves as the conduit, but micturition requires coordination of urethral and bladder functions. Urethral muscular components which affect urinary continence include an outer layer of striated muscle arranged in a circular pattern (external urethral sphincter [EUS]). Internal to the striated component of the urethral sphincter is a circular layer of smooth muscle, which in turn surrounds a well-developed layer of inner longitudinal muscle (internal urethral sphincter [IUS]). Deep to these layers is a prominent vascular plexus that is believed to contribute to continence by forming a watertight seal via coaptation of the mucosal surfaces. Distally the fibers of the compressor urethrae pass over the urethra to insert into the urogenital diaphragm near the pubic ramus. Urethral function is also impacted by the relatively static supportive layer beneath the vesical neck, which provides a backstop against which the urethra is compressed during increased intra-abdominal pressure.
- **Neurophysiology of the lower urinary tract** (Table 28-1).
- **Micturition cycle.** The bladder has two basic functions: storing urine (sympathetic) and, when socially appropriate, evacuating urine (parasympathetic). Bladder filling occurs with relaxation of the detrusor muscle and contraction of the IUS. With bladder filling, afferent activity via baroreceptors triggers the storage reflex to maintain sympathetic tone in the IUS. When the bladder is full, afferent activity in the pelvic nerve stimulates the micturition reflex.

LOWER URINARY TRACT SYMPTOMS (LUTS) AND OVERACTIVE BLADDER

Disorders of the lower urinary tract can be categorized as abnormalities of bladder storage or emptying:
- **Frequency**—The complaint by the patient that she voids too often.
- **Urgency**—The complaint of a sudden compelling desire to pass urine which is difficult to defer.

TABLE 28-1	Neuroanatomy of the Bladder and Urethra	
Muscle	**Innervation**	**Neurotransmitter receptors**
External urethral sphincter (EUS)	Perineal branch of pudendal nerve	Nicotinic acetylcholine
Internal urethral sphincter (IUS)	Sympathetic fibers from hypogastric plexus	Muscarinic acetylcholine, alpha- and beta-adrenergic, and others
Detrusor relaxation	Sympathetic fibers	Beta-adrenergic
Detrusor contraction	Parasympathetic fibers from sacral plexus	Muscarinic acetylcholine

Adapted from de Groat WC. Integrative control of the lower urinary tract: preclinical perspective. *Br J Pharmacol* 2006;147(S2):S25–S40.

- **Nocturia**—The complaint that the individual has to wake at night one or more times to void.
- **Nocturnal enuresis**—The complaint of loss of urine occurring during sleep.

Overactive Bladder

- **Overactive bladder (OAB)** is a clinical diagnosis used to describe bothersome symptoms of urinary urgency with daytime frequency or nocturia. OAB often results from inappropriate detrusor contraction. When spontaneous or provoked involuntary detrusor contractions are demonstrated on urodynamic testing, OAB is referred to as **detrusor overactivity (DO)**. DO may be neurogenic or idiopathic.

Medical Management of OAB

- Oral and transdermal medications are available (Table 28-2).
  - **Anticholinergics** inhibit involuntary detrusor contractions. Oxybutynin (Ditropan) and tolterodine (Detrol) are first line for OAB and do not differ in outcomes. Common side effects associated with oxybutynin include dry mouth, constipation, blurred vision, and gastritis. Tolterodine tartrate is more selective for muscarinic receptors in the bladder and better tolerated than oxybutynin. The most common side effects include constipation, interaction with warfarin, mental status changes, and dry mouth. For both medications, long-acting varieties are better tolerated but more expensive.
    - Newly introduced anticholinergic medications with potentially fewer side effects are now available. Trospium (Sanctura) is hydrophilic, and theoretically does not cross the blood-brain barrier, limiting central nervous system side effects. Darifenacin (Enablex) and solifenacin (Vesicare) are thought to cause less frequent dry mouth, a principal reason for noncompliance with treatment.
  - **Tricyclic antidepressants.** Imipramine improves bladder hypertonicity and compliance, suppressing involuntary detrusor contractions.

Behavioral Management of OAB

- Several behavioral strategies can help with DO.
  - **Bladder retraining drills** involve scheduled voiding with progressive increases in the interval between voids.

TABLE 28-2	Pharmacologic Treatment of Lower Urinary Tract Symptoms and Overactive Bladder	
Medication	**Dosage**	**Use**
Tolterodine immediate release	1–2 mg PO every 12 hr	OAB
Tolterodine long acting	2–4 mg PO once daily	OAB
Oxybutynin	2.5–10 mg PO every 8 hr	OAB
Oxybutynin extended release	5–30 mg PO once daily	OAB
Transdermal oxybutinin	3.9 mg/d patch; change twice weekly	OAB
Trospium	20 mg PO once or twice daily	OAB
Solifenacin	5–10 mg PO once daily	OAB
Darifenacin	7.5–15 mg PO once daily	OAB
Imipramine	25 mg PO 1–4 times daily	OAB, SUI, mixed UI, nocturnal enuresis
Flavoxate	100–200 mg PO every 6–8 hr	OAB, cystitis
Propantheline bromide	15–30 mg PO every 6–8 hr	Urinary nonobstructive retention
Duloxetine	20–80 mg once daily	SUI

OAB, overactive bladder; SUI, stress urinary incontinence; UI, urinary incontinence.

- **Biofeedback** is a form of patient reeducation in which a closed feedback loop is created so that one or more of the patient's normally unconscious physiologic processes is made accessible to her by auditory, visual, or tactile signals.
- **Pelvic floor muscle exercise (PFME),** requiring repeated voluntary pelvic floor muscle training (Kegel exercises), is more effective when associated with bladder training.
- **Functional electrical stimulation** and **weighted vaginal cones** are other alternatives that may be combined with the above modalities.

Surgical Management of OAB
- Surgical management of DO is reserved for intractable cases that have already failed multiple attempts at nonsurgical management. Procedures include **sacral nerve root neuromodulation, augmentation cystoplasty**, and **urinary diversion** via an ileal conduit. There is level I evidence supporting intradetrusor **botulinum toxin injections** in women with neurogenic and idiopathic urge incontinence; however, there is a high rate of associated urinary retention.

URINARY INCONTINENCE (UI)

The International Continence Society (ICS) defines **UI** as any involuntary leakage of urine. When a woman presents complaining of urinary leakage, this is a symptom of UI and should be distinguished from the sign of incontinence and from the diagnosis of UI, which has an extensive differential diagnosis. Although multiple etiologies exist for UI, the symptom falls into one of three types: **stress, urge,** and **mixed incontinence**. These types can present alone or in combination.

Types of Urinary Incontinence

- Urodynamic stress incontinence, or **stress urinary incontinence (SUI)**, is now the preferred term to "genuine stress incontinence." SUI is the most common type of UI among ambulatory incontinent women, accounting for 50% to 70% of cases. SUI occurs when abdominal pressure exceeds bladder pressure, for example, with coughing, sneezing, or laughing.
  - **Urethral hypermobility** is thought to occur due to loss of integrity of the fibromuscular tissue that supports the bladder neck and urethra.
  - **Intrinsic sphincter deficiency (ISD)** is diagnosed when the sphincteric mechanism is compromised and fails to close the urethrovesical junction. These patients are often severely incontinent.
- **Urge UI** is involuntary leakage accompanied by or immediately preceded by the urge to void. Many patients complain of inability to reach the toilet in time. Involuntary detrusor contractions are typically the cause.
- **Mixed incontinence** describes symptoms of both stress and urge incontinence.
- **Functional incontinence** is associated with cognitive, psychological, or physical impairments that make it difficult to reach the toilet, or interfere with appropriate toileting. A useful mnemonic is DIAPPERS: **D**elirium, **I**nfection, **A**trophy, **P**harmacology, **P**sychology, **E**ndocrinopathy, **R**estricted mobility, and **S**tool impaction.
- **Bypass incontinence** may be caused by urogenital fistulae or by congenital or acquired anatomic abnormalities.
  - In the United States, gynecologic surgery is the most common cause of a **urogenital fistula** (complicating 0.1% of hysterectomies). Other causes include radiation, trauma, and severe pelvic pathology. In developing countries, obstetric injuries are the most common cause. Patients often report painless and continuous vaginal leakage of urine, usually within the context of recent pelvic surgery (1 to 2 weeks).
    - **Evaluation.** Instillation of methylene blue dye into the bladder will stain a vaginal pack if a vesicovaginal fistula is present. Cystourethroscopy should be performed to determine the site and number of fistulae. Intravenous pyelography (IVP) or CT scan should be performed to locate ureterovaginal fistula.
    - **Treatment.** Postsurgical fistulae are usually repaired 3 to 6 months after diagnosis to allow inflammation to resolve and to attain optimal tissue vascularity. The Latzko procedure is most commonly used. Treatment of ureterovaginal fistulae depends on location. If close to the ureterovesical junction, ureteroneocystostomy can be performed. A psoas bladder hitch or Boari flap can be used to alleviate tension on this anastomosis.
  - **Ectopic ureter** may occur anywhere in the lower urinary tract but is more commonly opening to the urethra and is associated with urinary tract infections (UTIs) secondary to reflux.
  - **Suburethral diverticulum** is a fluid-filled mass along the anterior portion of the vagina in direct communication with the urethra. Presenting complaints often include dysuria and trouble voiding.

Risk Factors for UI

- **Gender.** UI is more common in women than in men.
- **Race.** Epidemiologic studies have not consistently demonstrated any racial difference in the prevalence of UI.
- **Age.** Bladder capacity, ability to postpone voiding, bladder compliance, and urinary flow rate decrease with age in both sexes; however, frequency, urgency, and incontinence are not a normal result of aging.
- **Hypoestrogenism.** Estrogen deficiency can result in urogenital atrophy with resultant thinning of the submucosa and a decrease in the functional urethral length. However, randomized trials have shown no association between estrogen deficiency and UI.
- **Parity.** The incidence of UI is higher among parous than nulliparous women.
- **Childbirth.** Damage to the pelvic tissues during a vaginal delivery is thought to be a key factor in the development of SUI and other pelvic support abnormalities, which is especially significant with operative delivery. Nevertheless, cesarean section has not been shown to be protective and pregnancy in and of itself may be detrimental to the pelvic floor, regardless of the route of delivery.
- **Underlying medical conditions** such as diabetes, obesity, dementia, stroke, depression, Parkinson's, or multiple sclerosis are risk factors for UI.
- **Previous pelvic surgery** with resultant scar formation.
- **Pharmacologic agents,** such as diuretics, caffeine, anticholinergics, and alpha-adrenergic blockers, may affect urinary tract function.
- Chronically **increased intra-abdominal pressure** (COPD, chronic constipation, obesity) is a risk factors for UI.

Diagnosis of UI

History and Physical Examination

- In addition to taking a thorough medical, surgical, gynecologic, and obstetric history, the clinician should gain an understanding of the duration, frequency, severity, precipitating factors, social impact, effect on hygiene, effect on quality of life, and measures used to avoid leaking in patients with UI.
  - **Urinary diary.** The patient records the volume and frequency of fluid intake and voiding as well as symptoms of frequency and urgency and episodes of incontinence for 1 to 7 days.
- A comprehensive **physical examination** should be performed at the first visit, including
  - Because UI may be the presenting symptom of neurologic disease, a screening **neurologic examination** to evaluate mental status and sensory and motor function of the lower extremities. Anal sphincter tone reflects pelvic floor innervation (i.e., pudendal nerve).
  - The **pelvic exam** includes a systematic evaluation of all components of the pelvic floor, including innervation, vulvar architecture, muscular and connective tissue support, and perineal scars. Particular attention should be given to urethral anatomy, exudate, diverticulum, and hypermobility (see Q-tip test below).
    - **Speculum exam,** using a Sims speculum or the posterior blade of a Graves speculum, is helpful to assess support and the presence of scarring.
    - The **bimanual exam** investigates the location, size, and tenderness of the bladder, uterus, cervix, and adnexa. The strength of the levator ani muscles is assessed by placing one or two fingers in the vagina and asking the patient to squeeze. The firm muscular sling of the posterior puborectalis should be readily palpable.

- **Sacral nerve roots** and the **sacral reflex** (also called the bulbocavernosus reflex) should be evaluated. If afferent and efferent pathways are intact, when the clitoris or the area lateral to the anus is lightly scratched, an ipsilateral contraction of the anal sphincter should occur. In older patients, this reflex may be absent.
- The **Q-tip test** evaluates urethral support. A cotton swab is placed in the urethra to the level of the vesical neck, and the change in axis on straining is measured with a goniometer to assess urethral hypermobility. Angular measurements of >30 degrees are generally considered abnormal.
- A **rectal examination** can further assess pelvic pathology as well as evaluate the presence of fecal impaction.
- A positive result on a **stress test** is essential to the diagnosis of SUI. The stress test is performed by looking for urine leakage from the urethral meatus when abdominal pressure is increased. It can be done while standing or in the dorsal lithotomy position and is very specific for SUI. False-negative results can be explained by low bladder volume or patient cooperation.

Diagnostic Tests
- UTI should be ruled out by microscopic analysis, urinalysis, or urine culture.
- **Postvoid residual (PVR)**—measurement can aid in diagnosing overflow incontinence and eliminating it from the differential diagnosis. It should be <100 mL.
- **Cystourethroscopy** is used to assess the anatomy and function of the lower urinary tract.
- **Urodynamic studies** can be used to assess the physiologic function of the bladder. Simple cystometric testing can be performed in the office using a straight catheter and syringe to fill the bladder with a known volume of sterile water. At maximum capacity, the patient is asked to cough and Valsalva in an attempt to demonstrate SUI or induce a detrusor contraction.

Treatment of SUI

- **Pharmacologic.** The limited available medications for SUI are aimed toward increasing urethrovaginal sphincter tone (see Table 28-2).
- **Pelvic muscle exercise.** Limited long-term prospective studies of this low risk intervention suggest effectiveness, which is dependent on patient adherence.
- **Continence pessaries.** In a prospective study following women successfully fitted with pessaries for pelvic organ prolapse (POP), after 2 months SUI improved in 45% of women.
- **Surgery.** The etiology of SUI may be multifactorial and may not always be able to be corrected by surgery. Reported cure rates vary widely, often depending on parameters used to define cure of SUI. The two basic techniques currently used for the treatment of SUI are the retropubic colposuspension and the suburethral sling.

Surgical Procedures for SUI
- **Cystocele repair** was described by Howard Kelly in 1913 as a surgical treatment for SUI. The objective cure rate of cystocele repair for SUI has been shown to be significantly lower than that of Burch colposuspension, and should be considered for treatment of anterior vaginal prolapse and not SUI.
- **Retropubic urethropexy** procedures are indicated for women with SUI and a hypermobile proximal urethra and bladder neck.
  - The **Burch retropubic colposuspension** is a well-established surgery for SUI. Permanent sutures are placed in the fibromuscular tissue lateral to the bladder

neck and proximal urethra, and the urethrovesical junction is supported by attaching the suture to the ileopectineal line (i.e., Cooper's ligament). Reported 5-year success rates have been over 80%.

- The **Marshall-Marchetti-Krantz** procedure supports the bladder neck and urethra similar to the Burch, except the permanent stitches are placed through the periosteum of the pubic symphysis instead of Cooper's ligament. This technique is seldom used now due to the risk of osteitis pubis.

- **Suburethral slings** are performed to support the urethra or bladder neck in a hammock providing static stabilization of the urethra at rest and dynamic compression of the urethra with increased abdominal pressure. Suburethral slings can be created using various biologic and synthetic materials.
  - **Tension-free vaginal tape (TVT).** A polypropylene mesh is placed without tension at the midurethra through the retropubic space. Cystoscopy is warranted. Bladder perforation is the most common complication (5%), with bowel or vascular injuries being the most serious complications (both <1%). Other risks include graft exposure and urinary retention. Success rates are similar for the use of TVT and the use of Burch colposuspension.
  - **Tension-free obturator tape (TOT).** The TOT is passed through a midurethral vaginal incision medial to the obturator foramen instead of through the retropubic space.

- **Urethral bulking agent injections** are appropriate in patients with ISD or refractory UI in the absence of urethral hypermobility. Complications are less frequent than with other surgical techniques for treating SUI but include transient urinary retention, irritative voiding, and UTI. While most patients have symptomatic improvement, recurrence of symptoms within months is been common.

URINARY RETENTION

- **Neurogenic bladder** is involuntary retention of urine associated with overdistention of the bladder due to bladder atonicity. Patients have absent or delayed sensation to void, increased bladder capacity, and high PVRs. The patient may be incontinent with dribbling, hesitancy, frequency, and nocturia. The condition is frequently associated with diabetes and neurologic diseases.
- **Detrusor sphincter dyssynergia** is a specific type of neurogenic bladder in which there is a lack of coordination between bladder contraction and urethral sphincter relaxation.
- **Bladder outlet obstruction**—may occur as a result of previous anti-incontinence surgery, urethral diverticulum, anterior vaginal wall prolapse, or malignancy.
- **Treatment for urinary retention.**
  - **Intermittent self-catheterization** is safe and can be used for transient or long-term conditions.
  - **Pessaries**. In women fitted with pessaries for prolapse, after 2 months 50% of urinary symptoms improved, but occult SUI (SUI with prolapse reduction) was a common side effect.
  - **Urethrolysis** can be performed after anti-incontinence surgery has resulted in voiding dysfunction and urinary retention secondary to obstruction.
  - **Sacral root neuromodulation** is approved for idiopathic voiding dysfunction.
  - **Resection of urethral diverticula** usually results in relief of obstructive or irritative voiding symptoms.

PAINFUL BLADDER SYNDROME (PBS)

Formerly known as **interstitial cystitis (IC)**, **PBS** is a chronic inflammatory condition with irritative voiding symptoms of urgency, frequency, pelvic, and lower urinary tract pain (70% of cases). Dyspareunia, sleep disturbance, and UI may be present. The prevalence of PBS in the United States is 5 to 500 per 100,000. PBS is more common in young, Caucasian (91%) women in their 40s. It is a frequent cause of chronic pelvic pain. See Chapter 27.

- The clinical presentation is highly variable. Irritative urinary symptoms initially dominate, but they are replaced by pain in the long-term.
- PBS is a **clinical diagnosis** of exclusion. The initial evaluation should be oriented to identify other causes of the patient's symptoms. Characteristic findings on cystoscopy include urothelial glomerulations (i.e., petechiae) after hydrodistension.
- **Treatment** is oriented to symptom control because no cure currently exists.
  - **Pharmacologic:** The best results have been obtained with multiple drug therapy. Oral combinations of pentosan polysulfate and hydroxyzine or triple therapy with pentosan, hydroxyzine and amitriptyline have shown success but may require prolonged treatment.
  - **Diet modification** has been useful for specific patients.
  - **Support groups** are helpful.
  - **Bladder instillation therapy.** This may need to be repeated weekly for up to 6 weeks before significant improvement is seen.
  - **Hydrodistention.** Cystoscopy with hydrodistention should be considered in cases refractory to treatment or when the diagnosis is not clear. About 90% of patients with PBS will show glomerulations.
  - **Other novel treatments** are botulinum toxin injection and sacral root neuromodulation.

PELVIC ORGAN PROLAPSE

Pelvic organ prolapse (POP) is defined as protrusion of the pelvic organs into or out of the vaginal canal. More specifically, POP refers to loss of support of the anterior or posterior vaginal wall or the vaginal apex, which permits the bladder, rectum, small bowel, sigmoid colon, or uterus to protrude into the vagina or, in its most severe form, through the vaginal introitus. POP includes anterior vaginal prolapse (previously known as cystocele), apical or uterine prolapse, and posterior vaginal prolapse (previously known as rectocele, enterocele, and perineal descent). It does not include rectal prolapse.

- POP is the indication for more than 300,000 surgeries annually in the United States, at a cost of $1 billion. Up to 11% of women have surgery for POP or related conditions by the age of 80 years. Twenty nine per cent of cases have a repeat surgery.

Etiology of Pelvic Floor Damage

- Pelvic floor damage may occur when normal pelvic organ supports are chronically subjected to increased intra-abdominal pressure. Pelvic floor damage is often associated with UI and occasionally with urinary retention or bowel dysfunction.
- Most women with severe POP have multiple risks which can be categorized as predisposing, inciting, promoting, and decompensating (Table 28-3). The multifactorial etiology helps explain why women with support defects following vaginal delivery frequently do not become symptomatic until later in life.

TABLE 28-3	Risk Factors for Pelvic Organ Prolapse		
Predisposing	**Inciting**	**Promoting**	**Decompensating**
Congenital defect	Pregnancy	Occupational/	Aging
Acquired tissue	Parity	recreational	Debilitation/
abnormalities	Denervation	Chronic abdominal	immobility
Race	Surgery	pressure	Menopause
Previous POP	Hysterectomy	Smoking	Myopathy
repair		Constipation	Neuropathy
		Obesity	
		Lung disease	

Adapted from Bump RC, Norton PA. Epidemiology and natural history of pelvic floor dysfunction. *Obstet Gynecol Clin North Am* 1998;25:723–746.

- The association of vaginal parity with POP implicates obstetric trauma as an etiology. Women with >1 vaginal delivery have a twofold increased risk, whereas women with >4 deliveries have an 11-fold risk for POP. Cesarean section appears to be protective if performed without labor. Data also suggest that pregnancy itself may injure endopelvic fascial support.
- History of previous surgical procedures for POP is a strong predictor for new pelvic support defects. Recurrence after POP surgical repair is between 10% and 30%.
- Patients with muscular dystrophy, myelodysplasia, meningomyelocele, spina bifida, and bladder exstrophy may develop POP more frequently.
- Other risk factors are similar to those for UI and include increasing age, hypoestrogenic states, high impact occupational and recreational activities, chronic illnesses or treatments that raise intra-abdominal pressure, and Caucasian race.

Specific Support Defects
- **Uterovaginal prolapse** occurs secondary to damage of the cardinal-uterosacral ligament complex.
- **Vaginal vault prolapse** refers to descent of the vaginal apex in a woman who has had a hysterectomy and is usually associated with an enterocele. The turning completely inside out of the vagina is called vaginal eversion or procidentia.
- **Anterior wall defects (cystoceles)** are present when descent of the anterior vaginal wall occurs. They are caused by separation of the paravaginal attachment of the pubocervical fascia from the arcus tendineus fascia pelvis or by tearing in the pubocervical fascial sheet, resulting in herniation of the bladder into the vagina. See Chapter 23 for anatomy.
- **Posterior wall defects (rectoceles)** occur at lateral, superior, and inferior attachments, as well as within the rectovaginal fascia itself, resulting in herniation of the rectum or small bowel into the posterior wall of the vagina.
- **Enterocele** is the result of detachment of the rectovaginal septum at the level of uterosacral ligaments, with small bowel filling the hernia sac between rectum and vagina.
- **Perineal descent** occurs when the perineal body becomes detached from the rectovaginal septum and becomes mobile (>2 cm).

Evaluation and Diagnosis

- The clinical evaluation focuses on eliciting the patient's complaints, defining the location and severity of support defects, and eliminating other potential etiologies of pelvic floor symptoms.
- Symptoms can be grouped into four main categories, which are directly related to the prolapse or may result from the prolapse:
  - **Bulge.** Patients may complain of pelvic pressure, heaviness, protruding tissues, bulging, and pelvic or back pain.
  - **Voiding dysfunction.** Patients may have symptoms associated with urethral obstruction secondary to prolapse, especially with anterior compartment prolapse. They may have urinary hesitancy, incomplete emptying, or the need for splinting, Valsalva, or prolapse reduction before successfully passing urine. Patients may have associated recurrent or persistent UTIs secondary to urinary retention. They may also demonstrate irritative voiding symptoms such as urgency, frequency, and urge incontinence. They may demonstrate occult stress incontinence when prolapse is reduced (e.g., after surgery or with pessary placement).
  - **Defecatory dysfunction.** Patients may have symptoms with defecation, especially with apical and posterior compartment prolapse. These include symptoms of incomplete defecation, required splinting or straining, pain with defecation, and anal incontinence (AI) of flatus, liquid, or formed stool.
  - **Altered sexual functioning.** Patients may complain of dyspareunia, avoidance of intercourse, decreased libido, and decreased self image.
- There are many validated and reliable surveys that can aid in eliciting a symptom history from patients, such as the Pelvic Floor Distress Inventory, the Pelvic Floor Impact Questionnaire, and the POP and Incontinence Sexual function Questionnaire.
- **Differential diagnosis.** Pelvic support defects are rarely localized to one anatomic compartment and are often multifactorial (Table 28-4). Of all complaints, herniation symptoms are the most specific for POP.
- **Physical examination.** To evaluate POP, four specific anatomic components should be assessed: (a) anterior vaginal wall, (b) uterus and vaginal apex, (c) posterior vaginal wall, and (d) presence or absence of an enterocele.
  - These compartments should be assessed both subjectively and objectively with a standardized system such as the Pelvic Organ Prolapse Quantification (POPQ) system. Additionally, pelvic muscle function should be assessed objectively with the Brink scale.
  - Examination of the anterior vaginal wall should evaluate the support of the urethra and bladder. With a speculum (or half of the speculum) used to depress the posterior vaginal wall, the patient is asked to strain, and any descent of the anterior vaginal wall is noted. Then, ring forceps, or a tongue depressor, may be used to support the anterior vaginal wall at midline to evaluate the support of the lateral sulci. Bulging limited to the lateral sulci indicates defects caused by lateral detachments of the pubocervical fascia from the arcus tendineus fascia pelvis (i.e., **paravaginal defects**).
  - Isolated evaluation of the posterior vaginal wall demonstrates rectoceles and enteroceles. With a speculum retracting the anterior vaginal wall, the posterior wall of the vagina can be inspected. A **rectocele** is present when the posterior vaginal wall and underlying rectum protrude toward the hymenal ring on straining. Rectovaginal examination helps demonstrate anterior displacement of the anterior-rectal wall. An **enterocele** is suspected with a bulging of the apical posterior vaginal wall

TABLE 28-4 Differential Diagnosis for Prolapse-Associated Symptoms

Symptom Group	Symptom	Differential Diagnosis
Herniation symptoms	Pelvic pressure Vaginal protrusion	Rectal prolapse

Voiding symptoms	Urinary hesitancy
	Incomplete emptying
	
	Required splinting
		Detrusor dysfunction
		Detrusor sphincter
		  dyssynergia
		Behavioral voiding
		  disorders

Lower urinary tract symptoms	Urinary frequency Urinary urgency Dysuria	Overactive bladder Excessive fluid intake Interstitial cystitis Urinary tract infection
Urinary incontinence	Urinary incontinence	Stress incontinence Detrusor overactivity
Defecatory dysfunction	Dyschezia Incomplete defecation Required splinting	Irritable bowel syndrome Colonic inertia Anismus
Fecal incontinence	Fecal urgency Fecal incontinence	Irritable bowel syndrome Diarrhea External anal sphincter dysfunction
Sexual dysfunction	Dyspareunia	Levator ani syndrome Libido dysfunction

Adapted from Cundiff GW. An 80-year-old woman with vaginal prolapse. *JAMA* 2005;293:2018–2027.

outward or when peristalsis is seen. On rectovaginal examination, small bowel can be palpated between the vagina and rectum with the patient straining.

- The ICS, American Urogynecologic Society, Society of Gynecologic Surgeons, and the National Institutes of Health recommend the standardized **POPQ** system for grading support defects (Fig. 28-1; Table 28-5). Many staging systems exist, but the POPQ system is widely accepted, easily learned, and reproducible.
  - The POPQ uses the hymen as a fixed point of reference and describes six specific topographic points on the vaginal walls (Aa, Ba, C, D, Bp, and Ap) and three distances (genital hiatus, perineal body, total vaginal length).
  - The prolapse of each segment is measured in centimeters during Valsalva relative to the hymenal ring with points inside the vagina reported as negative numbers and outside as positive. The numeric values are then translated to a stage as described in Table 28-5.
  - The perineal body is normally at the level of the ischial tuberosities. Descent of >2 cm below this level with flattening of the intergluteal sulcus indicates **perineal descent.**
- To fully evaluate POP, the patient may need to perform a Valsalva maneuver in lithotomy or strain while seated or standing while being examined by the provider. Pelvic floor muscle strength can be assessed, as outlined above.

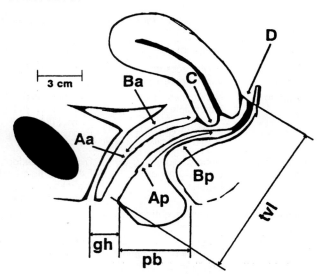

Figure 28-1. The Pelvic Organ Proplase Quantification (POPQ) system components and anatomic reference points. For explanation of terms, see Table 28-5. (From Bent AE, Ostergard DR, Cundiff GW, et al., eds. *Ostergard's Urogynecology and Pelvic Floor Dysfunction,* 5th Ed. Philadelphia: Lippincott Williams & Wilkins, 2003:97, with permission.)

- **Diagnostic tests** (e.g., urodynamics, cystoscopy, MRI) should be considered if the patient's symptoms could be consistent with another cause.

Treatment of POP

- The goal of treatment for POP is relief symptoms. The three therapeutic categories are expectant management, nonsurgical, and surgical.
- Although **expectant management** seems contradictory, it is not unreasonable for mildly symptomatic POP, especially given the reported 1-year regression rate of 48% for uterine POP and reoperation rate of up to 30%. Providers can offer reassurance that treatment is available if and when prolapse becomes bothersome. Risks of expectant management include UTI and vaginal mucosal erosion.
- The **nonsurgical approach** is especially useful in patients with a mild degree of prolapse, who desire future childbearing, have frail health, or are unwilling to undergo surgery.
  - **Pelvic muscle exercises** can alleviate the symptoms of prolapse. Kegel originally proposed the exercises that bear his name as a method to strengthen pelvic support.
  - **Pessaries.** The two basic types are supportive (most commonly a ring, with or without support) and space occupying (most commonly a Gellhorn). Pessaries can decrease symptom frequency and severity and delay or avoid surgery. Treatment with estrogen, either locally or systemically, helps the vaginal mucosa tolerate the foreign body. Because pessaries can cause vaginal wall erosion or ulceration and fistula formation, patients should be examined periodically. Complications

TABLE 28-5	Description and Staging of the POPQ System
Point/Distance	**Description**
Aa	Midline anterior vaginal wall, 3 cm proximal to the urethral meatus
Ba	Anterior vaginal wall, most distal point between Aa and anterior fornix (cuff)
C	Edge of the cervix (or vaginal cuff in posthysterectomy patients)
D	Posterior fornix. Not used in patients with hysterectomy
Ap	Midline posterior vaginal wall, 3 cm proximal to the hymenal ring
Bp	Posterior vaginal wall, most distal point between Ap and posterior fornix (cuff)
Genital hiatus	Middle of the urethral meatus to posterior midline hymenal ring
Perineal body	Posterior margin of genital hiatus to the middle anus
Total vaginal length	Greatest depth of vagina with C or D reduced to its normal position
Staging of the POPQ System	
Stage 0	Perfect support; Aa, Ap at −3. C or D within 2 cm of TVL from introitus.
Stage 1	Most distal portion of prolapse is −1 (or more negative) proximal to introitus.
Stage 2	Most distal portion within 1 cm of the hymenal ring (between −1 and +1).
Stage 3	Most distal portion >+1 cm but <(TVL-2) cm distal to introitus.
Stage 4	Complete prolapse; most distal portion between TVL and (TVL-2) cm distal to introitus.

are minimized by avoiding excessive pressure on the vaginal epithelium and by emphasizing proper pessary care, including regular surveillance, cleansing, and the use of estrogen replacement therapy. Poor candidates for pessary use include those who are unable to clean their pessaries, those who come for routine cleaning visits, and patients with a large genital hiatus.

- The goal of **surgery** is relief of prolapse symptoms. Overcorrection must be avoided because it can lead to new support problems. Although the uterus itself does not contribute to POP, many surgeons feel that removing the uterus concomitantly with repair maximizes the opportunity to correct apical support. The three categories of POP repair are obliterative, restorative, and compensatory (Table 28-6).

Surgical Procedures for POP

- Obliterative procedures include **colpocleisis** and **colpectomy**. They are useful for patients in frail health. A **partial colpocleisis (LeFort)** involves leaving the uterus in place with lateral drainage channels for cervical secretions. In a **total colpectomy,**

TABLE 28-6	Reconstructive Pelvic Surgeries by Anatomic Site and Type of Repair		
Site	**Compensatory**	**Restorative**	**Obliterative**
Vaginal apex	Abdominal sacrocolpopexy	Iliococcygeus suspension Sacrospinous fixation McCall's culdoplasty	Lefort colpocleisis Partial colpocleisis
Anterior vaginal wall	Anterior fascial replacement	Anterior colporrhaphy Defect-directed repair Paravaginal repair	Colpectomy
Posterior vaginal wall	Posterior fascial replacement	Posterior colporrhaphy Defect-directed repair Enterocele repair Perineal reconstruction	

the vaginal epithelium is removed and the vault is closed in sequential purse-string closure.
- Preoperative evaluation should include a Pap smear, pelvic sonogram, endometrial biopsy, and an understanding that the procedure precludes sexual intercourse. Cure rates for colpocleisis range from 86% to 100%, with the most common complication being SUI (9%) and regret (5% to 10%).
- **Sacrospinous ligament suspension** anchors the vaginal apex to the sacrospinous ligament. This approach is faster, less expensive, and is associated with earlier return to daily activities than the abdominal approach. There are high rates of anterior vaginal prolapse, thought to be due to the pronounced posterior deviation of the vaginal axis (37%). There is a 63% to 97% success rate. Complications include hemorrhage, nerve injury, stress incontinence, dyspareunia, and buttock pain.
- **Iliococcygeus fascial suspension**, performed in patients who have suboptimal uterosacral ligaments, attaches the vaginal apex to the iliococcygeal fascia just below the ischial spine.
- **Uterosacral ligament suspension** with fascial reconstruction suspends the apex of the vagina to the uterosacral ligaments. There is an 80% to 100% success rate. Complications include ureteral kinking.
- **Anterior colporrhaphy** reduces the protrusion of the bladder and vagina. In this procedure, layers of the vaginal muscularis and pubocervical fascia are plicated. The 5-year success rate is 30% to 40%.
- **Defect-directed repair** is a procedure in which isolated defects in the pubocervical fascia are identified and reapproximated, so that normal anatomy is restored.
- **Paravaginal repair** is performed for anterior vaginal wall prolapse and is a type of defect-directed repair. Reattaching the anterolateral vaginal attachments, and the

endopelvic fascia, to the arcus tendineus fascia pelvis is the goal. There is a 76% to 96% success rate.

- **Posterior colporrhaphy** is the plication of the pararectal and rectovaginal fascia over the rectal wall. A common complication is dyspareunia.
- **Defect-directed repairs** isolate defects in the rectovaginal fascia and reapproximate normal anatomy.
- **Perineorrhaphy** is the reconstruction of the elements of the perineal body. The goal is to build up the perineum and decrease genital hiatus caliber, but it has been associated with subsequent dyspareunia.
- Enterocele repair/prophylaxis procedures include the following:
  - The **Moschcowitz procedure** (abdominal) is performed by placing concentric purse-string sutures around the cul-de-sac, including the posterior vaginal wall, right pelvic sidewall, the serosa of the sigmoid, and the left pelvic side wall.
  - The **Halban procedure** (abdominal) obliterates the cul-de-sac via longitudinally placed sutures between the uterosacral ligaments.
  - Transverse **plication of the uterosacral ligaments** (abdominal) can also be used to obliterate the cul-de-sac.
  - In **McCall's culdoplasty** (vaginal) procedure, an enterocele is surgically corrected at the time of a vaginal hysterectomy. Some recommend this procedure with all vaginal hysterectomies.
- Circumstances occur in which surgeries that use native tissues may be insufficient, and a **compensatory procedure** is indicated. This usually means supplementing the native tissues with grafts. Grafts can be harvested from native fascia, or purchased commercially as synthetic materials, allografts, and xenografts.
  - The compensatory repair for apical POP is the **abdominal sacral colpopexy (ASC)**, which replaces the normal apical support with interposition of a suspensory bridge between the prolapsed or everted vagina and the anterior sacral promontory.
    - Success rates are 95% to 100%, both for correction of the anatomic deficits as well as relief of associated symptoms. It has a lower rate of recurrence, dyspareunia, and is more durable than other restorative procedures. Its complications include rare intraoperative hemorrhage and a 3% to 4% prevalence of vaginal mesh erosion.
  - The **sacral colpoperineopexy** is a modification of the sacral colpopexy developed to treat perineal descent with concurrent posterior and apical POP.
  - Anterior and posterior **vaginal wall fascial replacement**. Various graft materials and meshes have been used to try and strengthen repairs. The purpose of the graft is often twofold: via replacing the fascia and acting as an absorbable "collagen scaffold" for fibroblast infiltration and scar formation. If the repair is too tight, the loss of flexibility can lead to fecal urgency and dyspareunia.
  - There are many mesh "kits" and grafts for anterior and posterior repairs and for apical suspension. There are ongoing trials looking at outcomes; currently, data are limited to short-term follow-up.

DISORDERS OF ANORECTAL FUNCTION

Anal Incontinence (AI)

- **AI** includes loss of voluntary control of flatus or stool. **Fecal incontinence (FI)** is the loss of control over solid or liquid stool. AI can be a psychologically devastating and socially incapacitating condition.

- The prevalence of AI has been estimated to range between 2% and 24%. Like UI, the prevalence of FI has consistently been observed to increase with age.
- Anal continence is the end result of orchestrated functioning of the cerebral cortex, along with sensory and motor fibers innervating the colon, rectum, anus, and pelvic floor. Anal sphincter disruption with childbirth and pudendal nerve damage that occurs with pelvic floor weakening both may impair normal continence physiology.
  - Known risk factors for AI include aging, trauma, increasing parity, menopause, obesity, neurologic conditions, colorectal disease, congenital anomalies, and history of SUI. The etiology usually is multifactorial.
- Detachment of the rectovaginal fascia from the perineal body can compromise the support of the perineum, resulting in perineal descent. Lacerations of the internal and external anal sphincters at the time of vaginal delivery, even following repair, can result in impaired sphincter strength and AI.

Evaluation and Diagnosis
- **Medical history.** Patients will rarely volunteer symptoms of AI; consequently, all women should be asked about AI, especially those at risk or with symptoms of UI, diarrhea, or constipation.
- **Specific physical examination** begins with inspection of the perineal area for evidence of skin irritation or stool on the skin. One should also note the presence of gaping levator ani muscles or scarring. A focused sensory and motor neurologic examination should be performed.
- Several **diagnostic techniques** may be helpful in the workup of AI:
  - **Enema.** If the patient can hold approximately 100 mL of a tap water enema for more than a few minutes, then AI is not severe.
  - **Anorectal manometry** provides quantitative information regarding sphincter squeeze strength and progress with biofeedback therapy.
  - **Endoanal ultrasonography.** The value of endoanal ultrasound lies in its ability to locate defects in the internal or external sphincter to facilitate planning for surgical correction.
  - **MRI** evaluates the pelvic floor and anal sphincter without radiation.
  - **Defecography.** During a defecating proctogram, the patient's pelvis is imaged using fluoroscopy as she defecates while sitting after an enema is used to infuse contrast material.
  - **Anoscopy, proctoscopy, sigmoidoscopy,** or **colonoscopy** is indicated in patients with diarrhea or bloody stool, especially when taking biopsies is necessary to exclude cancer or mucosal disease.

Treatment of AI
- **Nonsurgical treatment** should be attempted with all patients before surgical reconstruction. The first step is to eradicate treatable underlying causes, such as transient neurologic conditions, inflammatory bowel disease, fecal impaction, metabolic disorders, or inadequate diets.
  - **Environmental** adjustments are necessary to decrease social isolation and anxiety, and to improve quality of life.
  - **Skin care** is important to prevent associated morbidities.
  - **Pelvic muscle–strengthening exercises and behavioral therapy.** All patients should undergo a pelvic muscle–training program before contemplating surgery. Improvement is seen in 63% to 90% of patients.

- **Pharmacologic** agents that slow motility and reduce frequency (e.g., loperamide hydrochloride [Imodium], diphenoxylate hydrochloride [Lomotil]) may help some patients exercise more control over their stool.
- **Dietary change.** In patients who do not have severe incontinence, increasing ingestion of natural fiber or the use of bulking agents, such as psyllium preparations (Metamucil), can change the consistency of stool, making it firmer and more easily controlled. Reduced caffeine intake will decrease colonic motility.
- **Surgical.** Patients with FI should try nonsurgical treatment before pursuing surgical management. The procedures performed include **sphincteroplasty, muscle transposition** (neosphincter), **artificial sphincter implantation**, and **colonic diversion**. **Sacral neuromodulation** is being studied, but not yet FDA approved, as a potential surgical therapy for FI.

Defecatory Dysfunction (Abnormal Evacuation)

- The term **constipation** has limited clinical use due to its broad meaning. The term **defecatory dysfunction** is a preferable diagnostic term, which refers to any difficulty with defecation, excluding FI.
  - The definition of defecatory dysfunction is: frequency of bowel movements of two or less per week, incomplete evacuation, hard stools, and delayed colonic transit.
- Etiology is frequently multifactorial and may be caused by systemic, neurologic, or psychiatric disorders, dietary habits, and various medications.

Evaluation, Diagnosis, and Treatment

- **Physical exam.** The pelvic examination is performed in the dorsal lithotomy position but may be changed to evaluate in sitting or standing positions. The rectovaginal exam helps in the diagnosis of high enteroceles. The presence of fecal material in the anal canal may suggest fecal impaction or neuromuscular weakness.
- **Ancillary tests.** Include barium enema or colonoscopy, colonic transit studies, neurophysiologic testing, and defecography.
- Women with motility disorders are best treated with dietary or pharmacologic modalities. Pelvic support defects can be managed surgically (e.g., rectocele repair, perineorrhaphy, rectopexy), whereas pelvic floor dyssynergia responds best to pelvic floor physical therapy with biofeedback.

SUGGESTED READINGS

Albo ME, Richter HE, Brubaker L, et al. Burch colposuspension versus fascial sling to reduce urinary stress incontinence. *N Engl J Med* 2007;356(21):2143–2155.

Barber MD, Kleeman S, Karram MM, et al. Transobturator tape compared with tension-free vaginal tape for the treatment of stress urinary incontinence: a randomized controlled trial. *Obstet Gynecol* 2008;111(3):611–621.

Brubaker L, Cundiff GW, Fine P, et al. Abdominal sacrocolpopexy with Burch colposuspension to reduce urinary stress incontinence. *N Engl J Med* 2006;354:1557–1566.

Nygaard IE, Heit M. Stress urinary incontinence. *Obstet Gynecol* 2004;104:607–620.

Nygaard IE, McCreery R, Brubaker L, et al. Abdominal sacrocolpopexy: a comprehensive review. *Obstet Gynecol* 2004;104(4):805–823.

Ulmsten U, Henriksson L, Johnson P, et al. An ambulatory surgical procedure under local anesthesia for treatment of female urinary incontinence. *Int Urogynecol J Pelvic Floor Dysfunct* 1996;7(2):81–85; discussion 85–86.

29 Fertility Control: Contraception, Sterilization, and Abortion

S.J. Hanson and Anne E. Burke

Family planning is an integral part of the health care of women. Prevention of unplanned pregnancies and access to family planning services have been one of the greatest advances in health care in the 20th century. However, access to and information about contraception and family planning services does not reach all women. Political climate and issues of social justice, in the United States and especially in the developing world, limit reproductive health services to women. This affects maternal mortality rates, population growth, and the status of women in society.

CONTRACEPTIVE METHODS

- Ninety-eight percent of US women have used some form of contraception during their lives. Sixty-two percent women of reproductive age in the United States are currently using birth control methods.
- The leading method of contraception in the United States is the oral contraceptive pill, used by 11 million women, followed by female sterilization, used by 10 million. The intrauterine device (IUD) is commonly used in many countries around the world and is the most common form of contraception used among female OB/GYN physicians.
- An estimated 50% of pregnancies in the United States are unintended. In 60% of these unintended pregnancies, the women used some form of birth control during the month of conception.
- Dissatisfaction with, and inconsistent or incorrect use of the various methods of contraception may result in unintended pregnancies. In methods requiring patient compliance, effectiveness can be compromised by user error. Appropriate patient counseling and history are important in selection of contraception. This includes physical examination, medical history, consideration of ethical and religious concerns, the patient's short- and long-term childbearing plans, and prior contraceptive use history.
- See Table 29-1 for failure rates of various contraceptive methods.

Voluntary Sterilization

Tubal Ligation
- Tubal ligation is a surgical procedure in which the fallopian tubes are permanently occluded, preventing sperm from reaching the ovum and causing fertilization. The

TABLE 29-1	Efficacy of Various Contraceptive Methods	
	% with Unintended Pregnancy	
Method	**Typical Use**	**Perfect Use**
No method	85	85
Spermicides	29	18
Withdrawal	27	4
Periodic abstinence		
Calendar	25	9
Standard days method	12	5
Ovulation method	25	3
Symptothermal	25	2
Postovulation	25	1
Diaphragm with spermicide	16	6
Condom		
Female	21	5
Male	15	2
Pill (combined)	8	0.3
Mini-pill (progestin-only)[a]	13	1.1
Patch (Ortho Evra)	8	0.3
Vaginal ring (NuvaRing)	8	0.3
Depo Provera	3	0.3
Implant (Implanon)	0.05	0.05
IUD		
Copper T (ParaGard)	0.8	0.6
Levonorgestrel IUS (Mirena)	0.2	0.2
Female sterilization	0.5	0.5
Male sterilization	0.15	0.10

Values are the percentage of women who experience an unintended pregnancy within the first year of typical use and first year of perfect use for each listed method. From Trussell J. Contraceptive efficacy. In Hatcher RA, Trussell J, Nelson AL, et al., eds. *Contraceptive Technology: Nineteenth Revised Edition.* New York, NY: Ardent Media, 2007. [a]From McCann MF, Lotter LS. Progestin-only oral contraception: a comprehensive review. *Contraception* 1994;50:SI195.

procedure can be performed postpartum (within 48 hr postvaginal delivery), at the time of cesarean delivery, or as an interval procedure (>6 weeks postpartum) via laparoscopy.
- Technique for sterilization depends on timing of surgery and the surgeon. The Parkland and Pomeroy are the most common methods used for postpartum/intrapartum salpingectomy. Banding, clipping, or burning is used most commonly via the laparoscopic approach.
- Sterilization is highly effective with no long-term side effects.
- Tubal ligation decreases the risk of ovarian cancer. This may be due to decreased risk of ascending carcinogens from the fallopian tubes.
- Associated risks should be discussed with the patient. Sterilization requires anesthesia. Abdominal approaches should consider factors such as prior abdominal surgery and pelvic adhesive disease before being performed.
- Tubal ligation offers no protection against sexually transmitted diseases (STDs).

| TABLE 29-2 | Failure Rates for Female Sterilization Methods |

Method	% Pregnant in 10 years
Postpartum salpingectomy	0.75
Interval partial salpingectomy	2.0
Unipolar cautery	0.75
Bipolar cautery	2.48
Spring clip (Hulka clip)	3.65
Silastic bands (Falope ring)	1.77
Filshie clip[a]	0.9–1.2

Data from Peterson HB, Xia Z, Hughes JM, et al. for the U.S. Collaborative Review of Sterilization Working Group. The risk of pregnancy after tubal sterilization: findings from the U.S. Collaborative Review of Sterilization. *Am J Obstet Gynecol* 1996;174:1161–1170. [a]Not studied in CREST. Data from Kovacs GT, Krins AJ. Female sterilizations with Filshie clips: What is the risk failure? A retrospective survey of 30,000 applications. *J Fam Plan Reprod Health Care* 2002:28:34–35.

- All women counseled on the risks of tubal ligation should be informed of the possibility of failure, ectopic pregnancy, and regret.
  - The Collaborative Review of Sterilization (CREST) study compared the long-term effectiveness of numerous methods of sterilization and found a rate of 18.5 pregnancies per 1,000 procedures overall (Table 29-2).
  - Failure rates are higher for women under the age of 30, because of higher fecundability.
  - The CREST study reported a 10-year cumulative probability of ectopic pregnancy for all sterilization methods of 7/1,000, with greater risk of ectopic pregnancy in younger women.
  - Twenty percent of women less than age 30 at the time of sterilization express regret, compared with 5% of women over age 30.

Hysteroscopic Tubal Sterilization (Essure *Micro Insert*)
- *Essure* is an irreversible form of tubal occlusion that can be performed in the operating room or in the office, taking <1 hr.
- Hysteroscopically, a 4 cm × 1 cm spring-loaded stainless steel and nickel titanium-coated expanding coil is released bilaterally into the tubal ostia.
- Tubal blockage occurs by tissue growth and scarring over time.
- A hysterosalpingogram is required 3 months after the procedure to confirm tubal occlusion.
- Failure rate from clinical trial research is <1%.
- This method may be preferred over tubal ligation in women who are obese or who have had prior abdominal operations resulting in adhesions.
- Expulsion of one or both devices occurs 3% of the time, and there is a 14% chance of inability to place one or both inserts.

Vasectomy
- Vasectomy involves surgical occlusion of the vas deferens, preventing sperm from being ejaculated. Up to 20 ejaculations are required before the procedure becomes effective (as determined by two azoospermia results on semen analysis).

- This method is highly effective, has no long-term side effects, is less expensive, and has fewer complications than tubal ligation.
- Vasectomy requires a surgical procedure, is permanent, offers no protection against STDs, and is not immediately effective.

Hormonal Contraceptives

- Hormonal contraceptives have been used routinely for almost 50 years in the United States. Contraceptives are among the safest and most effective medications prescribed.
- Hormonal contraceptives all include a progestin that prevents pregnancy by suppressing ovulation (inhibiting release of luteinizing hormone and follicle-stimulating hormone [LH/FSH] from the pituitary), thickening the cervical mucus, and altering the endometrium.
- Either combined (estrogen and progesterone) or progestin-only forms are available.
  - Combined methods include the pill, patch, and vaginal ring.
  - Progestin-only methods include the mini-pill, injection, patch, implant, and progesterone-containing IUD.

Combined Hormonal Contraceptives

- These are preparations of synthetic progestin and estrogen. Progestin performs the majority of the contraceptive effect, with estrogen added only to maintain the stability of the endometrium (and minor contribution to ovulation inhibition). This allows for monthly withdrawal bleeding and decreases irregular vaginal bleeding.
- Estrogen confers the majority of the medical risk associated with contraceptive use in women with medical problems.
- The WHO Medical Eligibility Criteria for Contraceptive Use can be consulted when weighing the risks associated with estrogen-containing hormonal contraception (e.g., pill, patch, ring) provision to patients (Table 29-3).
- As with all estrogen-containing medications, rare but serious side effects such as thromboembolism may occur, even in women with no known history. This must be considered in context.
  - Risk of venous thromboembolism (VTE) in women per year is
    - 4/100,000 at baseline
    - 10/100,000 in women using combined oral contraceptives (COCs)
    - 20/100,000 in women using patch
    - >100/100,000 in pregnant women
    - 550/100,000 in postpartum women
- These methods are highly effective and tolerated well by patients, but do not protect against STDs.
- Side effects:
  - *Estrogen*: bloating, headache, nausea, mastalgia, leukorrhea, hypertension (HTN), melasma, and telangectasia
  - *Progestin*: mood changes, fatigue, mild weight gain, and libido decrease

Combined Oral Contraceptives (COCs, "The pill")

- COCs are all low-dose, with <50 μg of ethinyl estradiol (20 to 35 μg preparations), and consist of varied doses of different progestins. Three weeks of active hormones are followed by 1 week of placebo. During the week off active pills, withdrawal bleeding will occur.
- COCs are highly effective but require the patient to remember pills daily. Failure rate increases if pills are missed.

TABLE 29-3	Contraindications to Estrogen-Containing Hormonal Contraception

Moderate or severe uncontrolled HTN
History of CVA or MI
Multiple risk factors for CAD: age, smoking, HTN, DM
History of or current DVT/PE
Migraines with aura or focal neurologic symptoms
Active hepatoma or liver cirrhosis or unexplained elevation of liver enzymes
Known or suspected breast cancer
Smoking >15 cigarettes per day and age >35
Breast-feeding <6 wk postpartum (theoretic risk of growth restriction)
Diabetic neuropathy, retinopathy, neuropathy, or other vascular disease
Valvular heart disease, complicated (SBE, pulmonary HTN, or atrial fibrillation)
Known thrombogenic mutation
Migraines without aura and age >35
Symptomatic gallbladder disease
Undiagnosed vaginal bleeding
Non–breast-feeding <3 wk postpartum

Category 4 (i.e., unacceptable risk) contraindications are listed. HTN, hypertension; CVA, cerebrovascular accident; MI, myocardial infarction; CAD, coronary artery disease; DVT, deep vein thrombosis; PE, pulmonary embolism; SBE, subacute bacterial endocarditis. World Health Organization. WHO Medical Eligibility Criteria for starting contraceptive methods (2004). Updates available at www.who.int/reproductive-health (last updated 2008).

- Besides providing contraception, COCs may be used to manage dysmenorrhea, menorrhagia, metrorrhagia, premenstrual symptoms, and mild acne.
- All brands of COCs have essentially equivalent efficacy and side effect profiles. Monophasic pills are associated with less breakthrough bleeding.
- Use of hormonal contraception decreases the risk of ovarian and uterine cancer.
- COC use does not increase risk of breast cancer.
- COCs may have decreased efficacy in obese women.
- Multiple methods may be used to start COCs:
  - "Quick start" method—starting on the day of counseling
  - "Sunday start" method—starting on the 1st Sunday after starting menses
  - "Day one start" method—starting the pills on the first day of menses
  - A week of backup contraception is recommended after all initiation methods
- Spotting, irregular menses, and nausea are common with initiation of hormonal contraception and generally resolve within the first 1 to 3 months.
- Also available are extended-use or continuous COCs (e.g., *Seasonale, Lybrel,* or standard monophasic pills continuously) that decrease the number of placebo pills and therefore decrease or eliminate withdrawal bleeding. These extended-use preparations may improve menorrhagia, dysmenorrhea, endometriosis, chronic pelvic pain, migraines, and epilepsy. Spotting or breakthrough bleeding may increase. There are no medical advantages to maintaining withdrawal bleeding.

Combined Transdermal Hormonal Contraceptive (Ortho Evra)
- The contraceptive patch contains norgestimate (progestin) and ethinyl estradiol and works in the same way as COCs.

- It is applied weekly to any body location (other than the breast) for 3 weeks, followed by a patch-free withdrawal bleeding week. This weekly use may increase compliance over the daily dosing of COCs.
- Transdermal delivery avoids hepatic first-pass metabolic effects and maintains steady serum hormone levels without the peaks and troughs seen with pills.
- Local adhesive reactions to the patch are rare (<5%), and adhesion is reliable.
- The patch is less effective in women who weigh >90 kg (198 pounds). Therefore, another method should be prescribed to obese women.
- An FDA "black box" warning states that the patch provides approximately 60% more total estrogen than a typical birth control pill containing 35 μg ethinyl estradiol, warning of increased VTE risk. Nonetheless, the daily peak in estrogen is approximately 25% less with the patch compared to pills. The clinical significance of this finding is unclear, especially because studies have not shown an increased risk of fatal blood clots compared to COCs. Therefore, patch use should not be restricted in women without contraindications.

The Combined Hormonal Vaginal Ring (NuvaRing)
- This flexible ring, 5 cm diameter and 4 mm thickness, releases ethinyl estradiol and etonogestrel (progestin). It is placed in the vagina for 3 weeks, then removed for 1 week, during which withdrawal bleeding occurs.
- The ring may be removed for up to 3 hr, including during intercourse. If the ring is out of the vagina for >3 hr, backup contraception should be used until the ring has been back in place for 7 days.
- Patients report increased satisfaction and compliance and a lower incidence of side effects and breakthrough bleeding than COCs and the patch.
- The lowest, steady-state hormonal level of estrogen is achieved with the ring, compared to the patch and COCs.
- Coital problems and expulsion of the device are rare.
- Patients must feel comfortable enough to place and remove the ring.
- May decrease vaginal yeast and bacterial infections due to local estrogen effect; however, may increase leukorrhea.

Progestin-Only Methods
- These are synthetic progestin preparations that prevent pregnancy without the use of estrogen; therefore, they can be used in many women with contraindications to combined contraceptive use (e.g., history of thromboembolic disease).
- Bleeding patterns with progestin-only methods are more variable.
- They may be used in breast-feeding women without causing a decrease in breast-milk production.
- Progestin-only methods decrease menorrhagia and associated anemia, decrease cramps, offer some protection against endometrial cancer, and may reduce the risk of pelvic inflammatory disease (PID) secondary to cervical mucus thickening.

Progestin-only Pills (Micronor, Ovrette)
- Taken daily with no hormone-free interval.
- Lower doses of progestin than COCs.
- Must be taken at the same time each day. More than 3 hr of delay should be considered a missed pill, and backup method should be used.

Progestin-only Injectable Contraceptives (DepoProvera)
- Every 11 to 13 weeks, 150 mg medroxyprogesterone acetate (DMPA) is injected intramuscularly by a medical provider.
- Menometrorrhagia is common after the first injection; however, 50% of women become amenorrheic after the first year of use and 80% after 5 years.
- Return of fertility may be delayed after discontinuation. Average delay is 6 to 10 months after last injection; up to 18 months is possible.
- Patients with sickle cell disease on DMPA have fewer crises and improvement in anemia.
- DMPA may increase seizure threshold and can therefore be recommended to patients with a history of seizure disorder.
- Overall 5 to 8 pounds/year (compared to 5 pounds/year COCs) of weight gain is reported to be associated with DMPA. In studies, this weight gain has not proven significant and may reflect overall weight change with age and the US obesity epidemic, especially in adolescents.
- DMPA has been associated with hair loss in some patients.
- A "black box" FDA warning states that DMPA may decrease bone mineral density (BMD), especially in adolescents. Studies have also shown this decrease in BMD after one injection, which continued with each subsequent injection. This does not reflect an increase in fracture risk. Additionally, this decrease in BMD is largely reversible and comparable to that which occurs with breast-feeding. Access to injected contraceptives should therefore not be restricted based on the time of use or the age of the user.

Progestin-only Implants (Implanon)
- The only implant currently available in the United States is Implanon.
- A single rod, 4 cm × 2 mm (the approximate size of a match), releases etonogestrel for 3 years.
- It is placed under the skin of the upper (usually nondominant) arm and injected from a preloaded syringe. FDA-mandated training is required for clinicians before placement and removal can be performed.
- A 5-year (two-rod) implant (*Jadelle*) is approved for use but not yet available in the United States. The prior implant used in the United States, *Norplant*, had multiple rods (six).
- The implant is extremely effective.
- This method is good for women who would like long-term reversible contraception but who may not want to be candidates for intrauterine contraception.
- Menstrual disturbances are common. Intolerance of bleeding may lead to discontinuation and patients should be counseled appropriately.

Progestin-Releasing Intrauterine Contraceptive System (Mirena-IUS)
- See IUDs, below.

Barrier Methods
Male Condom
- The male condom is made of latex, although nonlatex condoms are also available. They should be applied before vaginal penetration and should cover the

entire length of the erect penis. They should not be applied too tightly or loosely (a reservoir should be left to retain the ejaculate).

- Adequate lubrication should be used, and the condom should be removed immediately after ejaculation. Condoms with spermicidal lubricant are more effective at preventing pregnancy. No data exist to indicate that condoms lubricated with spermicides are more effective than other lubricated condoms in protecting against the transmission of HIV and other STDs. Thus, the CDC currently suggests that women who are at high risk for HIV infection should not use nonoxynol-9 spermicides.
- Condoms decrease sexual transmission of HIV and other infections (e.g., gonorrhea, chlamydia, trichomonas). However, because condoms do not cover all exposed areas, they may not be as effective in preventing infections transmitted by skin-to-skin contact (e.g., herpes simplex virus, HPV, syphilis, chancroid).

Female Condom
- Female condoms consist of a polyurethane sheath with two flexible rings at either end. The closed end with the upper/inner ring is applied against the cervix, and the open end with the lower/outer ring rests against the labia minora outside the introitus. Adequate lubrication is important for function and comfort.
- Like male condoms, this method decreases sexual transmission of HIV infection and other STDs. It also provides extra protection on the outside of the body that may decrease infections transmitted by skin-to-skin contact.

Diaphragm
- Diaphragms are barrier devices that are inserted into the vagina and prevent sperm from entering the upper genital tract.
- The diaphragm is a rubber or latex cup with a flexible ring. The edges of the diaphragm should lie just posterior to the symphysis pubis and deep into the cul-de-sac so that the cervix is completely covered behind the center of the diaphragm.
- The largest diaphragm that comfortably fills this space should be selected during an office exam and fitting. Diaphragms range in size from 50 to 105 mm in diameter, with the most commonly prescribed diaphragms being 65 to 75 mm.
- Clinical practice has been to recommend concurrent use of a spermicide with the diaphragm. A Cochrane review showed that studies have neither proved nor disproved the contraceptive contribution of concurrent spermicide use.
- If spermicide is used, it should be applied to the inside of the rubber cup before each coitus. The diaphragm should be left in place for a minimum of 6 hr after the last coital act but not >24 consecutive hours. It may be placed hours before intercourse.
- Women with uterine prolapse or structural abnormalities of the reproductive tract may not be able to use a diaphragm.
- A diaphragm should be inspected regularly for holes. It should be replaced at least every 2 years.
- Diaphragms may decrease STD transmission. They increase the risk of urinary tract infection.

Cervical Cap
- Round rubber cap with an inside rim that fits snugly against the outer cervix adjacent to the vaginal fornix; it has decreased efficacy in parous women.

Intrauterine Devices (IUD) or Systems (IUS)

- IUDs are flexible plastic devices that are inserted into the uterus and cause an alteration in the uterine environment.
- They are one of the most effective methods of long-term reversible contraception.
- Two types of intrauterine contraception are currently commercially available in the United States:
  - Copper-containing (*ParaGard T380A IUD*)
    - Works by causing a sterile inflammatory reaction in the uterus and interferes with sperm transport into the uterine cavity.
    - Effective for at least 10 years.
    - There is no change in the timing of menstrual bleeding; however, menses may be slightly heavier and longer, at least in the initial months.
    - Can also be used as postcoital contraception (see "Emergency Contraception," below).
  - Progestin (levonorgestrel)-releasing (*Mirena IUS*)
    - Works by the same means as other progestin-only contraceptives. Confers the same benefits as other above-mentioned progestin-only contraceptives.
    - Approved for 5 years in the United States.
    - Mirena IUS may also reduce menstrual blood loss and may decrease risk for endometrial cancer.
- IUDs should not be used if pregnancy is suspected, if anatomical uterine abnormalities are present distorting the cavity, if there is unexplained vaginal bleeding, or if pelvic malignancy is suspected.
- Overall, IUD use does not increase risk of PID. Progestin IUS may decrease risk by decreasing ascending infection due to the progestational effect on the cervical mucus. The Copper IUD does not decrease or increase risk. The *Dalkon Shield* was an IUD with a braided filament string used in the 1970s. This IUD was associated with some increase risk of PID. Modern IUDs have monofilament strings that do not share this risk.
- Placement of an IUD at the time of an active pelvic infection increases risk of PID. Women at high risk for sexually transmitted infections should be screened for STDs and have these treated before having IUDs placed. Otherwise, low-risk patients need not be screened before placement.
- History of PID or ectopic pregnancy is not a contraindication to IUD use. Instead, current risk factors should be considered.
- PID infection with an IUD in place should be treated, and the IUD left in situ. A desired intrauterine pregnancy with an IUD in place should have the IUD removed if possible.
- Immunocompromised women, including those with HIV/AIDS can safely have IUDs placed.
- Immediate postpartum and postabortal IUD placement is safe and may lead to a substantial decrease in unplanned pregnancy. Expulsion risk increases, however, from 2% to 20%.
- The risk of uterine perforation with insertion is 1/1,000.
- There is a higher relative risk of ectopic pregnancy, if pregnancy does occur, with an IUD in place.

Natural Family Planning (Rhythm Method)

- Natural family planning is a method in which a couple voluntarily avoids or interrupts sexual intercourse during the fertile phase of the woman's menstrual cycle.

Effectiveness varies significantly based upon the individual as this method relies upon regular menses, cooperation of both partners, and abstinence at times.
- Natural family planning methods include
  - Symptothermal—basal body temperature is taken, a spike occurs with ovulation, and intercourse is avoided then.
  - Cervical mucus—the usual tacky white-yellow cervical mucus changes viscosity into clear, slippery, stretchy discharge at ovulation. Intercourse is avoided then but allowed when the discharge is tacky or during menses.
  - Calendar—counts from last period to predict next ovulation, avoiding intercourse during the predicted week.

Lactational Amenorrhea Method

- During breast-feeding, suckling causes hormonal changes at the level of the hypothalamus that interrupt the pulsatile release of gonadotropin-releasing hormone. This, in turn, impairs LH surge and ovulation does not occur.
- This method is effective only if strict criteria are followed. Women must be exclusively or nearly exclusively breast-feeding. Feedings must be every 4 hr during the day and every 6 hr at night. Supplemental feedings should not exceed 5% to 10% of the total. This method is more successful if the infant is <6 months old.

EMERGENCY CONTRACEPTION

Emergency contraception (EC), or postcoital contraception, may be used after unprotected intercourse to prevent pregnancy. This works mainly through ovulation prevention. IUD EC may disrupt implantation. EC does not affect a pregnancy that has already implanted and is therefore not an abortifacient.

Hormonal EC

- Two options exist for hormonal EC: progestin-only and the Yuzpe regimen (estrogen and progestin). Plan B (levonorgestrel only) is the only dedicated EC product available in the United States.
- Plan B includes a total of 1.5 mg levonorgestrel that may be taken in two doses (0.75 mg 12 hr apart) or one dose (1.5 mg). The single dose regimen has better compliance with fewer side effects and increased efficacy. Plan B is available without a prescription for women over the age of 18. In younger women, advance prescription provision is mandated by the FDA.
- The Yuzpe regimen uses prescription COCs at increased dose. Four to five pills are taken after unprotected sex, with repeat dosing 12 hr later. The Yuzpe method has decreased efficacy and increased side effects relative to Plan B.
- Effectiveness is inversely related to time since coitus but may work up to 120 hr after intercourse.
- Contraindication to the use of EC is pregnancy; however, the use will not cause termination of existing pregnancy and is not teratogenic.
- This method is not ideal as routine contraception for those having regular intercourse, because it is less effective than other methods.
- Irregular bleeding and change in menses may also occur.
- Patients are encouraged to take a pregnancy test if menses have not resumed within 1 week after expected menstrual timing.

IUD as EC

- The Copper IUD may be inserted within 5 days of unprotected intercourse to decrease the chance of implantation.
- Pregnancy rate of 0.1% to 0.2% if inserted within 5 days.

ELECTIVE PREGNANCY TERMINATION

Epidemiology and History

- Forty-one million abortions occur each year worldwide. Half of these are unsafe, resulting in 67,000 maternal deaths from abortion and related complications around the world annually. This accounts for 13% of maternal mortality.
- Abortion is very safe in the United States, with the legal abortion mortality rate of 0.6/100,000.
- Roe v. Wade was a landmark Supreme Court Decision in 1973 that made access to abortion a federal right. In 1993, Planned Parenthood v. Casey further clarified that access should not pose an undue burden on women seeking induced abortion.
- Extensive study has shown that an abortion does not increase the risk of infertility, breast cancer, or future miscarriage.
- Long-term negative psychological effects have not been shown to occur in women who have had an abortion.

Evaluation, Counseling, and Follow-up

- Providers caring for women with unplanned and undesired pregnancy should be able to counsel patients on all the options available to them, including induced abortion.
- A nondirective counseling approach should be taken with the patient to ensure that she is confident in her decision.
- Those who decide not to provide this service because of a moral objection should be able to counsel patients, make appropriate referrals, and manage postabortal complications.
- Confirmation of intrauterine pregnancy and pregnancy dating should be performed.
- Maternal Rh status should be obtained, as Rh-negative women should receive Rhogam (see Rh alloimmunization, Chapter 18).
- STD screening should be offered.
- Contraception should be discussed with all women, as fertility can return immediately. Women can ovulate within 2 weeks of an abortion procedure.
- Pregnancy symptoms usually resolve within 1 week. Normal menses may take up to 6 weeks.
- Follow-up is usually recommended within 2 to 4 weeks to assess for complications, confirm resolution of pregnancy, and readdress contraception.

Surgical Termination in the First trimester

- By convention, abortion at <14 weeks performed surgically is referred to as Dilation and Curettage (D&C). This is the most common method of first-trimester abortion.
- First-trimester surgical abortion complication rates are very low. Failure is <1%.
- Prior to the procedure, the cervix must be opened. Very early pregnancies (e.g., <7 weeks) may not require additional cervical dilation. In pregnancies >7 weeks, the cervix can either be mechanically dilated or opened using osmotic or medical dilators. It is imperative that adequate, careful cervical dilation be performed to avoid cervical injury and excessive blood loss.

- Mechanical dilation uses surgical instruments that have progressively increasing diameters (e.g., Pratt, Hegar, or Denniston dilators) to open the cervix.
- Osmotic dilators, such as Dilapan (polyacrylonitrile) or laminaria (dried seaweed *Laminaria japonica*), absorb cervical moisture and gradually enlarge the endocervical canal and soften the cervix. They also cause the release of prostaglandin, which ultimately disrupts the stroma of the cervix and results in a soft, flaccid cervix that is easy to dilate. Osmotic dilators must be placed several hours before the procedure to give them time to effect cervical change, unlike manual dilation that is performed at the start of the surgical procedure.
- Medical ripening agents, including misoprostol and mifepristone, can also be used preoperatively to both soften and dilate the cervix.
- A paracervical block with local anesthesia is frequently given. Intravenous sedation may also be given.
- To empty the uterus of the products of conception (POCs), electric or manual vacuum aspiration (MVA) can be performed.
  - Electric vacuum aspiration (EVA) uses a suction curette attached to an electrically powered vacuum canister. The cannula of the curette should be approximately the same diameter (in millimeters) as the weeks' gestation. This gentle suction removes the POCs.
  - Sharp curettage can be used to ensure that all uterine contents have been evacuated, but is not necessary if completion can be confirmed with the suction cannula. The use of sharp curettage increases the pain of the procedure. It should be avoided in cases where infection is suspected.
  - MVA is safe and effective and has been in use for >30 years. A specially designed, handheld 60-mL syringe is attached to either a flexible or rigid cannula, of a diameter appropriate for gestational age. The apparatus is advanced through the internal os into the uterine cavity. Uterine contents can then be aspirated by manually generating negative air pressure into the syringe, collecting the POCs.
- After aspiration, the tissue should be washed and inspected to verify that the POCs are consistent with the gestational age. This includes placental villi and gestational sac, as well as fetal calvarium at greater gestational age.
- Doxycycline should be administered for infection prophylaxis.
- IUDs may be safely placed immediately after surgical abortion.

Surgical Termination in the Second Trimester

- By convention, surgical termination at >14 weeks is referred to as Dilation and Evacuation (D&E).
- D&E is considered the preferred method of second-trimester termination when highly experienced personnel are available and autopsy of an intact fetus is not required. In experienced hands, D&E is the safest method of second-trimester termination.
- Less than 5% of abortions are done by D&E. Complication rates from abortion in the second trimester of pregnancy increase with gestational age.
- Complications, such as cervical trauma, uterine perforation, hemorrhage, and retained products, are more common after 18 weeks' gestation and may result in significant morbidity.
- The procedure for surgical termination between 14 and 22 weeks' gestation is similar to the first-trimester procedure, with some caveats:
  - Ultrasonographic confirmation of gestational age is essential

- Preoperative cervical preparation is mandatory and is often carried out over 1 to 2 days before the procedure to maximize cervical dilation. Sequential insertion of osmotic dilators is most frequently used with or without manual and medical dilation
- The procedure may be routinely carried out under ultrasound guidance
- In addition to the application of the vacuum aspirator, instrumental removal of the POCs is usually required. It is essential to examine and account for all fetal parts and a volume of placental tissue consistent with the gestational age

Medical Termination in the First Trimester

- Medical abortion is safe and effective, generally used up to 63 days of gestation. At later gestations, there is a higher failure rate or more bleeding.
- Medical abortion may cause more pain and bleeding than surgical abortion.
- The procedure takes longer to complete than surgical termination and requires multiple visits.
- A reliable patient is required, as follow-up is essential. If medical termination fails or results in incomplete abortion or excessive bleeding, uterine evacuation is required.
- Medical abortion can be performed using mifepristone (RU-486) and misoprostol, or methotrexate and misoprostol.
  - Mifepristone works as a progesterone antagonist and alters the endometrial blood supply, blocking the support of pregnancy and softening the cervix
  - Methotrexate inhibits DNA synthesis and affects rapidly dividing cells, including trophoblast
  - Misoprostol is a prostaglandin that is used to induce uterine contractions after administration of either mifepristone or methotrexate, thus promoting expulsion of the POCs
- Mifepristone/misoprostol medical abortion is 94% to 98% effective, depending on gestational age and misoprostol dose, and is faster and associated with less bleeding than methotrexate/misoprostol medical abortion.
- Evidence-based recommendations support the use of mifepristone and misoprostol up to 63 days of gestation and with a lower mifepristone dose, than the FDA-approved regimen, which has a gestational age limit of 49 days.
- Methotrexate/misoprostol medical abortion may be slower and less effective (94% to 96%).
- Where access to methotrexate or mifepristone is limited, misoprostol alone can be used in repeat 24-hr dosing intervals for medical abortion. Effectiveness may vary from 47% to 96%.
- Side effects following administration of mifepristone and misoprostol consist primarily of pain, bleeding, and gastrointestinal (GI) upset.

Medical Termination in the Second Trimester

- Medical termination offers several advantages over D&E because it does not require anesthesia, a skilled operator is not required, and fetal examination can be performed on an intact fetus, such as in cases of genetic termination.
- However, as compared with D&E, the procedure can take 24 hr or longer, major complications and mortality are higher, and fever and severe GI side effects are common when prostaglandins are used.

- The overall goal is to administer medications that cause uterine contractions and lead to the expulsion of the POCs. Medications include high-dose intravenous oxytocin and different preparations of vaginally administered prostaglandins (prostaglandin E_2 [Prostin E_2] and misoprostol). Less commonly, hypertonic solutions (saline or urea) may be administered intra-amniotically to induce second-trimester abortions. Antiprogestins, such as mifepristone, may also be used.

Abortion Complications

- Complications with medical abortion generally stem from retained POCs, bleeding, and infection.
- Perforation is also a risk of surgical abortion. If perforation is suspected, the procedure is stopped, suction is not applied, and the patient should be examined with ultrasound and observed. If the patient shows signs of bleeding or instability, surgical management (laparoscopy vs. laparotomy) should be performed.
- Excess uterine bleeding or hemorrhage can be managed with postpartum uterotonics.
- Hematometra should be suspected if a patient has intense pain and an enlarged boggy uterus immediately after surgical abortion. Methergine should be given, and aspiration of the uterine clot performed.
- Postabortal endomyometritis is suspected in patients with fever postabortion. Oral or intravenous doxycycline and a cephalosporin, with or without metronidazole, should be administered.
- Retained POCs after abortion can also result in fever. This can lead to fatal sepsis if not recognized and treated.
- Oral prophylactic doxycycline administration, before or after surgical abortion, can reduce the risk of postabortion endomyometritis by 40%.
- There is also a rare risk of fatal sepsis resulting from medical abortion related to *Clostridium sordellii*. Buccal (vs. vaginal) administration of misoprostol, with or without prophylactic antibiotics, may decrease this risk further.
- The major complications of second-trimester termination include cervical or uterine lacerations and injury, uterine atony with subsequent hemorrhage, retained placental tissue, and electrolyte imbalance leading to disseminated intravascular coagulation in cases in which hypertonic solutions are used.

SUGGESTED READINGS

Blumenthal P, Edelman A. Clinical expert series: hormonal contraception. *Obstet Gynecol* 2008;112(3):670–684.

Chervenak FA, McCullough LB. The ethics of direct and indirect referral for termination of pregnancy. *Am J Obstet Gynecol* 2008;199(3):232–233.

Clark MK, Sowers MR, Nichols S, et al. Bone mineral density changes over two years in first-time users of depot medroxyprogesterone acetate. *Fertil Steril* 2004;82:1580–1586.

Grimes DA, Lopez LM, Manion C, et al. Cochrane Systematic review of IUD trials lessons learned. *Contraception*. 2007;75(6 Suppl):S55–S59.

Jabara S, Barnhart K. Is Rh immune globulin needed in early first-trimester abortion? A review. *Am J Obstet Gynecol* 2003;188:623–627.

Morrison CS, Bright P, et al. Hormonal contraceptive use, cervical ectopy, and the acquisition of cervical infections. *Sex Transm Dis* 2004;31:561–567.

Mosher WD, Martinez GM, Chandra A, et al. Use of contraception and use of family planning services in the United States: 1982–2002. *Advanced Data* 2004;350:1–36.

30 Domestic Violence and Sexual Assault

Amy S.D. Lee and Judy M. Lee

DOMESTIC VIOLENCE

Domestic violence is any intentional controlling behavior against an intimate acquaintance. This behavior may involve sexual assault, physical and/or emotional abuse, financial control, or isolation. Clinicians may fail to ask patients about abusive relationships and may ignore subtle or even overt clues. Victims of abuse usually keep their problems hidden but, if specifically questioned, may be more willing to share the details of their relationships.

- Domestic violence affects women of all ages, races, educational, and economic backgrounds. Cultural, social, and historical factors are determinants of domestic violence.
- Domestic violence is the single most common cause of injury to women in the United States.

Epidemiology of Domestic Violence

- Twenty-five to thirty-three percent of women have been assaulted or raped during their lifetime.
- Approximately, 25% of women in the United States will be abused by a current or former partner sometime during their lifetime.
- The majority (85%) of domestic violence victims are women. Women of all races are equally vulnerable. Abuse occurs with the same frequency in homosexual and heterosexual relationships.
- More than 30% of all emergency room visits by women in the United States can be attributed to domestic violence.
- In primary care practices, 20% of women revealed a history of abuse when specifically asked, whereas 5% reported being in a current abusive relationship. The incidence is higher in gastroenterology clinics, where up to 50% of women report a childhood or adult history of sexual and/or physical abuse. Up to 66% of women who suffer from chronic headaches and seek treatment with a neurologist report a history of abuse.
- Fifty-four percent of intimate partner violence is reported to police; only 24% of sexual assault is reported. One third of murdered women in the United States are murdered by an intimate partner.

Domestic Violence and Pregnancy

- Domestic violence may begin in pregnancy. If already ongoing, abuse often escalates during the course of the pregnancy and postpartum. The CDC reports 4% to 8% of pregnant women report suffering abuse during pregnancy.
- One in six abused women report their partner was first abusive in pregnancy. Twenty-five percent of all domestic violence victims are pregnant when abused.

- Domestic violence can result in poor pregnancy outcomes, such as miscarriage, preterm labor, low birth weight, and fetal injury or death.
- Women with an unintended pregnancy have a threefold higher risk of abuse than those women whose pregnancy was planned, and pregnant women have a threefold higher risk of being victims of attempted or completed homicide.

Evaluation and Intervention for Domestic Violence

- Although some women are victims of an acute attack or rape, others find themselves in long-standing abusive and destructive relationships. Such relationships tend to develop a cycle in which a violent episode is followed by a period reconciliation and apology. A tension-building phase soon begins and culminates in a repeat violent attack and the cycle begins anew. Over time, the degree of violence may escalate. Escape from the relationship is difficult for the victim because of fear, shame, powerlessness, and social isolation.
- Domestic violence is all-encompassing. Muelleman defines it as "the exercise of emotional intimidation, psychological abuse, social isolation, deprivation, nonconsensual sexual behavior, physical injury by a competent adult to maintain coercive control in an intimate relationship with another competent adult/adolescent."
- Women are more likely to be injured, raped, or even killed by a current or former male partner than by all other types of assailants combined. Women who are injured as a result of domestic violence are more likely to suffer serious injury than victims of violence by strangers.

Screening

- Ask about domestic violence as part of routine patient evaluation during office visits and emergency room evaluations. The majority of women report that they would reveal abuse history *only* if specifically asked.
- Routinely asking patients about domestic violence significantly increases detection. In a study of trauma victims, the institution of a screening protocol increased detection from 5.6% to 30%.
  - Interview the patient in private. The setting is very important. The patient must feel that she is in a safe and comfortable environment. It should be done without her partner, children, or other relatives present. Be aware that the batterer often accompanies the woman to the appointment and wants to stay close at hand to monitor what she says to the physician.
  - Assure patient confidentiality.
- Never ask what the patient did wrong or why she remains with her partner. Avoid judgment or value-laden terms, such as "abused" and "battered."
  - You can begin with an objective statement that demonstrates that your screening is universal and necessary to provide comprehensive health care. An example of an opening question would be, "Because violence is so common in many women's lives and there is help available for women being abused, I now ask every patient about domestic violence." This type of introduction increases the detection rate and helps the patient feel that she has not been singled out.
- Several useful questionnaires have been developed to address abuse. The SAFE questions can be used (Table 30-1). The three-question Abuse Assessment Screen has been shown to be useful in identifying physical or sexual abuse in pregnancy (Table 30-2).
- Initially, a patient may deny abuse if she is not emotionally ready to admit it, if she fears for herself or her family, or if she fears rejection from the physician. If

TABLE 30-1	SAFE Questionnaire

- **S**tress/safety: Do you feel safe in your relationship?
- **A**fraid/abused: Have you ever been in a relationship in which you were threatened, hurt, or afraid?
- **F**riends/family: Are your friends or family aware that you have been hurt? Could you tell them, and would they be able to give you support?
- **E**mergency plan: Do you have a safe place to go and the resources you need in an emergency?

Based upon Neufeld B. SAFE questions: overcoming barriers to the detection of domestic violence. *Am Fam Physician* 1996;53:2575–2582.

the provider suspects abuse and the patient initially denies it, the provider should readdress the issue during a subsequent visit.
- Most important, regardless of the method, make time to screen. Asking about domestic violence early and often takes less time than visits for premenstrual syndrome and pelvic pain.

Diagnosing Domestic Violence
- Some clues may be present in the patient's history or presentation that may lead a provider to suspect an abusive relationship. Typically, a battered woman has numerous emergency room visits for injury. There may be an inconsistent explanation for the injuries or a delay in seeking treatment. The injuries classically involve multiple sites, such as three or more body parts; affect the head, back, breast, and abdomen (accidental injuries are more likely to be peripheral); and are in various stages of healing. Patients who are abused tend to report somatic complaints, such as fatigue, headache, and abdominal pain. They are also more likely to suffer from eating disorders, gastrointestinal complaints, psychiatric disorders, and substance abuse.
  - Gynecologic and obstetric clues to the presence of abuse include increased prevalence of sexually transmitted disease, chronic pelvic pain, premenstrual syndrome, unintended pregnancy, and late prenatal care (Table 30-3).
- In the case that the patient reveals that she has been battered, the clinician should attempt to elicit the degree of risk to the patient. Specific questions include the following:
  - How were you hurt?
  - Has this happened before?

TABLE 30-2	Abuse Assessment Screen

- Within the last year, have you been hit, slapped, kicked, or otherwise physically hurt by someone?
- Since you've been pregnant, have you been hit, slapped, kicked, or otherwise physically hurt by someone?
- Within the last year, has anyone forced you to have sexual activities?

Based upon McFarlane J, Parker B, Soeken K, et al. Assessing for abuse during pregnancy. *JAMA* 1992;267:3176–3178.

- When did it first happen?
- How badly have you been hurt in the past?
- Have you ever needed to go to the emergency room for treatment?
- Have you ever been threatened with a weapon, or has a weapon ever been used on you?
- Have you ever tried to get a restraining order against a partner?
- Have your children ever seen or heard you being threatened or hurt?
- Do you know how you can get help for yourself if you are hurt or afraid?
- Is the violence getting worse?
- Are there threats of suicide or homicide?
- Is there a gun at home?

Interventions for Domestic Violence
- Most victims of abuse are not ready to leave their abusers. They may rely on their abuser for financial support and shelter or may have a fear of repercussions. In one study, only 45% of abused women who initially agreed to undergo treatment actually finished the program.
  - Empowerment of the patient is the first step.
  - Discuss the gravity of the situation and assess immediate safety needs.
  - Reinforce that the patient is not to blame.
  - Treat the patient's injuries and screen for suicidal tendencies, depression, and substance abuse.
  - Empower the woman to be able to protect herself and her children.
  - Discuss court restraining orders and laws against stalking.
  - Provide the patient with phone numbers of resource agencies.
  - Review an exit plan or exit drill (Table 30-4).
  - Provide continued ongoing support, and offer referrals for counseling.
  - Provide documentation, including direct quotations and photographs.

TABLE 30-3	Gynecologic and Obstetric Clues to Presence of Abuse

Chronic pelvic pain
Severe premenstrual syndrome
Multiple or recurrent sexually transmitted infections or recurrent vaginitis
Medical noncompliance
Sexual dysfunction
Abdominal pain
Unintended pregnancy
Late registration for prenatal care, no prenatal care
Noncompliance and missed appointment
Fetal or maternal injury (violence is often directed toward the woman's abdomen during pregnancy)
Spontaneous abortion or stillbirth
Vaginal bleeding in the second or third trimester
Preterm labor
Infection
Anemia
Poor weight gain
Low birth weight infants

TABLE 30-4	Exit Plan for Domestic Violence Intervention

The following exit plan has been proposed for a woman who feels that she or her children are in danger from her partner:

1. Have a change of clothes packed for herself and her children, including toiletries, necessary medications, and an extra set of house and car keys. These can be placed in a suitcase and stored with a friend or neighbor.

2. Cash, a checkbook, and savings account information may also be kept with a friend or neighbor.

3. Have available identification papers, such as birth certificates, social security cards, voter registration card, utility bills, and a driver's license, because children will need to be enrolled in school, and financial assistance may be sought. If available, also take financial records, such as mortgage papers, rent receipts, or an automobile title.

4. Take something of special interest to each child, such as a book or toy.

5. Have a plan of exactly where to go, regardless of the time of day or night. This may be a friend or relative's home or a shelter for women and children.

Modified from Helton A. Battering during pregnancy. *Am J Nurs* 1986;86:910–913.

- Providers need to know the resources and referral systems within their institution.
- Remember that the social worker is the key for referrals in a hospital.
- Some states require mandatory reporting of domestic violence. Each state differs in its reporting criteria. Providers should be familiar with the legal requirements of the state where they practice.

SEXUAL ABUSE

Suspected Child Sexual Abuse

- The majority of **childhood sexual abuse** occurs between ages 6 and 14, and especially between ages 12 and 14. The perpetrator is usually a relative or an acquaintance. Unlike in cases of physical abuse, physical or laboratory findings of trauma are rare. It is the child's word that is the indicator of the abuse. Some signs, however, can be used as diagnostic clues for childhood sexual abuse, especially if the abuse is recent or repetitive and leaves physical stigmata

- Definition: Child sexual abuse is defined as contact or interaction between a child and an adult in which the child is being used for sexual stimulation of that adult or another person. Abuse may also be committed by another minor either when that person is significantly older than the victim or when the abuser is in a position of power or control over the child. Sexual abuse also encompasses nonsexual contact, such as pornography or exhibitionism.

  - Sexual abuse should be considered in any child found to have a vaginal foreign body. Children and adolescents may suffer sex-related trauma at the perineal area. This may be difficult to diagnose, especially if the patient is embarrassed or if the trauma is related to abuse.

Evaluation for Pediatric Sexual Abuse

- In general, children suspected of being victims of abuse should be evaluated by professionals trained in conducting interviews, documenting questions and responses, and collecting necessary evidence. Centers designed for a multidisciplinary approach are ideal for these evaluations.
  - **History**
    - Establish rapport with the child.
    - Information must be recorded in the child's own words; for young children with limited verbal skills, techniques such as play-interviews or drawings have been used to promote communication.
    - When obtaining a history from the victim is impossible, the information may come from relatives, other household members, neighbors, or police officers.
    - Note the child's composure, behavior, and mental state, as well as interactions with parents and other people.
    - Nonspecific symptoms include night terrors, changes in sleeping habits, and clinging behavior.
  - **Examination**
    - A repeating theme in distinguishing abusive events from legitimate genital accidents is a mismatch between the history and the physical findings.
    - The examination should be complete, extending from head to toe, allowing the child to become accustomed to the touch of the evaluator and establishing trust.
    - Specific findings include pregnancy, presence of sperm, or sexually transmitted infections (oral, vaginal, rectoanal). Nonspecific findings must be interpreted with caution and include redness, irritations, abrasions, and bruising. Unfortunately, the absence of physical findings is common because healing is often complete by the time the child is evaluated. Colposcopic exam of the hymen can aid in the evaluation, but a normal exam does not exclude abuse.
  - **Evidence collection**
    - If the assault occurred within 72 hr of the examination, samples should be collected for the forensic laboratory and handled separately.
    - Items that can be collected for evidence include the clothing that was worn at the time of the assault and combings of pubic hair for the perpetrator's hair.
    - All collected specimens must be individually packaged, labeled, sealed with special evidence tape and signed by the appropriate people.
  - **Evaluation for semen**
    - A Wood's light can be used to examine the body for secretions on skin and clothing.
    - The most commonly used marker for the presence of semen is the enzyme acid phosphatase, but the activity of this enzyme decreases rapidly in the vagina and becomes indistinguishable after 72 hr.
    - Motile sperm can be recovered up to 8 hr after an assault.
    - Nonmotile sperm can be found up to 26 hr after an incident.
    - If oral sex was forced, separate swabs should be taken from the perioral skin, gums, tongue, and pharynx.

Treatment

- Treatment consists of addressing immediate medical needs as well as providing protection and psychological support for the victim and her family.

- **Injuries**
  - Emphasize good perineal hygiene with sitz baths.
  - All wounds should be well irrigated.
  - Vaginal and rectal lacerations can be sutured under anesthesia for good hemostasis.
  - Small hematomas can be controlled by pressure with an ice pack. Expanding hematomas may require incision, evacuation, and ligation for hemostasis.
  - Most of these wounds should be left open. A noninfected, fresh wound can be primarily closed. Any necrotic tissue should be debrided. After 3 to 5 days, a secondary debridement may be required.
  - If the child is not already immunized, she should be given a tetanus immunization.
- **Infection**
  - Screen for gonorrhea, syphilis, *Chlamydia, Trichomonas,* human immunodeficiency virus, and hepatitis B.
  - Antibiotic therapy can be instituted empirically at initial assessment, with or without symptoms.
  - A repeat rapid plasma reagin (RPR), human immunodeficiency virus, and hepatitis B panel should be performed in 6 weeks to rule out seroconversion.
- **Safety**
  - All suspected victims of child abuse should be referred to child protective services (CPS). Until the question of protection can be answered, providing temporary placement for the child is advisable.

Counseling
- A trained therapist should be available to assist both victim and family with the evaluation process, medical treatment, and encounters with CPS and law enforcement agencies.
- **Pregnancy:** If the child is peripubertal, the option of emergency conception should be addressed. A follow-up pregnancy test may be appropriate.
  - Former victims of childhood sexual abuse are at increased risk for conception during adolescence.
- Child's parent in abusive relationship
  - Forty-five to fifty-nine percent of mothers of abused children have been abused or raped themselves. Evidence or suspicion of child abuse must be reported by the licensed provider to the police or specified social agencies in all 50 states.

Suspected Adolescent Sexual Abuse

- More than 75% of **adolescent rapes** are committed by an acquaintance of the victim. These include date rape, statutory rape, and incest.
- Teenagers are still learning to establish social boundaries, and they bring various expectations to dating situations. Some adolescents believe that violence is acceptable in some social situations. Furthermore, adolescents may use alcohol and illicit drugs, which alter judgment. A history of nonvoluntary sexual activity has been associated with early initiation of voluntary sexual activity, unintended pregnancy, poor use of contraceptives, and involvement with a significantly older man (i.e., ≥5 years older).
- As part of routine screening, all teenagers should be asked direct questions regarding their sexual experiences and any incidence of coercion. This is an opportunity to identify adolescent victims and initiate discussion of contraception and STDs.

- Providers can offer education, counseling referrals, community resource information, and prevention messages. Some teenage empowerment messages include the following:
  - You have the right to say *no* to sexual activity.
  - You have the right to set sexual limits and insist that your partner honor them.
  - Be assertive. Stay sober. Recognize and avoid situations that may put you at risk.
  - Never leave a party with someone you don't know well.
  - No one should ever be forced or pressured into engaging in any unwanted sexual behavior.

Suspected Elder Abuse

- **Elder abuse** is a type of domestic violence, typically at the hands of adult family members or caregivers, that affects as many as 2 million Americans. Disabled adults are also at risk.
- Providers should apply the same criteria in assessing older or disabled individuals as they would in assessing a younger woman for domestic violence.
- Elder abuse must be reported to the state Elder Abuse Hotline, and abuse of disabled persons must be reported to the Disabled Persons Protection Commission.

RAPE EVALUATION AND TREATMENT

Rape is defined as any sexual act performed without consent. About one in four women will experience a rape during college years but only 10% to 15% will be reported to police. Approximately 50% of rape victims know their attacker, and these attacks are less likely to be reported.

Evaluation

- Assessment of physical injuries, with a focus on the genitalia
- Psychological assessment
- Pregnancy assessment and prevention
- STD evaluation and treatment
- Forensic evaluation
- When possible, evaluation should be performed by trained providers. Many institutions now have Sexual Assault Nurse Evaluation (SANE) in place. These professionals have been specially trained to care for sexual assault victims. If there is access to a SANE, emergency care should be provided to the patient but further evaluation should be done by the SANE so as to minimally interfere with evidence collection.

Patient Statement

- Make sure a chaperone who is the same sex as the patient is present at all times for the history and examination.
- Ask about injuries; this will help tailor your examination.
- Ask specifically about the nature of the violation. Elicit specifics regarding oral, vaginal, or rectal penetration as well as condom use.
- Ask what the patient has done since the event (e.g., showering, bathing, douching, voiding, defecating, changing clothes).
- Do not impose interpretation on the description—document the patient's exact description.
- Take a thorough sexual and gynecologic history, including history of infections, pregnancy, use of contraception, and last consensual intercourse.

- Obtain informed consent to proceed with the examination. This should be done for legal purposes and because it may help the victim regain autonomy.

Physical Examination
- Perform the exam with a chaperone. Be sensitive and gentle.
- The patient should undress with a sheet beneath her to capture any debris or evidence. Collect appropriate clothing from the patient and give it to the proper personnel.
- Document the patient's emotional state. Be thorough and systematic, and record all evidence of injury; use drawings and photographs as needed.
  - Perform a full skin examination and evaluate all orifices for evidence of laceration, bruising, bite marks, or use of foreign objects. A Wood's lamp and colposcope can be used to identify semen and subtle signs of trauma. Perform an overall general examination for any other injuries, such as abdominal trauma or broken bones.
- Collect dry and wet swabs of secretions to evaluate for semen and hair (evidence of coitus will be present in the vagina for up to 48 hr after the attack and in other orifices for up to 6 hr). Perform wet preparation to identify sperm. Collected samples are sent for acid phosphatase to identify semen or DNA in situ hybridization to identify a Y chromosome.
- Collect oral, cervical, and rectal culture specimens for testing for sexually transmitted diseases.
- Take samples of and perform combings of the patient's genital hair, and obtain fingernail scrapings.
- Maintain the chain of evidence—give samples directly to rape crisis personnel.

Laboratory Testing
- Radiographic imaging, if necessary, should be obtained.
- Gonorrhea and *Chlamydia* tests should be sent from any sites of contact
- Wet prep to look for *Trichomonas*
- Pregnancy test
- Baseline HIV counseling and testing
- Drug screening for the "date rape drugs" flunitrazepam (Rohypnol) and gamma-hydroxy butyrate (GHB)
- Obtain baseline specimens for herpes simplex virus, hepatitis B and C, and syphilis.

Treatment
- Suture lacerations as needed.
- Treat presumptively for STDs. Approximately, 43% of sexual assault victims have at least one preexisting STD. The risk of acquiring an STD from a sexual assault is as follows: gonorrhea, 6% to 12%; syphilis, 3%; HIV infection, <1%. See Chapter 25.
  - Treatment options for STDs include ceftriaxone 125 mg intramuscularly combined with metronidazole 2 g oral dose and doxycycline 100 mg orally twice daily for 7 days to provide coverage for gonorrhea, trichomoniasis, and *Chlamydia*. Azithromycin 1 g orally may be substituted for doxycycline and can improve patient compliance.
  - Provide hepatitis B vaccine if the victim has not received it already.
  - Sufficient evidence is not available on the efficacy of HIV antiretrovirals; however, they are usually offered if <72 hr has passed since the assault and thought to be more effective if started within 4 hr of the assault.

- Provide emergency contraception. The chance of pregnancy after the assault varies according to timing of the menstrual cycle but is generally reported to be 2% to 4% in victims not protected by some form of contraception.

Psychosocial Sequelae and Followup

- Victims may experience the **rape-trauma syndrome**, which includes feelings of anger, fear, shame, nightmares, and physical symptoms.
- Victims may develop posttraumatic stress syndrome, depression, and anxiety.
- Acute counseling should include safety planning. Victims should be referred to rape crisis programs.
- Follow-up in 1 to 2 weeks for psychological evaluation and a repeat pregnancy test.
- Follow-up in 4 weeks for repeat hepatitis B testing, collection of specimens for test of cure, and repeat pregnancy test.
- Follow-up at 3 to 6 months for repeat HIV, hepatitis B, and syphilis testing.
- Provide 24-hr hotline numbers and social work resources.
- The CDC recommends testing for RPR at 6, 12, and 24 weeks; HIV at 6, 12, and 24 weeks; and hepatitis B vaccination at 1- and 6-month intervals.

SUGGESTED READINGS

Muelleman RL, Reuwer J, Sanson TG, et al. An emergency medicine approach to violence throughout the life cycle. *Acad Emerg Med* 1996;3:708–715.

National Institute of Justice and Centers for Disease Control and Prevention. Prevalence, incidence, and consequences of violence against women: findings from the National Violence Against Women Survey. November, 1998.

National Center for the Prosecution of Violence Against Women at American Prosecutors Research Institute (APRI): Reporting Requirements for Competent Adult Victims of Domestic Violence, 2006. Available at www.usmc-mccs.org/famadv/restrictrpt.cfm (Accessed September 9, 2010).

Tjaden P, Thoennes N. National Institute of Justice and the Centers for Disease Control and Prevention. Extent, nature, and consequences of intimate partner violence, 2000.

U.S. Department of Justice, Bureau of Justice Statistics. Intimate partner violence, 1993–2001. February 2003.

U.S. Department of Justice, Office of Justice Programs, Bureau of Justice Statistics. Homicide trends in the U.S. July 11, 2007.

Websites
The National Coalition Against Domestic Violence: www.ncadv.org
The National Domestic Violence Hotline: www.ndvh.org
The U.S. Department of Justice: www.usdoj.gov, www.ndvh.org

Pediatric Gynecology

Maureen Grundy and Meredith Buonanno Loveless

Pediatric gynecology presents many challenges to the general obstetrician-gynecologist unaccustomed to dealing with these young patients. Most of the obstacles may be overcome by communicating effectively and allowing the patient to feel "in control."
- The interview is the most important aspect in determining the true reason for the visit. Due to different levels of maturity in each age group of children, considering different approaches to communication is important. Including parental figures in the discussion is key.
- Gynecologic problems experienced by the pediatric patient include vulvovaginitis, vulvar diseases, prepubertal vaginal bleeding, abnormal pubertal development, urogenital abnormalities, genital tumors, trauma, foreign bodies, and sexual abuse.

GYNECOLOGIC EVALUATION OF A CHILD

- The examination presents a unique set of difficulties that may be overcome by following a few key guidelines:
  - Give the patient a sense of control.
  - Display a caring and gentle attitude at all times; the initial evaluation can set the tone for all future examinations.
  - The physical exam should include an overall assessment of other organ systems. This allows the patient to feel more comfortable in the exam room and the examiner to gain an overall appreciation of height, weight, skin disorders, hygiene, and other indicators of pubertal development.
  - If the child is very young or has suffered physical abuse, she may need to be evaluated under anesthesia.
  - Make it clear to the child that the examination is permitted by her caregiver and that if anyone else tries to touch her genital area, she should tell her caregiver.
  - A chaperone should be present during the physical exam.

General Pediatric Physical Exam

- The abdominal exam can be facilitated by placing the child's hand over the examiner's hand.
- Palpate the inguinal regions to identify potential hernias or gonadal masses.
- Tanner classification of the external genitalia and breast development should be used to quantify pubertal changes (Fig. 31-1).

Pediatric Pelvic Exam: Positioning

- **Frog-leg posture:** child supine with feet together and knees bent outward. Commonly used in the younger patient.
- **Knee-chest position:** when combined with a Valsalva maneuver allows for assessment of the introital area. Using an otoscope for magnification or nasal speculum may help with visualization when the primary complaint is vaginal discharge or foreign bodies.

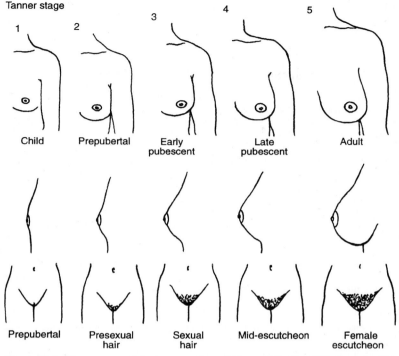

Figure 31-1. Tanner stages of development. (From Beckmann CR, Ling FW, Barzansky BM, et al. *Obstetrics and Gynecology*, 2nd Ed. Baltimore: Williams & Wilkins, 1995:8, with permission.)

- **Supine lateral-spread method:** often sufficient enough to allow for visualization of the vestibular structures
- **Mother's lap positioning:** allow the patient to sit in her mother's lap, knees bent, heels on mom's knees; combine with lateral traction of the labia for adequate exposure
- When a child is uncooperative or evaluation of the genitalia is not optimal, an **exam under anesthesia** or a return visit may be necessary.

Pediatric Pelvic Exam: Assessment

- Note perineal hygiene, presence of pubic hair, hymenal configuration, size of the clitoris, and the presence of vulvovaginal lesions.
- Specimens may be collected using a small urethral dacron swab. A second technique employs an empty butterfly catheter attached to a syringe and saline is flushed and aspirated to obtain a mix of secretions. A pediatric feeding tube attached to a 20-mL syringe also allows for vaginal irrigation.
- Lateral downward traction of the labia allows visualization of the hymen in prepubertal girls.
- Careful inspection of the hymen must be completed before pelvic examination. A Foley catheter balloon can be placed behind the hymen and filled to visualize a redundant hymen.

- Use of "extinction stimuli" can greatly facilitate a first pelvic exam. Use a distracting stimulus to draw attention from a second stimulus. For example, press a nonexamining finger into the patient's perineum before touching the introitus and allow the patient to acknowledge the presence of its pressure.
- Proper instrument selection is important. Speculum exams are rarely appropriate in the prepubertal patient. Often the hymenal ring is too tight to accommodate even a pediatric speculum. A nasal speculum can be used for an exam under anesthesia if speculum exam is necessary. A Huffman speculum (1/2 × 4 in) or Pederson (7/8 × 4 in) is appropriate for exams in adolescents.
- Rectoabdominal examination may aid in examination of the uterus in a patient who cannot tolerate a vaginal exam.
- Common exam findings:
  - Newborn child: It is important to recognize that maternal estrogen influences physical development of the newborn child. Vulvar edema, whitish pink vaginal mucosa, vaginal discharge, and breast enlargement may be normal in the newborn and should regress in the first 8 weeks of life.
  - Toddler-prepubertal child: Unestrogenized vaginal mucosa appears thin, hyperemic, and atrophic. Capillary beds may appear like roadmaps and are often mistaken for inflammation, especially around the sulcus of the vestibule and in the periurethral area.
  - Adolescent child: Vaginal mucosal is again estrogenized, and the tissue is easily distended. In early puberty, a thick white physiologic discharge is often present, as a result of unopposed estrogen causing vaginal and cervical secretions.

Documentation
- A labeled sketch of the external genitalia should be included in the medical record with a diamond-shaped space used to represent the vestibule of a child in the supine position. Twelve o'clock should represent the clitoris and 6 o'clock should represent the posterior fourchette.
- Key components include assessing Tanner stage, description of labia majora; labia minora; urethral meatus; hymen; and the presence of any discolorations, hemangiomas, or vulvovaginal lesions.

COMMON PEDIATRIC GYNECOLOGY COMPLAINTS

Vulvovaginitis
- Vaginal discharge is the most common gynecologic complaint in the prepubertal girl and accounts for 40% to 50% of visits to a pediatric gynecology clinic.
- Presents as vaginal discharge that can stain the underclothing.
- Bloodstains can occur if *Shigella*, group A beta-hemolytic *Streptococcus,* foreign body, or trauma is present.
- Vulvar burning or stinging may occur when urine comes into contact with irritated, excoriated tissues.

History: Key Points
- Note the duration, consistency, quality, and color of the discharge.
- Anaerobic infections may have a foul odor.
- Poor hygiene; back to front wiping; use of harsh soaps, bubble baths, and lotions; trauma associated with play; genital manipulation with a foreign body or

contaminated hands; close fitting, poorly absorbent clothing, including prolonged exposure to a wet bathing suit; thin, unestrogenized, alkaline vaginal mucosa; and lack of labial development may predispose to vulvovaginitis.
- Ask the child to demonstrate proper front to back wiping.
- Note the type of diaper and frequency of changes in younger children.
- Ask about recent systemic infections, new medications, bed-wetting, dermatosis, and nocturnal perianal itching.

Physical Examination
- Presentations for vulvovaginitis are extremely variable, ranging from no discharge to copious secretions. Erythema, edema, and excoriations are commonly noted. Evidence of poor perineal hygiene may be evident, with stool seen on the vulva or between the labia.
- Collect a sample of any discharge for microscopic examination and culture. Avoid contact with the hymen in prepubertal children.
- Carefully note the configuration of the hymen and evaluate for any signs of trauma. The perianal skin should also be examined.
- Vaginoscopy should be considered to exclude a foreign body, neoplasm, or abnormal connection with the gastrointestinal or urinary tract, especially in recurrent cases or those associated with bleeding.

Etiologies of Vulvovaginitis

Infection
- Normal prepubertal vaginal flora includes lactobacilli, α-hemolytic streptococci, *Staphylococcus epidermidis*, diphtheroid, and Gram-negative enteric organisms, especially *Escherichia coli*.
- While many cases of vulvovaginitis may be nonspecific, the most common pathogenic bacteria causing vulvovaginitis include Group A streptococcus, *Hemophilus influenzae*, *Staphylococcus aureus*, *S. pneumoniae*, and *E. coli*.
- Children may pass respiratory flora from the nose and oropharynx to the genitalia area, making this a possible etiology of vulvovaginitis.
- Children with chronic, nightly episodes of vulvar or perianal itching should be evaluated for *Enterobius vermicularis*.
- Shifts in flora resulting from inoculation by bacterial, viral, and yeast can result in inflammation and discharge. Several of these pathogens may be indicative of sexual activity or abuse.
- Treatment with antibiotics is indicated when an infectious pathogen is identified (Table 31-1).

Anatomic Abnormalities
- Ectopic ureter: May result in urinary leakage. Use an intravenous pyelogram (IVP) for diagnosis.
- High hymenal opening: may impair vaginal drainage; hymenectomy is curative in these cases.
- Urethral prolapse (see below).

Chemical Vaginitis
- Related to the use of new lotions, bubble baths, or harsh soaps that can cause irritation of the perineal and vulvar skin.
- Treatment includes discontinuation of the causative agent, perineal hygiene, and sitz baths.

TABLE 31-1	Treatment of Specific Vulvovaginal Infections in the Prepubertal Child

Etiology	Treatment
Streptococcus pyogenes	Penicillin V potassium 250 mg bid–tid × 10 d
Haemophilus influenzae	Amoxicillin 40 mg/kg/d × 7 d Alternate: amoxicillin/clavulanate, cefuroxime axetil, trimethoprim-sulfamethoxazole, erythromycin-sulfamethaxazole
Staphylococcus aureus	Cephalexin 25–50 mg/kg/d × 7–10 d Amoxicillin-clavulanate 20–40 mg/kg/d (of the amoxicillin) × 7–10 d Cefuroxime axetil suspension 30 mg/kg/d divided bid (max 1 g) × 10 d (tablets: 250 mg bid) Dicloxacillin 25 mg/kg/d × 7–10 d
Streptococcus pneumonia	Penicillin, amoxicillin, erythromycin, trimethoprim-sulfamethoxazole, clarithromycin
Shigella	Trimothoprim/sulfamethoxazole or ampicillin × 5 d For resistant organisms: ceftriaxone
Chlamydia trachomatis	≤45 kg: Erythromycin 50 mg/kg/d (divide in 4 doses/d) × 14 d ≥45 kg, <8 y: Azithromycin 1 g once ≥8 y: Azithromycin 1 g once OR doxycycline 100 mg bid PO × 7 d
Neisseria gonorrhoeae	<45 kg: Ceftriaxone 125 mg IM Alternate: Spectinomycin 40 mg/kg (max 2 g) IM once PLUS treat for *chlamydia* as above ≥45 kg: treated with adult regimens (see Chapter 25)
Candida	Topical nystatin, miconazole, clotrimazole, or terconazole cream; fluconazole orally
Trichomonas	Metronidazole 15 mg/kg/d given tid (max 250 mg tid) × 7 d
Enterobius vermicularis (pinworms)	Mebendazole (Vermox), 1 chewable 100-mg tablet, repeated in 2 wk

Modified from Emans SJ, Laufer MR, Goldstein DP, eds. *Pediatric and Adolescent Gynecology,* 5th ed. Philadelphia: Lippincott Williams & Wilkins, 2005:98, with permission. Data from Sexually Transmitted Disease Treatment Guidelines, 2006. *MMWR Recomm Rep* 2006;55(R11):1–94.

Systemic Illness
- Varicella, measles, Epstein-Barr virus, Crohn's disease, Stevens-Johnson syndrome, diabetes mellitus, Behçet's syndrome, and Kawasaki's syndrome may all result in vaginal discharge, vesicles, fistulas, ulcers, and inflammation.

Dermatologic Conditions
- Lichen sclerosis, psoriasis, atopic dermatitis, and contact dermatitis of the vulva may all present with symptoms similar to vulvovaginitis. These conditions may respond to topical corticosteroids.

Treatment
- Treatment depends on the etiology but almost always involves improving perineal hygiene.
  - Sitz or tub baths twice a day for half an hour help eliminate the vaginal discharge.
  - Nonirritating soaps and white cotton underpants should be recommended.
  - Nylon tights, tight blue jeans, prolonged wearing of wet bathing suits, and bubble baths should be discouraged.
  - Both the caregiver and child should be instructed on proper front to back wiping.
  - The child should be instructed to urinate with her knees apart to reduce urinary reflux into the vagina.
- Persistent symptoms after therapy (>2 weeks) warrant reexamination.
- In rare idiopathic persistent cases, vaginal irrigation with a 1% solution of povidone-iodine (Betadine) may help.
- Alternate approaches to persistent cases include a 2-month course of antibiotics or 2 to 4 weeks of estrogen cream.
- Recurrence often points to continued improper hygiene. Obese girls are at higher risk for recurrence.

Prepubertal Vaginal Bleeding

Vulvovaginitis
- May result in vaginal bleeding.

Urethral Prolapse
- Increased abdominal pressure can cause the urethral mucosa to protrude through the meatus, forming an annular, hemorrhagic mass that bleeds easily.
- Average age of onset is 5 years, and occurrence is more common in African Americans.
- Medical treatment consists of a short-term course of estrogen cream. Topical antibiotics and sitz baths may also be beneficial.
- Urinary retention or a large mass may require resection of the prolapsed tissue and insertion of an indwelling catheter may be warranted.
- Differential diagnosis includes urethral polyps, caruncles, cysts, and prolapsed ureteroceles.

Abnormal Uterine Bleeding
- See Chapter 37.

Endometrial Shedding
- Causes of endometrial shedding are outlined in Table 31-2.
- Precocious puberty is often associated with endometrial shedding in this population (see below, "Disorders of Puberty").

Labial Adhesions

- In the low estrogen environment of childhood, the labia may fuse in response to any genital trauma, even diaper rash.
- Adhesive vulvitis caused by chronic irritation is common between ages 2 and 6.
- Asymptomatic labial adhesions do not require treatment and will resolve spontaneously with increasing estrogen levels in puberty.
- If urinary retention or urinary tract infections (UTIs) occur, treatment is required and involves application of estrogen cream along the white line of the adhesion, with gentle traction twice daily for 2 to 6 weeks.

| TABLE 31-2 | Causes of Endometrial Shedding in Children |

- Physiologic neonatal withdrawal bleed in the first 2 wk of life secondary to maternal estrogen withdrawal
- Isolated premature menarche
- Iatrogenic or factitious precocious puberty caused by medications that contain exogenous estrogens
- Idiopathic precocious puberty
- Functional ovarian cysts
- Ovarian neoplasms
- McCune-Albright syndrome
- Central nervous system lesions
- Hormone-producing neoplasms

- Recurrence is common after treatment. Acute urinary retention requires surgical excision.

DISORDERS OF PUBERTY

Puberty is a result of pulsatile gonadotropin releasing haromone (GnRH) secretion and activation of the hypothalamic–pituitary–gonadal axis. The onset of puberty is generally between 8 and 13 years old in girls. Tanner stages are used to describe pubertal development.

Delayed Puberty
- Delay of puberty can be caused by anatomic abnormalities, chromosomal disorders, neoplastic growths, or nutritional deficiencies.
- Commonly presents as a physical delay in maturation combined with amenorrhea.
- Causes of delayed puberty can be classified, based on the level of follicle-stimulating hormone (FSH) present, as outlined in Table 31-3.

Hypergonadotropic Hypogonadism (High FSH)
- A sufficient amount of gonadotropins are present, but the ovaries are not responsive and therefore do not produce sex steroids.

Gonadal Dysgenesis
- Presents as a phenotypic female with persistent prepubertal development.
- May have some secondary sex characteristics and spontaneous menstruation. Most often associated with primary amenorrhea.
- **Turner's syndrome** (45, X) occurs in 1 in 2,000 to 2,500 girls. Phenotype includes primary amenorrhea and short stature.
- Patients with **Swyer's syndrome** (46, XY) often have a normal-to-tall stature. It is caused by a mutation or structural abnormality of the Y chromosome.

Primary Ovarian Failure
- Ovaries develop but do not contain oocytes; may be associated with chemotherapy, radiation, galactosemia, gonadotropin resistance, autoimmune ovarian failure, or ovarian failure secondary to previous infection.
- Treatment involves administration of exogenous estrogen and progesterone to avoid osteoporosis and facilitate development of secondary sexual characteristics.

TABLE 31-3	An Overview of Causes of Delayed Puberty

FSH Level	Differential Diagnosis
High >30 mIU/mL	• Gonadal dysgenesis syndromes: Turner's syndrome, Sweyer's syndrome • Primary ovarian failure
Low <10 mIU/mL	• Constitutional delay • Intracranial neoplasms • Isolated gonadotropin deficiencies • Hormone deficiencies • Kallmann's syndrome • Prader-Willi syndrome • Laurence-Moon-Biedl syndrome • Chronic disease and malnutrition
Normal	• *Anatomic deformities* result in normal development with primary amenorrhea. • Imperforate hymen • Transverse vaginal septum • Mullerian agenesis

Hypogonadotrophic Hypogonadism (Low FSH)
- An insufficient level of gonadotropins is present to permit follicular development, and, therefore, sex steroids are not produced.
  - **Chronic disease:** Conditions including states of malnutrition (e.g., starvation, anorexia nervosa, cystic fibrosis, Crohn's disease, diabetes mellitus, and hypothyroidism) may disrupt GnRH production.
  - **Constitutional delay**: A delay in the GnRH pulse generator postpones the normal physiologic events of puberty.
  - **Intracranial neoplasms**: Craniopharyngiomas and pituitary adenomas may cause delayed puberty. Visual symptoms are often associated with these tumors, as is short stature and diabetes insipidus. Diagnosis is by CT or MRI of the head.
  - **Isolated gonadotropin deficiencies:** often secondary to abnormalities in genes encoding proteins related to GnRH, FSH, or luteinizing hormone (LH).
  - **Hormone deficiencies:** Aberrations of growth hormone, thyroid hormone, or prolactin can affect puberty.
  - **Kallmann's syndrome:** Presents with a classic triad of anosmia, hypogonadism, and color blindness. The hypothalamus cannot secrete GnRH due to dysfunction in the arcuate nucleus. Few or no secondary sexual characteristics are present.
  - **Prader-Willi syndrome:** An autosomal deletion and imprinting disorder associated with obesity, emotional instability, and delayed puberty due to hypothalamic dysfunction.
  - Other uncommon causes include **Laurence-Moon** and **Bardet-Biedl syndromes**.

Eugonadism (Normal FSH)
- In cases of eugonadal pubertal delay, the hypothalamic-pituitary-gonadal axis remains intact, but primary amenorrhea occurs secondary to anatomic abnormalities in the genitourinary tract, androgen insensitivity, or inappropriate positive feedback mechanisms.

- Anatomic abnormalities: see "Congenital Anomalies" (below).
- Androgen insensitivity: see "Ambiguous Genitalia" (below).
- Other causes of primary amenorrhea with eugonadism include anovulation, androgen-producing adrenal disease, and polycystic ovarian syndrome.

Precocious Puberty

- **Precocious puberty** occurs in only 1 of 10,000 girls and is defined as the presence of secondary sexual characteristics at an age >2.5 standard deviations below the mean (i.e., 6 years old in African Americans and 7 years old in Caucasians).
- Accelerated growth velocity and rapid bone growth can result in short adult stature.
- Causes are divided into GnRH-dependent disorders and GnRH-independent disorders.

GnRH Dependent Disorders—Central Precocious Puberty

- Most commonly **idiopathic**; secondary sexual characteristics progress in normal sequence but more rapidly than in normal puberty and may fluctuate between progression and regression.
- Related to premature development of the hypothalamic-pituitary axis.
- Characteristic signs and symptoms include breast development without pubic hair development, an increase in height, acne, oily skin/hair, and emotional changes.
- May be transmitted in an autosomal recessive fashion.
- Often ovarian follicular cysts are present due to elevated levels of LH and FSH.
- Other causes involve **central nervous system disease**, particularly mass effects near the hypothalamus. The most common neoplasm is a hamartoma in the posterior hypothalamus.
  - Disease often involves areas surrounding the hypothalamus; mass effect, radiation, or ectopic GnRH-secreting cells are thought to cause premature activation of pulsatile secretion of GnRH from the hypothalamus.
  - Diagnosis by CT or MRI of the head; history may be significant for headache, mental status changes, mental retardation, dysmorphic syndromes, along with the premature development of secondary sexual characteristics.
  - Treatment should be directed at the underlying cause; the location of many of such tumors makes resection difficult, and, as a result, chemotherapy or radiation may be indicated.
  - GnRH agonist administration results in a short burst of gonadotropin release, followed by downregulation and a decrease in the level of circulating gonadotropins. Follow estradiol levels to make appropriate dose adjustments.

GnRH Independent Disorders—Pseudoprecocious Puberty

- Differential diagnosis includes estrogen-secreting tumors, benign follicular ovarian cysts, McCune-Albright syndrome, Peutz-Jeghers syndrome, adrenal disorders, and primary hypothyroidism.

Estrogen-Secreting Ovarian Tumors

- See Chapter 45.

Benign Ovarian Cysts

- Most common form of estrogen-secreting masses in children.
- May require a diagnostic laparoscopy or possibly exploratory laparotomy to differentiate from a malignant tumor. Removal of the cyst may be therapeutic.

McCune-Albright Syndrome

- Triad: café au lait spots, polyostotic fibrous dysplasia, and cysts of skull and long bones; precocious puberty is present in 40%.

- Associated with rapid breast development and early occurrence of menarche.
- Sexual precocity results from recurrent follicular cyst. Removal of cyst is not helpful.
- Aromatase inhibitors may help control symptoms.
- Evaluate with serial pelvic sonograms to detect the presence of gonadal tumors.

Peutz-Jeghers Syndrome
- Commonly characterized by mucocutaneous pigmentation and GI polyposis.
- Also associated with rare sex cord tumors, including epithelial tumors of the ovary, dysgerminomas, or Sertoli-Leydig cell tumors, whose estrogen secretion may result in feminization and incomplete sexual precocity.
- Girls with Peutz-Jeghers syndrome should be screened with serial pelvic sonograms.

Adrenal Disorders
- Some adrenal adenomas secrete estrogen and may result in sexual precocity.

Primary Hypothyroidism
- Characterized by premature breast development and galactorrhea without an associated growth spurt. See Chapter 13.

Key Points in Evaluation and Management of Precocious Puberty
- Perform a detailed evaluation with Tanner staging.
- Laboratory data should include LH, FSH, prolactin, estradiol, progesterone, 17-hydroxyprogesterone, DHEA, DHEAS, TSH, T4, hCG.
- A GnRH stimulation test can definitively diagnose central precocious puberty.
- Obtain an x-ray to determine bone age. Head CT or MRI can rule out an intracranial mass. Abdominal/pelvic ultrasound can be used to evaluate the ovaries.
- Goals for management include maximizing adult height and delaying maturation. Treat the intracranial, ovarian, or adrenal pathology if present and attempt to reduce associated emotional problems.

Premature Thelarche

- **Premature thelarche** is defined as bilateral breast development without other signs of sexual maturation in girls before age 8.
- Commonly occurs by age 2 and is rare after age 4.
- The etiology is unclear, but exogenous estrogen must be excluded.
- Precocious puberty must be ruled out.
  - Document the appearance of the vaginal mucosa, breast size, and presence or absence of a pelvic mass.
  - Obtain bone age. It is within normal range in premature thelarche.
  - Perform pelvic ultrasonography, which should exclude ovarian pathology.
  - Obtain plasma estrogen levels. They may be mildly elevated; significant elevations suggest another etiology.
- In idiopathic cases, regression often occurs after a few months but may persist for several years.

AMBIGUOUS GENITALIA

Male Feminization

- Genetic males (XY) undergo feminization related to androgen insensitivity.
- **Complete androgen insensitivity** or **"testicular feminization"**
  - Transmitted in a maternal X-linked recessive fashion

- Pathophysiology: Androgen presence is incapable of inducing maturation of the Wolffian duct. Antimüllerian hormone is present, and Müllerian duct formation remains inhibited. The resulting phenotype is female, with a vagina derived from the urogenital sinus that ends in a blind pouch and testes that often descend through the inguinal canal.
- Clinical presentation: primary amenorrhea, Tanner stage V breast development, scant axillary, and pubic hair.
- Management: gonadectomy is recommended once sexual maturation is complete secondary to an increased incidence of malignancy; exogenous estrogen therapy is also recommended.
- **Incomplete androgen insensitivity**
  - Less common with presentation ranging from near complete masculinization to near complete failure of virilization.
  - As minimal sensitivity to androgens is present, the Wolffian duct system develops to some extent, although spermatogenesis usually remains absent.
  - Physical exam may include a range of clitoromegaly or ambiguous genitalia.
  - Sex assignment depends on the degree of masculinization.
- **5-alpha reductase deficiency**
  - Genotypic males (XY) who are phenotypically female in the prepubertal state and become phenotypically men at puberty. Testicular function is normal and there is no breast development.

Female Virilization

- Genetic females (XX) are exposed to increased androgen levels that lead to inappropriate virilization, most often an indicator of organic disease in girls.
- Virilizing **congenital adrenal hyperplasia (CAH)**: most commonly associated with deficiency of 21-hydroxylase, an autosomal recessive disorder. May present in a newborn with ambiguous genitalia and possible salt wasting due to mineralocorticoid deficiency. Virilization may also be delayed until later childhood in less severe forms
- **Cushing's disease:** can manifest as growth failure, with or without virilization, obesity, striae, or moon facies.
- **Ovarian tumors:** Sertoli-Leydig cell tumor (e.g., arrhenoblastoma) is the most common virilizing ovarian tumor. Others include lipoid cell tumor and gonadoblastoma.

CONGENITAL ANOMALIES OF THE FEMALE REPRODUCTIVE TRACT

Anatomic disorders may present as primary amenorrhea, chronic pelvic pain, mucocolpos, hematocolpos, or hematometria.
- **Imperforate hymen**: may present as bulging, translucent mass at the introitus in the newborn or as cyclic pain, abdominal mass, hematocolpos, and/or a bluish perineal bulge after menarche. Imperforate hymen may regress as the girl enters childhood. In cases where there is no regression, surgical intervention is required to incise the hymen and allow stored debris to escape.
- **Transverse vaginal septum**: Due to failure of canalization of mullerian tubules and the sinovaginal bulb, leaving a membrane present. Presentation and examination may be similar to an imperforate hymen. If the membrane is thin, it can be incised and dilated. If thick, surgical incision with a skin graft may be required.

- **Longitudinal vaginal septum:** This is often associated with uterine and/or renal anomalies. Complaints include persistent bleeding despite the use of a tampon. Surgical correction is indicated.
- **Mullerian agenesis:** failure of the müllerian tract to develop results in a blind vaginal pouch without uterus or fallopian tubes present. Ovaries are not of mullerian origin and puberty progresses as usual with primary amenorrhea as a presenting complaint. This must be distinguished from androgen insensitivity, as described previously. One third of these patients have associated urinary tract anomalies, and 12% have skeletal anomalies. A neovagina can be created by progressive dilation or surgery.
- **Vaginal atresia/agenesis:** will present similarly to a transverse septum in adolescent girls. Treatment may involve progressive vaginal dilation or surgical reconstruction.

GENITAL TUMORS

- Genital tumors are uncommon in the prepubertal girl but need to be considered in a patient with a chronic genital ulcer, tissue protruding from the vagina, a malodorous or bloody discharge, or an atraumatic swelling of the external genitalia. Causes are outlined in Table 31-4.

FOREIGN BODIES AND TRAUMA

Foreign Bodies

- Most common at ages 2 to 4. The foreign bodies can vary from wads of toilet paper, buttons, or coins to peanuts and crayons.
- Retained foreign bodies in the vagina often present with bloody, brown, or purulent discharge of several weeks duration.
- Genital pruritus, abdominal pain, or fever may be present.
- Can be an indicator of sexual abuse.
- Persistent vaginal discharge in a toddler or young girl warrants an exam under anesthesia. Antibiotics should be started before removal. If the object remains undetected, peritonitis can develop from the ascension of purulent secretions into the fallopian tubes. A careful examination of the vaginal wall for any defects or additional embedded foreign bodies should be performed after the object has been removed. If the rectovaginal septum is involved, a temporary colostomy with delayed repair of the vaginal and rectal tissues may be indicated.

Traumatic Injuries

- The period of highest incidence is between ages 4 and 12, with 75% of all genital injuries occurring in young girls. Because of differences in anatomy between a child and an adult, a seemingly innocuous lesion can suggest serious injury. Common injuries include:

Straddle Injuries
- Most present as a swollen area of painful ecchymosis or hematoma over the labia; the mons, clitoris, and urethra can be involved.
- If hematuria is present, consider a voiding cystourethrogram to rule out bladder or urethra injury.
- Periurethral injuries can result in swelling and urinary retention. Early placement of a urinary catheter is advised.

TABLE 31-4 Malignant Genital Tumors in Pediatric Gynecology

Tumor	Characteristics	Treatment
Sarcoma botryoides (Rhabdomyosarcoma)	• Most common malignant tumor of the genital tract in girls • Fast-growing, aggressive • 90% before age 5, peak incidence age 2 • Arises in submucosa of vagina • Hallmark polypoid mass passing from the vagina, vulva, or urethra, usually anterior • Vaginal bleeding, abdominal pain	• First, stage with CXR/CT scan • Chemotherapy followed by surgery (type of procedure depends on stage of disease) • Possible radiotherapy • Follow-up (tends to recur locally) • Improved treatment regimens have led to more conservative surgical options and improved survival
Clear cell adenocarcinoma	• Often seen with maternal diethylstilbestrol exposure • Abnormal vaginal bleeding and discharge	• In early stages, conservative approach involves wide local excision, with lymph nodes dissection followed by local radiation • Advanced disease may require whole pelvic radiation
Germ cell tumors	• Most common ovarian neoplasm in pediatric population • Arises from primitive germ cells; two types—dysgerminomas and embryonal carcinoma • Presents as complex pelvic masses • Tumor markers: AFP, hCG, CEA	• Management is surgical and involves at least unilateral oophorectomy and staging if needed • Dysgerminomas respond to radiation, but future fertility should be taken into consideration

CXR, chest radiograph; CT, computed tomography; AFP, alpha-fetoprotein; hCG, human chorionic gonadotropin; CEA, carcinoembryonic antigen.

- Treat with observation and cold compresses for the first 6 hr. If the hematoma remains the same size or becomes smaller, warm sitz baths are often all that are required.
- Analgesics and prophylactic antibiotics can be used when a hematoma at the urethral orifice is causing pain and poor urination.

Accidental Penetration
- Most frequently seen between ages 2 and 4, often the result of falling on a sharp object (e.g., pen or pencil).
- Presentation often includes hematuria, vaginal discharge, or bleeding. A puncture wound may be intraperitoneal with rectal pain or bleeding as the presenting complaint.
- In an unstable patient with an injury above the hymen, laparoscopy or laparotomy should be performed.
- Workup involves examination with abdominal radiography, anoscopy, and sigmoidoscopy. Microscopic hematuria warrants careful urethral catheterization. Resistance to the passage of a catheter requires a voiding cystourethrogram. Catheterization should not be attempted with gross hematuria.

Lacerations
- Often secondary to forceful abduction of the legs, gymnastic exercise, water-skiing, bicycle accidents, or major motor vehicle accidents.
- Lacerations of the vaginal orifice frequently extend into the fornix.
- Examination under anesthesia must be performed to determine the extent of the injury and rule out involvement of the rectovaginal septum or peritoneal cavity.

Clitoral Strangulation or Ischemia
- Difficult to diagnose; symptoms may include irritability and engorgement and cellulitis of the clitoris.
- Often results when an entrapped hair from a caretaker accidentally becomes wrapped around the base of the organ. Treatment is removal of the stricture.

SUGGESTED READINGS

American Academy of Pediatricans. Management of urinary tract infections. *Pediatrics* 1999;103(4):843–852.

Antoniazzi F, Zamboni G. Central precocious puberty: current treatment options. *Pediatr Drugs* 2004;6(4):211–231.

Carel JC, Leger J. Precocious puberty. *N Engl J Med* 2008;358:2366–2377.

The initial reproductive health visit. ACOG Committee Opinion Number 335. American College of Obstetricians and Gynecologists. *Obstet Gynecol* 2006;107:745–747.

Lara-Torre E. Physical exam of pediatric and adolescent patients. *Clin Obstet Gynecol* 2008;51(2):205–213.

Merritt D. Genital trauma in children and adolescents. *Clin Obstet Gynecol* 2008;51(2):237–248.

Miller RJ, Breech LL. Surgical corrections of vaginal anomalies. *Clin Obstet Gynecol* 2008;51(2):223–236.

Shulman L. Mullerian anomalies. *Clin Obstet Gynecol* 2008;51(2):214–222.

IV Reproductive Endocrinology and Infertility

32 Infertility and Assisted Reproductive Technologies

Mindy S. Christianson and Edward E. Wallach

INFERTILITY

Definitions

- **Infertility:** failure of a couple of reproductive age to conceive after at least 1 year of regular coitus without contraception.
  - **Primary infertility:** infertility in a woman who has never been pregnant.
  - **Secondary infertility:** infertility in a woman who has had one or more previous pregnancies.
- **Fecundability:** probability of achieving pregnancy within one menstrual cycle. For a normal couple, this is approximately 25%.
- **Fecundity:** ability to achieve a live birth within one menstrual cycle.

Incidence

- Data from the 2002 National Survey of Family Growth revealed that 2% of women of reproductive age in the United States had an infertility-related medical appointment within the past year.
- Additionally, 11.9% of women of reproductive age reported having received infertility services at some point in their lives.
- Seven percent of couples with women of reproductive age reported they had not used contraception in the past year and the woman had not become pregnant.
- Demand for infertility services has increased in recent years. Reasons include the following:
  - Delayed childbearing in women due to career demands and marriage at a later age.

TABLE 32-1	Differential Diagnosis of Infertility	
Diagnosis	**Percent**	**Basic Evaluation**
Male factors	30	Semen analysis
Tubal/uterine/peritoneal factors	25	HSG, laparoscopy, chromopertubation
Anovulation/ovarian factors	25	BBT chart, midluteal progesterone level, endometrial biopsy, luteinizing hormone testing
Cervical factors	10	Postcoital test
Unexplained infertility	10	All of the above

HSG, hysterosalpingogram; BBT, basal body temperature. Adapted from Speroff L, Fritz MA. *Clinical Gynecologic Endocrinology and Infertility*, 7th Ed (Chapter 27). Philadelphia, PA: Lippincott Williams and Wilkins, 2005:1013–1067.

- An increase in variety and effectiveness of assisted reproductive technology (ART) treatments and an increased public awareness of these treatments, including in vitro fertilization (IVF).
- An increase in tubal factor infertility as a consequence of sexually transmitted diseases.
- Relative scarcity of babies placed for adoption due to effective contraception and increased availability of abortion services.

Differential Diagnosis

- The **differential diagnosis** of infertility encompasses five principal categories (Table 32-1):
  - Male factor
  - Ovulatory dysfunction
  - Structural (tubal/peritoneal and uterine)
  - Cervical factors
  - Unexplained causes

EVALUATION

- Evaluation is indicated for women who fail to conceive after one or more years of regular, unprotected intercourse.
- Women over the age of 35 should be evaluated sooner (i.e., after 6 months of regular, unprotected intercourse.)
- No woman should be denied her request for infertility services or counseling, regardless of duration.
- Successful reproduction requires proper structure and function of the entire reproductive axis, including hypothalamus, pituitary gland, ovaries, fallopian tube, uterus, cervix, and vagina.
- **Infertility evaluation** comprises eight major elements:
  - History and physical examination
  - Semen analysis
  - Sperm—cervical mucus interaction (postcoital testing [PCT])—for select patients
  - Assessment of ovarian reserve
  - Tests for occurrence of ovulation
  - Evaluation of tubal patency

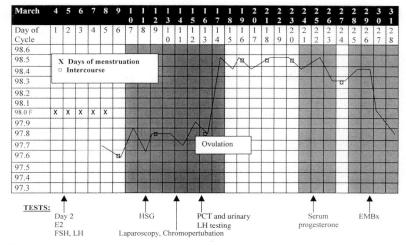

Figure 32-1. Sample basal body temperature (BBT) chart with complete infertility evaluation within one menstrual cycle. E_2, estradiol level; EMBx, endometrial biopsy; FSH, follicle-stimulating hormone level; LH, luteinizing hormone level; HSG, hysterosalpingogram; PCT, postcoital test.

- Detection of uterine abnormalities
- Determination of peritoneal abnormalities
- With proper coordination, the evaluation can be completed within one menstrual cycle (Fig. 32-1). No abnormality or cause of infertility can be identified in 10% to 15% of couples. This group comprises a category known as "unexplained infertility."

History and Physical Examination

- The initial assessment involves an extended and complete history from both partners and a complete physical examination.
  - Physical examination of the male partner can be deferred pending the results of the semen analysis and is usually performed by a urologist.
- History elicited from both male and female partners should include the following:
  - Duration of infertility, methods of contraception, previous evaluation and treatment, prior reproductive history, sexual dysfunction, sexually transmitted infections, tobacco and alcohol use, caffeine use, family history of mental retardation, and birth defects.
- History elicited from the female partner should include the following:
  - Complete menstrual history, dysmenorrhea or menorrhagia, pelvic or abdominal pan, dyspareunia, symptoms of thyroid disease, galactorrhea, symptoms of hirsutism, exercise habits, and indices of stress.
- Components of the female physical exam should include the following:
  - Weight and body mass index, thyroid exam, breast exam, signs of hirsutism, pelvic or abdominal tenderness, uterine size and mobility, adnexal masses and/or tenderness, cul-de-sac tenderness, or nodularity.
- Baseline labs may include the following: TSH, prolactin, FSH, 17-hydroxyprogesterone, serum testosterone, progesterone, dehydroepiandrosterone (DHEAS), semen analysis, and hysterosalpingogram (HSG).

Male Factor Infertility Evaluation

- The semen analysis is the cornerstone of male factor infertility evaluation.
  - Semen sample should be collected after at least 48 to 72 hr abstinence and is best evaluated within 1 hr of ejaculation.
  - Obtained either by masturbation or by sexual intercourse with a silicone condom, because latex condoms are spermicidal.
- Normal parameters according to the World Health Organization (WHO) are as follows:
  - Ejaculate volume between 1.5 and 5.0 mL
  - Semen pH above 7.2
  - Sperm concentration above 20 million/mL
  - Greater than 50% motility
  - Greater than 14% normal morphology.
- Semen analysis terminology:
  - **Azoospermia:** absence of sperm in the ejaculate.
  - **Oligospermia:** a concentration of fewer than 20 million sperm/mL.
  - **Asthenospermia:** reduced sperm motility.
- Men with an abnormal semen analysis should be referred to a urologist, especially in cases of oligospermia or azoospermia. Causes of male factor infertility include the following:
  - **Kleinefelter's syndrome**
    - Karyotype is 47,XXY.
    - Most common genetic anomaly in azoospermic men.
    - Found in 1:500 to 1:1000 live male births.
    - Incidence: 3% of infertile men, 3.5% to 14.5% of azoospermic men, 1% of couples referred to intracytoplasmic sperm injection (ICSI).
  - **Congenital absence of the vas deferens (CAVD)**
    - Associated with cystic fibrosis gene mutations in the *cystic fibrosis transmembrane conductance regulator* (CFTR) gene.
    - Partners of men with CAVD must be tested for the CFTR gene mutation before pursuing infertility treatment with retrieved sperm.
  - **Y-chromosome microdeletions**
    - May be found in up to 7% of men with male factor infertility
    - While these men may be able to father children via IVF/ICSI, male offspring will inherit the Y-chromosome microdeletion and be infertile.

EXCLUSION OF OVULATORY FACTOR INFERTILITY

To exclude ovulatory dysfunction, the presence of ovulation must be confirmed. In addition, ovarian reserve should be assessed to exclude oocyte depletion and premature ovarian failure.

Confirmation of Ovulation

- The basal body temperature (BBT) chart (Fig. 32-1) is a simple means of determining whether ovulation has occurred.
  - The woman's temperature is taken daily on awakening, before any activity, and recorded on a graph.
  - After ovulation, rising progesterone levels increase the basal temperature by approximately 0.4°F (0.22°C) through a hypothalamic thermogenic effect.

- Because the rise in progesterone may occur anytime from 2 days before ovulation to 1 day after, the temperature elevation does not predict the exact moment of ovulation but offers retrospective confirmation of its occurrence.
- A temperature elevation is usually sustained for 14 ± 2 days. One that persists for <11 days is suggestive of a luteal phase defect.
- Midluteal phase progesterone level is another test to assess ovulation.
  - A concentration >3.0 ng/mL in a blood sample drawn between days 19 and 23 suggests ovulation has occurred. Normal adequate luteal support usually produces a progesterone concentration >10 ng/mL.
- Daily monitoring of urinary LH is now widely used, given the proliferation of commercial tests for home use.
  - Using a threshold concentration of 40 mIU/mL, positive testing for urinary LH correlates well with the surge of serum LH levels that trigger ovulation.
  - Exclusive reliance on urinary LH testing to detect ovulation is discouraged. Seven to eight percent of women—both fertile and infertile—have false positive tests by this means.

Assessment of Ovarian Reserve

- Depleted ovarian reserve adversely impacts fecundability given the inferior quantity and quality of remaining oocytes. The following tests help identify both a depleted reserve and the likelihood of response to controlled ovarian hyperstimulation (COH) during assisted reproduction:
- Day 3 FSH concentration: Values below 10 to 15 mIU/mL suggest adequate ovarian reserve. The exact cutoff depends on the particular laboratory reference standards.
- Clomiphene citrate challenge test (CCCT): The administration of clomiphene citrate (CC) 100 mg orally on menstrual cycle days 5 to 9 with measurement of day 3 and day 10 FSH. An exaggerated FSH response portends poorly for spontaneous or assisted conception.
- Imaging of antral follicle counts by ultrasonography.

EXCLUSION OF STRUCTURAL FACTORS (TUBAL/ PERITONEAL AND UTERINE)

- Tubal/peritoneal factors include endometriosis, pelvic adhesion disease, or previous bilateral tubal ligation. Uterine factors include leiomyomata, intrauterine synechiae (Asherman's syndrome), septae, and other Mullerian anomalies.
- **Hysterosalpingogram (HSG)** assesses uterine and fallopian tube contour and tubal patency (Fig. 32-2).
  - HSG shows appreciable Mullerian anomalies as well as most endometrial polyps, synechiae and submucosal fibroids. It can also determine tubal patency.
  - Performed in the early follicular phase, within 1 week of cessation of menstrual flow, to minimize chances of interrupting a pregnancy.
  - The procedure is performed by injecting a radiopaque dye through the cervix. As more dye is injected, the dye normally passes through the uterine cavity into the fallopian tubes and then spills into the peritoneal cavity.
  - X-ray films are taken under fluoroscopy to evaluate tubal patency.
  - Nonsteroidal anti-inflammatory drugs may be given to prevent cramping.
  - HSG may have therapeutic effects. Several studies have indicated increased pregnancy rates for several months after the procedure.

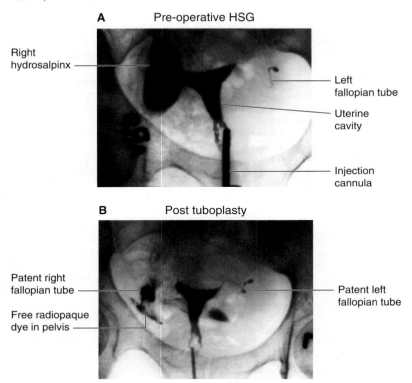

Figure 32-2. Hysterosalpingogram showing large right hydrosalpinx (**A**) that is resolved following successful tuboplasty (**B**). Real-time radiographs are obtained as radiopaque dye is injected through a cannula inserted in the cervical canal. Normal patent tubes demonstrate bilateral spillage from the fallopian tubes into the pelvis. (Original images courtesy of Dr. Edward Wallach, Johns Hopkins Hospital, Department of Gynecology and Obstetrics, Division of Reproductive Endocrinology and Infertility.)

- Prophylactic antibiotics (doxycycline, 100 mg orally twice daily for 5 to 7 days) are advisable when the patient has a history of pelvic inflammatory disease or when hydrosalpinges are identified during the study.
- **Saline infusion ultrasonography** (Sonohysterography [SHG])
  - SHG involves transvaginal ultrasound after the introduction of sterile water or saline into the uterine cavity.
  - Useful in assessment of uterine cavity abnormalities such as polyps or submucosal fibroids.
- **Hysteroscopy**
  - Definitive method to evaluate the intrauterine cavity.
  - Reserved for those patients with HSG or SHG results that merit further evaluation. It offers the possibility of minimally invasive treatment at time of the procedure.
- **Diagnostic laparoscopy**

- Assesses peritoneal and tubal factors, such as endometriosis and pelvic adhesions and can provide access for simultaneous corrective surgery.
- Laparoscopy should be scheduled in the follicular phase. This is the final and most invasive step in the patient's evaluation.
- Findings on HSG correlate with laparoscopic findings 60% to 70% of the time.
- Chromopertubation: Dye (usually a dilute solution of indigo carmine) instilled through the fallopian tubes during laparoscopy to visually document tubal patency.
- Hysteroscopy may also be included to ensure that no intrauterine abnormalities were missed on the HSG.

EXCLUSION OF CERVICAL FACTOR INFERTILITY

- The PCT or Huhner's test allows direct analysis of sperm and cervical mucus interaction and provides a rough estimate of sperm quality.
- The test is done between days 12 and 14 of a 28- to 30-day menstrual cycle (after 48 hr of abstinence) when maximum estrogen secretion is present.
- The mucus is examined within 2 to 12 hr.
- Because interpretation of the PCT is subjective, the validity of the test is controversial, despite its long history of use.
- The test's utility is most valuable for patients with history or physical exam findings suggestive of cervical factor, when the results will help direct treatment.
- However, a finding of 5 to 10 progressively motile spermatozoa per high-power field and clear acellular mucus with a spinnbarkeit (the degree to which the mucus stretches between two slides) of 8 cm generally suggests normal cervical function.
- Fecundity rates do not correlate directly with the number of motile sperm seen. The most common cause of an abnormal PCT is poor timing. Other causes include cervical stenosis, hypoplastic endocervical canal, coital dysfunction, and male factors. The sample can also be assessed for pH, mucus cellularity, WBC, and ferning. Clumping and flagellation of sperm without progression are often suggestive of antisperm antibodies.

ENDOMETRIAL BIOPSY AND THE LUTEAL PHASE DEFECT

- Endometrial biopsy can document ovulation by histologic demonstration of decidualized stroma, assess for endometritis, and allows for histologic dating of the endometrium within 2 to 3 days.
- Usually performed between days 24 and 26 of a 28-day menstrual cycle or 2 to 4 days before anticipated menstruation.
- Dates of the biopsy and subsequent menstrual cycle have been used to determine whether a luteal phase deficiency—insufficient progesterone support for the purported histologic date of the endometrium—is present.
- Recent reports have demonstrated that fertile women were at least as likely as their infertile counterparts to have an out-of-phase endometrial biopsy suggestive of a luteal phase defect.

TREATMENT FOR INFERTILITY

Anovulation

The vast majority of anovulatory women of reproductive age fall into WHO class II and, fortunately, this class proves responsive to ovulation induction. The agents most commonly used to stimulate multiple ovarian follicles are clomiphene citrate (CC), human menopausal gonadotropins (hMG), and purified follicle-stimulating hormone (FSH). The WHO stratifies anovulatory women into three classes

- WHO Class I: Hypogonadotropic hypogonadal anovulation
  - Hypothalamic amenorrhea attributable to low GnRH levels or pituitary unresponsiveness to hypothalamic GnRH, with resultant low FSH and serum estradiol levels.
  - Causes include excessive weight gain or loss, exercise or emotional stress.
- WHO Class II: Normogonadotropic normoestrogenic anovulation
  - Normal levels of estradiol and FSH; LH levels, however, are elevated. This class includes the polycystic ovarian syndrome (PCOS).
- WHO Class III: Hypergonadotropic hypoestrogenic anovulation
  - Main causes include premature ovarian failure (no follicles due to early menopause) or ovarian resistance.
  - These patients rarely respond to treatment for anovulation.
  - Donor eggs may be best option for these patients in achieving pregnancy.

Clomiphene Citrate (CC)

- Mechanism of action: synthetic, nonsteroidal estrogen agonist-antagonist that increases the release of gonadotropin-releasing hormone (GnRH) and subsequent LH and FSH release (antiestrogenic effect in hypothalamus results in increased GnRH secretion).
- Useful in women with oligomenorrhea and amenorrhea, with intact hypothalamic-pituitary-ovarian axes.
- Patients who are overweight and hyperandrogenic or hypoestrogenic have decreased responsiveness to CC.
- Initiated on day 3, 4, or 5 in the menstrual cycle, usually at a starting dose of 50 mg for 5 days.
- Adverse effects: vasomotor symptoms such as headache and mood change; rarely, visual symptoms such as transient blurry vision or scotomata have been reported.
- Complications: cystic ovarian enlargement and multifetal gestations (5% to 10% of pregnancies).

Exogenous Gonadotropins

- GnRH, hMG, and FSH are used primarily in women who fail to respond to CC or who have hypogonadotropic amenorrhea or unexplained infertility.
  - Prescription of these expensive drugs, which are used in the more complicated protocols for IVF (see below), should be left to specialists trained in their use.

Hyperprolactinemia

- Bromocriptine is used to induce ovulation in patients with hyperprolactinemia.
- Bromocriptine is a dopamine agonist that directly inhibits pituitary secretion of prolactin, which restores normal gonadotropin release.
  - The usual starting dose is 2.5 mg at bedtime to prevent dopaminergic side effects, which include nausea, diarrhea, dizziness, and headache.
  - If oral administration cannot be tolerated, vaginal administration is recommended.
- A response is usually seen in 2 to 3 months, and 80% of hyperprolactinemic patients ovulate and become pregnant.

- CC is added if ovulation does not occur within 3 months after beginning treatment.
- Cabergoline is an alternative for those who do not tolerate bromocryptine. See Chapter 13.

Thyroid Dysfunction
- See Chapter 13.

Hypothalamic-Pituitary Axis Dysfunction
- Hypothalamic-pituitary axis problems including extreme weight gain or loss, excessive exercise, and emotional stress can all impact the secretion of GnRH from the hypothalamus and cause ovulatory dysfunction. These must be addressed by appropriate behavioral or psychological intervention.

Male Factor Infertility
- Although the gynecologist does not directly treat male patients, therapies to treat male factor infertility often involve hormonal manipulation in the female partner. The evaluation is analogous to that in the woman, with examination of the hypothalamic-pituitary-testicular axis, outflow tract, and testicular function.
- Toxins, viruses, sexually transmitted diseases, varicoceles, and congenital problems can all influence infertility.
- The procedure of ICSI has revolutionized treatment of male infertility. As long as viable sperm can be retrieved by ejaculation, epididymal aspiration, or testicular biopsy, successful fertilization and pregnancy can be achieved. The fertilization rate is 95%, and the pregnancy rate is comparable to that of IVF.

Endometriosis
- Endometriosis is the ectopic growth of hormonally responsive endometrial tissue, and accounts for 15% of female infertility. Surgical treatment may be effective, though management by an infertility specialist for IVF may be necessary. See Chapter 35.

Luteal Phase Defects
- Luteal phase defects occur in both fertile and infertile women, and treatment is highly controversial. Nevertheless, in a couple with documented infertility, it is not unreasonable to treat a presumed luteal phase deficiency with intramuscular or intravaginal progesterone in the postovulatory phase of the cycle and, if pregnancy occurs, until the luteoplacental shift occurs.

Uterine Factors
- Uterine factors, such as submucous leiomyomas, intrauterine synechiae (Asherman's syndrome), and uterine deformities or septa, cause approximately 2% of infertility. The mainstay of treatment for these conditions is surgical correction, frequently via a hysteroscopic approach.

Infections
- Infections of the female and male genital tracts have been implicated as causes of infertility. *Chlamydia* infection and gonorrhea are the major pathogens and should be treated appropriately. *Ureaplasma urealyticum* and *Mycoplasma hominis* have also been implicated, and, if positively identified by culture, they should be treated with

oral doxycycline, 100 mg twice daily for 7 days. This has been shown to increase the pregnancy rate in patients with primary infertility.

Tubal Factor Infertility

- Tubal factor infertility has become more prevalent with the increased incidence of salpingitis. The frequency of tubal occlusion after one, two, and three episodes of salpingitis is reported to be 11%, 23%, and 54%, respectively. Appendicitis, previous abdominopelvic surgery, endometriosis, and ectopic pregnancy can also lead to adhesion formation and damaged tubes.
- Proximal tubal obstruction is identified on HSG. Tubal spasm may mimic proximal obstruction, however, and obstruction should be confirmed by laparoscopy. Treatment consists of tubal cannulation, microsurgical tubocornual reanastomosis, or IVF.
- Distal tubal disease or distortion can be seen on HSG and laparoscopy. The success of corrective surgery (neosalpingostomy) depends on the extent of disease.
- If IVF is pursued in patients with tubal factor infertility, several studies have shown that success rates of IVF are improved if hydrosalpinges are removed.
- For patients with a history of a prior bilateral tubal ligation who desire fertility, options include microsurgical sterilization reversal as well as IVF.
    - Success of tubal reanastomosis depends on age, type, and location of the sterilization procedure and final lengths of repaired fallopian tubes.
    - IVF may be a better option for patients who desire only a single additional child.

ASSISTED REPRODUCTIVE TECHNOLOGIES

- Since the first successful IVF pregnancy delivered in 1978, several techniques have been developed that enhance our ability to overcome infertility.
- Among them are the capabilities for embryo cryopreservation and ovum donation.
- Of all IVF procedures nationwide using fresh nondonor eggs or embryos, 34.9% resulted in pregnancy according to the 2006 National Fertility Clinic data, with 81.8% of these pregnancies resulting in a live birth of one or more infant.
- The majority (over 53%) of IVF pregnancies resulted in single live births, whereas 25.1% resulted in multiple-infant births. Miscarriages occurred in 15%, ectopic pregnancies in 0.7%, and stillbirths in 0.7%. The following types of procedures are currently used in ART.

Intrauterine Insemination (IUI)

- May increase cycle fecundity when semen analysis contains decreased numbers of total motile sperm (<20 million).
- IUI bypasses the inability of the uterus to tolerate large amounts of unprocessed seminal plasma by washing semen to maximize the number of motile sperm.
    - Components of the ejaculate removed include seminal fluid, excess cellular debris, leukocytes, and morphologically abnormal sperm.
- Best results are achieved when the final specimen contains 10 million total motile sperm.
- Timing of IUI is critical and should optimally occur as follows:
    - The day after detection of the midcycle urinary LH surge in spontaneous or clomiphene-induced ovulatory cycles.

- Thirty-six hours after administration of exogenous human chorionic gonadotropin (hCG) in cycles stimulated with gonadotropins.
- An IUI cannula is used to deliver sperm into the endometrial cavity. Following IUI, the patient remains in the recumbent position for 10 minutes.

In Vitro Fertilization (IVF)

- IVF refers to controlled ovarian hyperstimulation followed by aspiration of oocytes under ultrasound guidance, laboratory fertilization with prepared sperm, embryo culture, and transcervical transfer of the resulting embryos into the uterus. Although most IVF procedures use fresh oocytes from the patient, transfer of frozen oocytes and transfer of donor eggs are also options.
- The overall 2006 live birth/transfer rate for IVF was 35.4%. For patients undergoing IVF, the pregnancy success rate varies little by cause of infertility, with a success rate approximating the overall national rate in women with most diagnoses except for diminished ovarian reserve (Table 32-2).
- Several trends demonstrated in the 2006 data on IVF are worth noting: live birth rates decline progressively in women above age 35 attempting IVF using fresh nondonor eggs; use of ICSI is increasing with 62.2% of ART cycles using IVF with ICSI while 37.5% use IVF without ICSI; blastocyst transfer (day 5) confers an advantage in live birth rate over day 3, cleavage-stage embryo transfer; live birth rate per transfer was 35.4% for fresh nondonor embryos, 28.9% for frozen nondonor embryos; 53.7% for fresh donor embryos, and 32.1% for frozen donor embryos. This highlights the dependence of fertility on the age of the oocyte (donor), not on the age of the uterus (receiver or carrier).

TABLE 32-2	IVF Success Rates by Diagnosis	
Diagnosis of Patients Undergoing IVF	Percentage of Total Cases	Live Births Per Cycle (%)
Tubal factor	9.8	30.0
Ovulatory dysfunction	6.4	36.3
Diminished ovarian reserve	9.2	14.4
Endometriosis	5.1	33.1
Uterine factor	1.4	26.8
Male factor	18.3	35.7
Other causes	8.3	24.8
Unexplained cause	12.0	31.7
Multiple factors, female only	11.3	22.6
Multiple factors, female + male	18.3	27.7

The total does not equal 100% due to rounding. Success rates are for fresh nondonor eggs or embryos. Data from Centers for Disease Control and Prevention, American Society for Reproductive Medicine, Society for Assisted Reproductive Technology, 2006 Assisted Reproductive Technology Success Rates: National Summary and Fertility Clinic Reports, Atlanta: U.S. Dept of Health and Human Services; 2008. Access online at: http://www.cdc.gov/art/art2006.

Intracytoplasmic Sperm Injection (ICSI)

- In ICSI, a single spermatozoon is injected microscopically into each oocyte, and the resulting embryos are transferred transcervically into the uterus. The advent of ICSI has revolutionized fertility treatment for couples confronting male factor infertility refractory to IUI or IVF.
- The 2006 data demonstrate that approximately half of ICSI cycles were used for a diagnosis of male factor infertility while half were used for patients without a diagnosis of male factor infertility.
- Success rates of ICSI for male factor infertility compare favorably to routine IVF without ICSI performed for nonmale factor infertility.

Gamete Intrafallopian Transfer (GIFT) and
Zygote Intrafallopian Transfer (ZIFT)

- GIFT is extraction of oocytes followed by the transfer of gametes (sperm and oocyte) into a normal fallopian tube by laparoscopy.
- ZIFT refers to placement of embryos into the fallopian tube via laparoscopy after oocyte retrieval and fertilization.
- Both procedures are rarely used today.

INDICATIONS FOR IN VITRO FERTILIZATION

- **Tubal conditions**: large hydrosalpinges, absence of fimbria, severe adhesive disease, repeated ectopic pregnancies, or failed reconstructive therapy. Also, women with previous bilateral tubal ligation who chose IVF over reanastomosis.
- **Endometriosis**: if other forms of treatment have failed
- **Unexplained infertility**
- **Male factor infertility:** low sperm count, low sperm motility, and abnormal morphology associated with reduction in fertilizing ability
- **Uterine malformations:** related to diethylstilbestrol exposure
- **HIV-positive serodiscordant couples**: use of ICSI or sperm washing techniques has enabled HIV-negative women to safely achieve pregnancy using the sperm of their affected male partners.
- **Men and women seeking fertility preservation**: patients about to undergo chemotherapy or irradiation of their pelvic regions can consider cryopreservation of gametes, embryos, or ovarian tissue for subsequent childbearing via ART.
- **Couples seeking preimplantation genetic diagnosis (PGD:** see following).

CONTROLLED OVARIAN HYPERSTIMULATION (COH) AND PROTOCOLS FOR IN VITRO FERTILIZATION

The agents most commonly used to stimulate multiple ovarian follicles are CC, hMG, and purified FSH. The particular products and protocols used may be tailored as the treatment progresses, to boost the chances of an adequate response and increase the pregnancy rate.

Clomiphene-Only Regimens

- These regimens are generally given on days 5 to 9 of the menstrual cycle.
- Response may be followed by BBT measurement, ultrasonography, and measurement of LH and estradiol levels.

- CC is inexpensive and has a low risk of ovarian hyperstimulation syndrome (OHSS). However, it creates a low oocyte yield (one or two per cycle) with frequent LH surges that lead to high cancellation rates in IVF cycles and low pregnancy yield.
- Most treatment regimens start with 50 mg/day for 5 days beginning on cycle day 3 or day 5. If ovulation fails to occur, the dose may be increased to 100 mg/day.
- hCG, 5,000 IU to 10,000 IU, may be used to simulate an LH surge. Eighty percent of properly selected couples will conceive in the first three cycles after treatment. Potential side effects are vasomotor flushes, blurring of vision, urticaria, pain, bloating, and multiple gestation (5% to 7% of cases, usually twins).

Gonadotropin Regimens

- These regimens increase the number of recruited follicles in patients who do not achieve pregnancy with CC and in those patients with endometriosis or unexplained infertility.
- The hMG, which is a combination of LH and FSH, is usually given for 2 to 7 days.
- Although gonadotropin injections prove more effective at COH than clomiphene, they are more expensive and can lead to life-threatening OHSS.
- Trade names for hMG include Humegon, Pergonal, and Repronex.
- Attempts to minimize the potentially deleterious LH component of hMG have led to the manufacture of purified urinary FSH and, more recently, recombinant FSH.
- The purity and consistency associated with recombinant FSH argue for its exclusive use, but evidence of its superior efficacy has been conflicting and inconclusive. Follicle maturation during COH is monitored using sonography and serial measurement of estradiol levels.
- To complete oocyte maturation, hCG is administered once the follicles have reached 17 to 18 mm in diameter.
- Potential disadvantages of gonadotropin use include premature luteinization, spontaneous LH surges resulting in high cancellation rates, multiple gestations, and ovarian hyperstimulation.

GnRH Agonists (GnRHa)

- These are used via a flare-up protocol or a luteal phase protocol.
- The flare-up protocol causes an elevation of FSH in the first 4 days, which increases oocyte recruitment.
- After 5 days of administration, the GnRH agonist downregulates the pituitary to prevent premature luteinization and a spontaneous LH surge.
- The luteal phase protocol involves starting GnRHa administration on the 17th to 21st menstrual day in the cycle before IVF.
- GnRHa increase the number, quality, and synchronization of the oocytes recovered per cycle and thereby improve the fertilization rate, the number of embryos, and the pregnancy rate.
- Lupron is the most commonly used GnRH agonist in the United States.

GnRH Antagonists

- These block LH secretion, and the premature LH surges that force cycle cancellation without causing a flare-up effect.
- They are administered in a single dose on the 8th menstrual day or in smaller doses over 4 days.

- Because they block the periovulatory LH surge, less gonadotropins are required to stimulate ovulation and side effects are decreased.
- Trade names include Antagon and Cetrotide.

OOCYTE RETRIEVAL, CULTURE FERTILIZATION, AND TRANSFER

The two major techniques of oocyte retrieval are ultrasonographically guided follicular aspiration and laparoscopic oocyte retrieval. The former is the most widely used.

Ultrasonographically Guided Oocyte Retrieval
- A 17-gauge needle passed through the vaginal fornix to retrieve oocytes.
- Performed 34 to 36 hr after hCG injection under sedation.
- Potential complications include risk of bowel injury and injury to pelvic vessels.

Oocyte Fertilization
- Sperm are diluted, centrifuged, and incubated before 50,000 to 100,000 motile spermatozoa are added to each Petri dish containing an oocyte.
- Fertilization is documented by the presence of two pronuclei and extrusion of a second polar body at 24 hr.

Embryo Transfer
- Performed 3 to 5 days after oocyte insemination.
  - Day 5 blastocyst transfer is becoming more common today due to higher live-birth rates compared to cleavage-stage (day 3) embryos.
- Excess embryos not used for transfer can be cryopreserved for an unlimited period, with a survival rate of 75%.
- The actual number of embryos transferred depends on the individual's age and other risk factors for multiple pregnancy.
- The common practice is to supplement the luteal phase with progesterone given intramuscularly or by vaginal suppository, beginning the day of oocyte release and continuing into the 12th week of pregnancy.

MATERNAL, FETAL, AND LONG-TERM EFFECTS OF ART

Ovarian Hyperstimulation Syndrome (OHSS)
- OHSS can be a life-threatening complication of COH characterized by ovarian enlargement and increased capillary permeability.
  - Potentiated by COH cycles using GnRH analogs for downregulation or hCG to trigger oocyte maturation.
- Presentation: Abdominal bloating, ascites, decreased urine output, hemoconcentration, hypercoagulability, hydrothorax, acute respiratory distress syndrome, electrolyte imbalance, and multiple organ failure.
  - Classified as mild, moderate, or severe according to the presenting symptoms.
- Pathophysiology: Thought to be mediated by vascular endothelial growth factor, produced by the ovary in response to LH or hCG.
- Risk factors: Young age, pregnancy, low body weight, high or rapidly climbing estradiol levels, large size and number of follicles, and the presence of PCOS.
- Treatment: Moderate-severe cases of OHSS should be managed as an inpatient.

- Includes close monitoring of fluid and renal status, frequent evaluation of electrolytes and coagulation studies, intravascular resuscitation, thrombosis prophylaxis and paracentesis, and/or thoracentesis, as indicated.
- Prevention: If impending OHSS is suspected, prevention can be attempted by lowering or withholding ("coasting") the hCG triggering dose, postponing embryo transfer, or canceling the cycle.
  - OHSS is an entirely iatrogenic entity that is usually avoidable by vigilance and judicious execution and alteration of COH regimen.

Multiple Gestation

- 2006 data demonstrate that 31.8% of clinical pregnancies involved multiple gestation: 28.0% were twin pregnancies and 3.8% were triplet or higher order pregnancies.
- In attempting to limit the prevalence of multiple gestation, the American Society for Reproductive Medicine (ASRM) has issued practice recommendations governing the number of embryos transferred. These recommendations are stratified depending on whether cleavage-stage embryos or blastocysts are transferred.
  - Women <age 35: Strong consideration to transfer just one embryo if a favorable prognosis; no more than two embryos (cleavage stage or blastocyst) should be transferred.
  - Women aged 35 to 37: Two cleavage-stage embryos if a favorable prognosis, otherwise three cleavage-stage embryos may be transferred. No more than two blastocysts may be transferred.
  - Women aged 38 to 40: Three cleavage-stage embryos or two blastocysts if a favorable prognosis, otherwise four cleavage-stage embryos or three blastocysts may be transferred.
  - Women >age 40: Should receive no more than five cleavage-stage embryos or three blastocysts.
- Should multiple gestation ensue, recourse to selective fetal reduction is available for patients who are comfortable with the ethics and risks of that procedure.

Heterotopic Pregnancy

- Occurs in up to 1% of pregnancies after ART.
- This incidence is dramatically higher than the corresponding ratio in the general population (1 in 30,000).
- The finding of an intrauterine pregnancy (IUP) in a woman who has undergone ART should not be automatically considered a reassuring finding as the presence of a coexisting ectopic pregnancy is possible.
- Women after ART who display signs or symptoms suggesting ectopic pregnancy must be closely followed despite confirmation of an IUP.

Effects of IVF

- Inconsistent and equivocal evidence links IVF to increased risks of neonatal morbidity, birth defects, developmental disabilities, or certain childhood cancers.
- Conclusive evidence, however, does link IVF to an increased risk of low birth weight deliveries even amongst full-term, singleton neonates.

Effects of ICSI

- ICSI has been associated with a significant increase in sex and autosomal chromosome abnormalities and, potentially, with an increased risk of imprinting disorders, such as Beckwith-Wiedemann or Angelman syndromes.

- If a male with a Y chromosome microdeletion undergoes ICSI/IVF, male offspring will inherit the same microdeletion and, thus, also have male factor infertility.

SOCIAL IMPLICATIONS

The advent of ART has raised unique ethical and social implications for couples undergoing such treatments.

Embryo Cryopreservation

- It is now common practice to cryopreserve excess embryos not used during an embryo transfer cycle.
- While many couples will use these embryos for future cycles, the number of cryo-preserved embryos in the United States is estimated to be over 400,000.
- Disposition options for excess cryopreserved embryos include use, discard, donation to research (including stem cell research), donation to other couples, future embryo transfer, or continued storage.
- It is imperative that couples be aware that excess embryos could result from ART and that a plan be discussed in advance for these embryos.

Third-Party Reproduction

- Includes donor oocytes and sperm, donated embryos, and gestational carriers (sur-rogates).
- Ethical issues involved include the following:
  - Disclosure to children conceived by these technologies regarding their genetic origin.
  - Privacy issues for donors.
  - Compensation for oocyte donors and gestational carriers.

Preimplantation Genetic Diagnosis (PGD)

- PGD allows couples with various single-gene disorders and X-linked genetic diseases to avoid transmission of the disorder of offspring.
- Proceeds by biopsy and genetic analysis of one of the following specimens:
  - 1 to 2 blastomeres of a cleavage-stage (days 2 to 3) embryo derived from IVF.
  - Polar body biopsy from a metaphase II oocyte obtained after COH.
  - Trophectoderm tissue from a blastocyst-stage (day 5) embryo.
- Single-Gene Disorders
  - Using the polymerase chain reaction (PCR), DNA extracted from the biopsy specimen is used to screen for a known hereditary disorder—for example, cystic fibrosis, muscular dystrophy, and Huntington's disease.
  - Only unaffected preimplantation embryos would be transferred to the woman's uterus.
- Aneuploidy Testing
  - Fluorescence in situ hybridization (FISH) is a molecular technique that uses chromosome-specific sequences that can be hybridized to complementary probes attached to differentially colored fluorochromes.
  - FISH has been used for the PGD of aneuploidy and chromosomal abnormalities, such as translocations.
  - Such aneuploidy testing is implemented during the IVF cycles of women who are of advanced reproductive age, have a history of recurrent pregnancy losses, or have undergone multiple failed IVF cycles.

- Controversy persists as to both the efficacy of PGD for these indications and the extent to which accurate diagnosis of aneuploidy is confounded by rampant mosaicism (existence of blastomeres with both diploid and nondiploid chromosomal complements) in a cleavage-stage embryo.
- Sibling HLA-Matching
  - PGD was first used in 2000 to screen for Fanconi's anemia and simultaneously to select for a preimplantation embryo that was HLA matched to a preexisting sibling afflicted with this disorder.
- Elective Sex Selection
  - PGD, via either PCR or FISH, enables efficient and accurate gender selection by screening selectively for the Y chromosome.
  - Sharp debate over the propriety of such nonmedical use of reproductive technology has limited the prevalence of this application.

SUGGESTED READINGS

Blake DA, Farquhar CM, Johnson N, et al. Cleavage stage versus blastocyst stage embryo transfer in assisted conception. *Cochrane Database Syst Rev* 2007;(4):CD002118.

Centers for Disease Control and Prevention, National Center for Health Statistics. 2002 National Survey of Family Growth. U.S. Department of Health and Human Services Web site. Available at: http://www.cdc.gov/nchs/nsfg.htm

Centers for Disease Control and Prevention, National Center for Health Statistics. 2006 Assisted Reproductive Technology Report. Available at: http://www.cdc.gov/art/ART2006/index.htm

Legro RS, Barnhart HX, Schlaff WD, et al. (Cooperative Multicenter Reproductive Medicine Network) Clomiphene, metformin, or both for infertility in the polycystic ovary syndrome. *N Engl J Med* 2007;356(6):551–566.

Practice Committee of the American Society for Reproductive Medicine. Preimplantation genetic diagnosis: a practice committee opinion. *Fertil Steril* 2008;90:S136–S140.

Practice Committee of the American Society for Reproductive Medicine. Guidelines on numbers of embryos transferred. *Fertil Steril* 2009;92(5):1518–1519.

Speroff L, Fritz MA. *Clinical Gynecologic Endocrinology and Infertility,* 7th Ed. Philadelphia: Lippincott Williams and Wilkins, 2005.

33 Miscarriage and Recurrent Pregnancy Loss

Tiffany McNair and Kristiina Altman

FIRST-TRIMESTER MISCARRIAGE

Miscarriage, or spontaneous abortion, is generally defined as the spontaneous loss of a previable pregnancy. Previability refers to a fetus weighing <500 g or at gestational age (GA) <20 weeks.
- Miscarriages are classified according to the GA at which they occur.
  - Preclinical or **subclinical miscarriages** happen at or before 5 weeks' GA.
  - Clinical miscarriages include the following:
    - **Embryonic miscarriage** occurs at 6 to 9 weeks' GA or crown rump length (CRL) ≥5 mm without cardiac activity.
    - **Fetal miscarriage** occurs at 10 to 20 weeks' GA or CRL >30 mm without cardiac activity.

Incidence and Risk
- Thirty to forty percent of all conceptions result in miscarriage.
- Ten to fifteen percent of clinically recognized pregnancies end in first-trimester and early second-trimester losses (<20 weeks' GA).
  - Nearly 80% of sporadic losses occur during the first trimester and typically manifest before 12 weeks' GA.
- The risk of preclinical miscarriage is estimated as approximately 25% in women less than age 35. Among clinical miscarriages, this risk increases significantly with advanced maternal age (AMA) from 8% to 12% in women under age 35 to as high as 45% in those older than age 40. This increase is thought to be related to the increased risk of aneuploidic pregnancies in older women.
- Though maternal age probably has the greatest impact, several other factors carry an increased risk of sporadic first or early second trimester clinical miscarriage. See Table 33-1.
  - Previous obstetrical history: Risk of miscarriage increases from 20% to 43% in women with a history of one miscarriage and three or more, respectively.
  - Tobacco: Smoking and exposure to second-hand smoke increase the risk.
  - Observational and population-based studies have also implicated the following risk factors: alcohol and illicit drug use, NSAID use, fever, caffeine, and low folate levels.
- Common causes of sporadic losses include the following:
  - Chromosomal abnormalities account for approximately 50% of miscarriages.
    - Incidence is inversely related to GA.

TABLE 33-1	Risk Factors for Miscarriage

Increasing maternal age (>35 years old)
History of previous miscarriage
Tobacco
Alcohol
Illicit drug use (e.g., cocaine)
NSAID use
Caffeine (high intake)
Low folate levels/intake
Maternal fever/febrile illness
Maternal obesity
Maternal medical conditions (e.g., diabetes)

- 90% in anembryonic products of conception (sometimes referred to as "blighted ovum")
- 50% in embryonic abortuses
- 30% in fetal abortuses
○ Typically autosomal trisomies, monosomies, or polyploidies.
○ Maternal conditions, including uterine anomalies, endocrinopathies, hypercoagulable state, infection, and teratogen exposure.

Presentation

- The hallmark complaint of a pregnant woman experiencing a miscarriage is painful or painless **vaginal bleeding** after a missed period. The types of spontaneous abortion include the following:
  - **Threatened:** often painless, cervix closed, uterine size consistent with GA.
  - **Inevitable:** painful, cervix open, uterine size consistent with GA.
  - **Complete** (usually *before* 12 weeks' GA): mild pain, cervix closed, uterus small, contracted, and empty.
  - **Incomplete** (usually *after* 12 weeks' GA) painful, cervix open often with tissue in os or vagina, uterus small and not well contracted, with products of conception (POCs) still in the uterus.
  - **Missed** (intrauterine fetal demise at <20 weeks' GA): retained nonviable pregnancy in which the embryo or fetus lacks heartbeat but symptoms of miscarriage have not developed. Also called delayed miscarriage. The patient typically presents due to cessation of the normal symptoms of pregnancy (i.e., nausea, vomiting, breast tenderness) or receives the diagnosis unexpectedly during ultrasound evaluation.
  - **Septic:** painful, purulent discharge, cervix open, cervical motion tenderness, tender uterus, constitutional symptoms (e.g., fever, malaise), tachycardia, tachypnea. The infectious source is often *Staphylococcus aureus*. Septic miscarriage is frequently a complication of unsafe induced abortion as opposed to the sequela of spontaneous loss.

Assessment

- The **differential diagnosis** for early pregnancy bleeding includes the following:
  - Physiologic
  - Ectopic pregnancy

- Gestational trophoblastic disease
- Anatomic pathology of the vagina, cervix, or uterus
- The gold standard for diagnosis is imaging, usually with transvaginal ultrasound (TVUS). This modality is especially useful in differentiating intrauterine and ectopic pregnancies.
  - Viability can be determined through the appearance of a gestational and/or yolk sac and with measurement of the CRL.
  - In diagnosing a missed clinical miscarriage, the operator can use several sonographic criteria: (a) absence of fetal cardiac activity with a CRL >5 mm and/or (b) absence of a fetal pole in the presence of a mean sac diameter of >18 mm transvaginally or >25 mm transabdominally.
- The early presence of fetal cardiac activity in women of AMA is not necessarily reassuring. One series demonstrated an increased risk of miscarriage from 4% in women less than age 35% to 29% in women older than age 40.
- Evaluation also includes a complete blood, a type and screen, serum progesterone, and serial beta hCG measurements. The last is most useful in conjunction with imaging.

Management and Complications

- If bleeding is minimal or symptoms have resolved, a threatened miscarriage can be managed expectantly.
- Similarly, complete abortions often require no intervention other than evaluation of passed tissue to confirm POCs. In such cases or with expectant management, patients should be advised to bring POCs to the hospital for evaluation.
- Miscarriage carries a 1.5% to 2% risk of alloimmunization. Any Rh(D)-negative woman who experiences a spontaneous loss or has a threatened miscarriage should receive anti-D immune globulin (Rhogam). See Chapter 18.
- Incomplete, inevitable, or missed miscarriages can be managed via three methods, whose outcomes have been extensively studied and compared. Selecting an option is based on a combination of patient wishes, stability, and stage of miscarriage.

Expectant Management (EM)

- **EM** is an ideal option for women who present during the first trimester, are clinically stable, and would prefer no intervention.
- The success of EM is greatest in incomplete (91%) compared to missed (76%) or preclinical (66%) miscarriages. The average time to miscarriage completion is 2 weeks to 1 month.
- Surgical or medical intervention is indicated for failure of EM.

Medical Management

- **Medical management** is an effective method for women who decline surgery and would prefer not to wait for natural miscarriage completion (Table 33-2).
  - The World Health Organization (WHO) recommends either 800 μg vaginal or 600 μg sublingual misoprostol, to be repeated after 3 days. This results in a completion rate of 79% by 7 days and 87% by 30 days. Of note, the oral route tends to cause less desirable side effects, such as uterine cramping and gastrointestinal effects.
  - Several trials have included the combination of a progesterone antagonist (mifepristone) and misoprostol. There is an FDA-approved regimen (600 mg mifepristone and 400 μg misoprostol orally 48 hr later), though an alternative recommendation (200 mg mifepristone per mouth with 800 μg misoprostol per vagina) appears to have greater efficacy (92% compared to 95% to 99%) as well as fewer side effects and lower cost.

TABLE 33-2	Options for Medical Treatment of Miscarriage

Regimen	Directions
Misoprostol 800 μg (vaginal) or 600 μg (sublingual)	Give every 3 hr, may repeat twice
Misoprostol 400 μg (vaginal)	Give every 4 hr, may give four doses
Mifepristone 200 mg (oral) and misoprostol 800 μg (vaginal)	Give mifepristone followed by misoprostol 48 hr later
Mifepristone 600 mg (oral) and misoprostol 400 μg (vaginal)	Give mifepristone followed by misoprostol 48 hr later

Adapted from Dempsey A, Davis A. Medical management of early pregnancy failure: how to treat and what to expect. *Semin Reprod Med* 2008;26:401–410.

Surgical Management

- **Surgical management** via dilation and curettage (D&C) or dilation and evacuation (D&E) is the traditional approach in both first- and early second-trimester losses. This option is especially suitable for unstable patients or women who would prefer not to wait for completion.
- The surgical method carries an increased risk of uterine perforation, cervical trauma, and anesthesia complications.
- Perioperative doxycycline (100 mg given 12 hr apart on the day of surgery) is recommended for prevention of infection and sepsis.
- The management of septic abortions involves a combination of medical and surgical interventions. The patient must be stabilized, cultures (blood and endometrial) are obtained, and broad-spectrum antibiotics are then administered. Finally, uterine contents are removed via surgical evacuation.

SECOND TRIMESTER MISCARRIAGE

Incidence and Risk

- Second-trimester losses (13 to 27 weeks' GA) are rare and are often mistakenly grouped with their earlier counterparts. One to 5% of pregnancies result in miscarriage between 13 and 19 weeks' GA while only 0.3% spontaneously end between 20 and 27 weeks' GA. "Stillbirth" the customary term after 20 weeks' GA.
- Compared to first- and early second-trimester losses, there are similar etiologies to later second-trimester losses, such as chromosomal abnormalities, maternal medical conditions, and teratogenic exposures.
- Causative factors more specific to second-trimester miscarriage include: cervical insufficiency (CI), thrombophilia, maternal infection or exposures, and placental abruption.

Presentation, Assessment, and Management

- History should include the following: maternal symptoms of pregnancy loss, obstetric history, past medical and gynecologic history, family history, teratogenic exposures, drug use, and trauma.
- Initial assessment should also include a review of the pregnancy development, such as sequential vital signs, weight progression, sonographic data, and antenatal testing.

- There are several clinical scenarios associated with second-trimester loss:
  - **Cervical insufficiency (CI)** presents as painless cervical dilatation. On ultrasound, findings include cervical shortening, dilatation of the internal os, or funneling of the fetal membranes. These abnormalities can lead to bulging membranes with eventual preterm rupture, preterm contractions, and early labor. See Chapter 8 for full discussion of CI. Cerclage is not indicated for shortened cervix incidentally found on imaging.
  - **Placental abruption** may present with vaginal bleeding and uterine contractions but can also be occult. Early delivery is recommended and often performed by Cesarean section. Ultrasound does not necessarily diagnose abruption as a retroplacental clot can be obscured by the placenta itself.
  - **Preterm premature rupture of membranes** is a significant contributor to second-trimester loss. See Chapter 9.
- Postmiscarriage care is also a vital component of the plan. Patients should be instructed to rest the pelvis with nothing in the vagina for at least 2 weeks. They should also be advised to call a doctor for heavy bleeding, fever, or persistent abdominal pain.
  - There is no evidence to suggest restrictions on contraceptive use or to recommend future conception delay immediately following miscarriage.
  - Patients should be counseled on their risk of recurrence. These risks are a function of the underlying etiology.
  - Finally, acknowledgement of parental grief with provision of emotional support and professional counseling is encouraged.

RECURRENT MISCARRIAGE

Recurrent miscarriage (RM) has traditionally been defined as three or more consecutive losses of clinically recognized pregnancies <20 weeks' GA. In more recent literature, it is classified as two or more losses at any GA.
- Recurrent preclinical and embryonic miscarriages are more frequent, while recurrent fetal losses (particularly after 14 weeks) are less common.
  - Primary RM represents women with recurrent pregnancy loss without a previous viable pregnancy.
  - Secondary RM indicates women with recurrent pregnancy loss who have previously delivered a live infant.

Incidence and Risk

- 0.5% to 2% of all women will experience RM, the risk of which also significantly increases with AMA.
- Risks of RM include genetic factors, uterine pathology, endocrine factors, immunologic causes, thrombophilias, and, possibly, environmental factors and infectious agents. Fifty percent of all cases remain undiagnosed.
- Testing for RM may be initiated after two consecutive losses, especially in older couples. A detailed history and physical examination should be the initial step followed by more specific testing.

Etiologies and Management (Table 33-3)

Genetic Aberration
- The incidence of chromosomal abnormalities in RM depends on the GA of the pregnancy. It is thought that these abnormalities account for 70% of preclinical RM and 50% of clinical RM, similar to spontaneous miscarriages.
- The most common chromosomal abnormalities are autosomal trisomies (in descending frequency—16, 22, 21, 15, and 13), comprising 56% of clinical RM

TABLE 33-3	Management of Recurrent Miscarriage	
Etiology	**Evaluation**	**Treatment**
Genetic	Karyotyping (parental, products of conception)	Genetic counseling Donor gametes as needed
Uterine pathology	Hysteroscopy Hysterosalpingogram Sonohysterography TVUS (including 3D)	Hysteroscopic septoplasty, myomectomy, polypectomy Hysteroscopic adhesiolysis Cervical cerclage
Endocrine	Endometrial biopsy or midluteal progesterone level (neither reliable) Thyroid-stimulating hormone Serum luteinizing hormone Blood glucose and insulin levels Prolactin	Progesterone Levothyroxine Metformin Bromocriptine
Immunologic	Lupus anticoagulant Anticardiolipin antibody Anti-$\beta 2$ glycoprotein antibody	Aspirin, heparin (unfractionated or low-molecular weight)
Thrombophilias	Factor V Leiden Prothrombin gene mutation MTHFR gene mutation (serum homocysteine)	Aspirin, heparin Folic acid
Environmental	Review exposures, toxins	Environment and/or behavior modification
Infectious	Clinical evaluation, culture	Antibiotics

TVUS, transvaginal ultrasound; MTHFR, methylene tetrahydrofolate reductase. Adapted from Stephenson M, Kutteh W. Evaluation and management of early recurrent pregnancy loss. *Clin Obstet Gynecol* 2007;50(1):132–145; Reddy UM. Recurrent pregnancy loss: nongenetic causes. *Contemp Obstet Gyn* 2007;63–70.

cases. Other chromosomal abnormalities in clinical RM cases include polyploidy 20%, monosomy 18%, and unbalanced translocations 4%.
- Parental karyotyping may be indicated in couples with RM, particularly in those with three or more clinical miscarriages. When karyotyping is done, one partner in <10% of couples will be diagnosed with a chromosomal abnormality, usually a balanced translocation. A small percentage of abnormal parental karyotypes include inversions, microdeletions, and mosaicisms.
  - Balanced translocations most commonly appear in the mother. Given this increased prevalence, it is more beneficial to test the mother first followed by the father as needed.

- For evaluation of POCs, gestational tissue with the most successful cell culture growth are placenta, fascia lata, skin from nape of neck, tendons and blood.
  - These tissues should be placed in normal saline and *not* in formalin.
  - The approximate laboratory cost for routine tissue culture, chromosome analysis, and karyotyping of POCs is approximately $1,400.

Uterine Pathology
- Uterine malformations are noted in 13% to 17% of women who experience RM, compared to approximately 7% in the general population.
- **Congenital anomalies** involve developmental defects of the Müllerian duct system, including septate, arcuate, bicornuate, unicornuate, and didelphic uteri. Septate and bicornuate uteri are most commonly associated with RM and especially with embryonic losses.
- A variety of imaging modalities are used in the evaluation and diagnosis of uterine pathology in relation to reproductive loss. While two-dimensional abdominal or TVUS and hysterosalpingography (HSG) are popular screening tools, they have relatively low rates of accuracy.
  - HSG aids in examination of the intrauterine cavity, but it is unable to reliably detect subtle uterine pathology.
  - Sonohysterography, or saline-infused hysterography, is a more accurate diagnostic tool than plain ultrasound.
  - Combined hysteroscopy and laparoscopy remain the most definitive diagnostic approach by providing examination of both internal and external abnormalities. This method is also therapeutic as it permits septal resection as needed.
  - 3D transvaginal US and MRI are also promising tools to aid in displaying uterine morphology in women with RM.
  - In the office, flexible hysteroscopy is a minimally invasive and convenient method of diagnosing patients with congenital anomalies.
- **Acquired conditions** that cause abnormalities within the uterus and cervix include uterine synechiae, leiomyoma, polyps, and cervical laxity or shortening.
  - Uterine fibroids may be submucosal, intramural, serosal, or pedunculated. Some studies show that submucosal fibroids may be associated with RM. Vascular supply to the placenta may be affected due to an unfavorable implantation site while large fibroids may distort the uterine cavity.
  - Intrauterine synechiae may occur following instrumentation of the uterus. Aggressive postpartum curettage may lead to significant synechiae formation, or Asherman's syndrome, that interfere with placentation.
  - CI may be the result of obstetric lacerations, loop electrosurgical excision, cone biopsy, or aggressive dilation in association with D&Cs.
    - Patients with three or more unexplained second-trimester losses may be treated with elective cerclage placement at 13 to 16 weeks if ultrasound reveals a viable fetus.
- Resection of uterine septa (septoplasty), hysteroscopic lysis of adhesions, myomectomy, polypectomy, and cervical cerclage placement are all treatments for congenital and acquired uterine abnormalities.

Endocrine Dysfunction
- Endocrine factors are implicated in 15% to 30% of RM cases.
- Poorly controlled diabetes mellitus, obesity, and luteal phase deficiency (LPD) have been associated with more frequent miscarriages. See Chapter 13.

Luteal Phase Deficiency

- Functional corpus luteum defects or abnormal endometrial progesterone receptors contribute to the RM rate, especially embryonic losses. Currently, there is no reliable means to diagnose LPD using either serum progesterone measurements or serial endometrial biopsies.
- Progestational agents are available in various preparations, including oral, vaginal, and intramuscular (IM) formulations.
  - Oral supplementation has proven to be the most convenient but less efficacious due to its rapid metabolization and inability to bolster the progestational effect at the level of the uterus.
  - Studies comparing the efficacy of IM versus vaginal routes in LPD and in vitro fertilization have thus far shown no significant statistical difference in clinical pregnancy or miscarriage rates.
  - However, given the less appealing side-effect profile of IM agents (e.g., pain, risk of bleeding and abscess formation, oil allergy, inconvenience), trials are underway to compare several vaginal options (usually 25 to 100 mg twice daily), including the gel (Crinone) and micronized insert (Endometrin).
- Although studies have shown no statistically significant difference in the miscarriage rate between women "all-comers" receiving progesterone and those receiving placebo, there is a significant difference when stratified for obstetric history (i.e., three or more previous consecutive losses).

Polycystic Ovarian Syndrome (PCOS)

- An increased risk of miscarriage has been noted in this population of women. Hyperandrogenism, elevated luteneizing hormone levels, obesity, and hyperinsulinemia have all been proposed as explanations for RM among these women. Some evidence also suggests that insulin resistance is associated with increased plasma homocysteine levels.
- Metformin has been shown to decrease the miscarriage rate in the PCOS population, but no randomized controlled trials examining its use in women with PCOS and RM offer definitive evidence.
  - The presumed mechanism of action in this cohort is related to insulin lowering and improved oocyte quality.
  - Existing prospective studies show no evidence of teratogenicity or developmental problems in the first 18 months of life in the infants of mothers who used metformin in early pregnancy.
  - Certain authors advocate using metformin 500 to 2,500 mg by mouth daily through the first trimester in affected women.

Thyroid Dysfunction

- Hypothyroidism is thought to have an association with RM, but causation has not been proved. See Chapter 13 for thyroid disorders. Thyroxine therapy should be initiated in hypothyroid patients in early pregnancy, if not prior to conception.

Immune Dysfunction

- Autoimmune and alloimmune factors have been implicated in up to 15% of women with RM.
- **Antiphospholipid syndrome (APS)**
  - Antiphospholipid antibodies (e.g., lupus anticoagulant and anticardiolipin antibodies) are formed against vascular endothelium and platelets, eventually leading

to vascular constriction and thrombosis. Thrombus may lead to placental infarction and second-trimester fetal losses.

- Criteria for APS include at least one clinical and one laboratory data point.
  - Clinical criterion:
    - one or more episodes of arterial, venous, or small vessel thrombosis;
    - one or more unexplained pregnancy loss of morphologically normal fetus of greater than or equal to 10 weeks' GA;
    - one or more premature births of morphologically normal fetus at less than or equal to 34 weeks' GA due to pregnancy-induced hypertension or placental insufficiency;
    - three or more consecutive miscarriages before 10 weeks' GA excluding anatomic, hormonal, parental genetic factors.
  - Laboratory criterion:
    - Positive titers of moderate to high dilution at least 12 weeks apart of anticardiolipin antibody;
    - anti-β2 glycoprotein antibody;
    - or lupus anticoagulant.
- Routine testing for lupus anticoagulant (Russell's viper venom test) and anticardiolipin antibodies (IgG and/or IgM) in medium or high titers should be performed in women with suspected prothrombotic states. If antibody levels are elevated, they should be drawn twice at least 6 weeks apart and in the nonpregnant state.
- Studies have shown improved pregnancy outcome in women with APS who receive antithrombotic therapy.
  - Treatment with unfractionated heparin and low-dose ASA is more effective than ASA alone in increasing the live birth rate—80% compared to 40%, respectively.
  - Heparin, which does not cross the placenta, is also demonstrated to be more effective than intravenous immunoglobulin IVIG therapy.
  - Several pilot studies suggest low-molecular weight heparin (LMWH) may be equivalent in its efficacy compared to the unfractionated variety.
  - LMWH carries a decreased risk of heparin-induced thrombocytopenia, heparin-induced osteopenia, and maternal bleeding.
  - LMWH offers the added benefit of once daily dosing, and therefore increased tolerability.

Alloimmunity

- This concept reflects the theory that pregnancy survival depends on maternal tolerance to foreign fetal antigens instead of maternal sensitization leading to activation of the immune response.
- Attempted therapies include leukocyte immunization, IVIG, third party donor cell immunization, and trophoblast membrane immunization.
- These treatments are not routinely recommended due to lack of significant evidence to support decreased miscarriage rates.

Hereditary Thrombophilias

- Though studies have been inconclusive regarding causality, thrombophilias are regarded as significant risk factors for RM.
- These maternal conditions encompass autosomal dominant mutations in genes whose byproducts regulate the clotting cascade, causing a hypercoagulable state. The most frequently occurring mutations are Factor V Leiden deficiency and Prothrombin G20210A mutation. See Chapter 17.

- Adverse outcomes of pregnancies in women with these abnormalities include pre-eclampsia, IUGR, and fetal demise.
- Miscarriage risk is highest in the second and third trimesters. It is hypothesized that spiral artery thrombosis precedes the cascade of events leading to late fetal loss.
- The return on testing for inherited thrombophilias is greatest in cases of fetal death due to greater incidence of second-trimester RM with thrombophilias.
- Mutations in the methylene tetrahydrofolate reductase (MTHFR) gene, resulting in hyperhomocysteinemia, are also associated with increased risk of RM. Mutations are autosomal recessive, placing only homozygotes at increased risk.

Infection and Environmental Exposures
- Infectious agents are known causes of miscarriage, but their responsibility for RM is controversial and studies are lacking.

Psycho-Social-Spiritual Support
- Parental stress and anxiety should be considered while caring for couples who experience RM.
- Studies have shown that emotional support, close surveillance with frequent office visits, phone calls, and even serial ultrasound studies improve pregnancy outcomes.
- These strategies have been shown in controlled studies to halve the RM rate (from >50% to 25%) in the absence of any medical or surgical intervention.
- Depending on patients' desires and beliefs, referral to psychological support and pastoral care services is also important in the setting of RM.
- An empathetic attitude with supportive care throughout the process can have a major impact on the well-being and future pregnancy outcomes of this patient population.

SUGGESTED READINGS

Jauniaux E, Farquharson RG, Christiansen OB, et al. Evidence-based guidelines for the investigation and medical treatment of recurrent miscarriage. *Hum Reprod* 2006;21(9):2216–2222.
Michels TC, Tiu AY. Second trimester pregnancy loss. *Am Fam Phys* 2007;76(9):1341–1346.
Zhang J, Gilles JM, Barnhart K, et al. A comparison of medical management with misoprostol and surgical management for early pregnancy failure. *N Engl J Med* 2005;353(8):761–769.

34 Uterine Leiomyomas

Sarah Cohen and Catherine Sewell

Uterine leiomyomas, also known as myomas or fibroids, represent the most common pelvic tumors in women. As benign smooth muscle neoplasms, leiomyomas only rarely undergo malignant transformation (<0.5%).

- While traditionally described as present in 20% of women over age 35, postmortem examinations suggest a frequency of 50%.
- The majority of patients with fibroids are asymptomatic. Symptoms may include pelvic pressure, urinary or fecal complaints, and abnormal bleeding.
- Leiomyomas represent the single most common indication for hysterectomy, but there are now several medical and minimally invasive options for treatment.

ETIOLOGY AND PATHOPHYSIOLOGY

- Leiomyomas originate from smooth muscle cells of the uterus or less commonly from the smooth muscle cells of uterine blood vessels. Thought to be clonal in origin, they range in size from millimeters in diameter to large tumors reaching the costal margin. These tumors may be solitary or multiple and are classified by location within the uterus.
- **Submucosal fibroids** develop from myometrium just deep to the endometrial lining and can often protrude into the endometrial cavity or even outside the cervical os if pedunculated. **Intramural fibroids,** located within the uterine corpus wall, may distort the uterine cavity. **Cervical fibroids** are similarly intramural but are found instead in the uterine cervix. **Subserosal fibroids** develop below the serosal layer, are often pedunculated, and occasionally extend between folds of the broad ligament.
- A genetic basis for the presence and growth of uterine leiomyomas appears likely. Family history of leiomyomas increases an individual's risk 1.5- to 3.5-fold. It has been suggested that up to 40% of leiomyomas have associated chromosome abnormalities, including deletion of portions of 7q, trisomy 12, or rearrangements of chromosomes 6, 10, and 12. The incidence of leiomyomas is estimated to be two to three times greater among African American women and often occur at a younger age in this population.
- The growth of uterine leiomyomas is related to circulating estrogen exposure. Progesterone may exert an antiestrogen effect on the growth of leiomyomas. They are most prominent and demonstrate maximal growth during the reproductive years and tend to regress after menopause. Whenever leiomyomas grow after menopause, malignancy must be considered. The growth of leiomyomas during pregnancy is common and likely related to the enhanced uterine blood supply that accompanies pregnancy and edematous changes in these tumors.
- As leiomyomas grow, they risk diminution of blood supply, which leads to a continuum of degenerative changes, including calcium deposition. Calcific change

can be appreciated radiographically as a diffuse honeycomb pattern, a series of concentric rings, or a solid calcific mass. Necrosis, cystic changes, and fatty degeneration are manifestations of compromised blood supply secondary to growth or to infarction from torsion of a pedunculated leiomyoma. Histologically, degenerative changes in myomas may also be seen with progesterone stimulation or, less frequently, malignant transformation.

- Malignant degeneration of leiomyomas is possible, although most **leiomyosarcomas** are thought to arise de novo. Leiomyosarcomas are diagnosed on the basis of counts of ten or more mitotic figures per ten high-power fields (HPFs). Those tumors with 5 to 10 mitotic figures per 10 HPFs are referred to as smooth muscle tumors of uncertain malignant potential. Tumors with <5 mitotic figures per 10 HPFs and little cytologic atypia are classified as cellular leiomyomas.

CLINICAL MANIFESTATIONS AND DIAGNOSIS

Signs and Symptoms

- Most patients with leiomyomas are symptom free. The most commonly experienced symptoms (pain, pressure, and menorrhagia) are related to the size and location of the fibroids or to compromise of blood supply with degeneration.
- Uterine fibroids may be found on routine pelvic exams when an enlarged or irregularly shaped uterus is palpated. Various radiologic modalities may be useful for the diagnosis and/or characterization of uterine fibroids (Table 34-1).
- **Excessive menstrual bleeding** is the most frequently encountered symptom and may be due to vascular alterations in the endometrium. The obstructive effect on uterine vasculature produced by intramural tumors has been associated with the development of endometrial venule ectasia. As a result, leiomyomas give rise to proximal congestion of the myometrium and endometrium. The engorged vessels in the

TABLE 34-1	Diagnostic Imaging for Uterine Leiomyomas
Diagnostic Modality	**Strengths/Weaknesses**
Hysterosalpingography	• Evaluates the contour of uterine cavity and patency of fallopian tubes • Does not evaluate the exact location of fibroids
Sonohysterography	• Characterizes the location and amount of endometrial cavity distortion caused by submucosal fibroids
Transvaginal ultrasound	• Useful for detecting fibroids and following their growth • Not as accurate as MRI at determining the precise location or size of fibroids, especially in larger uteri or those with multiple fibroids
Magnetic resonance imaging	• Identifies size and location of fibroids • Used before uterine artery embolization

thin atrophic endometrium that overlies submucosal tumors contribute to excessive bleeding during cyclic sloughing. The increased size of the uterine cavity also gives rise to the increased volume of menstrual flow.

- Patients may also present with **pressure** and **increased abdominal girth**. Pressure on the bladder customarily provokes **urinary frequency**. When the leiomyoma is adjacent to the bladder neck and urethra, stress incontinence or acute urinary retention with overflow incontinence may occur. Ureteral obstruction is a rare complication of larger leiomyomas extending to the pelvic sidewall. Posteriorly located fibroids may produce **constipation**, rectal pressure, or tenesmus.
- **Chronic pain** symptoms may include dysmenorrhea, dyspareunia, and noncyclic pelvic pain. Acute pain may be a consequence of torsion of the stalk of a pedunculated leiomyoma, cervical dilation by a submucosal leiomyoma protruding through the lower uterine segment, or degeneration of a leiomyoma.
- Submucosal and intramural fibroids are associated with a higher rate of spontaneous miscarriage and **infertility** due to impaired implantation, tubal function, or sperm transport. Although it has been shown that removal of submucosal fibroids significantly improves fertility outcomes, there is conflicting evidence regarding the effect of intramural myomectomy on future fertility. Subserosal fibroids are not associated with subfertility.
- **Obstetrical complications** that are associated with a fibroid uterus include preterm labor, malpresentation, cesarean delivery, postpartum hemorrhage, and peripartum hysterectomy. Less common adverse outcomes that may be related to fibroids include intrauterine growth restriction, abnormal placentation, first trimester bleeding, preterm rupture of membranes, abruption, and labor dystocia.

TREATMENT FOR LEIOMYOMAS

Observation

- No standard size of an asymptomatic myomatous uterus has been invoked as an absolute indication for treatment. In a patient with a large asymptomatic myomatous uterus in whom dimensions have not increased and malignancy is unlikely, the patient's age, fertility status, and desire to retain the uterus or avoid surgery must be factored into the treatment plan. Physical and ultrasonographic examinations should be performed initially and may be repeated in 6 to 8 weeks to document the size and growth pattern. If growth is stable, the patient may be followed clinically with annual pelvic examination and imaging as indicated.
- Rapidly growing fibroids raise concern for malignancy; however, the definition of rapid growth is highly variable. One commonly accepted definition is an increase of 6 weeks size over 1 year. Postmenopausal uterine growth or bleeding increases the suspicion for malignancy; however, premenopausal women with rapid growth do not necessarily require surgical excision.

Medical Therapy

- **Nonhormonal** medical therapy is aimed at controlling the symptoms of leiomyomas, specifically excessive menstrual flow or pain. Such therapies include nonsteroidal anti-inflammatory drugs, although there are little data regarding their effects on menorrhagia or dysmenorrhea specifically due to fibroids.
- **Hormonal** therapy for fibroids includes contraceptive steroids, progestational compounds, and gonodotropin-releasing agonists or antagonists. Investigations

are underway regarding treatments such as aromatase inhibitors, selective estrogen receptor modulators, gonadotropin-releasing hormone antagonists, and selective progesterone receptor modulators.

- Similar to the nonhormonal medical options, combinations of estrogen and progesterone may control bleeding symptoms while not promoting leiomyoma growth. There is conflicting evidence regarding the effect of **progestational therapy** on change in fibroid or uterine volume, with some small studies showing decrease in leiomyoma size during treatment. Conversely, use of mifepristone, an **antiprogestin**, has been associated with decrease in the size of leiomyomas with slow rate of regrowth following treatment cessation.
- The **levonorgestrel-releasing intrauterine system (LNg-IUS)** slowly delivers progesterone directly to the uterus and significantly reduces menstrual bleeding. The effect of the LNg-IUS on myoma-mediated menorrhagia depends on the size of uterine cavity and patient characteristics of blood loss. No significant decrease of fibroid or uterine volume has been demonstrated.
- **Gonadotropin-releasing hormone analogs (GnRHa)** have been used successfully to achieve hypoestrogenism in various estrogen-dependent conditions. Reduction in tumor size of approximately 50% on average has been observed with the use of GnRHa over a 3-month course of treatment. The effects of hormonal treatment are transient, and within 6 months after withdrawal of hormonal therapy leiomyomas return to pretherapy state.
  - These agents are useful as a conservative therapy in perimenopausal women or as an adjunct to surgical treatment. Longer than 6 months of GnRHa therapy in young patients is neither practical nor desirable because of the possibility of bone loss. Common side effects of GnRHa include hot flashes, nausea, vomiting, diarrhea, constipation, rash, dizziness, acne, breast tenderness, and headaches.
  - Concomitant treatment with a low dose of steroid hormone, referred to as **add-back therapy**, can be used to minimize the adverse affects of GnRHa in patients who benefit from continued therapy after the initial 3-month course.
  - Adjunctive presurgical therapy with a 3- to 4-month course of GnRHa should reduce tumor size and thereby decrease operative time and blood loss. By producing amenorrhea, GnRHa therapy enables a patient to preoperatively restore her own hemoglobin levels from baseline menorrhagia-related iron deficiency anemia. However, when GnRHa is used before myomectomy, it may result in a less distinct plane between the fibroid and surrounding myometrium.

Surgical Therapy
Myomectomy
- **Myomectomy**, or surgical excision of the fibroid tissue, should be considered whenever preservation of the uterus is desired for its childbearing function. The location and size of the myoma(s), along with surgical expertise of the operator, dictate the approach to myomectomy. Subserosal or intramural fibroids may be resected abdominally, laparoscopically, or with robotic assistance. Submucosal myomectomy may be performed hysteroscopically or vaginally.
- For patients who wish to conceive, a delay of 4 to 6 months before attempting pregnancy is advisable after the surgical procedure, especially if significant myometrial disturbance was created. Cesarean section is generally the procedure of choice for the delivery of patients who have undergone a myomectomy with extensive myometrial dissection, due to an increased risk of uterine rupture with labor.

- Complications of myomectomy include substantial blood loss, paralytic ileus, and pain. The risk of postoperative adhesive disease following abdominal myomectomy may be as high as 90%. A laparoscopic approach or use of adhesion barriers at time of surgery may reduce this risk. The need for future surgery due to recurrence of leiomyomas is roughly 20% to 25% following myomectomy.

Hysterectomy

- Removal of the uterus is the **definitive procedure** for treatment of symptomatic leiomyomas. Hysterectomy should also be considered in the event of a rapidly enlarging tumor, in which case a reasonable likelihood of malignancy exists. Surgical approaches to hysterectomy include abdominal, vaginal, laparoscopic, laparosocopic-assisted, and robotic-assisted. Similar to myomectomy, the method of approach is dictated by size, location, number, and surgical expertise.
- Patient satisfaction with symptom relief from hysterectomy is very high but accompanied by the surgical morbidity of a major operation. Some women have been found to express posthysterectomy regret regarding loss of fertility, therefore adequate preoperative counseling is essential.

Minimally Invasive Techniques

Uterine Artery Embolization

- **Uterine artery embolization (UAE)** decreases the blood supply to the uterus and ultimately causes ischemic necrosis of leiomyomas. The procedure is performed by interventional radiologists and involves catheterization of the femoral artery to gain access to the hypogastric arteries. Under fluoroscopic guidance, the uterine arteries are occluded with substances such as Gelfoam, absolute alcohol, Ivalon particles (polyvinyl alcohol), and metal coils. This procedure is generally reserved for intramural myomas.
- The benefits of UAE include short operating and recovery time, use of local anesthesia, and minimal blood loss. Risks of the procedure include infection (4%), complications of angiography (3%), and uterine ischemia or nontarget embolization. Premature ovarian failure secondary to compromise of the ovarian circulation has been reported. Patients typically experience cramping for the first 12 to 18 hr after the procedure. Postembolization syndrome (fever, nausea, vomiting, and at times, severe abdominal pain) has been observed in approximately 30% of patients.
- Outcomes of UAE include 40% to 60% reduction in uterine size and decreased menstrual bleeding with high rates of patient satisfaction. Patients have significantly less postoperative pain and return to work sooner compared to those undergoing hysterectomy but have increased rates of minor complications. Long-term outcomes may be inferior to myomectomy, with the rate of reoperation in patients undergoing UAE as high as 30%. The reoperation rate is age dependent, with higher likelihood of success in women over age 40.
- The impact on fertility postprocedure has not been well-defined and is not generally recommended in patients who desire future fertility. Initial case reports of pregnancy after UAE seem to indicate an increased risk of obstetric complications, such as preterm labor, miscarriage, and malpresentation.

Magnetic Resonance Imaging–Guided Focused Ultrasound Surgery (MRgFUS)

- With MRgFUS, fibroid tissue is heated and destroyed using targeted ultrasonic energy passing through the anterior abdominal wall. This procedure is performed with MRI thermal mapping and conducted over several outpatient visits. MRgFUS is not appropriate for pedunculated myomas or those adjacent to bowel or bladder. Although the procedure is currently FDA approved for pre-menopausal women who do not desire future fertility, outcome data beyond 24 months is lacking. Potential side effects include skin or nerve burns.

- Studies are being performed to investigate similar MRI-guided radiofrequency ablation or laser photocoagulation techniques.

Myolysis/Cryomyolysis

- **Laparoscopic coagulation** of a leiomyoma, or myolysis, is performed with a neodymium: yttrium-aluminum-garnet laser by causing degeneration of protein and destruction of vascularity. Dense pelvic adhesions have been found on follow-up. Bipolar coagulation and cryomyolysis effect similar results using radiofrequency energy or supercooling, respectively. There is limited long-term efficacy or safety data for these methods, and they are not recommended for women desiring future fertility.

Laparoscopic Uterine Artery Occlusion

- **Laparoscopic uterine artery occlusion (LUAO)** is a technique that may represent a new alternative to UAE. In this procedure, the uterine arteries are accessed retroperitoneally and surgically occluded. Similar short-term outcomes to UAE have been shown; however, there is limited longitudinal data.

Doppler-Guided Uterine Artery Occlusion

- **Doppler-guided uterine artery occlusion (D-UAO)**, currently in development, utilizes a transvaginal vascular clamp with Doppler-guidance to ligate the uterine arteries and may be a future alternative to UAE.

SUGGESTED READINGS

Alternatives to hysterectomy in the management of leiomyomas. ACOG Practice Bulletin Number 96. American College of Obstetricians and Gynecologists. *Obstet Gynecol* 2008;112:387–400.

Breech LL, Rock JA. Leiomyomata uteri and myomectomy. In: Rock JA, Jones HW, eds. *Telinde's Operative Gynecology*, 10th Ed. Philadelphia, PA: Lippincott Williams & Wilkins. 2008;687–727.

Cheng MH, Wang PH. Uterine myoma: a condition amenable to medical therapy? *Expert Opin Emerg Drugs* 2008;13(1):119–133.

Goodwin SC. Uterine artery embolization for treatment of leiomyomata: long-term outcomes from the FIBROID Registry. *Obstet Gynecol* 2008;111(1):22–33.

Hodge JC. Genetic heterogeneity among uterine leiomyomata: insights into malignant progression. *Hum Mol Genet* 2007;16 Spec No 1:R7–R13.

Levy BS. Modern management of uterine fibroids. *Acta Obstet Gynecol Scand* 2008;87(8):812–823.

Pritts EA, Parker WH, Olive DL. Fibroids and infertility: an updated systematic review of the evidence. *Fertil Steril.* 2009;91(4):1215–1223.

35 Menstrual Disorders: Endometriosis, Dysmenorrhea, and Premenstrual Dysphoric Disorder

Camille Gunderson and Melissa Yates

ENDOMETRIOSIS

Endometriosis is defined as the extrauterine presence of functioning endometrial glands and stroma. Most commonly found in the ovaries but also located in the pouch of Douglas, vesicouterine space, uterosacral ligaments, and surrounding pelvic peritoneum. Less commonly seen in laparotomy and episiotomy scars, appendix, pleural and pericardial cavities, and the cervix.

Theories of the Pathogenesis of Endometriosis
- The etiology of endometriosis is unknown. Several theories involving anatomic, immunologic, hormonal, and genetic factors have been postulated.
- **Retrograde menstruation:** Sampson's original theory suggests that endometriosis is related to retrograde menstruation of endometrial tissue via the fallopian tubes into the peritoneal cavity. Support for this theory is as follows:
  - Blood flow from the fimbriated ends of fallopian tubes has been visualized during laparoscopy (seen in 90% of women with patent fallopian tubes).
  - Endometriosis is most often found in the dependent portions of the pelvis.
  - Incidence of endometriosis is higher in women with obstruction to normal outward menstrual flow (e.g., cervical stenosis).
  - Endometriosis is more common in women with shorter menstrual cycles or longer duration of flow, providing more opportunity for endometrial implantation.
- **Immunologic factors:** Increasing data suggest that specific immunologic factors at the site of endometrial implants play a major role in determining whether and to what extent a patient will develop the disease. These factors are thought to explain the attachment and proliferation of the endometriotic cells.
- **Inflammatory factors:** Elevated levels of interleukin-6 and tumor necrosis factor-α have been noted in the peritoneal fluid of endometriosis patients. Interleukin-8 may help in the attachment of endometrial implants in the peritoneum and is also an angiogenic agent.
- **Hormonal factors:** Unlike normal endometrial tissue, endometriotic implants can produce aromatase, leading to extraovarian estrogen production. This may explain why endometriosis can recur in women who have undergone hysterectomy and bilateral

salpingo-oophorectomy. Prostaglandin E_2, a proinflammatory compound, has been shown to be a powerful inducer of aromatase activity in endometriotic implants.

- **Coelomic metaplasia:** This theory postulates that totipotential cells of the ovary and peritoneum are transformed into endometriotic lesions by repeated hormonal or infectious stimuli. This may explain the finding of endometriosis in mature teratomas and extraperitoneal sites.
- **Lymphatic spread:** One study showed that 29% of women with endometriosis at autopsy had positive pelvic lymph nodes for the disease. Thus, lymphatic spread may be another mechanism to explain why endometriotic implants can be found in remote anatomic areas, such as the lung.
- **Genetic factors:** Women who have a first-degree relative with endometriosis have a sevenfold greater risk of developing endometriosis. The mode of inheritance is most likely multifactorial.

Patient Characteristics

- Mean age at diagnosis is 25 to 30 years. The greatest incidence has been observed in nulliparous women with early age at menarche and shorter menstrual cycles. Increased parity and greater cumulative lactation have been shown to be protective factors in development of endometriosis.
- Although some women with endometriosis are asymptomatic, the most common symptoms are dysmenorrhea, infertility, pelvic pain, and dyspareunia.
  - **Dysmenorrhea:** Incidence of endometriosis in patients with dysmenorrhea is believed to be 40% to 60%. One study found endometriotic implants in approximately 70% of teenagers who underwent laparoscopy for chronic pelvic pain. Dysmenorrhea often starts before the onset of menstrual bleeding and continues until bleeding abates.
  - **Infertility:** Incidence of endometriosis is believed to be 20% to 40% among infertile couples, with some studies showing endometriosis to be seven to ten times more likely in this patient group. Often, asymptomatic patients undergoing laparoscopy for infertility often will be diagnosed with mild endometriosis.
  - **Pelvic pain:** The severity of pelvic pain does not correlate with the amount of endometriosis present. The pain typically associated with endometriosis is central, deep, and often in the rectal area. Unilateral pain may be compatible with lesions in the ovary or pelvic sidewall. Forty to fifty percent of patients with deep dyspareunia have been found to have endometriosis. This pain can be especially prominent during the premenstrual and menstrual phases of the cycle. Dysuria or dyschezia can result from urinary or intestinal tract involvement.

Abnormal Clinical Findings Associated with Endometriosis

- Nodularity of the uterosacral ligaments, which are often tender and enlarged
- Painful swelling of the rectovaginal septum
- Pain with motion of the uterus and adnexa
- Fixed retroverted uterus and large immobile adnexa are indicative of severe pelvic disease

Confirmation of Diagnosis

- **Pelvic ultrasonography:** May be useful in suggesting the presence of endometriomas at a cost significantly less than CT or MRI.
- **Diagnostic laparoscopy:** Definitive diagnosis can be made only through laparoscopy and histologic examination, which reveals both endometrial glands and stroma. Hemosiderin-laden macrophages have been identified in 77% of endometriosis biopsy specimens.

- Experienced clinicians often presumptively diagnose endometriosis based on a classic blue-black powder-burn visual appearance; however, nonclassic lesions may appear vesicular, red, white, tan, or nonpigmented. Red lesions are considered to be the more active form of endometriosis. The presence of defects in the peritoneum (usually scarring overlying endometrial implants) is known as Allen-Masters syndrome. Endometriomas can also be visualized during laparoscopy and may be referred to as "chocolate cysts" due to their dark brown appearance.

Staging System—American Society for Reproductive Medicine Classification of Endometriosis

- See Table 35-1.

Medical Treatment

- Estrogen stimulates the growth of endometriotic implants similar to its effect on normal endometrial tissue. Medical therapy is aimed at suppressing ovarian estrogen

TABLE 35-1	American Fertility Society Classification of Endometriosis		
Endometriosis	<1 cm	1–3 cm	>3 cm
Peritonium			
Superficial	1	2	4
Deep	2	4	6
Ovary			
Right superficial	1	2	4
Right deep	4	16	20
Left superficial	1	2	4
Left deep	4	16	20
Posterior			
Cul-de-sac	Partial		Complete
Obliteration	4		40
Adhesions	<1/3 Enclosure	1/3–2/3 Enclosure	>2/3 Enclosure
Ovary			
Right filmy	1	2	4
Right dense	4	8	16
Left filmy	1	2	4
Left dense	4	8	16
Tube			
Right filmy	1	2	4
Right dense	4[a]	8[a]	16
Left filmy	1	2	4
Left dense	4[a]	8[a]	16

Determination of the stage or degree of endometrial involvement is based on a weighted point system. The following categories have been established: stage I (minimal disease) 1–5 points; stage II (mild disease) 6–15; stage III (moderate disease) 16–40 points; stage IV (severe disease) >40 points.
[a]If the fimbriated end of the fallopian tube is completely enclosed, change the point assignment to 16.
From American Society for Reproductive Medicine. Revised classification of endometriosis: 1996. *Fertil Steril* 1997;67(5):817–821.

stimulation by interrupting the hypothalamic-pituitary-ovarian axis. Inhibition of ovulation by gonadotropin suppression removes the stimulation of endometriosis by cycling sex steroids.

- **Oral contraceptive pills (OCPs):** These pills cause anovulation and decidualization, which results in atrophy of endometrial tissue. Symptomatic relief of pelvic pain and dysmenorrhea is reported in 60% to 95% of patients. However, the estrogenic component may potentially stimulate growth and increase pain during the first few weeks of treatment. The recommended dose is a 20- to 30-μg ethinyl estradiol pill. Continuous use is a viable alternative for patients who experience the majority of their symptoms during menses. The side effect of this treatment is irregular bleeding but this is generally well tolerated in patients who desire symptom relief.

- **Gonadotropin-releasing hormone (GnRH) agonists:** When given over the long-term, suppress pituitary function by downregulating pituitary GnRH receptors. This interruption of the hypothalamic-pituitary-ovarian axis produces a "medical oophorectomy" or "pseudomenopause." Three available agents are leuprolide acetate (Lupron Depot), 3.75 mg by intramuscular injection every month for 6 months; nafarelin acetate nasal spray, 200 μg twice daily for 6 months; and goserelin acetate (Zoladex), 3.6 mg subcutaneous implants at 28 day intervals for 6 months. Side effects are related to the hypoestrogenic state. Treatment is usually limited to 6 months to avoid the long-term consequences of the hypoestrogenic state on bone metabolism and lipid profile changes.

  - **Add back therapy:** Largely used for minimization of side effects. Numerous studies have demonstrated the efficacy of adding back combined estrogen/progesterone to patients on GnRH agonist therapy. Patients receiving add-back therapy have significantly less vasomotor side effects and bone mineral density loss over a 6-month period while still benefiting from pain improvement from their endometriosis. Vaginal bleeding is a side effect of add-back therapy and is dose dependent. A postmenopausal estrogen-progesterone add-back regimen can be used, such as daily conjugated estrogen 0.625 mg together with medroxyprogesterone acetate 2.5 mg. An alternate regimen is 2.5 mg norethindrone acetate daily.

- **Progestins:** Progestins inhibit ovulation by luteinizing hormone (LH) suppression and, eventually, may induce amenorrhea (Table 35-2). They also suppress endometriosis through decidualization and atrophy of endometrial tissue. Progesterone therapy can be continued for suppression of endometriosis symptomatology; however, health care providers should be aware of the potential for bone demineralization with long-term progesterone use.

- **Danazol (Danocrine):** A derivative of the synthetic steroid 17α-ethinyltestosterone. It suppresses the midcycle LH surge, inhibits steroidogenesis in the human corpus luteum, and produces a high-androgen and low-estrogen environment that does not support the growth of endometriosis. Approximately 80% of patients experience relief or improvement in symptoms within 2 months of beginning danazol treatment. Androgenic side effects greatly reduce compliance. Recurrence of symptoms is almost 50% within 4 to 12 months after discontinuation of therapy. Adverse side effects occur in approximately 15% of women taking danazol.

- **Aromatase inhibitors:** Recent studies have evaluated the third-generation aromatase inhibitors, letrozole and anastrozole, for treatment of endometriosis refractory to other modalities. They are used alone or combined with GnRH agonists. These medications have been shown to decrease circulating estrogen levels by 50%. The most significant side effect is decreased bone density, which is not necessarily ameliorated with the use of calcium and vitamin D; however, evidence at this point is conflicting with regard to the overall decrease in bone density, requiring further study.

TABLE 35-2	Medical Management of Endometriosis		
Drug	**Mechanism**	**Dosage**	**Side Effects**
Gonadotrophin-releasing hormone analogs	Down-regulation of pituitary receptors, inhibition of the hypothalamic-pituitary-ovarian axis leading to ovarian suppression.	Lueprolide acetate (Lupron): 3.75–7.5 mg IM qmo × 6 Nafarelin acetate (Synarel): 200–400 μg intranasally bid × 6 mo Goserelin acetate (Zoladex): 3.6 mg implant SC q12wk × 6 mo	Hot flashes, vaginal dryness, bone demineralization, insomnia, libido changes, fatigue
Oral contraceptives	Anovulation, atrophy and decidualization of endometrial tissue	Monophasic pill	Weight gain, breakthrough bleeding, breast tenderness, bloating, nausea
Progestins	Atrophy and decidualization of endometrial tissue, suppression gonadotropins, inhibition of ovulation, amenorrhea	Medroxyprogesterone acetate: 150 mg IM q3mo × 4 or 30 mg PO qd × 90 d Megestrol acetate: 40 mg PO qd × 6 mo	Weight gain, fluid retention, breakthrough bleeding, depression Possible bone demineralization with long-term use
Danazol	Anovulation by decreasing the midcycle luteinizing hormone surge Inhibition of steroidogenesis, creation of high-androgen and low-estrogen environment	Megestrol acetate: 400–800 mg PO qd × 6 mo	Amenorrhea, virilization, acne, hirsutism, atrophic vaginitis, decrease in breast size, hot flashes, deepening of voice.

Adapted from Management of endometriosis. ACOG Practice Bulletin Number 114. American College of Obstetricians and Gynecologists. *Obstet Gynecol* 2010;116:223–236.

Additional side effects include vaginal spotting, hot flushes, headaches, and mood swings, which are better tolerated compared to the side effects of GnRH agonists.
- Pain control with **nonsteroidal anti-inflammatory drugs (NSAIDs)** inhibits prostaglandin production by ectopic endometrium. NSAIDs are a good first-line agent, especially when the diagnosis of endometriosis has not been firmly established.

Surgical Treatment

- Ideal for patients with infertility or symptoms that are refractory to medical treatment. Surgical management can be subdivided into definitive surgery and conservative surgery.
  - **Definitive surgery** entails total abdominal hysterectomy with bilateral salpingo-oophorectomy, excision of peritoneal surface lesions or endometriomas, and lysis of adhesions. This definitive treatment is not always an option, however, if the patient wishes to maintain reproductive capacity or to conserve ovarian tissue. A "semidefinitive" procedure that preserves an uninvolved ovary is usually discouraged because of the sixfold increased risk of developing recurrent symptoms and an eightfold reoperation rate to remove the remaining ovary.
    - Hormone replacement therapy (HRT) after definitive surgery: Patients who have undergone hysterectomy and bilateral salpingo-oophorectomy may receive postoperative replacement estrogen.
  - **Conservative surgery** is usually achieved with laparoscopic excision or destruction of endometrial implants via laser vaporization, electrocoagulation, thermal coagulation.

Endometriosis and Infertility

- Exact incidence of infertility caused by endometriosis is unknown.
- Theories on the physiologic changes caused by endometriosis that affect fertility potential include abnormal folliculogenesis, elevated oxidative stress, altered immune function, alterations in peritoneal fluid cytokines, and decreased presence of integrins during the implantation phase, thus decreasing endometrial receptivity. Together these factors decrease oocyte quality and impair fertilization and implantation.
- Fewer oocytes are retrieved when an endometrioma is present but the pregnancy rate with in vitro fertilization (IVF) is not greatly altered.
- Conservative surgery to excise rectovaginal endometriosis does not improve future pregnancy rates although it does yield significant pain relief.

Endometriosis and Ovarian Malignancy

- The prevalence of endometriosis in patients with epithelial ovarian carcinoma, especially in endometrioid and clear cell types, is higher than that of the general population. Conversely, ovarian carcinoma has been documented in 0.3% to 0.8% of patients with endometriosis.
- The pathology of endometriosis exhibits many of the characteristics of neoplastic lesions: reduced cell cycle inhibitor activity, ability to resist apoptosis, angiogenic potential similar to malignant neoplasms, and ability to invade surrounding tissue.
- Endometriosis implants may represent a precancerous state. Endometriosis is related to a chronic inflammatory state involving cytokine release, which can lead to malignant mechanisms. Both atypical endometriosis and ovarian cancers associated with endometriosis have p53 overexpression; the Ki-67 index was noted to be three times higher in atypical endometriosis.
- Clear cell and endometrioid carcinoma are the most common histologies associated with ovarian endometriosis. Numerous studies reviewing the histologic slides of endometriosis demonstrate simultaneous atypical endometriosis and malignancy.
- Endometriosis-associated ovarian carcinoma is found at an earlier stage and lower grade and is associated with a better overall survival rate than sporadic ovarian cancer.
- There is a definite causal relationship between endometriosis and specific histologic types of ovarian cancer. However, the low magnitude of the conferred risk is

consistent with the view that ectopic endometrium undergoes malignant transformation with a frequency similar to its eutopic counterpart.

- At present, malignant transformation of endometriotic lesions is a recognized mechanism in the development of ovarian cancer. However, definitive surgery to remove all visible evidence of endometriosis is not recommended as a prophylactic means of reducing the development of ovarian malignancy. Rather, long-term use of oral contraceptives is the preferred method of cancer risk reduction as an 80% lower occurrence of ovarian cancer in women with endometriosis has been shown in patients using the drug for >10 years.

DYSMENORRHEA

- Primary dysmenorrhea is painful menstruation with no evident hormonal or anatomic pathology. Secondary dysmenorrhea has a demonstrable cause.
- Risk factors include young age (<20 years), heavy menstrual flow, smoking, weight loss attempts, nulliparity, and psychiatric disorders such as depression and anxiety. Prevalence progressively decreases beyond age 24, and symptomatic improvement may occur after childbirth. Parity has no effect once age is factored in.
- Primary dysmenorrhea presents within 6 months of menarche. It only occurs during ovulatory cycles, which may or may not be present at menarche. If dysmenorrhea does not appear until more than a year after menarche, secondary dysmenorrhea should be suspected.
- See Chapter 27 as well.

Pertinent Findings in History and Physical Exam

- Defined as spasmodic cramping ("labor-like" pains) beginning a few hours before or simultaneous with the onset of menses, which are often accompanied by nausea, vomiting, backache, irritability, fatigue, diarrhea, and headache.
- Symptoms with primary dysmenorrhea last only 2 to 3 days; however, pelvic pain and tenderness persist beyond this interval with secondary dysmenorrhea. Pain is most intense during first 24 to 36 hr of menstrual flow, which is consistent with the time of maximal prostaglandin release into the menstrual fluid.
- Clinical presentation with secondary dysmenorrhea varies considerably with its cause. Endometriosis is the most common cause, but other possibilities are pelvic inflammatory disease, pelvic adhesions, and uterine fibroids.
- Pelvic examination is not required to assess primary dysmenorrhea; it is diagnosed solely on the basis of symptom description and chronology.
- Evaluation of secondary dysmenorrheal requires a complete pelvic exam. The use of microbiologic cultures, ultrasound, and other imaging modalities may be required to identify the etiology of secondary dysmenorrhea.

Treatment of Dysmenorrhea

- Three modalities exist: pharmacologic, nonpharmacologic, and surgical. Pharmacologic is preferred for primary dysmenorrhea.
- NSAIDs are the gold standard of treatment of primary dysmenorrhea. No specific NSAID is most efficacious, but older and generically available NSAIDs are preferred. They relieve primary dysmenorrhea by reducing endometrial prostaglandin production and by exerting a central nervous system analgesic effect. They do not affect menstrual flow volume but do reduce the amount of menstrual fluid prostaglandin level to below that of normal pain-free cycles.

- Combined OCPs reduce menstrual fluid volume and prostaglandins to within, or even below, normal range with concomitant clinical relief during that cycle. Monophasic and triphasic pills are equally effective.
  - There is insufficient research regarding pain relief in primary dysmenorrhea with low-dose estrogen OCPs or progesterone only OCPs.
- Glyceryl trinitrate, magnesium, calcium channel antagonists, and vitamin B_6 have been shown to have varying beneficial effects on symptom reduction with primary dysmenorrhea.
- Nonpharmacologic treatment includes transcutaneous nerve stimulation (TENS), acupuncture, acupressure, and heat-wrap therapy. High-frequency TENS offers significant pain relief via raising pain threshold and increasing the release of endorphins from the spinal cord and peripheral nerves. While acupressure only has a suggestive role in the reduction of dysmenorrhea, acupuncture has been shown to be equally beneficial to ibuprofen in pain reduction. Continuous suprapubic heat application has been shown more therapeutic than acetaminophen during the initial 8 hr of application.
- Surgical interventions including nerve ablation (uterosacral nerve ablation and presacral neurectomy) and spinal manipulation have shown no long-lasting therapeutic benefit according to Cochrane meta-analyses. Additionally, they carry significant risk of adverse events.

PREMENSTRUAL SYNDOME AND PREMENSTRUAL DYSPHORIC DISORDER

- **Premenstrual syndrome (PMS)** is a cluster of mood, cognitive, and physical disturbances with the hallmark symptom of irritability. It is distinct from depression or anxiety disorders.
  - Mood symptoms include irritability, mood swings, depression, and anxiety; cognitive disturbances may be confusion or poor concentration. Physical problems consist of bloating, breast tenderness, appetite changes, hot flashes, insomnia, headache, and fatigue.
- **Premenstrual dysphoric disorder (PMDD)** represents the more severe end of the spectrum. It is comprised of the same blend of symptoms but involves an increased severity in perceived symptoms and a marked impairment in daily life.
  - Symptom onset occurs anytime in the 2 weeks prior to the onset of bleeding, continues to the start of bleeding, and resolves after a day or two of menstrual flow.
- In order to make the diagnosis, the symptoms must be characteristic of PMS/PMDD, limited to the luteal phase, and not attributable to a general medical condition.
- A critical reduction in serotonergic function during the luteal phase is the likely underlying mechanism of PMS/PMDD.

Evaluation and Diagnosis

- Dysmenorrhea, depression and anxiety disorders, menstrual migraine, cyclic mastalgia, irritable bowel syndrome, and hypothyroidism may all present with mood or physical disturbances similar to those that manifest with PMS/PMDD. See also Chapter 27.
- The diagnostic process can be completed in two clinic visits separated by two menstrual cycles. At the initial visit, symptoms are evaluated and a differential diagnosis is formulated. The patient should be instructed to keep a symptom

log. Two months later, the information is reviewed and a management plan is made.
- There are no laboratory or physical exam findings required to make the diagnosis. Rather, these tests are used to rule out other causes of similar symptoms. Hormone levels (estrogen, progesterone, LH, follicle-stimulating hormone [FSH]) do not vary between women with and without PMS/PMDD; thus, there is no use in obtaining these values.

Symptom Diary
- Timing of symptoms and menstrual flow is confirmed by a prospective record (symptom diary) maintained for at least two cycles.
- Patients are asked to record their five most bothersome symptoms and to indicate each evening the presence and the severity of each.
- Such logs are helpful for clinicians in order to determine whether the reported symptoms are limited to the luteal phase or are present throughout the cycle, suggesting a general medical condition. Additionally, they are helpful for patients for instituting self-help strategies and for anticipating symptoms.

Treatment
- Since PMS/PMDD is a chronic problem, adverse effects, cost, and severity of symptoms should all be considered before employing a specific treatment.
- Lifestyle changes are probably most appropriate for mild-to-moderate PMS/PMDD. Regular aerobic exercise, dietary limitation of caffeine, alcohol, and salt, and increased consumption of complex carbohydrates during the luteal phase have been shown to reduce the severity of symptoms.
- Dietary supplements (especially St. John's wort, but also ginkgo and kava) are somewhat effective for mild-to-moderate PMS but ineffective for PMDD. However, patients should be aware of their potential adverse effects. (Especially the affect of St. John's wort on the effectiveness of OCPs).
- Mineral supplements can reduce both emotional and luteal phase symptoms. In a randomized trial of 497 women, there was a reduction of 48% of symptom scoring in women taking 1,200 mg calcium carbonate daily versus a 30% reduction in women taking placebo after 3 months.
- In several small randomized trials, NSAIDs taken in the luteal phase have been shown to decrease all physical symptoms with the exception of breast tenderness.
- Yaz, the combined OCP containing drosperinone and 20 µg of ethinyl estradiol, was recently approved by the FDA for treatment of PMDD and has been shown effective in treating mood, physical and behavioral symptoms of PMDD.
- SSRIs are the most effective pharmacologic treatment for moderate-to-severe PMS and PMDD. Continuous dosing exerts a greater inhibition of symptoms than intermittent dosing. Fluoxetine, sertraline, citalopram, and paroxetine all demonstrated a statistically significant improvement in symptoms.

SUGGESTED READINGS

Allen C, Hopewell S, Prentice A, Non-steroidal anti-inflammatory drugs for pain in women with endometriosis. *Cochrane Database Syst Rev* 2005; (4):CD004753.

Barbieri RL, Niloff JM, Bast RC Jr, et al. Elevated serum concentrations of CA-125 in patients with advanced endometriosis. *Fertil Steril* 1986;45(5):630–634.

Brosens I, Puttemans P, Campo R, et al. Non-invasive methods of diagnosis of endometriosis. *Curr Opin Obstet Gynecol* 2003;15(6):519–522.

Premenstrual syndrome. ACOG Practice Bulletin Number 15. American College of Obstetricians and Gynecologists. *Obstet Gynecol* 2000;95(4).

Sagsveen M, Farmer JE, Prentice A, et al. Gonadotrophin-releasing hormone analogues for endometriosis: bone mineral density. *Cochrane Database Syst Rev* 2003;(4):CD001297.

Sampson JA. Peritoneal endometriosis due to menstrual dissemination of endometrial tissue into the peritoneal cavity. *Am J Obstet Gynecol* 1927;71:422–469.

Somigliana E, Vigano' P, Parazzini F, et al. Association between endometriosis and cancer: a comprehensive review and a critical analysis of clinical and epidemiological evidence. *Gynecol Oncol*;101(2):331–341.

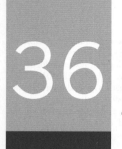

36 Evaluation of Amenorrhea

Sherrine A. Ibrahim and Samuel Smith

Amenorrhea is the absence of menses. It is physiologic during pregnancy, lactation, and menopause. Lack of regular, spontaneous menses for any other reason after the expected age of menarche is pathologic.

- **Primary amenorrhea:** No menstruation by age 14 in the absence of any secondary sexual development (i.e., thelarche, pubarche) or no menstruation by age 16 regardless of the presence of secondary sexual characteristics.
  - The following are common causes of primary amenorrhea: hypergonadotropic hypogonadism and primary ovarian failure, hypogonadotropic hypogonadism, outflow tract abnormalities/Müllerian anomalies, complete androgen insensitivity syndrome (CAIS), hypothalamic dysfunction, hyperprolactinemia, hypothyroidism, enzyme deficiencies (CYP17 deficiency), and pregnancy. See Table 36-1.
- **Secondary amenorrhea:** Lack of menses for 6 months or for three menstrual cycles in women who have experienced menarche. However, evaluation need not be deferred solely to conform to this definition.
  - The following are common causes of secondary amenorrhea: pregnancy, Asherman's syndrome, hypogonadotropism, hypothalamic dysfunction, Sheehan's syndrome, hyperprolactinemia, hypothyroidism, polycystic ovarian syndrome (PCOS), premature ovarian failure (POF) and hypergonadotropism, postpill amenorrhea, and menopause. See Table 36-1.

MENSTRUAL PHYSIOLOGY

- Spontaneous, cyclic menstruation requires an intact and functional hypothalamic-pituitary-ovarian axis (HPOA), endometrium, and outflow tract. Abnormalities in any of these structures may result in amenorrhea.
- Additionally, other endocrinopathies may cause perturbations in the HPOA and cause amenorrhea.
- Normal physiology of the HPOA: **Nucleus arcuatus** (medial basal hypothalamus) → pulsatile secretion (90 minutes) of **gonadotropin releasing hormone (GnRH)** → stimulates **gonadotrophs** in anterior pituitary to synthesize, store, and secrete gonadotropic hormones: **follicle-stimulating hormone/luteinizing hormone (FSH/LH)** → stimulate **ovarian follicle** development and estradiol secretion (negative feedback on HP initially then positive feedback to trigger LH surge) → inhibin secretion and **corpus luteum** secretion of progesterone at far greater levels than estradiol (negative feedback on HP axis; Fig. 36-1).

TABLE 36-1	Pathologic Causes of Amenorrhea

Etiology	Causal Factor	Primary/Secondary/Both
Reproductive Tract		
Mayer-Rokitansky-Küster-Hauser	Müllerian agenesis (MRKH) syndrome	Primary
Imperforate hymen	Failure of perforation during development	Primary
Transverse septum	Vertical fusion defect	Primary
CYP17 deficiency (46, XY)	Genetic male; Müllerian regression	Primary
Complete androgen insensitivity	Genetic male; mutation in androgen receptor	Primary
Asherman's syndrome	Endometrial scarring	Secondary
Ovarian		
Gonadal dysgenesis	Absence of two normal X chromosomes or mosaicism	Both
Pure gonadal dysgenesis	Insult during embryonic development	Primary
Premature ovarian failure	Idiopathic, chromosomal abnormality, autoimmune disease, infection	Both
CYP17 deficiency (46, XX)	Inability to synthesize sex steroids	Primary
Polycystic ovary syndrome	Inappropriate gonadotropin secretion, insulin resistance	Both
Pituitary		
Hyperprolactinemia	Lactotroph hyperplasia ± prolactinoma, drugs	Both
Pituitary adenomas	Thyrotroph, corticotroph, or other hyperplasia	Both
Sheehan's syndrome	Postpartum hemorrhage	Secondary
CNS		
Hypothalamic amenorrhea	Stress, eating disorders, weight loss, excessive exercise	Both
Kallmann's syndrome	Lack of functional GnRH-secreting neurons	Primary
Congenital GnRH deficiency	Lack of functional GnRH-secreting neurons	Primary
Brain injury	Interruption of HPOA	Both
Tumors	Interruption of HPOA	Both
Inflammatory or infiltrative process	Interruption of HPOA	Both
Other Endocrinopathies		
Hypothyroidism, Cushing's syndrome, late-onset adrenal hyperplasia		Both

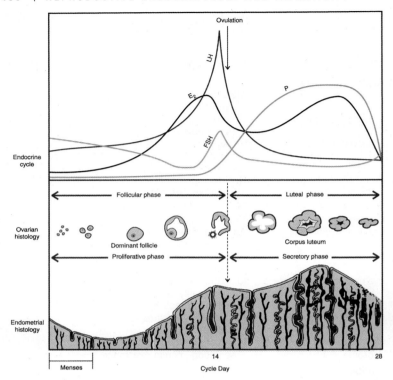

Figure 36-1. The normal menstrual cycle. Changes in serum hormones, ovarian follicle, and endometrial thickness during a 28-day menstrual cycle. Menses occur during the first few days of the cycle. E_2, estradiol; FSH, follicle-stimulating hormone; LH, luteinizing hormone; P, progesterone. From Berek and Novak. *Gynecology*, 14th Ed. Philadelphia: Lippincott Williams & Wilkins; 2007.

EVALUATION OF AMENORRHEA (Fig. 36-2)

Initial Evaluation of Primary Amenorrhea

- Check urine/serum human chorionic gonadotropin (hCG), check for signs of breast development (implies estrogen secretion was initiated) and whether there is a cervix and uterus present on clinical exam. FSH is the most important hormone to check if breast development is absent and the uterus is present. This allows you to determine if the hypogonadism is hypergonadotropic or hypogonadotropic. If breast development has occurred, but there is absent cervix/uterus you must distinguish between CAIS and Müllerian agenesis. If breast development has occurred and the uterus is present, then the evaluation will be the same as for secondary amenorrhea (check β-hCG, prolactin [PRL], TSH, and FSH).
- Outflow tract may be evaluated by clinical exam or ultrasound. Rarely, breast development is absent and cervix/uterus is absent, and in these instances, all patients will have a 46,XY karyotype (Table 36-2).

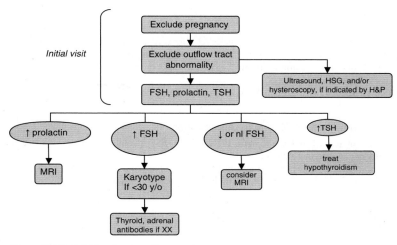

Figure 36-2. Initial evaluation of amenorrhea.

TABLE 36-2	Evaluation of Primary Amenorrhea	
	Breast Development Present	**Breast Development Absent**
Uterus is present	*Arrest in pubertal development.* Evaluate in the same way as for secondary amenorrhea—*β*-hCG, FSH, TSH, PRL, ultrasound	**Hypergonadotropic (high FSH)** Abnormal karyotype (e.g., 45,X or 46,XY) *Gonadal dysgenesis* Normal karyotype (46,XX) *17-hydroxylase deficiency Galactosemia*
		Hypogonadotropic (low FSH) *Gonadal dysgenesis GnRH deficiency (Kallmann's syndrome) Hypothalamic dysfunction Hypothalamic-pituitary tumors*
Uterus is absent	*Müllerian agenesis/MRKH syndrome Complete androgen insensitivity syndrome (CAIS)*	*Testicular regression Testosterone biosynthesis disorders*

- If hypergonadotropic (↑ FSH) check karyotype. Those with a Y cell line require gonadal removal.
- If hypogonadotropic (↓ FSH) check MRI to rule out HP tumors (e.g., craniopharyngioma) and then consider constitutional delay, Kallmann's syndrome, and hyperprolactinemia unless stigmata exist for anorexia nervosa or other syndromes (e.g., Prader Willi).
- If hyperprolactinemic check MRI for pituitary micro/macroadenoma, rarely suprasellar lesions.

Initial Evaluation of Secondary Amenorrhea

- Pregnancy test (β-hCG), prolactin (PRL), TSH, FSH for all patients.
- Consider progestin challenge.
- Evaluate for physiologic explanations for secondary amenorrhea by history, physical, and labs. Physiologic explanations include pregnancy, menopause, and postpartum lactation. Adolescents may have oligomenorrhea but amenorrhea usually lasts for <3 months.
- Evaluate for pathologic explanations.
  - If onset is related to pregnancy, abortion, or other surgical procedure, consider cervical stenosis or Asherman's syndrome. Evaluation includes some combination of hysterosalpingography (HSG), pelvic sono, hysteroscopy, sonohysterogram, or uterine sounding.
  - If signs/symptoms of androgen excess exist (e.g., hirsutism, androgenic acne), evaluate for PCOS and late-onset adrenal hyperplasia (LOAH). Elevated 17-hydroxyprogesterone is the serum marker for LOAH due to 21-hydroxylase deficiency. PCOS is common and affects ≥5% of women.
  - FSH—screens for POF.
  - TSH—screens for hypo-hyperthyroidism. Treat if diagnosed and then determine whether menses normalize.
  - PRL—screens for hyperprolactinemia. If present evaluate for primary hypothyroidism, pituitary micro/macroadenomas (by MRI), and for medications that can cause ↑PRL (including SSRIs).
- If FSH, LH, and E$_2$ are low/low normal and the evaluation is otherwise negative, the diagnosis of exclusion is hypothalamic dysfunction. MRI of sella turcica may be indicated to identify a tumor if amenorrhea is associated with headaches or visual field defects. Most patients will have negative MRI, particularly if otherwise asymptomatic and stresses that can interfere with pulsatile secretion of GnRH are identified (e.g., excessive dieting, extreme exercise, coexisting medical illness, psychological stress). Yield from MRI is extremely low if there is a positive withdrawal bleed to progestin challenge in hypothalamic amenorrhea patients.
- If FSH is high, suspect ovarian failure. If under 30 perform karyotype to look for a Y cell line, which would require gonadectomy.
- Clinical history dictates whether additional testing should be added to the above laboratory studies:
  - Long-standing oligoovulation and androgenic symptoms (acne/hirsutism): check 17-OH progesterone to rule out LOAH and serum androgens; check ultrasound to evaluate for polycystic appearing ovaries. If PCOS, check baseline metabolic evaluation minimally for FBS and lipids. May also check LH:FSH ratio, insulin levels.
  - Signs or symptoms of Cushing's syndrome: screen with late night salivary cortisol (easiest), 24 hr urinary free cortisol, 1 mg overnight dexamethasone suppression, or 2 day low-dose dexamethasone suppression screening tests.

• Progestin challenge: 10 mg Provera for 10 days. Positive response is withdrawal bleed within 2 to 7 days.
  • About 20% of patients with POF, hypothalamic amenorrhea, and hyperprolactinemia experience withdrawal flow depending upon the degree of hypoestrogenism. At least, 80% of PCOS patients will demonstrate withdrawal bleed.
  • If there is no withdrawal bleed, estrogen/progestin cycle was advised in the past but is seldom performed today. Failure to withdraw after sequential estrogen then estrogen/progestin is supportive of Asherman's syndrome or cervical stenosis, but these conditions are rarely seen in the absence of a previous surgical procedure and the amenorrhea can be temporally related to the procedure.

Important History for Amenorrhea

• **Present illness.** Does the patient experience cyclic pelvic or abdominal pain, headache, visual changes, hot flushes, or vaginal dryness?
• **Development.** What was the age of pubarche, thelarche, and menarche? Was menarche spontaneous or induced? Is there a history of hirsutism, virilization, or galactorrhea?
• **Medical.** Is she taking, or has she recently discontinued, any medications or supplements? Does she have any systemic illnesses? Has she experienced cranial or pelvic trauma or surgery? Were oral contraceptives (OCPs) recently discontinued?
• **Social.** Is she participating in athletic activities, diets, or experiencing stress?
• **Family history.** Is there a history of late pubertal development, early menopause, mental retardation, or short stature?

Physical Examination for Amenorrhea Should Include

• Height and weight as well as BMI and waist hip ratio if obese. Tanner stages of breast and pubic hair development for primary amenorrhea. Check BP.
• The internal and external genitalia must be examined. Establishing whether or not a uterus is present is especially important in a young woman with developed breasts who presents with primary amenorrhea.
• Consider an abdominal ultrasound study, if necessary, to confirm the presence of a uterus in primary amenorrhea.
• Look for signs of hirsutism, virilization, Cushing's syndrome, thyroid disease.

ETIOLOGIES OF AMENORRHEA

Outflow Tract Abnormalities

Outflow Tract Abnormalities Resulting in Primary Amenorrhea

• **Imperforate hymen** and **transverse vaginal septum** are outflow tract malformations that typically present with acute pain in an early teenager who has developed breasts but failed to menstruate.
• **Müllerian agenesis**, also known as Mayer-Rokitansky-Küster-Hauser (MRKH) syndrome, is a relatively common cause of primary amenorrhea. The incidence ranges from 1:4,000 to 1:10,000. Subjects with MRKH commonly present in their late teens with normal breast development, normal pubic hair development. Amenorrhea is generally the only complaint, although 2% to 7% may have rudimentary Müllerian structures with functioning endometrium, resulting in cyclic pain. Imaging of the urinary tract should be performed in all patients with vaginal agenesis, because approximately 30% have renal anomalies. Skeletal abnormalities are also commonly associated with MRKH, which is much more common than CAIS. Vaginal dilator therapy can usually create a functional vagina.

- **Complete androgen insensitivity syndrome**, previously known as testicular feminization, is an X-linked, recessive disorder that occurs in genetic men but results in phenotypic women. Testes are present and secrete normal male levels of anti-Müllerian hormone (AMH) and testosterone. AMH results in regression of Müllerian structures. Masculinization fails to occur because of an androgen receptor defect. Like MRKH, patients with CAIS typically present in the later teens with normal breast development and a chief complaint of amenorrhea. Physical exam can often differentiate the two conditions because pubic and axillary hair is sparse in CAIS, and testes are often palpable in the inguinal region, otherwise they are abdominal. The diagnosis is confirmed by documenting serum testosterone (T) in the normal male range (>200 ng/dL) or determining 46,XY karyotype. The incidence of gonadal neoplasia is 52%, and the incidence of gonadal malignancy is 22% in CAIS. Under these circumstances, gonadectomy must be performed. Since malignancy rarely occurs before age 20, deferring surgery until after pubertal maturation and epiphyseal closure have occurred is preferable. Vaginal dilator therapy can usually create a functional vagina.

Outflow Tract Abnormalities Resulting in Secondary Amenorrhea

- **Asherman's syndrome** is the only end-organ cause of secondary amenorrhea and accounts for 7% of cases in this population. Asherman's syndrome (i.e., intrauterine synechiae) is most commonly associated with aggressive postpartum curettage or abortion. Other risk factors include uterine or cervical surgeries, such as cesarean section, septoplasty, myomectomy, and cone biopsy procedures. Rarer causes include tuberculosis, schistosomiasis, infection associated with IUDs, and other severe pelvic infections. Diagnosis can be confirmed with HSG, sonohysterogram, or hysteroscopy. Hypomenorrhea is common if cervical stenosis is absent.

Diagnostic Tests for Outflow Tract Abnormalities

- Hysterosalpingography
- Ultrasonography/saline infusion ultrasonography
- Hysteroscopy
- MRI if clinical suspicion high for Müllerian anomalies.

Hypergonadotropic Primary Amenorrhea

- **Gonadal dysgenesis** is the most common cause of primary amenorrhea, accounting for 43% of such cases. Peripheral blood karyotype aids in diagnosis. Although **Turner's syndrome (TS)** is the most frequent cause of gonadal dysgenesis, any condition resulting in depletion of germ cells can cause gonadal dysgenesis and replacement of the gonads with fibrous streaks.
  - **TS** is a condition in which all or part of one of the X chromosomes is missing. Approximately, 60% of TS patients are 45,X. The other 40% include karyotype abnormalities such as 45,X/46,XX mosaics, 46,XXqi isochromosome, and 46,XXp-short arm deletion. Internal and external genitalia develop normally for females. The cohort of primordial follicles undergoes accelerated atresia so that oocytes are depleted long before the onset of puberty. A lack of gonadal estrogen production results in a failure of breast development.
    - Most patients with TS exhibit several cardinal features including webbed neck, shield chest, short stature, and sexual infantilism and are diagnosed long before seeing a gynecologist for primary amenorrhea. Some TS patients, especially those with mosaic karyotypes, can undergo spontaneous puberty and conception (16% and 3.6% of cases, respectively).

- **Mosaicism** involving partial deletions or rearrangements of one X chromosome can cause a wide range of gonadal dysfunctions, from gonadal dysgenesis to POF. Determining whether a Y chromosome is present in a mosaic is important since the presence of the SRY portion of the Y chromosome predisposes to tumor formation. Presence of a Y chromosome requires gonadectomy or removal of gonadal streak.

- **Pure gonadal dysgenesis** is a term used to describe 46,XX or XY individuals who experience dysgenesis of germinal tissue early in embryonic development. Such dysgenesis likely results from genetic, environmental, or infectious insults, though a specific cause is rarely identified. All subjects are phenotypic women of normal height who fail to undergo puberty. Patients with 46,XY gonadal dysgenesis, also known as **Swyer's syndrome**, require removal of their gonadal streaks to prevent malignant transformation.

- **CYP17 deficiency** is a rare disorder that can affect 46,XY, or XX individuals. The lack of 17α-hydroxylase and 17, 20 lyase activities results in both gonadal and adrenal insufficiencies. XY individuals are phenotypic women (due to lack of androgen production) but lack a uterus because AMH was secreted in fetal life. Subjects usually present at the time of puberty with hypertension (due to excess mineralocorticoid production), hypokalemia, and hypergonadotropic hypogonadism. CYP17 deficiency is autosomal recessive disorder.

Hypergonadotropic Secondary Amenorrhea

- **Premature ovarian failure (POF)**, also called premature ovarian insufficiency, is a term generally used to describe amenorrhea associated with depletion of oocytes before age 40. This definition includes the causes of primary gonadal failure discussed previously. In those with primary amenorrhea, approximately 50% will have an abnormal karyotype. Most cases of POF present as secondary amenorrhea, and up to 90% may be unexplained POF.

  - **X chromosome abnormalities**, such as short- or long-arm deletions or mosaicism, not severe enough to cause primary gonadal dysgenesis, may manifest as POF. Thirteen percent of women <30 years old with spontaneous POF have an abnormal karyotype.

  - **Spontaneous POF** is not induced by chemotherapy, radiation, or surgery. The majority of cases are idiopathic; 6% have premutations in the gene responsible for **fragile X syndrome (FMR1)**; 4% have **steroidogenic cell autoimmunity**, placing them at risk for adrenal insufficiency. Since 14% of patients with familial POF and 2% of isolated POF will have the FMR1 premutation, it is important to evaluate for the FMR1 gene premutation by obtaining a family history of POF, fragile X, unexplained MR, tremor/ataxia syndrome, and/or any developmental delay in children. In addition, about 20% of patients with POF develop autoimmune hypothyroidism. Therefore, women with POF should undergo adrenal and thyroid antibody testing. Those under age 30 should also have karyotyping performed. Inclusion of any Y chromosomal material is an indication for gonadectomy.

  - Radiation, chemotherapy (especially with alkylating agents), and removal of ovarian tissue are factors for iatrogenic premature follicular depletion.

  - POF can be associated with psychological distress, grief, anger, guilt, shame, etc. They may also suffer from vasomotor symptoms secondary to estrogen deficiency (i.e., vasomotor flushes, sleep disturbance, vaginal dryness, osteoporosis). Hormone therapy (HT) may be used for symptomatic relief (e.g., OCPs, progestins), but POF patients require twice as much estrogen than postmenopausal women to alleviate symptoms.

Hypothalamic Amenorrhea

- This is a common cause of both primary and secondary amenorrhea.
- The term **hypothalamic amenorrhea** applies to conditions in which GnRH secretion is diminished in the absence of any organic pathology.
- Physical or **psychological stress**, **anorexia nervosa**, **exercise**, and **weight loss** can contribute to dysfunctional hypothalamic GnRH secretion.
- Reduced pulsatile secretion of GnRH results in low levels of LH, FSH, and estrogen (hypogonadotropic hypogonadism). Absent pulsatile secretion of GnRH is uncommon except in Kallmann's syndrome and congenital GnRH deficiency.
- **Postpill amenorrhea** is rare and diagnosed if amenorrhea persists for 1 year after discontinuing contraception.
- **Kallmann's syndrome** is an inherited disorder resulting from a genetic mutation that causes failure of olfactory and GnRH neuronal migration from the olfactory placode. This syndrome is characterized by primary amenorrhea, absent breast development, presence of cervix and uterus, and anosmia.
- **Congenital GnRH deficiency** is a genetic condition resulting in the absence of functional hypothalamic neurons. Unlike Kallmann's syndrome, it is not associated with anosmia.
- **Other CNS pathologies**, such as hypothalamic neoplasms, trauma, hemorrhage, or cranial irradiation, can interrupt the function of the HPOA. **Craniopharyngioma** is the most common CNS neoplasm causing delayed puberty. An MRI should be ordered for any patient with hypogonadotropic amenorrhea when no obvious cause (e.g., excessive exercise or weight loss) is present.

Pituitary Disorders

- **Pituitary lesions** can present with amenorrhea and low or normal levels of gonadotropins. The most common pituitary lesion is the prolactinoma, but nonfunctioning adenomas, adenomas that secrete other pituitary hormones, or empty sella syndrome may also be present.
- **Hyperprolactinemia** accounts for 14% of secondary amenorrhea and a small portion of primary amenorrhea. When galactorrhea and amenorrhea are experienced simultaneously, the chance of being hyperprolactinemic is 90%. Hypothalamic GnRH secretion is suppressed by negative feedback of excess PRL, thereby lowering serum FSH and LH. Breastfeeding amenorrhea is a physiologic cause of hyperprolactinemia.
  - Medications that can cause hyperprolactinemia include most antipsychotics and antidepressants, H_2 receptor blockers, methyldopa, verapamil, reserpine, and metoclopramide.
  - A mildly elevated serum prolactin should be repeated in a fasting, nonstressed environment because PRL concentration can vary with time of day, level of stress, and other factors. A confirmed elevation in PRL prompts imaging of the pituitary gland, usually by MRI. At least 30% to 40% of women with hyperprolactinemia have a pituitary adenoma. The incidence of malignancy in prolactinomas is very rare; resection is rarely required.
  - Treatment of hyperprolactinemia is usually successful with dopamine agonist therapy (e.g., bromocriptine). See Chapter 13.

- **Galactorrhea** is mammary secretion of a milky fluid, excluding breastfeeding. Workup needed if nulliparous or if 12 months since childbirth/weaning. Careful physical exam of the breasts must be performed, with attempted expression of the nipples. Discharge may be white/clear in color but also greenish or even bloody. Bloody discharge suspicious for cancer requires mammography.
    - Differential diagnosis includes the following: increased PRL release as a consequence of a pituitary tumor, drugs that inhibit hypothalamic dopamine (e.g., phenothiazines, reserpine, amphetamines, tricyclic antidepressants), hypothyroidism, excessive estrogen via hypothalamic suppression, stress, hypothalamic lesions, increased PRL concentrations from nonpituitary sources (e.g., lung and renal tumors).
    - Dopamine agonist therapy is the treatment of choice.
    - Initial evaluation for hyperprolactinemia/galactorrhea is as follows:
        ○ Check TSH, PRL, progestin challenge (if amenorrhea)
            - If elevated TSH → hypothyroid
            - If withdrawal bleed and normal PRL/TSH → anovulation
            - If PRL >60 ng/mL × 2 samples → MRI of the brain
            - If no withdrawal bleed and normal PRL/TSH → estrogen/progestin cycle
            - If withdrawal bleed with OCPs → check FSH/LH
            - High FSH → ovarian failure
            - Low/normal FSH → order MRI
            - If MRI WNL → hypothalamic amenorrhea
- **Sheehan's syndrome** is a condition of pituitary necrosis and hypopituitarism following postpartum hemorrhage and hypotension. See Chapter 13.
- **Isolated gonadotropin (FSH/LH) deficiency** is a rare condition usually associated with thalassemia major, retinitis pigmentosa, or prepubertal hypothyroidism.

Polycystic Ovarian Syndrome

- Diagnostic criteria established by the National Institutes of Health in 1990 define **PCOS** as hyperandrogenism and chronic anovulation in cases in which secondary causes (e.g., adult-onset congenital adrenal hyperplasia, hyperprolactinemia, androgen-secreting neoplasms) have been excluded.
- The Rotterdam Consensus Conference in 2004 expanded the criteria so that PCOS is diagnosed when two of the following three criteria are present, and after other causes have been excluded:
    - Chronic oligoovulation
    - Chronic androgen excess
    - Polycystic appearing ovaries on ultrasound
- PCOS accounts for approximately 28% of secondary amenorrhea; however, it can also be a cause of primary amenorrhea.
- When signs or symptoms of hyperandrogenism are present, serum testosterone and DHEAS levels should be assessed to exclude the presence of adrenal or other androgen-producing tumors. Serum androgen levels are not sensitive or specific for tumors, however.
- PCOS is associated with an increased risk for Type 2 Diabetes, hypertension, lipid abnormalities, metabolic syndrome, and endometrial cancer. Insulin resistance is common in PCOS and is related to these medical sequelae. Metabolic evaluation should include assessment for lipid abnormalities, impaired glucose tolerance, or diabetes.

- Withdrawal bleeding should be induced every 1 to 2 months to prevent endometrial hyperplasia and malignancy. Oral contraception and cyclic progestins may be used.

Other Endocrinopathies

- Hypothyroidism or hyperthyroidism, Cushing's disease, or uncontrolled diabetes mellitus can alter the normal feedback mechanisms and functioning of the HPOA. See Chapter 13.
- **Hypothyroidism** accounts for only 1% to 2% of primary and secondary amenorrhea, but, because diagnosis and correction are relatively simple, including TSH in the initial battery of assays is justified.
- **Cushing's syndrome** is a clinical state resulting from prolonged, inappropriate endogenous hypercortisolism. It is characterized by loss of normal HPA feedback mechanisms and loss of the normal circadian rhythm of cortisol secretion. Screening tests include late night salivary cortisol (evaluated diurnal variation), 24 hour urinary free cortisol (evaluates secretion), and dexamethasone suppression testing (evaluates impaired feedback). Most cases are due to pituitary tumors.

Menopause

- **Menopause** occurs secondary to a genetically programmed loss of ovarian follicles. It is defined as 12 months of amenorrhea after the final menstrual period. It reflects complete, or near complete, ovarian follicular depletion and absence of ovarian estrogen secretion. Mean age of menopause is 51.4 years in American women. It is characterized by elevated FSH and low E_2. See Chapter 40.

TREATMENT OF AMENORRHEA

- **Surgery** may be required in patients with either congenital anatomic lesions or Y chromosome material (e.g., surgical correction of a vaginal outlet obstruction to allow passage of menstrual blood, creation of a neovagina for patients with Müllerian failure, hysteroscopic lysis of adhesions followed by long-term estrogen administration to stimulate regrowth of endometrial tissue for Asherman's syndrome, gonadectomy). In cases of symptomatic macroadenomas, referral to neurosurgery is indicated.
- **Psychological counseling** is important in patients with absent Müllerian structures or a Y chromosome, and in patients with POF.
- Women with prolonged hypoestrogenic amenorrhea resulting from conditions such as hypothalamic amenorrhea or POF should be counseled regarding the benefits and risks of estrogen/progesterone **HT and oral contraception**. Both therapies will help maintain or improve bone mineral density. The benefits and risks of HT are different when used for these conditions compared to menopausal women. Supplemental **calcium** (1,000 to 15,000 mg daily) and **vitamin D** should be encouraged to help offset risk of osteoporosis.
- Functional hypothalamic amenorrhea can be reversed by **decreasing stress, reduced exercise intensity, weight gain, cognitive behavioral therapy for anorexia, or resolution of illness**. When related to anorexia, comprehensive medical evaluation and intensive **psychotherapy** are usually required.
- Hyperprolactinemia, if idiopathic or due to pituitary adenoma, is treated with **dopamine agonists** such as bromocriptine and cabergoline.

- PCOS treatment is directed toward the symptoms of hyperandrogenism such as relief of hirsutism, and preventing the long-term consequences of PCOS (i.e., endometrial hyperplasia, obesity, and metabolic defects). **Oral contraceptives** are the mainstay of therapy since they reduce ovarian androgen secretion, protect against endometrial hyperplasia, and minimize dysfunctional uterine bleeding episodes.

SUGGESTED READINGS

Balen A. Polycystic ovary syndrome and cancer. *Hum Reprod Update* 2001;7:522–525.

Nelson LM, Covington SN, Rebar RW. An update: spontaneous premature ovarian failure is not an early menopause. *Fertil Steril* 2005;83:1327–1332.

Practice Committee of the American Society for Reproductive Medicine. Current evaluation of amenorrhea. *Fertil Steril* 2004;82:266–272.

Rebar RW, Connolly HV. Clinical features of young women with hypergonadotropic amenorrhea. *Fertil Steril* 1990;53:804–810.

Reindollar RH, Byrd JR, McDonough PG. Delayed sexual development: a study of 252 patients. *Am J Obstet Gynecol* 1981;140:371–380.

Reindollar RH, Novak M, Tho SP, et al. Adult-onset amenorrhea: a study of 262 patients. *Am J Obstet Gynecol* 1986;155:531–543.

Speroff L, Fritz MA. *Clinical Gynecologic Endocrinology and Infertility*, 7th Ed. Philadelphia, PA: Lippincott Williams and Wilkins; 2005.

Zacur HA. Indications for surgery in the treatment of hyperprolactinemia. *J Reprod Med* 1999;44:1127–1131.

37 Abnormal Uterine Bleeding

Amr Madkour and Dayna Finkenzeller

The evaluation of **abnormal uterine bleeding (AUB)** requires characterization and quantification of the bleeding, specifically the onset, duration, frequency, amount, and pattern.

MENSTRUAL DIMENSIONS

- The mean menstrual blood loss in women with normal hemoglobin and iron levels is 35 mL, with 95% of women losing <60 mL each menstrual cycle.
- **Menstrual frequency** may be characterized as:
  - Normal—24 to 35 days
  - Oligomenorrhea—menstrual intervals longer than 35 days
  - Polymenorrhea—menstrual intervals shorter than 24 days
- The **volume** of menstrual blood loss and **cycle regularity** should be determined.
  - Normal blood loss—5 to 80 mL
  - Regular cycles—2 to 20 days cycle-to-cycle variation over 12 months
  - Light cycle—<5-mL blood loss
  - Menorrhagia—heavy, regular periods with >80-mL blood loss
  - Metrorrhagia—irregular bleeding, especially between cycles
  - Menometrorrhagia—heavy, irregular bleeding that includes intermenstrual bleeding
  - Withdrawal bleeding—a predictable pattern of bleeding that occurs after the withdrawal of progestin therapy
  - Breakthrough bleeding—unpredictable bleeding that occurs while on hormonal contraception
- **Duration** of menstrual bleeding is defined as:
  - Normal—4 to 6 days
  - Prolonged— >7 days
  - Shortened— <3 days

DIFFERENTIAL DIAGNOSIS OF AUB

Causes of uterine bleeding can be organized by age groups (Table 37-1).

Prepubertal AUB

- Benign **prepubertal bleeding** may occur in the first few days of life due to the withdrawal of maternal estrogen, but all other cases of bleeding require evaluation.
- See Chapter 31.

Reproductive Age AUB

- AUB in the **reproductive years** is associated with pregnancy, anovulatory bleeding, and coagulation disorders.

TABLE 37-1 Differential Diagnosis of AUB by Age Group

Children	Adolescent	Reproductive	Perimenopausal	Menopausal
• Physiologic	• Anovulatory due to immaturity of hypothalamic-pituitary-ovarian axis	• Pregnancy related	• Anovulatory	• Atrophy
• Vulvovaginitis	• Coagulopathy	• Anovulatory	• Endometrial hyperplasia	• Endometrial carcinoma
• Trauma	• Pregnancy	• Vaginal/pelvic infection	• Endometrial polyps	• Endometrial hyperplasia
• Urethral prolapse	• Vaginal/pelvic infection	• Pelvic tumor	• Leiomyomas	• Endometrial polyp
• Endocrinopathies	• Benign lesions	• Endocrinopathies	• Adenomyosis	• Leiomyomas
• Precocious puberty	• Medications	• Coagulopathy	• Genital tract neoplasm	• Hormone replacement therapy
• Ovarian cyst	• Mullerian anomalies			
• Genital tract neoplasm	• Genetic abnormality			

Adapted from Shwayder JM. Pathophysiology of abnormal uterine bleeding. *Obstet Gynecol Clin North Am* 2000;27:219–234, with permission.

History and Physical Exam
- The patient's sexual history, past medical history, gynecologic and obstetric history, and contraceptive and medication regimens are pertinent. Any change in the patient's diet, weight, and exercise pattern is relevant.
- Family history should be reviewed for possible bleeding disorders.
- Adolescent girls should be screened for physical abuse.
- Inspection of the vaginal vault may reveal discharge suggestive of infection, or evidence of trauma, lesions, polyps, products of conception, or masses.
- A bimanual examination should be performed to evaluate the internal os, presence of cervical motion tenderness, size and contour of uterus and adnexa, and presence of any palpable masses, lesions, or tenderness.
- Tanner staging should be documented.

Diagnostic Testing
- Order laboratory serum testing for human chorionic gonadotropin (β-hCG), thyroid stimulating hormone (TSH), follicle stimulating hormone (FSH), prolactin, and complete blood count (CBC).
- In women with risk factors for neoplastic processes a tissue diagnosis is required.
- If anovulatory bleeding and pregnancy have been ruled out, evaluate for coagulation disorders.

Perimenopause AUB

- **Perimenopausal AUB** is most commonly due to anovulation and structural abnormalities (e.g., fibroids, polyps, hyperplasia).

History, Exam, and Testing
- In addition to history obtained for other women, menopausal symptoms should be explored.
- Order TSH, FSH, and prolactin.
- Imaging should evaluate for fibroids. See Chapter 34.
- Obtain tissue specimens/biopsies if needed.

Postmenopause AUB

- **Postmenopausal AUB** is primarily caused by endometrial and vaginal atrophy. However, as approximately 15% of these women will have some form of hyperplasia and 7% to 10% will have endometrial cancer, AUB in the age group suggests malignancy until proven otherwise.
- As with very young patients, careful attention should be paid to determine the source of bleeding, such as the rectum.
- Tissue sampling and imaging in this population are essential.

EVALUATION OF AUB

Ultrasonography

- **Transvaginal ultrasonography (TVUS)** is useful to evaluate for the presence of fibroids, polyps, intrauterine pregnancy, and ectopic pregnancy. In the workup for possible malignant processes, sonography can be used to search for a thickened endometrial stripe and masses within the uterus, adnexa, or cervix.
  - TVUS is a better diagnostic tool in postmenopausal than premenopausal women, with a sensitivity of 94% and specificity of 78% in diagnosing an endometrial abnormality using a cutoff of 5 mm for the endometrial echo.

- **Saline infusion sonography**, or sonohysterography, involves distention of the uterine cavity with sterile saline to enhance visualization of the endometrial surface during TVUS. Sonohysterography is the most sensitive noninvasive method of diagnosis for endometrial polyps and submucous myomata. However, it does not distinguish between benign and malignant processes.

Hysteroscopy

- The gold standard for evaluating the endometrial cavity is **hysteroscopy**. The advantage of this procedure is that it provides direct visualization of the endometrial cavity and can be performed in the office setting or operating room. It can be both diagnostic and operative, allowing for directed biopsies and excision of polyps and small myomas. Office hysteroscopy with targeted biopsies has a sensitivity and specificity of 98% and 95%, respectively, compared with histologic findings at the time of hysterectomy.

Magnetic Resonance Imaging (MRI)

- **Pelvic MRI** can be useful in the diagnosis of adenomyosis and can accurately localize and measure fibroids, facilitating determination of the best treatment (e.g., embolization, resection, hysterectomy).

Endometrial Sampling

- The American College of Obstetricians and Gynecologists (ACOG) recommends **endometrial sampling** in women over age 35 with anovulatory bleeding. Endometrial biopsy should also be considered in younger women with a history of chronic anovulatory bleeding or risk factors for endometrial carcinoma.
- Endometrial sampling is a rapid, safe, and cost-effective procedure that can be performed in the office to evaluate AUB. A potential drawback is that the biopsy does not sample the entire endometrium and a localized lesion may be missed.

Dilation and Curettage

- **Dilation and curettage (D&C)** can be both diagnostic and therapeutic but incurs the cost of an operating room and carries the risks of anesthesia. However, D&C may be indicated in women with nondiagnostic endometrial biopsies, biopsies with insufficient tissue for analysis, or women with cervical stenosis, making an office procedure unsuccessful.

SPECIFIC CAUSES OF AUB

Pregnancy Associated Bleeding

- **Pregnancy** should be suspected in any woman in her reproductive years.
- If urine β-hCG is positive, a pelvic examination must be performed and an ultrasonographic study obtained. The differential includes ectopic pregnancy or threatened, inevitable, incomplete, or missed abortion. A quantitative serum β-hCG test and Rh status are needed in all of these cases.
- Any patient who is hemodynamically unstable, bleeding heavily, or septic requires surgical intervention.
- Women with missed or incomplete abortions who are stable and not bleeding heavily may be treated medically with misoprostol, which has a success rate of approximately 84%. See Chapter 33.

Dysfunctional Uterine Bleeding

- **Dysfunctional uterine bleeding (DUB)** is a diagnosis of exclusion for AUB without a demonstrable pathologic cause and is found in approximately one third of all patients evaluated. The predominant causes of DUB are anovulation or oligoovulation. Anovulation is multifactorial and related to alterations of the hypothalamic-pituitary-ovarian axis.

- With long-term anovulation, estrogen production occurs without the progesterone produced from the corpus luteum, thus creating an unopposed estrogen state. Therefore, these women are at risk for endometrial hyperplasia. Anovulation is also associated with polycystic ovary syndrome, which also places women at risk for endometrial hyperplasia. Morbid obesity can also cause DUB. Peripheral conversion of androstenedione to estrone occurs in adipose tissue producing elevated estrogen levels. Occasionally, DUB may be associated with ovulatory cycles.

- The optimal treatment will relieve symptoms and improve quality of life with minimal side effects. It is directed toward stabilizing the endometrium and treating the underlying hormonal alterations. Treatment is usually long-term because symptoms tend to return when therapy is discontinued. Various medical therapies are available (Table 37-2).

  - Administration of progestins may be especially useful in patients with contraindications to combined oral contraceptive pills (OCPs), such as smokers over age 35. Although progestin therapy does not result in ovulation, it does prevent the negative sequelae of unopposed estrogen and regulates bleeding. However, very little data are available and no consensus exists on type of progestin or dosage. Side effects of progestins include breast tenderness, weight gain, and headaches. The levonorgestrel-releasing intrauterine system (Mirena) has been shown to decrease blood loss by up to 90% in women with menorrhagia.

  - OCPs also regulate menses and often decrease flow. Extended-use regimens may be especially useful in this population.

  - Nonsteroidal anti-inflammatory drugs (NSAIDs) may reduce menstrual volume in women with menorrhagia by at least 20% to 40% and need to be taken during menses only.

  - Danazol has been shown to significantly reduce menstrual blood loss (approximately 50%) and may induce amenorrhea. However, androgenic side effects limit its use.

  - Antifibrinolytic medications (e.g., tranexamic acid) decrease menstrual blood flow by 50%, and similar to NSAIDs, need to be taken during menses only. Practitioners have been reluctant to prescribe antifibrinolytics because of their pro-thrombotic potential; however, studies have not shown increased incidence of thrombosis in treated women versus the general population. Antifibrinolytics may be especially useful in women who cannot tolerate hormonal treatments.

  - Gonadotropin-releasing hormone (GnRH) agonists have limited use for treating AUB long-term and have significant side effects, such as hot flashes, osteopenia, and vaginal dryness. Symptoms return shortly after discontinuation. GnRH agonists can reduce uterine volume by 30% to 50%, which may facilitate less invasive surgery (i.e., vaginal vs abdominal hysterectomy). Add-back therapy, which typically includes a progestin or a progestin plus low-dose estrogen, alleviates menopausal symptoms. A progestin plus a bisphosphonate is recommended if GnRH agonists are used for over 6 months but may be initiated together.

| TABLE 37-2 | Pharmacologic Management of Abnormal Uterine Bleeding |

Hormonal Management

Progestins
Medroxyprogesterone (*Provera*) 10 mg 3×/d for 14 d (days 12–25);
   or for 5–10 d
Norethindrone acetate (*Aygestin*) 5 mg 3×/d for 14 d (days 12 and 25)
   for anovulatory bleeding; or on days 5–25 for ovulatory bleeding
Medroxyprogesterone acetate injection (*Depo Provera*) 150 mg IM every 12 wk
Levonorgestrel-releasing intrauterine system (*Mirena*)

Combined estrogen and progestins
Oral contraceptives
Transdermal preparations
Vaginal ring
Hormone replacement therapy

Androgenic steroids
Danazol 200 mg/d

Gonadotropin-releasing hormone (GnRH) agonists
Leuprolide (*Lupron*) 3.75 mg IM/mo or 11.25 mg every 3 mo
Goserelin (*Zoladex*) 3.6 mg SQ every 4 wk

Nonsteroidal Anti-inflammatory Drugs (NSAIDs)

Mefenamic acid 500 mg 3×/d
Ibuprofen 600–800 mg every 6 hr
Meclofenamate sodium 100 mg 3×/d
Naproxen sodium 550 mg × 1, then 275 mg every 6 hr

Antifibrinolytic Agents

Tranexamic acid 1 g 4×/d on days 1 to 5; or 1.5 g 3×/d

Adapted from Singh RH, Blumenthal P. Hormonal management of abnormal uterine bleeding. *Clin Obstet Gynecol* 2005;48:337–352; and Roy SN, Bhattacharya S. Benefits and risks of pharmacological agents used for the treatment of menorrhagia. *Drug Safety* 2004;27:75–90, with permission.

Surgical Treatment for DUB
- Surgical treatment may be warranted in patients who fail medical management.
  - D&C may be an initial step in treating AUB but does not typically have a sustained therapeutic effect.
  - Endometrial ablation is designed to ablate the full thickness of the endometrium. A variety of modalities are available, including thermal ablation, microwave, laser, cryocautery, and radiofrequency, each with its own advantages and disadvantages.
    - Before performing endometrial ablation in a woman with anovulatory bleeding, endometrial hyperplasia or carcinoma must be ruled out. It should be used to treat AUB in women with no intrauterine pathology, although some of the devices are approved for women with submucosal or intracavitary fibroids.

- ○ Across all methods, the overall success rate is approximately 80% to 90%, with 30% to 50% of women reporting amenorrhea 6 months postprocedure. Still, within 5 years, 15% will have a second ablation and 20% will have a hysterectomy. Endometrial ablation is not recommended in women who desire future fertility.
- Hysterectomy provides definitive treatment for menorrhagia and may be a reasonable option in women with severe menorrhagia, refractory to medical and less radical surgical therapy, who have completed their childbearing.

Coagulation Disorders

- Menorrhagia during adolescence should be attributed to a **coagulation disorder** until proven otherwise. Bleeding from multiple sites (e.g., nose, gingiva, intravenous sites, gastrointestinal, and genitourinary tracts) may suggest coagulopathy. There is a higher prevalence of bleeding disorders in women with menorrhagia.

Von Willebrand Disease

- **Von Willebrand disease** is the most common inherited bleeding disorder, affecting 1% to 2% of the population. Low, abnormal, or absent von Willebrand factor (vWF) leads to a spectrum of disease severity with three main types of von Willebrand disease (vWD; types 1, 2, and 3). In women with vWD, menorrhagia is the most common manifestation, occurring in 60% to 95% beginning at menarche.
- Women with vWD are also likely to report postpartum or postoperative bleeding. The frequency of vWD in women with menorrhagia is 5% to 20%.
- Other coagulopathies may also cause AUB, including platelet abnormalities, idiopathic thrombocytopenic purpura, and hematologic malignancy (e.g., leukemia).
- Testing for vWD should be considered in women with a history of unexplained menorrhagia beginning at menarche. ACOG recommends screening for vWD in adolescents with severe menorrhagia before starting hormonal therapy and in adult women with significant unexplained menorrhagia.
  - vWF levels vary over time and are affected by various physiologic, genetic, and pharmacologic factors. Several tests are performed to diagnose vWD: factor VIIIC activity, vWF antigen, ristocetin cofactor activity (i.e., vWF activity), platelet function tests, and bleeding time. vWF multimer tests are subsequently performed to distinguish among subtypes.
  - The ristocetin cofactor assay may be the best single screening test.
- Therapy usually involves treating the underlying cause and may require administration of blood products.
  - Little data are available regarding treatment of menorrhagia in women with vWD. Oral contraceptives, desmopressin, and antifibrinolytic agents are options. Nasal desmopressin appears to be an effective treatment for vWD.

Endocrine Disorders

- **Endocrinopathies** can cause anovulation, producing an environment of unopposed estrogen. In the absence of progesterone, the endometrium eventually breaks down, which may or may not lead to the formation of hyperplasia. Hypothyroidism and hyperprolactinemia are common disorders that can lead to anovulation.
- See Chapters 13 and 38.

Hepatic Dysfunction

- Decreased metabolism of estrogen and decreased clotting factor synthesis are common ramifications of **liver failure**. Anovulation may also ensue. Menometrorrhagia is common.

- Liver function tests are necessary to make the diagnosis. Physical examination findings of jaundice, ascites, hepatosplenomegaly, palmar erythema, pruritus, and spider angioma are suggestive of liver failure. See Chapter 16.
- If possible, the underlying cause should be treated. If the patient is coagulopathic and hemorrhaging, administration of packed red blood cells and fresh frozen plasma may be indicated. Progesterone therapy may also be beneficial.

Medication Side Effects

Psychotropic Medications

- Certain medications used in the treatment of psychiatric patients can affect the hypothalamic-pituitary axis and interfere with ovulation.
- Antipsychotic medications (i.e., dopamine antagonists) most commonly cause hyperprolactinemia and subsequent abnormalities in menstruation.
- Phenothiazines and antidepressants, particularly tricyclics, also interfere with the normal menstrual cycle.

Hormone Medications

- Medroxyprogesterone acetate. Approximately 50% of the patients taking medroxyprogesterone (Depo-Provera) experience amenorrhea after 1 year of use; 80% after 5 years. Irregular bleeding also may be experienced.
- Combination OCPs. Intermenstrual (breakthrough) bleeding is a side effect associated with OCP use that often leads to discontinuation. With long-term use, AUB may result from endometrial atrophy.
- Progestational agents. High doses of progesterone often are used in the treatment of AUB and endometrial hyperplasia. Prolonged use of these agents may result in endometrial atrophy, which itself can cause AUB.

Other Medications

- Anticoagulants. If the dosage of anticoagulants is too high, the patient can experience AUB.
- Digitalis, phenytoin, and corticosteroids have been implicated as causes of AUB.

Intrauterine Devices

- Copper-containing **intrauterine devices**, unlike the levonorgestrel-releasing Mirena intrauterine system, increase average monthly blood loss by approximately 35%.
- Such bleeding is often treated successfully with NSAIDs.

Genital Infection

- AUB is not a common presenting symptom of either **endometritis** or **cervicitis**. If present, bleeding associated with endometritis is most commonly intermenstrual, while bleeding associated with cervicitis is usually postcoital.
- Endometritis is diagnosed by fundal tenderness and fever. Any recent history of instrumentation of the uterus adds to the suspicion of endometritis. Cervicitis is diagnosed by clinical examination and results of cervical cultures. See Chapter 25.

Benign Pathology

Leiomyomata

- **Leiomyomata** (fibroids) are the most common uterine neoplasm, and is the number one indication for hysterectomy in the United States. See Chapter 34.
- AUB is the most common presenting symptom in women with leiomyomata.

- Although submucosal fibroids, followed by intramural fibroids, are most likely to cause bleeding, fibroids of any size and in any location can cause abnormal bleeding.

Endometrial Polyps

- Generally, benign endometrial lesions tend to be asymptomatic but may be present in 10% to 33% of women with complaints of bleeding, typically metrorrhagia.
- Diagnosis is by saline infusion sonogram and hysteroscopy.
- Polyps may respond to hormonal therapy. They should be removed via operative hysteroscopy when found in postmenopausal women. Cervical polyps can be removed by grasping them with forceps, twisting them off, and cauterizing the base.

Endometrial Hyperplasia

- **Endometrial hyperplasia**, a precursor to endometrial carcinoma, is classified into simple or complex, based on architectural features, and typical or atypical, based on cytologic features. Endometrial hyperplasia tends to occur during periods of long-term unopposed estrogen exposure, either secondary to anovulatory cycles or exogenous use. AUB is the most common presenting symptom.
- An endometrial tissue sample, either from an endometrial biopsy or D&C, is required to diagnose endometrial hyperplasia.
- Treatment depends upon age, desire for future fertility, surgical risk, and presence of atypia in the pathology specimen.
  - **Hyperplasia without atypia** may be managed by long-term follow-up with repeat endometrial sampling if abnormal bleeding recurs.
    - Cyclic medroxyprogesterone acetate is recommended (MPA 10 mg/day for 12 to 14 days/cycle for 3 to 6 months) in young anovulatory women to induce monthly withdrawal bleeding and subsequently normalize the endometrium, which occurs in approximately 86% of patients on this regimen.
    - Local progesterone administration via the levonorgestrel-releasing intrauterine system (Mirena) and combined oral contraceptives are also options.
    - Postmenopausal women with endometrial hyperplasia without atypia, on estrogen replacement therapy, should discontinue and may then be treated with medroxyprogesterone and repeat D&C.
  - **Atypical endometrial hyperplasia** is more likely to progress to carcinoma, and therefore, more aggressive treatment is needed. Atypical hyperplasia concomitantly exists with endometrial carcinoma in up to 25% to 50% of cases. Thus, a significant number of women diagnosed with atypical hyperplasia on curettage will be diagnosed with invasive carcinoma if hysterectomy is performed.
    - For patients who wish to retain their fertility, progestational therapy is an acceptable approach. Treatment with continuous regimens of megestrol acetate (40 mg two to four times daily) is associated with a regression rate of 94%. Treatment is continued for 6 months with endometrial biopsies performed at 3 and 6 months. Dosing is increased if regression is not observed. This approach also may be used in women who are poor surgical candidates. If regression does not occur, megestrol dose can be increased to 200 mg/day. Once regression occurs, maintenance therapy should begin with either megestrol, cyclic medroxyprogesterone acetate, or a levonorgestrel-releasing intrauterine system.
    - It must be emphasized that conservative therapy in women with complex atypical hyperplasia involves risk and close follow-up is necessary. Progesterone withdrawal regimens are not consistently effective and should not be used in the treatment of atypical hyperplasia. Also see Chapter 44.

Malignancy

Endometrial Cancer

• Endometrial carcinoma is rare in patients younger than age 40. Postmenopausal bleeding, however, should be assumed to represent endometrial cancer until proven otherwise.

• In a postmenopausal woman not receiving hormone replacement therapy (HRT), the presence of a thickened endometrial stripe (>5 mm) on ultrasonography is considered abnormal. Tissue sampling is then required. See Chapter 44 for further discussion.

Cervical Cancer

• Cervical carcinoma is a disease of both the relatively young and the old. Almost all cervical lesions that cause abnormal bleeding are visible on examination. The most common bleeding patterns associated with cervical carcinoma are intermenstrual and postcoital bleeding. See Chapters 42 and 43 for screening and treatment.

Ovarian Cancer

• Estrogen-producing ovarian tumors, such as a granulosa-theca cell tumor, can produce endometrial hyperplasia and AUB. See Chapter 35.

SUGGESTED READINGS

Management of Anovulatory Bleeding. ACOG Practice Bulletin Number 14. American College of Obstetricians and Gynecologists. *Int J Gynaecol Obstet* 2001;72(3):263–271.

Von Willebrand Disease in Women. ACOG Committee Opinion Number 451. American College of Obstetricians and Gynecologists. *Obstet Gynecol* 2009;114:1439–1443.

Lacey JV Jr, Chia VM. Endometrial hyperplasia and the risk of progression to carcinoma. *Maturitas* 2009;63(1):39–44.

Casablanca Y. Management of dysfunctional uterine bleeding. *Obstet Gynecol Clin North Am* 2008;35(2):219–234, viii.

Hyperandrogenism

Jennifer Ducie and Lisa Kolp

Androgens are necessary for normal ovarian and sexual function. They play an important role in cognition, bone health, muscle mass, body composition, mood, energy, and a woman's sense of well-being. The obstetrician/gynecologist must have a strong knowledge base regarding the role androgens play in normal female physiology.

- Androgens are precursors for estrogen synthesis.
- Although controversial, it has been proposed that androgens may be necessary for normal sexual desire in women.
- Androgens also affect skeletal homeostasis. They affect bone metabolism directly via androgen receptors expressed by osteocytes or indirectly via conversion of androgens to estrogen. Multiple studies have shown that women with low androgen concentrations have lower bone density and increased fracture risk.

ANDROGENS IN THE FEMALE

Androgens circulate in the body in various forms. Circulating androgens found in the blood of premenopausal women include dehydroepiandrosterone (DHEA), DHEA sulfate (DHEA-S), androstenedione, and testosterone. Androgens are produced by the adrenal glands, the ovary, and from peripheral conversion.

Androstenedione

- Produced in equal amounts by the adrenal glands (50%) and the ovaries (50%)
- Majority of androstenedione is converted to testosterone
- Less potent androgen than testosterone but can produce significant androgenic effects when present in excess amounts
- Normal serum concentration ranges from 60 to 300 ng/dL, often with a 15% increase at midcycle. Circulates in blood bound to both sex hormone–binding globulin (SHBG) and albumin.

Testosterone

- The most potent androgenic hormone
- In women, nearly 25% of testosterone is secreted from the ovaries and 25% is from the adrenal glands. The remaining one-half is produced from peripheral conversion of androstenedione to testosterone in the kidneys, liver, and adipose tissue.
- Normal circulating concentrations range from 20 to 80 ng/dL.
- Approximately 65% of testosterone in the circulation is bound to SHBG. Nineteen to thirty-three percent of testosterone is loosely bound to albumin. The remaining 1% of testosterone circulates in the free and active form (Fig. 38-1).
- Testosterone levels decrease by 50% from ages 20 to 40. Premenopausal production of testosterone decreases under the control of luteinizing hormone (LH).

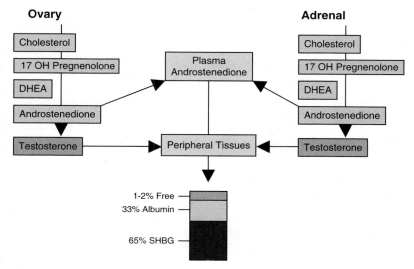

Figure 38-1. Endogenous production and secretion of testosterone in women. DHEA, dehydroepiandrosterone; SHBG, sex hormone binding globulin.

As menopause is entered, SHBG levels remain constant, yielding an even greater decrease in free testosterone. However, serum hormone concentrations of SHBG fall due to the lack of estrogen, finally resulting in an increase in bioavailable testosterone. Free testosterone levels in an 80-year-old woman are only 20% lower than those in a 20-year-old.

DHEA and DHEA-S

- Androgen precursors, much less potent than testosterone, produced predominantly by the adrenal glands, with some component of ovarian production and peripheral conversion.
- DHEA is metabolized quickly, thus measurement of its serum concentration does not reflect adrenal gland activity. DHEA-S has a much longer half-life than DHEA, and measurement of its serum level is used to assess adrenal function.
- Serum hormone concentrations of DHEA-S in women vary widely (normal range of 38 to 338 µg/dL).

Dihydrotestosterone

- Testosterone is converted to dihydrotestosterone (DHT) by 5-alpha-reductase, an enzyme found in many androgen-sensitive tissues.
- Very potent androgen primarily responsible for the androgenic effects on hair follicles.

Sex Hormone–Binding Globulins

- Androgenicity is determined by free hormone concentrations. Thus, SHBG influences the hormonal state. Testosterone and insulin both decrease SHBG levels, whereas estrogen and thyroid hormone increase its levels.

- Symptoms of hyperandrogenism may be seen in patients with a normal total testosterone level if the serum hormone concentration of SHBG is reduced to a level that significantly increases the free hormone.

CLINICAL FINDINGS IN HYPERANDROGENISM

Hyperandrogenism is characterized by an abnormally elevated serum concentration of androgens or physical findings consistent with androgen excess. Androgenic hormones in the female can stimulate abnormal terminal hair growth, voice and muscle changes, hair loss, clitoral enlargement, and reduction in breast size. Physical characteristics of hyperandrogenism are as follows:

Androgenic Hair Changes
- During gestation, the hair follicles of the developing fetus produce fine, unpigmented hair known as **lanugo**. The total number of hair follicles is determined late in the second trimester of pregnancy. With time, some of the hair follicles produce thick, darkly pigmented **terminal hair** in response to androgen exposure. The remaining hair follicles produce **vellus hair**, which is finer and not as darkly pigmented.
- **Normal hair growth cycle** follows three stages: **anagen** (growth phase) → **catagen** (involution phase) → **telogen** phase (rest phase).

Hirsutism
- **Hirsutism** is excessive male pattern hair growth in women. It refers to the growth of terminal hair on the face, chest, back, lower abdomen, and upper thighs caused by the overactivity or overexpression of circulating androgens. The abnormal hair growth is predominantly midline. Androgens stimulate hair growth, increase the diameter of the hair shaft, and deepen the pigmentation of the hair. In contrast, estrogens slow hair growth and decrease hair diameter and pigmentation.
  - **Idiopathic hirsutism** is the term used when a hirsute individual has normal levels of circulating androgens and has not been diagnosed with PCOS or another disorder.
  - **The Ferriman-Gallwey score** is an objective tool that may be used in the clinical setting to grade hair growth in women. This method evaluates nine different androgen-sensitive hair growth sites on a scale from 0 to 4. Ninety-five percent of women will have a score under 8. Scores >8 suggest an excess of androgen-mediated hair growth and this should be confirmed with a more extensive hormone evaluation.

Hypertrichosis
- **Hypertrichosis** is the generalized, excessive growth of vellus hair. It may be caused by genetic factors, underlying malignancy, or exposure to drugs such as phenytoin, penicillamine, diazoxide, cyclosporine, and minoxidil. It may also be seen with a number of medical conditions, including anorexia nervosa, hypothyroidism, malnutrition, porphyria, dermatomyositis, and paraneoplastic syndromes. Hypertrichosis should not be mistaken for hirsutism.

Hair Loss
- Recession of hair in the frontal and temporal regions of the scalp and the crown of the head (i.e., **male pattern baldness**) in response to androgens is common with aging. This is the most common pattern of hair loss and affects approximately 30% to 40% of men and women alike. However, hair loss is less evident

in women because it is typically more diffuse and rarely complete. The fact that excessive androgen activity stimulates hair growth on some parts of the body while causing hair loss from others remains unexplained.

- Young men and women with **androgenic alopecia** have higher levels of 5-alpha-reductase, increased androgen receptors, and lower levels of the enzyme cytochrome P-450 aromatase (which converts androgens such as testosterone and 4-androstene-dione to the estrogens estradiol and estrone, respectively).

Skin Changes

- Androgens stimulate secretions from pilosebaceous glands, resulting in oily skin. Severe acne is a manifestation of excessive androgenic hormone activity.

Voice Changes

- In response to excessive androgen exposure, the vocal cords undergo irreversible thickening, resulting in a lower tone of voice.

Male Body Habitus

- Hypertrophy of major muscle groups, such as arm and leg muscles, occurs in response to androgen exposure and may result in the development of a male body habitus.

Clitoromegaly

- Enlargement of the clitoris may occur in response to excessive androgen exposure. This is a dose-dependent event and is irreversible.

Virilization

- This is a more extreme state of excess androgenic activity than hirsutism. It refers to a constellation of symptoms, including deepening of the voice, male body habitus, male pattern baldness, clitoromegaly, and reduction of breast size.
- Virilization is very rare and may be associated with adrenal tumors and hyperplasia or ovarian tumors, such as theca-lutein cysts, luteomas, and Sertoli-Leydig cell tumors.

Acanthosis Nigricans

- Acanthosis nigricans is a gray-brown, velvety discoloration of the skin indicating hyperinsulinemia. Hyperandrogenism is associated with hyperinsulinemia and insulin resistance; obese patients with hirsutism may develop acanthosis nigricans in the groin, neck, axillary, and vulvar regions.

DIAGNOSIS OF HYPERANDROGENISM

History and Physical Examination

- Hyperandrogenism may be diagnosed if signs of androgen excess are present (above).
- A careful medical history should be taken, including a detailed menstrual history asking about age of menarche, regularity of menstrual cycles, pregnancies, oral contraceptive preparation (OCP) use, and presence of symptoms of ovulation or menstrual molima. Patients should be asked about a history of thyroid disease and hyperinsulinemia.

- A complete physical examination should be conducted, including evaluation for galactorrhea and acanthosis nigricans.
- Pay particular attention to medications (above) and family history.

Laboratory Evaluation

- Measurement of serum androgen levels may be obtained to diagnose hyperandrogenism (Fig. 38-2). The clinician should check the following:
  - **Testosterone** serum hormone concentrations
  - **DHEA-S** >700 ng/dL is consistent with abnormal adrenal function.
  - **17-alpha-hydroxyprogesterone (17-OHP)**; normal 100 to 300 ng/dL
  - **Prolactin** (normal range 1 to 20 ng/mL). Hyperprolactinemia can be associated with hyperandrogenism, as it is likely that prolactin receptors are located on the adrenal glands. When prolactin binds to these adrenal receptors, it stimulates the release of DHEA-S.
  - **Thyroid function tests**
  - Assessment of hyperinsulinemia:
    - Normal fasting glucose <100 mg/dL.
    - Impaired glucose tolerance indicated by fasting glucose 100 to 126 mg/dL.

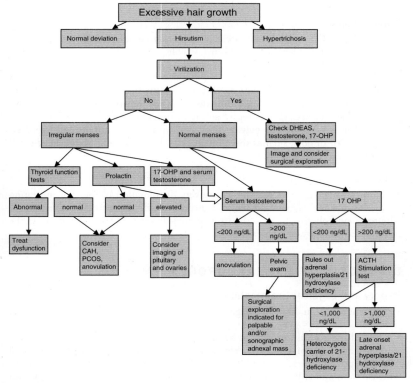

Figure 38-2. Algorithm for the diagnosis of hyperandrogenism.

○ Diabetes mellitus diagnosed with two fasting glucose levels >126 mg/dL.
○ Fasting glucose to insulin ratio of <4.5 is consistent with insulin resistance.

CAUSES AND TREATMENT OF HYPERANDROGENISM

Five major causes of hyperandrogenism have been identified
- PCOS
- Late-onset adrenal hyperplasia
- Tumors of the ovary or adrenal glands
- Cushing's syndrome
- Idiopathic or drug-induced processes

Polycystic Ovary Syndrome

- PCOS is the most common endocrine disorder among reproductive-age women. It affects approximately 5% to 10% of this population.
- In 1935, Stein and Leventhal described seven women who were amenorrheic, obese, and hirsute with cystic ovaries. From this initial description, the term **Stein-Leventhal syndrome** was originally used to identify other similarly affected women.
- Because of the cystic changes found within the ovaries of affected patients, the terms **hyperandrogenemic chronic anovulation syndrome, PCOS**, and **polycystic ovary disease (PCOD)** are now used to describe these patients.
- Individuals with PCOS do not have orderly follicular development. Most cycles fail to lead to the emergence of a dominant follicle or release of an oocyte. Although follicle development occasionally proceeds to ovulation, development of the follicle to only its initial growth stage is common. The ovarian cortex becomes populated with numerous small follicles, or "cysts." The hyperandrogenemic state is believed to be both a cause and effect of incomplete follicular development.
- PCOS is associated with amenorrhea, hyperandrogenism, hyperinsulinemia, and metabolic syndrome. In patients affected by this disorder, it is important to make the appropriate diagnosis early and to closely monitor these individuals, as they may be at risk for other comorbidities as a consequence of the underlying pathology.

Diagnosis of PCOS
- In May 2003, the Rotterdam ESHRE/ASRM-sponsored PCOS consensus workshop revised the diagnostic criteria to include two of the following three manifestations:
  - Oligomenorrhea and/or anovulation
  - Clinical and/or biochemical signs of hyperandrogenism
  - Polycystic ovaries and exclusion of other etiologies
- The revision of the diagnostic criteria for PCOS sparked debate as it created a "new" phenotype of patients affected by this pathology. This new subgroup of patients includes those individuals with anovulation and polycystic ovaries who have neither clinical nor biochemical evidence of androgen excess. The other phenotype is an ovulatory female with polycystic ovaries and hyperandrogenism.
- Patients with PCOS often present with oligomenorrhea, amenorrhea, hirsutism, obesity, and infertility. All or some of these symptoms may be present.
- Hyperandrogenism can be demonstrated by either hirsutism or elevated levels of androgens.

- Virilization is not a common finding and should raise doubt about the diagnosis of PCOS.
- Insulin resistance and a diagnosis of metabolic syndrome are often associated with PCOS.
- Polycystic ovaries are defined as 12 or more follicles in each ovary measuring 2 to 9 mm, or increased ovarian volume >10 mL.
- Tests for insulin resistance are not necessary for the diagnosis of PCOS.
- Obese women with PCOS should be screened for comorbid metabolic syndrome. Providers should check a cholesterol panel, blood pressure, fasting glucose, and 2-hr oral glucose tolerance test. Further studies are needed to determine the utility of these tests in nonobese women with PCOS.

Pathophysiology of PCOS
- The exact cause of PCOS remains unknown. Abnormalities of the hypothalamic-pituitary axis and the ovarian or adrenal steroidogenic pathway have been suggested as possible explanations.
  - **Pituitary and hypothalamus.** At the level of the hypothalamic-pituitary axis, increases in the frequency and amplitude of LH pulses have been recorded. A ratio of serum LH to follicle-stimulating hormone of >2 is observed in PCOS patients.
  - **Ovarian androgen production.** Increased secretion of androgens from the ovaries has been observed in patients with PCOS. Elevated LH levels may lead to increased activity of ovarian theca cells, thus producing androgens. Also, elevated insulin may stimulate androgen secretion from both the ovaries and adrenals.
  - **Adrenal androgen production.** Some PCOS patients have mild elevations of DHEA-S levels. Studies designed to detect adrenal gland enzyme deficiencies or excesses resulting in elevated androgens have been identified in only a few PCOS patients.
  - **Consequences of anovulation.** Ovulation for many women with PCOS may occur infrequently, but ovaries in these patients continue to secrete low levels of estrogen. Due to the lack of cyclic estrogen and progesterone withdrawal over time, unopposed estrogen can lead to proliferation of the endometrium that may result in abnormal bleeding and, if untreated, may progress to endometrial hyperplasia. Chronic anovulation is a risk factor for endometrial cancer.
  - **Hyperinsulinemia and insulin resistance.** Increased resistance to insulin is often observed in patients with PCOS, whether or not they are obese. Insulin may cause or contribute to the hyperandrogenic state by activating insulin receptors within the ovary, augmenting androgen secretion, or by acting on insulin-like growth factor receptors.

Treatment for Hyperandrogenism/PCOS
- Treatment of the patient with hirsutism, hyperandrogenism, or hyperandrogenic chronic anovulation depends upon the underlying etiology and the desire for pregnancy. Hirsutism is slow to respond to hormone suppression. Results may not be seen for up to 6 months. Unfortunately, androgen suppression will not alter previous hair growth patterns. Mechanical methods of hair removal, such as shaving, waxing, depilatories, and electrolysis, should also be considered.
  - **Lifestyle modifications** should be first line in the management of hyperandrogenism. For those individuals who suffer from hirsutism and obesity, weight loss of even 5% of original body weight can often improve symptoms related to PCOS. Weight loss may result in an elevation of SHBG, a decrease in bioavailable testosterone, and improvement in insulin sensitivity.

- **OCPs** reduce circulating gonadotropin levels and increase SHBG levels; both work to decrease circulating androgens. OCPs are the first line of treatment of oligomenorrhea caused by PCOS. Progestins decrease total androgen level by reducing the activity of 5-alpha-reductase. OCP usage results in an overall decrease in the formation of new androgen-dependent hair growth and androgen-stimulated acne. All low-dose OCP preparations are believed to have similar results. If therapy with OCPs is suboptimal, addition of an antiandrogen, such as spironolactone or finasteride, is recommended.
- If combination OCPs are contraindicated or not desired, **medroxyprogesterone acetate** may be administered (5 to 10 mg for 10 to 12 days) every month or every other month to produce regular withdrawal bleeding. Patients should be cautioned that, unless contraception is used, pregnancy is possible with cyclic progestin therapy.
- **Metformin hydrochloride** is a biguanide antihyperglycemic drug, FDA-approved for the management of type 2 diabetes mellitus. Metformin decreases hepatic gluconeogenesis, thus reducing the need for insulin secretion. It also decreases the intestinal absorption of glucose and improves insulin sensitivity in the peripheral system, including skeletal muscle, liver, and adipose tissue. In some studies, metformin has been shown to restore menses in approximately 50% of women with PCOS. Another trial showed that metformin, compared to placebo, can improve plasma insulin and insulin sensitivity, reduce serum free testosterone, and increase serum HDL cholesterol.
  - **Dosing:** The optimum dose of metformin for restoration of menses in women with PCOS ranges from 500 mg by mouth three times daily to 850 mg by mouth twice daily. Patients should be titrated onto the appropriate dose of this medication, starting at the lowest dose once daily, due to the GI side effects.
  - Metformin has a limited role in the treatment of hirsutism. Other agents may be added to metformin to improve these symptoms.
  - Metformin appears to be unique among insulin-sensitizing agents in that it can improve weight loss (particularly a greater reduction in abdominal fat), hyperandrogenism, and menstrual cycles in individuals with PCOS.
- **Spironolactone** therapy is often initiated if OCP use is not an option for the treatment of hirsutism or if results from OCP therapy are not optimal. An aldosterone antagonist, spironolactone, is an antihypertensive agent that was originally found to cause gynecomastia in men. Spironolactone directly inhibits 5-alpha-reductase and decreases androgen synthesis. The usual dose is 25 to 100 mg by mouth twice daily. After 6 months of therapy at 100 to 200 mg/day, there is a reduction in the diameter of terminal hair and cessation of new terminal hair growth. Doses are then tapered to a maintenance dose of 25 to 50 mg/day. Because of potential adverse effects on genitalia of male fetuses, spironolactone should be used with contraception in sexually active women. Other side effects include diuresis, orthostatic hypotension, fatigue, dysfunctional uterine bleeding, hyperkalemia, and breast enlargement.
- **Flutamide** is a nonsteroidal antiandrogen used for prostate cancer that blocks the binding of androgen to its receptor. When administered in a dosage of 250 mg/day, inhibition of new hair growth is observed. Side effects include dry skin, and, rarely, hepatotoxicity. Liver function should be monitored during treatment. Due to adverse fetal effects, effective contraceptive therapy is mandatory.
- **Finasteride.** An inhibitor of mostly type II 5-alpha-reductase, finasteride was developed initially as a treatment for prostate hypertrophy and cancer. By inhibiting 5-alpha-reductase, the drug decreases DHT activity at the level of the hair follicle.

Finasteride treatment prevents new hair growth and decreases the terminal hair shaft diameter. Finasteride is orally dosed at 5 mg daily. No major side effects have been associated with this drug. Again, due to adverse fetal effects, adequate contraception should be used.

- **Minoxidil** is the only drug approved by the FDA for treatment of androgenic alopecia in women. It promotes hair growth by increasing the duration of the anagen phase and enlarging miniaturized and suboptimal follicles. It is available over the counter as a 2% and 5% topical solution.
- **Corticosteroid therapy** is another alternative for the treatment of hirsutism and hyperandrogenism and is the primary mode of therapy for those individuals suffering from congenital adrenal hyperplasia (CAH). The steroids suppress the hypothalamic-pituitary-adrenal axis and can result in improved hirsutism and ovulatory function. Corticosteroid therapy should not be used for the long term in patients with PCOS, as it may result in debilitating osteoporosis and worsening glucose intolerance.
- **Eflornithine hydrochloride** is a cream that reduces unwanted facial hair. Eflornithine is a potent antagonist of ornithine decarboxylase, the enzyme necessary for the production of polyamines, organic compounds that stimulate and regulate the growth of hair follicles and other organs. Women who apply eflornithine hydrochloride (13.9% cream) to their faces twice daily have shown improvement after 24 weeks in some clinical trials. The benefit is usually first seen at 8 weeks.
- **Surgery.** Older women who have no desire for fertility and who do not desire continued hormonal therapy may consider bilateral oophorectomy, with or without hysterectomy.

Fertility Treatment for PCOS
- In PCOS patients, assistance with ovulation induction frequently is required.
- **Clomiphene citrate** is usually administered orally in dosages of 50 to 100 mg/day for 5 days on a monthly basis to induce ovulation in infertile women. It is not used for cycle regulation or as a primary treatment for hirsutism. Monitoring with a basal body temperature chart, LH levels, pelvic ultrasonography, or serum progesterone 14 days after the last clomiphene citrate dose may be used to confirm ovulation. For the patient resistant to clomiphene citrate, metformin hydrochloride (500 mg three times daily) may result in ovulation.
- Direct stimulation of the ovary may be used to induce ovulation through the intramuscular or subcuticular administration of gonadotropins in the treatment of anovulatory infertility. See Chapter 32.

Late-Onset or "Nonclassical" Adrenal Hyperplasia

- Excess androgen production is a common feature shared by most forms of **CAH**. Unlike typical CAH, symptoms of late-onset CAH are not evident until late childhood or adolescence.
- The most common adrenal enzyme defect and autosomal recessive disorder is 21-hydroxylase (21-OH) deficiency.
- Deficiencies of 11-beta-hydroxylase and 3-beta-hydroxysteroid dehydrogenase are rarely seen.
- 21-OH converts progesterone to 11-deoxycorticosterone, or 17-hydroxyprogesterone (17-OHP) to 11-deoxycortisol (Table 38-1). A decrease in the activity of this enzyme causes diminished cortisol production, resulting in increased pituitary secretion of adrenocorticotropic hormone (ACTH). ACTH stimulates the adrenal gland to produce increased precursor 17-OHP. Higher 17-OHP levels lead to secretion of androstenedione, which is converted to testosterone.

TABLE 38-1	Enzymes and Their Characteristics		
Deficient Enzyme	Androgen Levels	Mineralocorticoid Levels	Female Virilization at Birth
21-Hydroxylase	Excess	Deficiency	Yes
11-β-Hydroxylase	Excess	Excess	Yes
17-α-Hydroxylase	Deficiency	Excess	No

Diagnosis
- Measure the basal levels of 17-OHP in the morning. Levels of 17-OHP should be <200 ng/dL.
  - Levels that exceed 200 ng/dL but are <800 ng/dL require ACTH-stimulation testing (Fig. 38-2).
  - Levels over 800 ng/dL are virtually diagnostic of CAH.
  - Patients with late-onset hyperplasia have 17-OHP levels >1,500 ng/dL in response to a 250-μg ACTH stimulation challenge.
- Patients should be tested for 21-hydroxylase deficiency (CYP21A2 deficiency) especially when they present with symptoms of hyperandrogenism at a young age or if they have a known family history of CAH. Women of Hispanic or Eastern European Jewish descent should also be tested, as the prevalence of this disorder among these populations is greater than in the general population.

Treatment
- Individuals diagnosed with late-onset adrenal hyperplasia may be treated by the administration of glucocorticoid agents to restore ovulation. This treatment also reduces circulating androgen levels. Glucocorticoid administration is therefore appropriate therapy for infertility or hirsutism in individuals with late-onset adrenal hyperplasia. In patients with 21-OH deficiency, prednisone 5 mg before bedtime is used to suppress endogenous ACTH.
- Alternatively, OCPs or antiandrogens may be used successfully to treat hirsutism, alone or in combination with dexamethasone. Ovulation-inducing drugs may also be used to treat infertility.

Androgen-Producing Ovarian or Adrenal Tumors
- Tumors of the ovary or adrenal gland that secrete androgens are rare.
- The presence of an **androgen-producing tumor** is suspected on the basis of clinical findings.
- Palpation of an adnexal mass in a patient with symptoms of hyperandrogenism or rapid onset of virilization even in the presence of normal testosterone levels should prompt a workup for a pelvic tumor.
- Testosterone levels exceeding 200 ng/dL and DHEA-S levels >1,000 μg/dL are concerning for the presence of an ovarian or adrenal androgen-producing tumor.
- Surgical removal with or without adjuvant therapy is the treatment of choice.

Cushing's Syndrome
- Patients with **Cushing's syndrome** often exhibit specific physical findings. See Chapter 13.

Idiopathic and Drug-Induced Hirsutism

- **Idiopathic hirsutism** is diagnosed in hirsute individuals who have a negative workup for other causes of hirsutism. Studies show that 5% to 15% of hirsute patients may have idiopathic hirsutism. An alternative explanation is based on the hypothesis that patients with idiopathic hirsutism demonstrate increased skin sensitivity to androgens. One theory is that patients with idiopathic hirsutism convert testosterone to DHT in greater quantities than normal due to increased activity of 5-alpha-reductase.
- Occasionally, drugs may be causative. Danazol and methyltestosterone are two drugs that may cause iatrogenic hirsutism.
- The same medications used to treat hirsute PCOS patients, may be used to treat patients with idiopathic hirsutism.

SUGGESTED READINGS

Brodell LA, Mercurio MG. Hirsutism: diagnosis and management. *Gend Med* 2010;7(2): 79–87.

Ferriman D, Gallwey JD. Clinical assessment of body hair growth in women. *J Clin Endocrinol Metab* 1961 Nov;21:1440–1447.

Hock DL, Seifer DB. New Treatments of hyperandrogenism and hirsutism. *Obstet Gynecol Clin* 2000;27(3):567-581, vi–vii.

Polycystic Ovary Syndrome. ACOG Practice Bulletin Number 108. American College of Obstetricians and Gynecologists. *Obstet Gynecol* 2009;114:936–949.

39 Female Sexual Response and Sexual Dysfunction

Mary Kimmel and Linda Rogers

"In the human race the mind tends to rule the body, and [that] sex in the human being is even more a mental passion than a physical instinct."—From Elizabeth Blackwell's *The Human Element in Sex*. The text notes that **sexual function** is a "complex compound faculty," involving thoughts and feelings, social ties, conscience, and duty.

- Although Dr. Blackwell was writing and educating women utilizing these ideas in the 1800s, a complex model has only recently been developed and utilized to understand female sexual function, to define dysfunction, and to develop treatment. We are now beginning to understand the complexity of female sexual function and dysfunction and the need for new approaches to treatment.

EPIDEMIOLOGY

- In the 1999 National Health and Social Life Survey, 1,410 men and 1,749 women aged 18 to 59 were surveyed and 43% of women responded that they experienced sexual concerns. A British national survey found that 54% of women reported at least one sexual problem lasting at least 1 month but only 21% sought help.
- The most common female sexual problem in both studies was a lack of interest. Difficulty with orgasm was reported by 24%, difficulty with arousal by 19%, and pain with sex by 14%. Accurate assessments of female sexual dysfunction are hampered by the fact that many patients have more than one type of dysfunction. Additionally, many patients complaining of lack of interest actually have a problem with another phase of the sexual response cycle, in part because they lack familiarity with the terms.
- Multiple studies have found that female sexual dysfunction is associated with a decreased sense of physical and emotional satisfaction and a decreased sense of overall well-being.

DIAGNOSIS OF SEXUAL DISORDERS

Screening

- Many physicians infrequently discuss sexual dysfunction due to limited time and training, embarrassment, or absence of effective treatment options. A few simple questions can initiate the discussion:
  - Are you currently involved in a sexual relationship?
  - If yes, do you have sex with men, women, or both?
  - Do you have any concerns about or pain with sex?

- If no, do you have any concerns you would like to discuss?
- Once a dialogue has been initiated, a complete history is obtained. This should include the nature and frequency of the problem, the degree of distress, whether the problem is lifelong versus newly acquired, situational or generalized, partner's sexual problems or concerns, partner reaction, and history of previous treatment.
- It is important to elicit the patient's thoughts concerning the cause of the problems and their expectations from treatment. The physician must also get a medical history, a psychological/psychiatric history (e.g., mood disorders, body image disorders), sexual history including sexual abuse or violence, and a psychosocial history (e.g., relationship difficulties, cultural and religious beliefs that may affect function, work/finance/children and other life stressors). It is also important to ask about the use of soaps, laundry products, douches, or other possible skin irritants.

Physical Exam

- A thorough physical exam can help identify causes, address concerns, and educate the patient about her anatomy.
- During visual inspection of the external female genitalia and perineum, it is important to note any atrophy, lack of estrogenization, loss of architecture, scarring, hypopigmentation or hyperpigmentation, or possible infection. The exam should include the urethral meatus and anus. Wet prep and pH should be performed to evaluate signs of infection. Suspicious skin changes on the vulva warrant biopsy. Fungal cultures or polymerase chain reaction (PCR) testing should be sent if there is any doubt about the presence of yeast, as wet prep has a sensitivity of only 50%.
- A moistened cotton swab is then used to systematically examine the vulva and map any areas of pain. Tenderness is most commonly found adjacent to the hymenal ring, but it is important to check the rest of the vulva for more generalized tenderness.
- A speculum exam and gentle digital exam are then performed. Attention should be paid to tenderness, adnexal masses or nodularity, pelvic floor muscle tone, prolapse, and the anal reflex.
- Laboratory tests are rarely useful as they are poorly predictive of function and perception of function.

PHYSIOLOGY OF FEMALE SEXUAL FUNCTION

Female sexual function is a complex interplay of the central nervous system (CNS), the peripheral nervous system, and the end organs.

- In the CNS, the medial preoptic, anterior hypothalamic, and limbohippocampal areas are involved in sexual arousal. Dopaminergic stimulation of the peripheral nervous system modulates the vasculature and musculature.
- Estrogens, androgens, oxytocin, and dopamine are believed to promote female sexual response, and progesterone, prolactin, and serotonin are inhibitory.
- The autonomic nerves release nitric oxide and vasointestinal polypeptide that mediate vasodilatation.
- Increased blood flow causes labial engorgement, increased vaginal lubrication, vaginal lengthening and dilation, and increased length and diameter of the clitoris.
- Contraction of the pelvic floor muscles likely involves adrenergic and cholinergic mechanisms from the efferent pudendal nerve.
- The pelvic floor muscles, especially the levator ani and the perineal membranes, and the smooth muscle of the vagina spasm during orgasm.

- Estrogen primarily maintains the integrity of the tissues. Androgen levels correlate poorly, but are associated, with libido and arousal.
- The arousal response in women also involves changes such as increased heart rate, muscle tension, and changes in breast sensations and a subjective state of arousal.

THEORIES OF SEXUAL FUNCTION

For many years, female sexual function was described with a model more characteristic of men than of women, especially women in long-term relationships. Masters and Johnson, in 1966, defined the human sexual response as a sequential model including excitement (desire and arousal) → plateau → orgasm → resolution (Table 39-1).

- Recent research has found that the female sexual response is much more complex and is usually not linear.

TABLE 39-1	Physiologic Female Sexual Response	
Phase	**Sex Organ Response**	**General Sexual Response**
Excitement	Vaginal lubrication Thickening of vaginal walls and labia Expansion of inner vagina Elevation of cervix and corpus Tumescence of clitoris	Nipple erection Sex-tension flush
Plateau	Orgasmic platform in outer vagina Full expansion of inner vagina Secretion of mucus by Bartholin's gland Withdrawal of clitoris	Sex-tension flush Carpopedal spasm Generalized skeletal muscle tension Hyperventilation Tachycardia
Orgasm	Contractions of uterus from fundus toward lower uterine segment Contractions of orgasmic platform at 0.8-s intervals External rectal sphincter contractions at 0.8-s intervals External urethral sphincter contractions at irregular intervals	Specific skeletal muscle contractions Hyperventilation Tachycardia
Resolution	Ready return to orgasm with retarded loss of pelvic vasocongestion Return of normal color and orgasmic platform in primary (rapid) stage Loss of clitoral tumescence and return to position	Diaphoresis Hyperventilation Tachycardia

From Beckman CR, Ling F, Barzansky BM, et al. *Obstetrics and Gynecology*, 4th Ed. Philadelphia: Lippincott Williams & Wilkins, 2002:610, with permission.

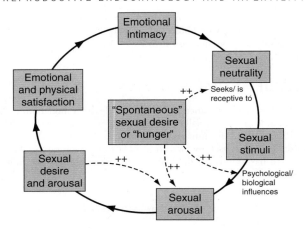

Figure 39-1. Basson's model of female sexual response. (From Basson R. Female sexual response: the role of drugs in the management of sexual dysfunction. *Obstet Gynecol* 2001;98:350–353, with permission.)

- A study of women's health including 2,400 multiethnic women (Hispanic, white non-Hispanic, African American, Chinese, and Japanese) in midlife in six US cities (the Study of Women's Health Across the Nation [SWAN]) found that 40% never or infrequently felt desire, but the majority of those women reported being capable of arousal and only 13% expressed discontent.
- Rosemary Basson developed a model in 2001 that incorporates psychological and social aspects (e.g., emotional intimacy and emotional satisfaction in addition to desire and physical satisfaction). In her model, desire does not always precede sexual arousal. Women often rather begin from a state of "sexual neutrality" (neither desirous of or aversive to), and respond to or seek sexual stimuli, based on many possible psychological motivations, including a need for intimacy, rather than a desire for physical release. The response to this stimulus is usually arousal, which then leads to desire, and hence, improved arousal. This model can be explained to patients concerned about lack of desire and can normalize what women commonly experience (a lack of spontaneous desire but the presence of reactive desire), and this can be a simple intervention to decrease a woman's anxiety (Fig. 39-1).

SEXUAL DYSFUNCTION DISORDERS

- The *Diagnostic and Statistical Manual of Mental Disorders*, fourth edition (DSMIV 2000), classifies sexual dysfunction into disorders of desire, arousal, orgasm, and pain.
  - **Hypoactive sexual desire disorder**—Persistent or recurrent deficient or absent sexual fantasies and desire for sexual activity that cause marked distress or interpersonal difficulty.
  - **Sexual aversion disorder**—Persistent or recurrent aversive response to any genital contact with a sexual partner and emphasizes the role of avoidance.

- **Female sexual arousal disorder**—Persistent or recurrent inability to attain or to maintain until completion of sexual activity an adequate genital lubrication-swelling response of sexual excitement that causes marked distress or interpersonal difficulty.
- **Female orgasmic disorder**—Persistent or recurrent delay in, or absence of, orgasm following a normal sexual excitement phase.
- **Sexual pain disorders**
  - **Vaginismus**—Persistent or recurrent involuntary spasm of the outer third of the vagina that interferes with sexual intercourse.
  - **Dyspareunia**—Genital pain associated with sexual activity that causes distress or interpersonal difficulty.
- The DSMIV definitions of women's sexual dysfunction are problematic because they are based on the sequential model of sexual function. The International Consensus Conferences developed a revised classification system.
  - **Hypoactive sexual desire disorder**—Absent or diminished feelings of sexual interest or desire, absent sexual thoughts or fantasies, and a lack of responsive desire.
  - **Female sexual arousal disorder**
    - **Subjective sexual arousal disorder**—Absence of or markedly diminished feelings of sexual arousal (sexual excitement and sexual pleasure) from any type of sexual stimulation. Vaginal lubrication or other signs of physical response still occur. This addresses research that shows that for women there can be a lack of correlation between feelings of subjective arousal and the genital changes associated with arousal.
    - **Genital sexual arousal disorder**—Absent or impaired genital sexual arousal (e.g., minimal vulval swelling or vaginal lubrication from any type of sexual stimulation and reduced sexual sensations from caressing genitalia). Often seen in women with autonomic nerve damage and in some estrogen-deficient women.
    - **Combined sexual arousal disorder**—Both subjective and genital arousals are lacking.
  - **Female orgasmic disorder**—Lack of orgasm (i.e., a variable, transient peak sensation of intense pleasure creating an altered sense of consciousness, usually accompanied by involuntary, rhythmic contractions of the pelvic, striated circumvaginal musculature often with concomitant uterine and anal contractions and myotonia that resolves the sexually-induced vasocongestion and usually includes an induction of well-being and contentment) or markedly decreased intensity of sensation or delay from stimulation, despite high arousal or excitement.
  - **Sexual pain**—See Chapter 27.
    - **Vaginismus**—Persistent difficulty to allow vaginal entry of a penis, finger, and/or any object, despite the woman's expressed wish to do so. There is variable involuntary pelvic muscle contraction, avoidance, and anticipation or fear of pain with intercourse. Structural or other physical abnormalities must be ruled out/addressed.
    - **Dyspareunia**—Persistent or recurrent pain with attempted or complete vaginal entry and/or penile vaginal intercourse. **Vulvodynia** is vulvar discomfort most often described as burning pain, occurring in the absence of relevant visible findings of a specific, clinically identifiable disorder; it can occur without sexual contact. Vulvodynia is thought to be a form of neuropathic pain. **Vestibulodynia** (formerly vulvar vestibulitis syndrome) is a subset of vulvodynia that

is characterized by severe pain during attempted vaginal entry and tenderness localized to the vulvar vestibule, which is thought to be due to proliferation of C-afferent nociceptors in the vestibular mucosa.

- One must define whether the patient's disorder is secondary or primary and whether it is situational or generalized. In reality, there is overlap among these disorders. Orgasm is impossible without arousal, and a lack of arousal commonly leads to a lack of desire because sexual activity is not enjoyable or reinforcing. Similarly, sexual pain makes sexual interaction uncomfortable and leads to lack of enjoyment. Insufficient arousal can also play a role in the etiology of pain syndromes—lack of vaginal lubrication and failure of "tenting" response of the distal vagina can lead to pain.

Vulvodynia and Vaginismus

- These disorders are especially important for the obstetrician/gynecologist to understand because patients typically present first to their gyn provider with their concern over introital dyspareunia. Unfortunately, it is still common for patients with these disorders to spend years going to multiple providers who tell them that there is "nothing wrong."
- It is imperative for the physician to understand that although there may be no visible physical changes or microbiological abnormalities, this disorder is now understood to involve changes in the nervous system, including an increase in nerve density and sensitivity in the vulva (peripheral sensitization), and changes in the CNS, which amplify the pain rather than diminish it (central sensitization).
- The currently accepted term for vulvodynia confined to the vulvar vestibule is vestibulodynia (about 12% lifetime incidence of women in a 2003 population-based study by Harlow). Pain confined to the clitoris is clitorodynia, and generalized vulvar pain is generalized vulvodynia (3% lifetime incidence).

Assessment of Vulvodynia and Vaginismus

- The highest incidence of vulvodynia is in ages 18 to 32. When perimenopausal or menopausal women present with these symptoms, treat vaginal atrophy, preferably with topical estrogen, prior to diagnosing vulvodynia.
- Patients with vulvodynia are more likely to have other pain disorders such as migraine headaches, fibromyalgia, irritable bowel syndrome, and interstitial cystitis. Allergies and endometriosis may also be more prevalent.
- See Chapter 27 for pelvic pain examination approach and technique.
- Patients who receive the diagnosis for vaginismus generally have a significant phobic component regarding penetration and usually have never experienced penetration. Their physical exam is frequently indistinguishable from the vulvodynia patient, and introital hypersensitivity and muscle hypertonicity are commonly identified.
- Question carefully about hygiene practices. Patients frequently attribute symptoms to uncleanliness and overwash with harsh soaps or use over the counter products with potential irritants or sensitizers such as benzocaine (Vagisil).

Treatment for Vulvodynia and Vaginismus

- Nearly all patients with these disorders benefit from **pelvic floor physical therapy**, which must be performed by a physical therapist with specialized training.
- **Mental health counseling** is helpful for most patients or couples, but it is important to stress that this is to help the individual or couple cope with the disorder, because the patient may assume that you are implying that her disorder is "purely psychological."

- **Vaginal dilator therapy**
  - This can be initiated and taught by the gynecologist, for those patients who are willing and exhibit identifiable introital muscle tightness. Begin by teaching Kegel exercises and relaxation, then helping patient to insert the smallest dilator while in the office. Patients may find using a mirror helpful.
  - Dilators can be purchased online, or other cylindrically shaped objects can be used, including culturette tubes, syringes (with the luer-lock tips removed), and candles.
  - Patients can be encouraged to use their own fingers, and later their partner's fingers, as dilators. This has the advantage of encouraging the patient's comfort with her own genitals.
  - Patients should understand that they are not actually physically dilating their vaginas but gradually desensitizing their reactions to vaginal penetration. The analogy of desensitizing the eye's reaction to the insertion of a contact lens may be useful.

Medical Treatments
- Many of the same **oral medications** that are used for other types of neuropathic pain are used. These patients tend to be anxious, hypervigilant, and sensitive to side effects, so start with a low dose and increase gradually.
  - Tricyclic antidepressants (e.g., amitriptyline, desipramine): 25 to 150 mg/day
  - Gabapentin 900 to 3,600/day
  - Topiramate 25 to 200 mg/day
  - Venlafaxine 37.5 to 150 mg/day.
- **Topical medications** are often preferred by patients. No randomized controlled trials exist, and medications must usually be compounded in a specialized pharmacy. The vehicle is important because many patients are prone to irritant reactions. Cellulose gel, acid-mantle cream, and stearin-lanolin are examples of vehicles which tend to be well tolerated. In general, gels and ointments are tolerated better than creams. Patients must be shown exactly where to apply the product, as they may lack knowledge of their own anatomy.
  - Lidocaine 2% to 5%, applied three times daily. This may cause stinging in some patients.
  - Gabapentin 6%, applied three times daily
  - Amitriptyline 2%/baclofen 2%
  - Estrogen is often tolerated better in a noncream base. Some patients may be prone to vulvovaginal thinning, especially on the more progestogen-dominant hormonal contraceptive methods, and may benefit from discontinuing the method or from the addition of topical estrogen.
  - Topical steroids are generally not recommended, especially for long-term therapy, because of the potential for tissue thinning and steroid rebound dermatitis.

Surgical Treatment
- Surgical management with **vestibulectomy** has an 85% success rate.
- Success rates are lower for women with vulvodynia or vaginismus who decline sexual counseling, those who have untreated hypertonicity, and those with longer lengths of time with symptoms.

Follow-Up for Vaginismus/Vulvodynia Patients
- Patients should be reevaluated periodically during treatment (e.g., every 4 to 8 weeks) to track their response to treatment and to check for emergence of other disorders, such as vulvovaginal candidiasis or other infections, dermatologic problems,

worsening pelvic floor muscle function, or relationship issues. Compliance with, and tolerance of medications, need to be reassessed periodically.

Treatments for Desire and Arousal Disorders

- Given that there is so much overlap among these disorders and that the female sexual response is a complex interaction, the treatment must often also be multifaceted.
  - Androgens—Androgens can be given in the form of DHEA, methyltesterone, and testosterone creams or gels (approved for men only) or in the form of transdermal patch (in development). Of women who have undergone oophrectomy and hysterectomy, those with a 300 μg transdermal testosterone patch had significantly increased numbers of sexual fantasies, amount of masturbation, and number of episodes of sexual intercourse. The positive well-being, depressed mood, and composite scores improved at 300 μg versus 150 μg and placebo. However, there are concerns about the lack of safety data and the risks of clitoromegaly, hirsutism, acne, hepatotoxicity, and lipid profile worsening. Androgens can masculinize a female fetus. Additionally, the risk for breast cancer with additional androgens is unknown. Some studies indicate a possible decrease in risk, while others point to an increased risk.
  - Estrogen—Improves atrophy, which has been found to increase the risk of dyspareunia, but the Women's Health Initiative trial showed no overall significant difference in satisfaction.
  - Tibolone—A compound with mixed steroid effects that has been shown to increase sexual function scores but is only available in Europe.
  - Sildenafil—A randomized trial of 781 women with arousal disorder showed no conclusive impact of sildenafil. This is likely related to the fact that women may have physical changes, but it does not affect the mental component and therefore women do not subjectively feel increased sexual arousal. It does appear to be beneficial for patients taking selective serotonin reuptake inhibitors (SSRIs) or those with spinal cord injury. There has been recent interest in the similar phosphodiesterase inhibitor *tadalafil* (*Cialis*), which may be better for women because it is longer acting.
  - L-Arginine—Precursor of nitric oxide and two small RCTs by the same author show increased desire, orgasm, and sexual function.
  - Counseling
  - Cognitive behavioral therapy—Identifies and modifies factors such as maladaptive thoughts, unreasonable expectations, behaviors that reduce trust, and insufficient stimuli. Works to increase communication among partners.
  - Sex therapy—Includes sensate therapy that initially starts with nonsexual intimacy and focuses on feedback on what is pleasurable. This technique is effective in reducing sexual anxiety and helps both partners avoid "spectatoring" or monitoring their own response during the encounter.
  - The suction vacuum device—The clitoral suction vacuum increases clitoral engorgement when the vacuum is applied and may lead to improved vascularization and sensation. This is currently the only FDA-approved treatment for female sexual dysfunction.
  - Buproprion—As a non-SSRI antidepressant with dopaminergic activity, it may help with mood disorders, and can be used instead of SSRIs, or may be used to counteract SSRIs effects on sexual function. There is some evidence that buproprion has prosexual effects in nondepressed women.

- Others treatments—Sublingual apomorphine is a dopamine agonist, and phentolamine is an adrenergic receptor antagonist. Zestra is available online and over the counter and has some research to support efficacy.

Treatment of Female Orgasmic Disorder

- Arousal, desire, and pain disorders should be ruled out or addressed.
- Orgasmic function can be treated as a learned skill, and cognitive behavioral treatments (generally directed masturbation) are highly effective.
- Self-treatment books such as *For Yourself* by Lonnie Barbach, or *Becoming Orgasmic* by Julia Heiman and Ray Lopiccolo, are useful.

SEXUAL FUNCTION AND SPECIAL POPULATIONS

- **Postpartum**—Fewer women with anal sphincter tears report sexual activity. Pain and healing scar, in addition to breast-feeding, new baby, fatigue, and hormone changes, affect sexual activity postpartum. Of 796 women, only 32% resumed intercourse within 6 months but 89% after 6 months.
- **Menopause/premature ovarian failure**—Dysfunction and dyspareunia are more likely in women with vulvovaginal atrophy. However, overall health status, mental health, and partner status have a greater impact on sexual function. Note that women aged 20 to 49 with premature ovarian failure are significantly affected.
- **Lesbians**—Strive for inclusive statements when addressing all patients and do not make assumptions. Strive to have forms that are gender neutral. If a patient identifies herself as a lesbian or as a woman who has sex with woman, ask the screening questions about whether she has concerns or pain. Women who have sex with women may identify themselves in different ways. Lesbian couples may have concerns about whether their partner will be included in decisions about care. Lesbian women may be more wary of health care providers. Lesbian women are at risk for the same things as heterosexual women. For example, lesbian women still need sexually transmitted disease screening because of past sexual encounter with a male or through female-to-female contact. Lesbian women are still at risk for domestic violence.
- **Medical disorders and medications**—Many medical disorders can affect sexual function. For example, diabetes and peripheral vascular disease may affect vasocongestion. Depression and substance and tobacco abuse can affect sexual function. Medications such as SSRIs, antipsychotics, antihypertensives, oral contraceptive pills, and medroxyprogesterone acetate are also known to affect sexual function.
- **Pelvic floor disorders**—Women with higher pelvic floor dysfunction scores are more likely to report decreased arousal, infrequent orgasm, and increased dyspareunia. Urinary incontinence can cause a fear of odor, loss of self-esteem, and embarrassment and may actually occur during sexual activity, and can decrease desire. There has been concern that treatments such as slings which come close to the dorsal nerve of the clitoris might adversely affect sexual function; however, surgical treatment of prolapsed or stress urinary incontinence has been found to increase sexual function.
- **Posthysterectomy**—There are theoretical concerns that surgery can disrupt the complex neurologic and vascular anatomy involved in sexual response. However, because female sexual response is a complex mix of mental and physical, hysterectomy has not been shown to compromise sexual function for most women—in fact, many have an increase in sexual function once issues such as menorrhagia are resolved. A recent study showed no difference in sexual function for patients who had total abdominal hysterectomy versus supracervical hysterectomy.

- **Breast cancer and gynecologic oncology patients**—Disease and treatment can cause changes such as postcoital bleeding and pain, decreased desire, arousal, opinion of self, and overall decreased quality of life. Radiotherapy, in particular, causes sexual side effects.
- **Infertility**—Many infertile couples think of sexual activity as goal oriented and the measure of success as the ability to produce a child. They can have trouble finding pleasure in sexual activity.

SUGGESTED READINGS

Basson R. Sexual desire and arousal disorders in women. *N Engl J Med* 2006;354(14): 1497–1506.

Carey JC. Pharmacological effects on sexual function. *Obstet Gynecol Clin North Am* 2006;33:599–620.

Haefner HK, Collins ME, Davis GD, et al. The vulvodynia guideline. *J Lower Genital Tract Dis* 2005;9(1):40–51.

Kammerer-Doak D, Rogers R. Female sexual function and dysfunction. *Obstet Gynecol Clin North Am* 2008;35:169–183.

Rosen R, Barsky J. Normal sexual response in women. *Obstet Gynecol Clin North Am* 2006;33:515–526.

Shifren JL, Braunstein GD, Simon JA, et al. Transdermal testosterone treatment in women with impaired sexual function after oophrectomy. *N Engl J Med* 2000;343(10):682–688.

Srivastava R, Thakar R, Sultan A. Female sexual dysfunction in obstetrics and gynecology. *Obstet Gynecol Surv* 2008;63(8):527–537.

40 Menopause

Mindy S. Christianson and Howard Zacur

DEFINITIONS AND EPIDEMIOLOGY OF MENOPAUSE

Menopause is the permanent cessation of menses, dated by the last menstrual period followed by 12 months of amenorrhea.
- The average age of menopause is 51 years, with a normal range of 43 to 57 years.
  - Can also be induced by oophorectomy or iatrogenic ablation of ovarian function.
- In 2001, the Stages of Reproductive Aging Workshop divided normal female reproductive aging into stages, with the goal of clarifying terminology relating to menopause (Fig. 40-1).
  - The transition from reproductive to postreproductive life is divided into several stages, with the final menstrual period (FMP) serving as an anchor.
    - Five stages (–5 to –1) precede the FMP and two stages follow (+1 and +2).
  - **Menopausal transition**, traditionally termed **perimenopause** or **the climacteric**, is the transition period from regular menstruation until menopause.
    - May last for 5 years or more, highly variable in duration.
    - Characterized by menstrual cycle changes that include variable cycle length, with skipped periods and increasingly longer intervals of amenorrhea.
    - Associated with the cessation of ovulation, a marked decline in estradiol production, and a modest decline in androgen production.
    - Early menopausal transition (–2) is depicted by variable cycle length (>7 days different from the norm) and increased FSH.
    - Late menopausal transition (–1) is characterized by ≥2 skipped cycles and an interval of amenorrhea >60 days.
- Diagnosis of menopause is clinical, without reliance upon hormonal measurements.
  - When any doubt exists about menopause, other causes of secondary amenorrhea must be ruled out. See Chapter 36.

PHYSIOLOGY OF MENOPAUSE

- Oocytes undergo atresia throughout a woman's life, with follicular quantity and quality undergoing a critical decline approximately 20 to 25 years after menarche. This follicular decline results in loss of ovarian sensitivity to gonadotropin stimulation.
- During perimenopause, follicular dysfunction can lead to variable menstrual cycle length. The follicular phase of the cycle is usually shortened due to the decreased number of functional follicles.
- The early menopause transition is typified by increased levels of FSH leading to overall higher estrogen levels.
- As follicular depletion continues, decreased inhibin produced by follicles leads to continued increased FSH. Follicular depletion also leads to recurrent anovulation and subsequent increase in FSH and LH levels.

				Final Menstrual Period (FMP)				
Stages:	−5	−4	−3	−2	−1	0	+1	+2
Terminology:	Reproductive			Menopausal Transition			Postmenopause	
	Early	Peak	Late	Early	Late*		Early*	Late
				Perimenopause				
Duration of Stage:	variable			variable			(a) 1 yr	(b) 4 yrs	until demise
Menstrual Cycles:	variable to regular	regular		variable cycle length (>7 days different from normal)	≥2 skipped cycles and an interval of amenorrhea (≥60 days)	Amenorrhea	none	
Endocrine:	normal FSH		↑ FSH	↑ FSH			↑ FSH	

*Stages most likely to be characterized by vasomotor symptoms ↑ = elevated

Figure 40-1. Stages/nomenclature of normal reproductive aging in women. (From Soules MR, Sherman S, Parrott E, et al. Executive summary: stages of reproductive aging workshop (STRAW). *Fertil Steril* 2001;76:874, with permission.)

MENOPAUSAL SYMPTOMS AND TREATMENT

Vasomotor Symptoms

- Seventy-five percent of menopausal women experience vasomotor symptoms such as hot flashes, hot flushes, and night sweats.
  - Symptoms begin an average of 2 years before the FMP.
  - Eighty percent of those who have hot flashes endure them for longer than 1 year and fifty percent for longer than 5 years.
- **Pathophysiology:** Due to vasomotor instability thought to be secondary to dysfunction of central thermoregulatory centers in the hypothalamus.
  - Characterized by a sudden reddening of the skin over the head, neck, and chest, accompanied by a feeling of intense body heat. Concludes with profuse perspiration.
  - Hot flashes may also cause sleep disturbance and irritability.
  - Norepinephrine and serotonin are the neurotransmitters thought to trigger hot flashes.
- **Risk factors:** Surgical menopause (up to 90% of women will have vasomotor symptoms), early menopause, low circulating levels of estradiol, smoking, and possibly low body mass index (BMI).
- **Treatment:** Hormone therapy (HT) is first line treatment.
  - **Estrogen** administration: The most effective treatment for hot flashes, given orally, transdermally, or vaginally (Table 40-1).
    - Oral dosing: Results in plasma level fluctuations and an estradiol to estrone ratio of <1.
    - Oral estrogen plus androgen combinations are available and may help with decreased postmenopausal libido, but this is somewhat controversial.
    - Transdermal estrogen: Delivers estrogen at a relatively constant rate of 50 to 100 μg/dL, comparable to premenopausal endogenous estrogen production.
      - Maintains the 1:1 ratio of estradiol to estrone that approximates the natural, premenopausal ratio.
      - Avoids first-pass liver metabolism effect, which prevents an effect on synthesis of clotting factors and decreases the effect on lipid metabolism.

TABLE 40-1	Hormone Replacement Therapies

Drug	Dosage
Oral estrogens	
Conjugated equine estrogens (Premarin)	0.3–2.5 mg daily
Synthetic conjugated estrogens (Cenestin, Enjuvia)	0.3–1.25 mg daily
Micronized estradiol (Estrace)	0.5–2 mg daily
Esterified estrogens (Menest)	0.3–2.5 mg daily
Estropipate (Ogen, Ortho-Est)	0.625–2.5 mg daily
Estradiol (Femtrace)	0.45–1.8 mg daily
Oral progestins	
Micronized progesterone (Prometrium)	200 mg for 12 d each month or 100 mg daily
Medroxyprogesterone acetate (Provera)	10 mg daily for 12 d each month
Norethindrone acetate (Aygestin)	2.5–10 mg for 12 d each month
Oral estrogen/progestin combinations (continuous)	
Conjugated estrogens/medroxyprogesterone acetate (Prempro)	0.3/1.5 mg/daily, 0.45/1.5mg/daily, 0.625/2.5 mg or 0.625/5mg/daily
Estradiol/norethindrone acetate (Activella)	1.0/0.5 mg daily
Estinyl estradiol/norethindrone acetate (FemHRT)	5 µg/1 mg daily, 2.5 µg/0.5g daily
Estradiol + drospirenone (Angeliq)	1 mg/0.5 mg daily
Cyclical oral	
Estradiol/norgestimate (Prefest)	1 mg estradiol for 15 d, and then 1 mg estradiol/0.09 mg norgestimate for 15 d
Conjugated estrogens/medroxyprogesterone acetate (Premphase)	0.625 mg conjugated estrogens for 14 d, then 0.625 mg conjugated estrogens/ 5 mg medroxyprogesterone for 14 d
Transdermal estrogen preparations	
Transdermal estradiol patch(Alora, Climara, Esclim, Estraderm, Menostar, Vivelle, Vivelle-Dot)	Variable dosing; apply twice weekly or weekly, depending on brand
Topical estradiol gel (Divigel, Elestrin, Estragel)	Variable dosing; apply once daily
Topical estradiol emulsion (Estrasorb)	1.74 g/pouch; two pouches applied daily
Topical estradiol spray (Evamist)	1.53 mg/spray; 2–3 sprays daily
Vaginal estrogen preparations	
Vaginal conjugated estrogens (Premarin)	0.625 mg/g; apply daily
Vaginal estradiol cream (Estrace)	0.01% cream; daily then 1–3 times/wk
Vaginal estradiol ring (Estring, Femring)	50–100 µg/d (Femring), 7.5 µg/d (Estring); Replace every 90 d
Vaginal estrodiol tablets (Vagifem)	10 µg daily for 2 wk, then twice weekly

(Continued)

TABLE 40-1	Hormone Replacement Therapies *(Continued)*
Drug	**Dosage**
Transdermal estrogen and progestin preparations	
Estradiol + levonorgestrel (Climara Pro)	0.45 mg/0.015 mg; apply weekly
Estradiol + norethindrone acetate (Combipatch)	0.05 mg/0.14 mg; 0.05 mg/0.25 mg; apply twice weekly
Oral estrogen and androgen combinations	
Esterified estrogens + methyltestoster- one (Estratest H.S.)	0.625 mg/1.25 mg daily
Esterified estrogens + methyltestoster- one (Estratest)	1.25 mg/2.5 mg daily

- Dosing of HT for vasomotor symptoms is listed in Table 40-1.
- In women with a uterus, **progestins** must be added to any estrogen regimen to prevent the increased risk of endometrial cancer associated with unopposed estrogen use.
  - The progestin is administered either continuously with daily dosing or cyclically with daily dosing only during the last half of each cycle.
- Current recommendations: Estrogen should be used at the lowest effective dose for the shortest duration possible for the relief of hot flashes.
- **Contraindications for HT:** History of venous thromboembolism or stroke or those at high risk for developing these conditions, history of breast cancer, or coronary heart disease (CHD).
- **Alternatives** to HT for vasomotor symptoms are for patients who feel estrogen produces unacceptable side effects or who have contraindications.
  - **Selective serotonin and norepinephrine reuptake inhibitors (SSRI, SNRI):**
    - **Venlafaxine** 150 mg QD reduces hot flashes by 61% over a 4-week treatment course, and **paroxetine** at either 12.5 mg or 25 mg/day has also reduces hot flashes by approximately 60%.
  - **Clonidine** (0.05 to 0.15 mg/day) and **gabapentin** (900 mg/day) are also used to treat side effect symptoms.
  - **Medroxyprogesterone acetate,** 150 mg intramuscularly per month, has been shown to be 90% effective in the treatment of hot flashes.
  - **Alternative therapies** such as soy, black cohosh, red clover, and dong quai may also be useful in the treatment of hot flashes. Further investigation is needed to clarify their role in the alleviation of hot flashes and their side effects.

Urogenital Atrophy

- **Pathophysiology:** The vagina, urethra, and bladder trigone have high estrogen receptor concentrations. Loss of estrogen that accompanies menopause thus leads to urogenital atrophy.
- Atrophic vulva loses most of its collagen, adipose tissue, and water-retaining ability and becomes flattened and thin. Sebaceous glands remain intact, but secretions decrease, leading to vaginal dryness.
- Vaginal shortening and narrowing occur, and the vaginal walls become thin, lose elasticity, and become pale in color.

- Dyspareunia is the most common complaint related to vaginal atrophy.
- Estrogen deficiency within the urethra and bladder is associated with urethral syndrome, which is characterized by recurrent episodes of urinary frequency and urgency with dysuria.
- **Treatment**
  - **Moisturizers and lubricants:** Include Replens, Astroglide, and K-Y jelly.
    - Used to relieve symptoms related to vaginal dryness and dyspareunia.
    - Astroglide and K-Y jelly are used at the time of coitus to alleviate dyspareunia, whereas Replens is used on a sustained basis.
  - **Local estrogen therapy:** Mainstay therapy for urogenital atrophy.
    - Local estrogen therapy improves vaginal atrophy and associated symptoms.
    - Can also relieve dysuria, and may protect against recurrent lower urinary tract infections.
    - Estrogen therapy does not improve urinary stress or urge incontinence.
    - Different forms of estrogen therapy are available.
    - Low-dose estrogen creams are applied intravaginally from daily to two times a week at doses of 0.3 mg of conjugated estrogens or 0.5 g of estradiol per application.
    - Estring is a silicone ring embedded with estrogen that releases 6 to 9 μg of estradiol daily and is kept in place for 3 months. It has minimal systemic absorption.
    - Vagifem tablets are given vaginally as one per day for 14 days followed by twice per week dosing. They have also been shown to estrogenize the vaginal mucosa without resulting in significant systemic absorption.

Menstrual Cycle Disturbances

- Because of the changing hormonal milieu, complaints of irregular bleeding are very common during the menopausal transition.
- If episodes of bleeding occur more often than every 21 days, last longer than 8 days, are very heavy, or occur after a 6-month interval of amenorrhea, evaluation of the endometrium must be undertaken to rule out neoplasm. This includes endometrial biopsy and possible dilation and curettage with hysteroscopy.
- **Oral contraceptive pills** can be used during the menopausal transition until the onset of menopause.
  - Benefits of this therapy, in addition to relief of vasomotor symptoms, include contraception, decreased risk of endometrial and ovarian cancers, establishment of regular menses, and increased bone density.

SPECIAL CONCERNS FOR MENOPAUSAL WOMEN

Osteoporosis

- **Osteoporosis** is the condition of decreased bone mass and bone microarchitectural deterioration with resulting increased risk of skeletal fractures.
- In the United States, 4 to 6 million women (13% to 18% of those over 50 years old) have osteoporosis, resulting in 1.5 million fractures per year.
- **Pathophysiology**
  - Estrogen deficiency causes an imbalance of skeletal remodeling, with an increase in resorption that is greater than bone formation.
  - Results from a dominance of osteoclasts, which break down bone, and a decrease in osteoblastic activity. Estrogen binds to receptors on osteoblasts and inhibits their activity.

- Decreased serum calcium levels lead to an increase in parathyroid hormone (PTH), which stimulates osteoclastic activity. Estrogen deficiency also leads to increased bone sensitivity to PTH.
- Bone resorption matches bone formation until approximately age 25 to 35 years old. Bone mass decreases after that at a rate of 0.4% per year.
- After menopause, bone mass decreases 2% to 5% annually for 10 years and then the rate stabilizes to 1% per year.
- Most common fracture sites include the lumbar vertebrae, wrist (distal radius), and hip (femoral neck).
- Known **risk factors** account for 30% of osteoporosis incidence (Table 40-2).
- **Prevention and treatment** guidelines are in Table 40-3.
- **Diagnosis** is determined by bone mineral density (BMD) with dual-energy x-ray absorptiometry being the preferred technique.
  - BMD is best measured at the hip and is predictive of hip fracture and fracture at other sites.
    - *T*-scores are standard deviations above or below the comparison mean BMD of young women aged 20 to 29 years.
    - *Z*-scores correspond to the same measurements using women of the same age as the reference.
      - Normal bone *T*-scores are above –1.0.
      - Osteopenia *T*-scores are between –1.0 and –2.5.
      - Osteoporosis *T*-scores are at or below –2.5.
      - For each reduction in bone mass of one standard deviation, the risk of fracture doubles.

TABLE 40-2	Risk Factors for Osteoporosis

Family history of osteoporosis
Current cigarette smoking
Low body weight: <127 pounds for average height or BMI <21
Estrogen deficiency due to menopause, especially early menopause (<45 yo)
Anorexia nervosa and other eating disorders
Insufficient Vitamin D intake
Prolonged premenopausal amenorrhea (>1 y)
Lifelong low calcium intake
Excessive alcohol intake
Current low bone mass
Inadequate physical activity
Medications, including glucocorticoids, gonadotropin-releasing hormone analogs, anticonvulsants, long-term heparin, excessive thyroid hormones, cholestyramine
Personal history of fracture as an adult
History of a fracture in a first-degree relative
Caucasian/Asian women
Advanced age
Numerous medical conditions (e.g., HIV/AIDS, Cushing's syndrome, hyperthyroidism, diabetes, rheumatoid arthritis)

BMI, body mass index. Adapted from National Osteoporosis Foundation. Risk Factors for Osteoporosis. Found at www.nof.org/prevention/risk.htm.

TABLE 40-3	Prevention and Treatment of Osteoporosis in Women After Age 50

Prevention

Calcium, 1,200 mg/d
Vitamin D, 800–1,000 IU/d
Regular weight-bearing, muscle-strengthening exercise
Smoking cessation
Moderate alcohol consumption

Treatment

Treatment for all women ≥50 years old with the following:
- Vertebral or hip fracture
- T-score ≤−2.5 at the femoral neck or spine
- T-score between −1.0 and −2.5 at the femoral neck or spine and 10-year hip fracture risk[a] ≥3%
- Ten year major osteoporosis-related fracture probability[a] ≥20%.

[a]Ten year fracture risk based on the US-adapted World Health Organization absolute fracture risk model, FRAX® (found at www.sheffield.ac.uk/FRAX). Adapted from National Osteoporosis Foundation. Clinician's Guide to Prevention and Treatment of Osteoporosis. Washington, DC: National Osteoporosis Foundation.

- **Screening** should be offered to any postmenopausal patient who presents with a fracture. Other candidates for BMD determination are women older than age 65.
  - The US Preventive Services Task Force recommends screening at age 60 for women who have risk factors for osteoporosis (Table 40-2).
    - The strongest risks for osteoporosis identified were low body weight, older age, weight under 70 kg (154 pounds), and not taking estrogen.
  - FRAX is a World Health Organization (WHO) funded, web-based program that calculates a patient's risk of osteoporotic fracture based on *T*-score and other variables.
- **Treatment:** Several medications are available to treat osteoporosis.
  - **Oral bisphosphonates:** A class of drug analogous to physiologically occurring inorganic pyrophosphates, inhibitors of bone resorption. They are generally considered first-line treatment for osteoporosis.
    - **Alendronate** sodium (Fosamax)
      - Mechanism: Oral bisphosphonate.
      - Dosing: 5 mg daily for prevention of osteoporosis and 10 mg daily or 70 mg weekly for treatment.
      - Treatment not only prevents bone loss but also progressively increases bone mass of the spine, hip, and total body.
      - Also reduces risk of vertebral fractures, progression of vertebral deformities, and height loss in postmenopausal women with osteoporosis.
    - **Risedronate** sodium (Actonel)
      - Mechanism: Oral bisphosphonate.
      - Dosing: 5 mg daily or 35 mg weekly for prevention and treatment of osteoporosis.

- Prospective studies of postmenopausal women with normal lumbar spine BMD values found that patients who received 5 mg daily had increased spine and femoral trochanter BMD, whereas patients in the placebo group experienced decreased BMD at both sites.
- Benefits of treatment are sustained—1 year after cessation of therapy, lumbar spine BMD was 2.3% lower than baseline in patients given risedronate but 5.6% lower in patients who received placebo.
- In women with osteoporosis, risedronate has been shown to reduce vertebral fractures.
  ○ **Ibandronate** (Boniva)
  - Mechanism: Oral bisphonate.
  - Dosing: 2.5 mg daily or 150 mg monthly.
  - Demonstrated to be effective at decreasing bone turnover in postmenopausal women but has not been shown to reduce hip fracture risk.
  ○ Bisphosphonate side effects:
  - Heartburn, esophageal irritation, esophagitis, abdominal pain, and diarrhea.
  - Oral calcium supplementation may interfere with the absorption of bisphosphonates.
  - Patient should take each dose after an overnight fast, while sitting in the upright position, and should follow by drinking a glass of water.
  - The patient must remain upright and not eat for 30 minutes after administration.
  - Long-term side effects are unknown.
- **Intravenous bisphosphonates** are an alternative for patients unable to tolerate the oral forms.
  ○ **Zoledronic acid** (Reclast) is given annually (5 mg IV) for treatment and every 2 years for prevention.
  ○ **Ibandronate** (Boniva) may be given 3 mg IV every 3 months.
  ○ IV Bisphophonate side effects include flu-like symptoms and hypocalcemia (more common in those with vitamin D deficiency). Check 25-hydroxy vitamin D level and treat as needed before infusion.
- **Selective estrogen receptor modulator**
  ○ **Raloxifene hydrochloride** (Evista)
  - Estrogen-like effects on bone and the cardiovascular system and antiestrogen effects on breast and uterus. It is FDA approved for the prevention and treatment of osteoporosis.
  - Dosing: 60 mg daily
  - A study involving postmenopausal women, both with and without osteoporosis, found that patients treated with raloxifene daily for 2 years had statistically significant increases in lumbar spine and hip BMD compared to patients who received placebo. Has not been shown to decrease risk of hip fracture.
  - Also has been shown to reduce vertebral fractures.
  - Side effects: hot flashes and leg cramps.
  - An increased risk of thromboembolic events is found with raloxifene use.
  - A trial involving postmenopausal women with osteoporosis found a decreased risk of breast cancer in these patients.
- **Peptide hormone**
  ○ Salmon **calcitonin**
  - Mechanism: Inhibits bone resorption by decreasing osteoclast activity. May also have an analgesic effect.

- Dosing: Nasal form, Miacalcin 200 IU daily, used effectively in the treatment of postmenopausal osteoporosis. Can also be administered subcutaneously or intramuscularly in a 100-IU dose every other day.
    - Calcitonin, in both injectable and nasal spray preparations, is effective in preventing early postmenopausal bone loss.
    - Side effects: Nausea and flushing. Rhinitis and epistaxis may occur with intranasal dosing. No long-term adverse effects are found.
  ○ **Synthetic PTH: Teriparatide** (Forteo)
    - Mechanism: A synthetic human PTH that stimulates bone formation during short term use.
    - Shown to reduce spine fractures by 65% and nonspine fractures by 54%.
    - A daily dose of 20 μg is injected subcutaneously.
    - Side effects: Nausea, leg cramps, and dizziness.
    - Use for longer than 24 months is not recommended because long-term side effects are unknown.
    - Usually given to patients who have a history of osteoporotic fracture and inability to take bisphosphonates.
  ○ Hormone therapy
    - Has been demonstrated to increase spine and hip BMD and decrease hip and vertebral fractures in women with osteoporosis and in those without osteopenia or osteoporosis.
    - Recent studies have suggested that lower doses of oral HT than previously used can also prevent bone loss.
    - FDA has approved a lower dose transdermal estrogen patch with 0.014 mg of estradiol (Menostar) for the prevention of osteoporosis.
    - HT combined with bisphosphonate treatment has been shown to result in a greater increase in bone density than either treatment alone.

Cognition and Dementia

- There is an accelerated deterioration of cognitive function once menopause begins.
- Alzheimer's disease is three times more common in women than in men.
- In cultured cells and animal models, estrogen has a protective effect on neurons.
- Limited evidence exists, however, regarding beneficial effects of estrogen on cognition.
  - The Baltimore Longitudinal Study of Aging showed women taking estrogen performed better on a short-term visual memory test.
  - The Women's Health Initiative Memory Study (WHIMS) noted a slightly increased risk of cognitive decline and dementia in women 65 years and older taking estrogen alone or with progestin.
  - Studies to date have lacked consistency in testing outcomes and specific aspects of memory function.

Cardiovascular Health

- Coronary artery disease (CAD) is the leading cause of death among postmenopausal women.
- Women lag 10 years behind men in terms of CAD risk prior to menopause.
- By age 70, a woman has the same risk of CAD as a male of the same age.
  - The Framingham study showed a two- to sixfold increased incidence of CAD in postmenopausal women compared to premenopausal women in the same age group.

- Premenopausal women have higher levels of high-density lipoprotein (HDL) and lower levels of total cholesterol and low-density lipoprotein (LDL) than their post-menopausal and male counterparts.
- Animal studies suggest that estrogen protects endothelial function and inhibits the oxidation of LDL.

Hormone Replacement Therapy

Hormone Therapy (HT) and Coronary Heart Disease (CHD)

- The first prospective trial to look at the effect of HT on CHD was the **Postmeno-pausal Estrogen/Progestin Interventions** or PEPI trial, which found that women on HT had greater high-density lipoprotein cholesterol levels than women taking placebo.
- The next large prospective trial was the **Heart and Estrogen/progestin Replace-ment Study (HERS)**. In postmenopausal women with established CHD, the use of estrogen plus progestin did not prevent further heart attacks or death from CHD. There were significantly more thromboembolic events in the HT users.
- The **Women's Health Initiative (WHI)** enrolled postmenopausal women aged 50 to 79 years (mean age 63). Women with severe menopausal symptoms were discouraged from participating.
  - Participants received either estrogen plus progestin (combined equine estrogens [CEE], 0.625 mg/day and medroxyprogesterone acetate [MPA], 2.5 mg/day), estrogen alone (CEE 0.625 mg/day) if they had a hysterectomy, or placebo.
  - The primary outcome was CHD, with fractures being a secondary outcome.
  - Adverse events monitored were breast cancer and venous thromboembolism.
  - After 5 years, the estrogen plus progestin arm of the study was stopped early because the number of cases of breast cancer in the treatment group exceeded the predetermined threshold for increased risk.
    - In one year, of 10,000 postmenopausal women who took estrogen plus proges-tin, 38 were diagnosed with breast cancer compared to 30 of 10,000 women who took placebo.
    - Women in the estrogen alone group have not shown increased rates of breast cancer.
  - Regarding CHD and other vascular events, results showed that per 10,000 women annually, the number of heart attacks, strokes, and blood clots were 37, 29, and 34 in the estrogen plus progestin arm compared to 30, 21, and 16 per 10,000 women taking placebo.
    - Women taking estrogen alone also showed increased risk of these events relative to placebo.
  - There were fewer bone fractures and diagnoses of colon cancer in both hormone groups.
  - A secondary analysis showed that women who initiated HT closer to menopause had reduced CHD risk compared to the increased risk of CHD among women more distant from menopause.
    - Lower risk was found for young women and higher risk for older patients.

HT and Dementia

- Together HERS and WHIMS suggest that HT does not decrease the risk of cogni-tive decline in postmenopausal women.

HT Conclusions

- HT remains the most effective treatment for menopausal signs and symptoms. It should not be used for the prevention of chronic diseases.

- Further study is required to determine the side effects of HT when given in early menopause as the WHI primarily included women over 10 years postmenopause. The recent studies on HT were based on one estrogen and progesterone formulation only, and results might not be applicable to other formulations, doses, or routes of administration.

SUGGESTED READINGS

Anderson GL, Limacher M, Assag AR, et al. Effects of conjugated equine estrogen in postmenopausal women with hysterectomy: the Women's Health Initiative randomized control trial. *JAMA* 2004;291:1701.

Barrett-Connor E, Grady D, Sashegyi A, et al. Raloxifene and cardiovascular events in osteoporotic postmenopausal women: four-year results from the MORE (Multiple Outcomes of Raloxifine Evaluation) randomized trial. *JAMA* 2002;287:847.

Bone HG, Hosking D, Devogelaer JP, et al. Ten years' experience with alendronate for osteoporosis in postmenopausal women. *N Engl J Med* 2004;350:1189.

Grady D. Management of menopausal symptoms. *N Engl J Med* 2006;355:2338.

Grady D, Herrington D, Bittner V, et al. Cardiovascular disease outcomes during 6.8 years of hormone therapy: Heart and Estrogen/progestin Replacement Study follow-up (HERS II). *JAMA* 2002;288:49.

Hormone therapy, Women's Health Care Physicians Executive Summary. American College of Obstetricians and Gynecologists. *Obstet Gynecol* 2004;104:1S.

Nelson HD. Commonly used types of postmenopausal estrogen for treatment of hot flashes: scientific review. *JAMA* 2004;291:1610.

Rossouw JE, Anderson GL, Prentice RL, et al. Risks and benefits of estrogen plus progestin in healthy postmenopausal women: principal results from the Women's Health Initiative randomized controlled trial. *JAMA* 2002;288:321.

Rossouw JE, Prentice RL, Manson JE, et al. Postmenopausal hormone therapy and risk of cardiovascular disease by age and years since menopause. *JAMA* 2007;297:1465.

The Writing Group for the PEPI Trial. Effects of estrogen or estrogen/progestin regimens on heart disease risk factors in postmenopausal women: the Postmenopausal Estrogen/Progestin Interventions (PEPI) Trial. *JAMA* 1995;273:199.

Vasomotor symptoms. American College of Obstetricians and Gynecologists. *Obstet Gynecol* 2004;104(4 suppl):106S.

V Gynecologic Oncology

41 Diseases of the Vulva and Vagina

Lauren Krill and Colleen McCormick

Vulvar and vaginal disease should be understood by its presentation, etiology, location, and associated systemic and laboratory findings. Clinicians should have a low threshold to biopsy any suspicious vulvar abnormalities, because the appearance of malignant lesions is often similar to that of benign processes. While the vulva is susceptible to the same pathologic processes that occur on all skin, it is also preferentially affected by some specific disorders.

ANATOMY OF THE VULVA AND VAGINA

- The **vulva** is that area of skin encompassing the labia majora to the hymen (Fig. 23-7). See also Chapter 23.
- The vulva is bordered laterally by the genitocrural folds, anteriorly by the mons pubis, and posteriorly by the perineal body. The medial side of the labia minora to the hymen is known as the vulvar vestibule.
  - Hart's line is the thin zone of color and texture change between the labia minora and the vestibule, marking the transition from the skin of the external genitalia to the mucosa of the vestibule.
  - Within the vestibule lie the urethral meatus, vaginal introitus, ostia of Bartholin's glands (major vestibular glands), minor vestibular glands, and Skene's ducts (Fig. 23-8).
- Branches of the external and internal pudendal arteries provide the vascular supply to the vulva (Fig. 41-1).
- Sensory innervation of the anterior vulva is via the genitofemoral nerve and the cutaneous branch of the ilioinguinal nerve, whereas the posterior vulva and the clitoris are innervated by the pudendal nerve.
- The medial group of superficial inguinal nodes collects the lymphatic drainage of the vulva (see Fig. 41-3).
- The **vagina** is a hollow viscus extending from the hymenal ring to the vaginal fornices surrounding the proximal cervix; it is lined by hormone-responsive nonkeratinized stratified squamous epithelium.

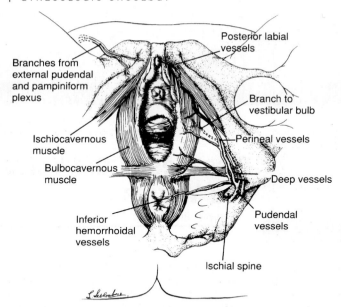

Figure 41-1. Superficial vulvar musculature and vascular supply of the vulva. (From Rock JA, Jones HW, et al. *Te Linde's Operative Gynecology,* 10th Ed. Philadelphia, PA: Lippincott Williams & Wilkins, 2008:505, with permission.)

- The vascular supply of the vagina is provided by the vaginal branch of the internal iliac artery and extensions of the uterine artery that form an anastomotic plexus along the lateral vaginal sulci. The distal vagina also receives blood from pudendal vessels, and the posterior wall receives contributions from the middle rectal artery.
- The vagina is innervated by fibers from the pudendal nerves and the vaginal plexus, which arises from the hypogastric plexus (sacral rami S2-4).
- The primary sites of lymphatic drainage for the vagina are the hypogastric, obturator, and external iliac lymph nodes via the lateral perivaginal plexus. The distal third of the vagina may also drain to the inguinal-femoral nodes, and the posterior vagina may drain to the inferior gluteal, presacral, or perirectal lymph nodes.

INFECTIOUS DISEASES OF THE VULVA

- Sexually transmitted, viral, and fungal infections, and parasite infestations of the vulva and vagina are discussed in Chapter 25.
- Bacterial skin infections of the vulva include **folliculitis** and **furunculosis**, most frequently caused by *Staphylococcus,* and **cellulitis** secondary to infection with *Staphylococcus* or *Streptococcus.*

- Treatment of initial infection: Cephalexin 500 mg PO qid, or dicloxacillin 500 mg PO qid, or clindamycin 300 to 450 mg PO tid.
- For recurrent infections: Add to previous regimen Hibiclens washes + 2% mupirocin ointment tid × 10 days.

INFLAMMATORY DISEASES OF THE VULVA

Behçet's Syndrome

- **Behçet's syndrome** is a rare chronic disease characterized by a triad of relapsing oral ulcers, genital ulcers, and ocular inflammation. The disease is most common in Japan and the Middle East.
- Other findings include acne, cutaneous nodules, thrombophlebitis, and colitis.
- Genital ulcers are small, painful, and deep and may result in fenestration of the labia. Ulcers generally heal in 7 to 10 days without scarring.
- Treatment options include topical (betamethasone valerate ointment 0.1%), intralesional (triamcinolone, 3 to 10 mg/mL, injected into ulcer base), or systemic corticosteroids (prednisone 1 mg/kg for severe involvement, especially CNS).

Hidradenitis Suppurativa

- **Hidradenitis suppurativa** is a chronic, painful apocrine gland disorder causing deep, suppurated subcutaneous nodules that form sinus tracts and confluent masses. The axillae and anogenital region are most frequently involved. The lesions wax and wane; flares are common with menstruation. The lesions ulcerate, resulting in draining sinuses and extensive scarring.
- Superinfection of hidradenitis suppurativa is polymicrobial and cultures help guide treatment. The effectiveness of medical therapy wanes as deeper tissues become involved.
- Treatment options are extensive and are approached in stepwise fashion.
  - Oral antibiotics: Empiric treatment with clindamycin in conjunction with a quinolone or broad-spectrum coverage is appropriate. For example, erythromycin (250 to 500 mg qid), tetracycline (250 to 500 mg qid), or minocycline (100 mg bid) until lesions resolve. Therapy for superinfections should be guided by culture results. Oral (prednisone 70 mg tapered over 14 days, for severe inflammation) or intralesional (triamcinolone 3 to 5 mg/mL) corticosteroids are helpful in hastening resolution of the lesions.
  - Isotretinoin (Accutane) has been effective in some cases, but precaution must be taken because of the toxicity and teratogenicity associated with this agent.
  - Surgery is reserved for severe cases resistant to medical management. Surgical debridement must be extensive; simple incision and drainage is not adequate. Patients should be counseled that postoperative recurrences at previously affected and new sites can occur and hence close surveillance is indicated.

Fox-Fordyce Disease

- **Fox-Fordyce disease** is a papular eruption caused by the occlusion of apocrine sweat glands in the axilla and anogenital region. Patients present with flesh-colored dome-shaped papules in clusters that are intensely pruritic. Lichenification is common.
- This disease is rare and predominantly affects African Americans. Exacerbations tend to occur before and during menses. Symptoms regress during pregnancy.
- Treatment is with oral contraceptives (high estrogen content), topical estrogen ointment (1 mg estrone in peanut oil [Theelin] per ounce of petrolatum), or antiacne topical agents.

VULVAR DERMATOSES

Atrophic Vulvovaginitis

- The hypoestrogenic state of menopause produces atrophy of the vulvar and vaginal epithelium. The mucosa becomes friable and easily irritated and is more prone to infection.
- Patients complain of vulvar dryness, pain and burning, pruritus, dyspareunia, and dysuria. The diagnosis is clinical.
- On physical examination, the labia majora appear lax while the labia minora are significantly atrophied. The mucosa is thin, pale, and smooth with loss of the normal rugae of the vagina. Fissures may be present.
- Avoid use of harsh soaps and hygiene products. Treatment with estrogen replacement therapy, either topical or oral, helps relieve symptoms.

Contact Dermatitis

- Soaps, detergents, hygiene products, vaginal creams, and clothing can all produce a local reaction on the vulva, which may last days to weeks.
- On physical examination, symmetric eczematous lesions are seen at the area of contact.
- Identify and remove the offending agent. Oatmeal soaks and sitz baths can be used to help control symptoms, and for severe reactions, a mild steroid ointment may be used sparingly.

Lichen Simplex Chronicus

- Characterized by intense and persistent pruritus. The rash often involves the perineum.
- Continual scratching of the vulva leads to lichenification, producing a thickened, leathery appearance with prominent skin markings.
- Foci of atypical hyperplasia or cancer can develop, with a 3% chance of developing invasive squamous cell carcinoma. Evaluation should include colposcopy and full-thickness biopsy.
- Initial treatment with topical tricyclic/antipruritic ointments (doxepin 5% ointment), antihistamines (hydroxyzine 25 to 50 mg nightly), or the use of an anxiolytic/sedatives may relieve pruritus.
  - Topical corticosteroid preparations covered by continuous dry occlusive gauze dressings (betamethasone valerate ointment 0.1%) or intralesional corticosteroids (triamcinolone 3 mg/mL) are effective for cases that are more difficult to treat.

Lichen Planus

- **Lichen planus** is an uncommon, papulosquamous eruption that can affect the genitalia and oral mucosa. The pathophysiology is thought to involve T-cell autoimmunity to basal keratinocytes.
- Patients present with complaints of itching, pain, and burning of the vulva.
- White papules in a linear or reticular pattern are often seen on the vulva (Wickham's striae).
- A wide range of morphologies are seen, the most common and most difficult to treat is the erosive form. When the erosive disease progresses, the vulva and vagina become denuded and scarred with loss of the clitoris and labia minora. Introital stenosis is present in severe disease.
- Lichen planus is a chronic recurrent disease, hence complete control is not typical and spontaneous remission is unlikely. The use of ultrapotent topical steroids is first-line treatment. Surgery is not curative and is reserved for treatment of postinflammatory sequelae, such as labial adhesions and introital stenosis.

Lichen Sclerosis

- **Lichen sclerosis** is of unknown etiology and is characterized by severe vulvar pruritus, atrophy, and scarring, with gradual loss of the labia minora and prepuce of the clitoris.
- The perirectal area is often involved. The disease is chronic and can occur at any age, but postmenopausal white women are most commonly affected.
- Women with lichen sclerosis have a 20% risk of having other autoimmune disease, most frequently alopecia areata, vitiligo, or thyroid disease.
- Patients have a 5% chance of developing vulvar squamous cell carcinoma, although lichen sclerosis is usually not considered a premalignant lesion.
- Vulvar punch biopsies should be performed to confirm the diagnosis.
- Treatment includes chronic use of ultrapotent topical corticosteroid (0.05% clobetasol propionate ointment). Topical estrogen (0.01% estradiol cream) is indicated for atrophic symptoms. Periodic clinical examinations should be performed and patients should return for biopsy if ulcerations persist or new lesions appear. Surgery is reserved for management of malignancy and postinflammatory sequelae, such as labial adhesions and introital stenosis.

VULVAR PAIN SYNDROMES

- See also Chapters 27 (chronic pelvic pain) and 39 (sexual dysfunction).

Vulvodynia

- **Vulvodynia** is defined as chronic vulvar discomfort, occurring in the absence of relevant visible findings, or a specific identifiable neurologic disorder. The pain is often described as burning, stinging, or throbbing. These symptoms interfere with the ability of women to have vaginal intercourse, wear tight clothing, exercise, or even sit down. Vulvodynia affects roughly 15% of the female population.
- Symptoms may be generalized, localized, provoked, unprovoked, or mixed. The cotton swab test has been described to systematically map affected areas of the vestibule, perineum, and inner thigh for initial evaluation, to differentiate localized from generalized vulvodynia, and to gauge treatment success. Vulvodynia is a diagnosis of exclusion and thorough evaluation is needed to rule out other pathologies.
- Often a combination of multiple treatments may be required to improve symptoms of vulvodynia. These include general vulvar care, topical local anesthetics and estrogen creams, oral medications (e.g. tricyclic antidepressants, gabapentin, carbamazepine), trigger point injections with combined steroids and local anesthetics, dietary changes, cognitive behavioral therapy, biofeedback and physical therapy, and surgery for resistant localized pain. See Chapter 39.

Vulvar Vestibulitis Syndrome

- **Vulvar vestibulitis syndrome** (VVS) is chronic inflammation of the vestibular glands and is characterized by erythema and severe pain elicited by touch only. The main presenting symptoms are dyspareunia and terminal dysuria.
- Patients with VVS usually benefit from pelvic rest, anti-inflammatory/antiallergenic therapy (e.g., Burow's soak baths/sitz baths, antihistamine therapy, Stearin-Lanolin cream application), and pelvic relaxation exercises. Infectious etiologies, if present, should be treated. Medical therapies as described above for vulvodynia may be appropriate (see Chapter 39).

- Surgical repair of the vulva and perineum is usually performed for patients who fail to respond to conservative therapy or those who suffer from scars and/or recurrent tears of the perineum.

Levator Ani Myalgia

- **Pelvic floor myalgia** is often the result of trauma or inflammation of the perineal branch of the pudendal nerve causing painful spasms of the affected muscles and fascia.
- Treatment of pelvic muscle myalgia may require pudendal block (triamcinolone + local anesthetic) and pelvic physiotherapy/biofeedback.

Vulvar Neuropathy

- The pudendal, genitofemoral, and ilioinguinal nerves are the main nerves serving the vulvovaginal area. Trauma to these nerves may result in continuous dull, aching, or burning neuropathic pain. See Chapter 27.
- Gabapentin 300 to 1,200 mg PO TID or amitriptyline 0.5 to 2 mg/kg PO qhs have been shown to be effective treatment.

BENIGN NEOPLASTIC VULVAR LESIONS

Urethral Caruncle

- **Urethral caruncle** is a benign, generally asymptomatic exophytic papule at the urethral meatus that may cause bleeding. It must be differentiated from malignancy. No treatment is required unless symptomatic, in which case topical estrogen therapy (0.01% Estrace cream, 2 to 4 g daily for 1 to 2 weeks) or destruction via cryosurgery or laser vaporization will control bleeding.

Acrochordon

- **Acrochodons** (i.e., skin tags) are common, frequently pedunculated fibroepithelial polyps that have a rubbery consistency. They often arise in areas of chronic irritation. Acrochordons do not need to be removed unless they are symptomatic.

Seborrheic Keratoses

- **Seborrheic keratoses** are flat to slightly raised pigmented lesions that have a characteristic waxy, "stuck-on" appearance. Although benign, all pigmented vulvar lesions should be carefully evaluated to rule out melanoma or squamous cell carcinoma. If suspicious for malignancy, evaluate with excisional biopsy.

Lipoma

- **Lipomas** are benign tumors composed of adipose tissue. They are soft and sometimes pedunculated. They commonly appear on the mons pubis and labia majora. No treatment is necessary unless the lipoma is bothersome, in which case it can be excised.

BENIGN VULVAR CYSTS

Bartholin's Cyst

- Bartholin's glands (greater vestibular glands) produce a clear, mucoid secretion that provides continuous lubrication for the vestibular surface. They are lined by transitional epithelium and are prone to obstruction, which results in **Bartholin's cyst** formation. Superinfection results in an abscess. Usually polymicrobial, approximately 10% of **Bartholin's abscesses** may be caused by *Neisseria gonorrhoeae*.

- Treatment of Bartholin's gland abscesses may include incision and drainage, marsupialization, or in case of recurrence, resection of the gland (Fig. 41-2). Attempts at incision and drainage are therapeutic only when the lesion becomes fluctuant. The incision is made near the hymenal ring (i.e., at the vaginal introitus near the duct orifice), and a Word catheter is inserted. In women age 40 or older, biopsy is recommended because of the risk of Bartholin's adenocarcinoma. Antibiotic therapy, even after incision and drainage, is not usually necessary unless cellulitis is also present. Simple Bartholin's cysts that are not infected and not causing symptoms may not need treatment.

Epidermal Cysts

- **Epidermal inclusion cysts** are seen frequently on the labia majora, containing a white or yellow material made up of keratin and lipid-rich debris. They arise from blockage of pilosebaceous ducts. If traumatized, they can become erythematous and tender. If symptomatic, cysts can be surgically excised.

Mucus Cysts

- **Mucus cysts** are found within the vestibule and develop from vestigial embryonic structures or from obstruction of the minor vestibular glands. They are lined by mucus-secreting simple columnar epithelium without myoepithelial cells.

Gartner's Cysts

- **Gartner's duct cysts** arise from remnants of the mesonephric ducts. They most often appear as multiple small cysts along the lateral vagina and hymenal ring. These

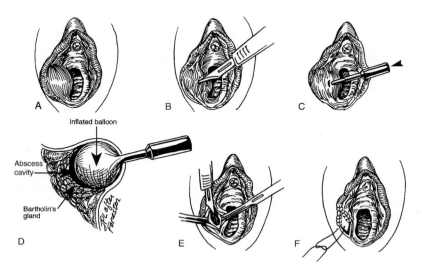

Figure 41-2. Surgical management of Bartholin abscess. (**A**), typical presentation of a Bartholin cyst or abscess; (**B**), small stab incision of the cyst near the hymenal ring; (**C**), insertion of a Word catheter which is inflated in (**D**), to allow fistula drainage tract formation; (**E**), opening of the cyst wall for marsupialization seen in (**F**). (From Beckmann CR, Ling F, Barzansky BM, et al. *Obstetrics and Gynecology*, 4th Ed. Philadelphia: Lippincott Williams & Wilkins, 2002:372.)

cysts are usually asymptomatic and are discovered incidentally. Treatment is not necessary unless cysts are very large, in which case they can be excised.

Cysts of the Canal of Nuck (Processus Vaginalis Peritonei)

- These peritoneal lined cysts are found in the superior aspect of the labia majora. They arise from inclusions of the peritoneum at the insertion of the round ligament to the labia majora. These cysts must be distinguished from an inguinal hernia.

MALIGNANT NEOPLASTIC DISEASES OF THE VULVA

Vulvar neoplasms represent an estimated 3% to 5% of all primary malignancies of the female genital tract. Squamous cell carcinoma is the most common histopathology found in vulvar cancer, followed by melanoma, basal cell carcinoma, and sarcoma. These lesions frequently present as pruritus and are often misdiagnosed by health care providers. The majority of patients experience symptoms for >6 months before diagnosis.

Squamous Cell Vulvar Neoplasia

- Vulvar squamous cell neoplasia may be intraepithelial or invasive.

Vulvar Intraepithelial Neoplasia (VIN)
- Histologic criteria for **VIN** include disordered maturation and nuclear abnormalities, loss of polarity, pleomorphism, mitotic figures, and coarsened nuclear chromatin. Cytologic atypia is present throughout the epithelium. The degree of maturation present in the surface epithelium defines the grade of dysplasia.
  - VIN 1 demonstrates squamous maturation in the upper two thirds of the epithelium.
  - VIN 2 shows loss of maturation in the lower two thirds of the epithelium. Surface maturation is present.
  - VIN 3 presents with full thickness loss of squamous maturation. Stromal invasion does not occur. Cytologic atypia may be severe.
- Younger patients tend to have multifocal disease linked to HPV types 16 and 18. As such, risk factors for VIN in this group are similar to those for developing cervical cancer. Lesions of VIN are flat-topped papules or plaques. Elderly patients who develop VIN 3 typically have a unifocal lesion associated with atrophy and are usually not infected with HPV. VIN associated with HPV tends to be multifocal and therefore colposcopic examination and directed biopsy of the entire lower genital tract are warranted.
- In 2004, a simplified classification system of VIN was introduced to reflect the malignant potential of the lesion. There are three subcategories: **VIN usual type** (warty, basaloid, or mixed), **VIN differentiated**, and **VIN unclassified**.
  - This system eliminates the VIN 1 category, and the term VIN is reserved for histologically high-grade squamous cell lesions. VIN 2 and VIN 3 are combined with the expectation that they are difficult to differentiate and would both be treated as high-grade preinvasive neoplasms.
- **Treatment.** Wide local excision of lesions should be performed if invasion cannot be excluded. Laser ablation performed properly results in less scarring and is an attractive option if no evidence of malignancy exists. Topical agents, such as imiquimod and 5-fluorouracil cream, are currently investigational therapies. Recurrence occurs in one third of women. Women younger than age 40 have a 5% risk of developing

invasive disease, whereas the risk for older women rises to 15% to 20%. Therefore, long-term surveillance of the lower genital tract is recommended every 3 months for the first 2 years and then 6 months for 3 years.

Invasive Squamous Cell Vulvar Cancer

- Squamous cell lesions account for 85% to 90% of vulvar malignancies. As with VIN, two subtypes of **invasive squamous cell carcinomas** exist.
  - The classic, warty, or Bowenoid type is identified in younger patients and is related to HPV. These lesions may be multifocal.
  - The keratinizing, differentiated, or simplex types occur in older women and is not associated with HPV. These lesions tend to be unifocal, and a significant number are associated with atrophic lesions, such as lichen sclerosis.
- Pruritus is the most common symptom associated with vulvar squamous cell carcinoma. Despite symptoms, most women delay enlisting the care of a medical practitioner. A high index of suspicion is required for all vulvar lesions and vulvar symptoms, with a low threshold for biopsy or referral to a specialist.
- Accurate **surgical staging** predicts prognosis, as nodal status has the most prognostic significance, and directs treatment for squamous cell carcinoma of the vulva. The International Federation of Gynecology and Obstetrics (FIGO) staging system was recently revised to reflect the risk of nodal metastases on survival (Table 41-1).
- **Treatment.** Vulvar carcinomas, especially early stage lesions, are treated surgically. Traditionally, these lesions were treated with a radical en bloc resection. Presently, management has shifted toward less radical procedures. Wide local excision of the primary lesion is typically performed with resection to the urogenital diaphragm and 1 cm margins.
  - Given the extremely low incidence of lymphatic involvement, lesions <2 cm with 1 mm or less invasion do not require lymphadenectomy. Unilateral lesions >2 cm from midline structures, without evidence of distant spread, may be treated with ipsilateral inguinofemoral lymphadenectomy (Fig. 41-3). The use of sentinel lymph node biopsy in early-stage vulvar cancer is currently under investigation.
  - If all nodes are negative, no further treatment is necessary; if the ipsilateral inguinal nodes are positive for metastasis, then bilateral groin dissection should be performed and possible pelvic lymph node dissection. Adjuvant pelvic radiation therapy should be considered for patients with affected groin lymph nodes.
  - Larger or more advanced stage lesions may be treated with radical vulvectomy with bilateral groin dissection, chemoradiation, or pelvic exeneration. Lesions close to the urethra, vagina, or rectum may be treated initially with chemoradiation, thus enabling more conservative surgery that preserves function and body image.
- Long-term **surveillance** is recommended every 3 months for the first 3 years and then 6 months for 2 years.

Verrucous Carcinoma

- **Verrucous carcinoma** is a variant of squamous carcinoma that occurs in postmenopausal women. These tumors are large, fungating masses that may be mistakenly diagnosed as condyloma acuminata resistant to treatment. Because the histologic appearance of verrucous carcinoma closely resembles normal squamous epithelium, a sufficiently deep biopsy must be obtained for diagnosis. Although lymph node metastasis is exceedingly rare, local destruction and tumor recurrence are common.
- **Treatment.** Treatment consists of radical local excision. Radiation therapy is contraindicated because it may induce increased aggression in malignant activity.

TABLE 41-1	FIGO Staging for Carcinoma of the Vulva (2009) and 5-Year Survival	
Stage	**Description**	**5-Year Survival[a]**
0	**Carcinoma in situ, intraepithelial neoplasia.**	
I	**Tumor confined to vulva or perineum.**	**98%**
IA	Tumor confined to vulva or perineum; lesion ≤2 cm with stromal invasion ≤1 mm, no nodal metastasis.	
IB	Tumor confined to vulva or perineum; lesion >2 cm or stromal invasion >1 mm, with negative nodes.	
II	**Tumor of any size with extension to adjacent perineal structures (lower 1/3 urethra, lower 1/3 vagina, anus) with negative nodes.**	**85%**
III	**Tumor of any size with or without extension to adjacent perineal structures with positive inguino-femoral lymph nodes.**	**74%**
IIIA	(i) With 1 lymph node metastasis (≥5 mm) or (ii) One to two lymph node metastasis(es) (<5 mm).	
IIIB	(i) With two or more lymph node metastases (≥5 mm) or (ii) Three or more lymph node metastases (<5 mm).	
IIIC	With positive nodes with extracapsular spread.	
IV	**Tumor invading other regional (upper 2/3 urethra, upper 2/3 vagina) or distant structures.**	**31%**
IVA	Tumor invading any of the following: (i) upper urethra and/or vaginal mucosa, bladder mucosa, rectal mucosa, or fixed to pelvic bone (ii) fixed or ulcerated inguino-femoral lymph nodes	
IVB	Distant metastasis to any site including pelvic lymph nodes.	

[a]Five-year survival data according to previous FIGO staging system. Adapted from Pecorelli S. FIGO Committee on Gynecologic Oncology. Revised FIGO staging for carcinoma of the vulva, cervix, and endometrium. *Int J Gynecol Obstet* 2009;105:103–104.

Basal Cell Carcinoma

- In contrast to other locations where **basal cell carcinoma** is the most common skin cancer, this malignancy constitutes only 2% to 3% of all vulvar carcinomas. They occur most commonly in postmenopausal white women. In contrast to other areas of skin, ultraviolet light exposure plays no role in the etiology of vulvar basal cell carcinoma.
- Grossly, these lesions appear as flesh colored to whitish nodules or plaques that are often ulcerated. The prognosis is good, despite a 20% risk of local recurrence. Metastases to the inguinal lymph nodes are rare.
- **Treatment.** Wide local excision.

Melanoma

- **Melanomas** constitute the second most common primary malignancy of the vulva, comprising 5% to 10% of vulvar neoplasms. Anogenital lesions account for 3% of

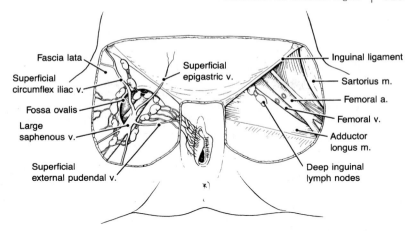

Figure 41-3. Superficial and deep lymphatic drainage of the vulva and femoral triangle. (From Rock JA, Jones HW, et al. *Te Linde's Operative Gynecology,* 10th Ed. Philadelphia: Lippincott Williams & Wilkins, 2008:85.)

all melanomas. Vulvar melanoma is a disease of the elderly, with peak frequency occurring in the sixth to seventh decades of life.

- Melanomas are typically raised lesions, with irregular pigmentation and borders. The lesions are found with approximately equal frequency on the labia majora and on mucosal surfaces. Prognosis depends primarily on tumor thickness and on the presence or absence of lymph node involvement.
- **Treatment.** Radical local excision is recommended for the primary lesion. Although nodal status has prognostic significance, the therapeutic role of regional lymphadenectomy is not well defined. Five-year survival rate is 35%.

Paget's Disease of the Vulva

- **Paget's disease of the vulva** is rare. Most affected patients are in their seventh or eighth decade of life and experience local irritation, pruritus, and bleeding.
- The lesion has slightly raised edges and is erythematous, with islands of white epithelium. Lesions are multifocal and are sharply demarcated and often have foci of excoriation and induration.
- Adenocarcinoma of the underlying sweat glands is found in 10% to 15% of patients who have intraepithelial Paget's disease. Ten percent of patients with vulvar Paget's disease are found to have associated breast, colon, or genitourinary cancer; thus, the workup should include colonoscopy, cystoscopy, mammogram, and colposcopy. If the disease is limited to the epithelium, its clinical course is usually prolonged and indolent.
- **Treatment.** Although radical surgery was formerly the mainstay of therapy, newer evidence suggests that local excision with 2- to 3-cm borders of all involved tissue carries similar prognosis. Local recurrence is common and can be treated with laser ablation. Five-year survival rates are high, and, because of the late age of onset of disease, patients usually die of illness other than Paget's disease. If an underlying adenocarcinoma is

identified, the patient should undergo radical excision and inguinal lymphadenectomy. The prognosis in patients with lymph node involvement is poor.

Bartholin's Gland Carcinoma

- Although primary vulvar adenocarcinomas are rare, the majority arise from the Bartholin's gland.
- Primary cancers of the Bartholin's gland include **adenocarcinomas and squamous cell carcinomas**. The latter may be associated with HPV. Bartholin's gland malignancies typically occur in the sixth decade of life, and biopsy of suspicious lesions is recommended in women age 40 and older.
- **Treatment.** Radical excision is recommended for the management of primary lesion. Unfortunately, given an extensive vascular and lymphatic supply, metastatic disease is common. Inguinofemoral lymphadenectomy is recommended.

Vulvar Sarcoma

- **Sarcomas** of the vulva are rare and account for 1% to 2% of vulvar malignancies. The age range is broader than for squamous cell carcinoma of the vulva. Lymphatic metastasis is uncommon.
- **Treatment.** Wide local excision is recommended, followed by adjuvant radiation, chemotherapy, or both.

MALIGNANT NEOPLASTIC DISEASES OF THE VAGINA

Vaginal cancer is rare and accounts for <2% of all primary malignancies of the female genital tract. Squamous cell carcinoma is the most common histopathology, followed by adenocarcinoma.

Squamous Cell Vaginal Neoplasia

- Vaginal squamous cell neoplasia may be intraepithelial or invasive.

Vaginal Intraepithelial Neoplasia (VaIN)

- **VaIN** is a preinvasive lesion defined by the presence of squamous cell atypia without invasion. Lesions are classified according to the depth of epithelial involvement.
  - Cytologic atypia is present throughout the epithelium involving the lower one third and two thirds of the epithelium, in VaIN 1 and 2, respectively.
  - VaIN 3 involves more than two thirds of the epithelium.
- Most disease is multifocal and found in the vaginal apex. VaIN is consistently associated with prior or concurrent neoplasia elsewhere in the lower genital tract. The majority are associated with either intraepithelial neoplasia or carcinoma of the cervix or vulva. The risk factors for VaIN are similar to those for CIN suggesting similar etiology, chiefly HPV infection.
- VaIN is usually asymptomatic, although patients can present with postcoital spotting or vaginal discharge. It is diagnosed by persistently abnormal pap smears with no evidence of cervical neoplasia. After VaIN is diagnosed, invasive disease must be excluded by colposcopy and biopsy, especially before undertaking nonexcisional therapy. VaIN progresses to invasive cancer in 3% to 7% of patients.
- **Treatment.** The management of VaIN depends on the grade of the lesion. Therapeutic techniques range from topical antineoplastic agents to excision and rarely radiotherapy. Surgical excision is the mainstay of therapy for high-grade lesions. Following therapy, gynecologic examination and vaginal cytology should be performed at 3-month intervals to evaluate for persistent or progressive disease.

Thereafter, patients can be followed at 6-month intervals for 3 years before return-ing to routine screening.

Invasive Squamous Cell Vaginal Cancer

- **Squamous cell carcinoma** accounts for 95% of vaginal malignancies. Patients may present with painless vaginal bleeding and discharge.
- Visual inspection of the vagina as the speculum is being inserted or removed may reveal a gross lesion. Often vaginal tumors are detected incidentally as a result of cytologic screening for cervical cancer. The posterior wall of the upper one third of the vagina is the most commonly affected site. Colposcopy is helpful for visualiza-tion. Definitive diagnosis is accomplished by biopsy.
- **Staging** is performed clinically, based upon findings from physical and pelvic examination, cystourethroscopy, proctosigmoidoscopy, and chest radiography. The prognosis of squamous cell carcinoma of the vagina depends on FIGO staging (Table 41-2). Lymphatic dissemination from lesions in the upper third of the vagina spreads to pelvic and paraaortic lymph nodes, while tumors in the distal third of the vagina spread to inguino-femoral and then pelvic nodes.
- **Treatment.** Treatment depends upon the location, size, and clinical stage of the tumor. Invasive disease can be treated with surgery and radiation.
  - In Stage I disease, surgery is preferred if negative surgical margins can be achieved. Disease limited to the vaginal fornix can be treated with radical hysterectomy, par-tial vaginectomy, and pelvic lymphadenectomy. Proximity of the bladder, urethra, and rectum to the vagina precludes the administration of high dose radiation. Radiotherapy can be delivered by external beam radiation or brachytherapy.
  - Radiation and concurrent cisplatin chemosensitization is used for advanced Stage III and IV disease. Carcinoma involving the distal third of the vagina necessitates dissection of groin nodes.

TABLE 41-2	FIGO Staging Classification of Vaginal Cancer and 5-Year Survival	
Stage	**Description**	**5-Year Survival**
0	Carcinoma in situ, intraepithelial neoplasia.	
I	The carcinoma is confined to the vaginal wall.	95%
II	The carcinoma involves subvaginal tissue but has not extended to the pelvic sidewall.	67%
III	The carcinoma extends to the pelvic sidewall.	32%
IV	The carcinoma extends beyond the true pelvis or involves the bladder or rectum; bullous edema as such does not permit a case to be allotted to Stage IV.	
IVA	Tumor invades bladder or rectal mucosa or there is direct extension beyond the true pelvis.	18%
IVB	Spread to distant organs.	Almost 0%

Adapted from FIGO Committee on Gynecologic Oncology. Current FIGO staging for cancer of the vagina, fallopian tube, ovary and gestational trophoblastic neoplasia. *Int J Gynecol Obstet* 2009;105:3–4.

- Treatment of recurrent disease may require pelvic exeneration or diverting surgeries.
- The desire to maintain a functional vagina is an important psychosexual issue that should be addressed on an individual basis. Treatment failure usually occurs in the first 2 years; therefore, **surveillance** involves follow-up every 3 months for 2 years, then 6 months intervals for 5 years, and annually thereafter.

Adenocarcinoma of the Vagina

- **Vaginal adenocarcinoma** is rare, accounting for <10% of vaginal cancers. Clear cell adenocarcinoma may arise from areas of adenosis in women exposed to diethylstilbestrol in utero. Screening in these patients should begin at menarche or 14 years of age. Prognosis of clear cell adenocarcinoma is good and the overall survival is 78%. However, primary non–clear cell adenocarcinoma of the vagina carries a worse prognosis than squamous cell carcinoma.
- **Treatment.** In general, adenocarcinoma is treated similarly to squamous cell carcinoma.

Melanoma

- Primary malignant **melanoma of the vagina** is rare. It presents as blue-black or black-brown masses, plaques, or ulcerations, commonly in the distal one third of the anterior vaginal wall. Symptoms include vaginal bleeding, mass, or discharge. Staging is based on tumor thickness.
- Historically, the **treatment** has been radical surgery and more recently has included wide local excision. Although generally thought to be radioresistant, radiotherapy may help with local control. Primary malignant melanomas of the urogenital mucous membranes may be aggressive. The 5-year survival rate for vaginal melanomas is usually <20%.

Embryonal Rhabdomyosarcoma (Sarcoma Botryoides)

- **Sarcoma botryoides** is a highly malignant tumor that occurs in the vagina during infancy and early childhood. Usually presents as soft nodules that resembles a bunch of grapes. The polypoid mass may fill or protrude from the vagina. See also Chapter 31.
- **Treatment.** Treated with multimodality chemotherapy with vincristine, dactinomycin, and cyclophosphamide (VAC) and limited surgery in order to preserve reproductive function.

SUGGESTED READINGS

Apgar B, Cook JT. Differentiating normal and abnormal findings of the vulva. *Am Fam Physician* 1996;53:1171–1180.

Barhan S, Ezenagu L. Vulvar problems in elderly women. *Postgrad Med* 1997;102:121–132.

Boardman L, Kennedy C. Diagnosis and management of vulvar skin disorders. ACOG Practice Bulletin Number 93. *Obstet Gynecol* 2008;111(5):1243–1253.

Duong TH, Flowers LC. Vulvo-vaginal cancers: risks, evaluation, prevention, and early detection. *Obstet Gynecol Clin N Am* 2007;34:783–802.

Foster D. Vulvar disease. *Obstet Gynecol* 2002;100:145–163.

Haefner HK, Collins ME, Davis GD, et al. The Vulvodynia guideline. *J Low Genit Tract Dis* 2005;9:40–51.

Larrabee R, Kylander D. Benign vulvar disorders. *Postgrad Med* 2001;109:151–164.

Van der Zee AG, Oonk MH, De Hullu JA et al. Sentinel node dissection is safe in the treatment of early-stage vulvar cancer. *J Clin Oncol* 2008;26:884.

42 Cervical Intraepithelial Neoplasia

Matthew W. Guile and Cornelia Liu Trimble

EPIDEMIOLOGY OF CERVICAL NEOPLASIA

- **Cervical cancer** is diagnosed in approximately 11,000 women annually in the United States, with 3,600 annual deaths attributable to the disease.
- Worldwide, cervical cancer is the second most common cancer in women.
- Infection by **human papillomavirus (HPV)**, of which >100 strains have been identified, is a necessary prerequisite for the development of cervical cancer.
- HPV types 16, 18, 31, 33, 35, 39, 45, 52, 56, 58, 59, and 68 are high-risk types, which are implicated in carcinogenesis. HPV types 6 and 11 cause benign genital warts. See Chapter 25.
- Approximately 80% of women will be infected by HPV at some point in their lives. The infection is transmitted through sexual intercourse and the majority of women will clear the infection immunologically.
- Persistent infection with a high-risk type of HPV is a risk factor for cervical cancer. Risk factors for persistent infection include smoking, immunocompromised status, increased parity, and increased age.
- The Pap smear is used as a screening test to identify the presence of visually abnormal cervical epithelial cells. Certain cytologic changes are associated with HPV infection.
- A second screening test is often used to verify the presence of HPV infection, the Digene Hybrid Capture test. This test detects the presence of high-risk HPV DNA.
- 4.8 million women a year have an abnormal Pap smear in the United States and these cytologic abnormalities are described using the Bethesda system (below).
- Histologic abnormalities are classified in a two tiered system, with low-grade lesions described as cervical intraepithelial neoplasia grade 1 (CIN 1) and high-grade lesions as (CIN 2/3).
- CIN 1 is associated with a high rate of spontaneous regression while CIN 2/3 persists much more frequently and is recognized as a cervical cancer precursor.
- Development of invasive cervical cancer from CIN 2/3 is estimated to take 8 to 12 years.

Primary Prevention

- Women who smoke have a fourfold increased risk of developing cervical cancer, and cessation should be stressed to all women with cervical lesions.
- All women with abnormal Pap smears should be offered HIV testing and testing for other sexually transmitted diseases.
- A quadrivalent HPV vaccine directed against HPV types 6, 11, 16, and 18 (Gardasil, Merck) was approved for use in 9- to 26-year-old females by the FDA in 2006.

- A large randomized clinical trial demonstrated that the vaccine was 99% effective in preventing CIN 2/3, adenocarcinoma in situ, and cervical cancer in HPV 16/18-naive women over a median follow-up of 3 years
- The vaccine is administered in three doses at 0, 2, and 6 months. See Chapter 1. HPV vaccination does not change screening recommendations.

DIAGNOSTIC CATEGORIES: CYTOLOGY

The 2001 revision of the Bethesda System is used to describe abnormal cervical cytology employing the following categories:
- Atypical squamous cells (**ASC**)
  - Of undetermined significance (**ASC-US**)
  - Cannot exclude high grade (**ASC-H**)
- Low-grade squamous intraepithelial lesion (**LSIL**)
- High-grade squamous intraepithelial lesion (**HSIL**)
- Atypical glandular cells (**AGC**)
  - Not otherwise specified (**AGC-NOS**)
  - Favor neoplasia (**AGC-favor neoplasia**)
  - Adenocarcinoma in situ (**AIS**)

SCREENING

- Cytologic changes associated with HPV infection can be identified on **Pap smear** and this serves as the basis of cervical cancer screening programs.
- Screening guidelines are formulated by the American Society for Colposcopy and Cervical Pathology (ASCCP). The first guidelines were issued in 2001, after a conference was convened to review the available data and make recommended changes in management. In 2006, the ASCCP revised the previous evidence-based consensus statement for appropriate triage of cytologic abnormalities. The American College of Obstetricians and Gynecologists further revised the guidelines in 2009.
  - Regular screening should now begin at 21 years of age, regardless of the age of first sexual intercourse. From age 21 to 29 years, screening may be conducted every two years. Immunosuppressed adolescents and young adults, however, should be screened annually.
  - In patients older than 30, screening can be performed every 3 years after three negative results provided there is no history of HIV, immunosuppression, CIN 2/3, or diethylstilbestrol exposure in utero. Women 30 and older who do not meet criteria for less frequent testing or those who have important risk factors, should continue to be screened on an annual basis.
  - Combined cervical cytology and HPV DNA testing is appropriate for women 30 years and older. Women with negative results on both tests should not be screened more frequently than every 3 years.
  - Screening can be stopped by age 65 to 70 years old, if there are no risk factors and ten years of negative screening that includes at least 3 negative test results. Screening may be reinstituted if risk factors change. Annual well-woman and pelvic exam are still recommended for all adult women.
  - Women who have had a total hysterectomy for benign indications do not require screening unless they have a history of CIN 2/3.

- HIV-positive or other immunosuppressed women should be screened at 6-month intervals for 1 year after the diagnosis of HIV and then may resume the annual screening schedule.
- Commercially available assays can reliably detect the presence of high-risk HPV in cervical cytology specimens.

Pap Smear

- Pap smear reports include specimen type, specimen adequacy, results, and any ancillary testing performed (i.e., high-risk HPV probe).
- Specimen type indicates whether test is a vaginal or cervical sample.
- Adequacy is reported as satisfactory, unsatisfactory, or endocervical cells not present/ lack of transformation zone.
  - Unsatisfactory Pap smears should be repeated in 2 to 4 months.
  - Pap smears, which lack an endocervical component can be repeated in 1 year or postpartum unless any of the following risk factors are present, all of which necessitate repeat screening in 6 months:
    ○ History of ASC-US or greater abnormalities in the past without three interval normal Pap smears
    ○ High-risk HPV positivity in the previous 12 months
    ○ Previous glandular abnormality
    ○ Immunosuppression
    ○ Inability to visualize the endocervical canal
  - Patient noncompliance
- The results section relays any cytologic abnormality.

Cytologic Abnormalities

ASC

- Approximately 2 million ASC Pap smears a year are recorded in the United States.
- ASC-US is present in 4.7% of samples and is associated with a 7% to 12% prevalence of CIN 2/3.
- ASC-H is present in 0.4% of samples and CIN 2/3 is present in 26% to 68% of women with this result.
- The risk of invasive cancer associated with an ASC Pap is 0.1% to 0.2%.

AGC

- AGC are found in 0.4% of Pap smears
- More common in women 40 years of age and older
- AGC are commonly associated with squamous abnormalities (20% to 30%) and malignancy or AIS (8% to 10%)
- AGC-favor neoplasia has a higher risk of malignancy than AGC-NOS

LSIL

- LSIL is reported in 2.1% of Pap smears and is strongly correlated with HPV infection.
- High-grade dysplasia or neoplasia is found in 12% to 17% of women who undergo colposcopy for LSIL.

HSIL

- HSIL is reported in 0.7% of Pap smears.
- CIN 2/3 is found in 53% to 97% of women with HSIL cytology, and invasive cancer is present in 2.0% of these women.

TREATMENT OPTIONS

- Treatment options can be classified as ablative or excisional.
- Ablative procedures do not obtain a sample for pathologic examination.
- Excisional procedures should be performed when invasive cancer cannot be ruled out, microinvasive cancer is suspected on a biopsy, a two-level discrepancy between cytology and histology exists, and whenever concern is raised for endocervical disease.

Ablative Methods

- **Cryotherapy** is performed with a super-cooled probe applied directly to the lesion. Not appropriate for endocervical disease.
- **Carbon dioxide laser** is used to vaporize the tissue to 7 mm depth. Special equipment is necessary, but more irregular areas can be treated.

Excisional Methods

- All excisional procedures increase a woman's risk of future preterm delivery and premature rupture of the membranes.
- **Loop Electrosurgical Excision Procedure (LEEP)** is an excisional procedure employing a wire with an electrical current. The shape and size of the loop can be altered, and a second "hat" can be done to obtain further endocervical tissue. Cautery artifact can make interpretation of margins difficult
- **Cold Knife Cone (CKC)** employs a scalpel to excise a cone-shaped wedge of the cervix. The size and shape of the cone can be tailored to the lesion, and this method allows for pathologic determination of margin status. CKC should be considered over LEEP for cases with AIS, suspected microinvasion, unsatisfactory colposcopy, or a lesion extending into the endocervical canal.

MANAGEMENT STRATEGIES: CYTOLOGIC ABNORMALITIES

ASC-US: Three Acceptable Management Options

- **Reflex testing for high-risk HPV.** This is the preferred management strategy. A positive result necessitates colposcopy, and a negative result allows for resumption of standard screening. The sensitivity for CIN 2/3 is 92% with this strategy (Fig. 42-1).
- **Repeat Pap smears at 6 and 12 months.** If either repeat Pap smear is abnormal, the patient is referred to colposcopy. Two consecutive negative results allow for resumption of standard screening. The sensitivity for CIN 2/3 is 95% with this method.

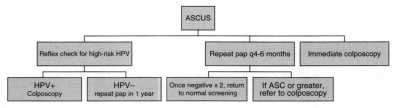

Figure 42-1. Triage strategy for ASC-US. (Adapted from Wright TC, Massad LS, Dunton CJ, et al. for the 2006 American Society for Colposcopy and Cervical Pathology-sponsored Consensus Conference. 2006 Consensus Guidelines for the Management of Women with Abnormal Cervical Cancer Screening Tests. *J Low Genit Tract Dis* 2007;11(4):201–222.)

- **Immediate colposcopy.** A single colposcopic examination will miss approximately 1/3 of CIN 2/3, and therefore a negative colposcopy requires repeat cytology in 12 months.

Special Populations
- Adolescents (between 13 and 20 years old) have a higher prevalence of HPV and are more likely to clear the infection.
  - The new guidelines to delay first testing until age 21 are designed to reduce unnecessary diagnosis and treatment of young women. It is further expected that this will reduce cervical procedures that can increase risk for future pregnancy complications.
- Pregnant women are managed identically to women older than 20 years, with the exception that colposcopy can be deferred to 6 weeks postpartum. Endocervical curettage is never acceptable in pregnancy.
- Immunosuppressed and postmenopausal women are managed identically to the general population.

ASC-H

- These patients require colposcopic examination. Negative colposcopy should be followed by cytology in 6 and 12 months or HPV DNA testing at 12 months.

AGC

- All women with AGC should undergo colposcopy with endocervical biopsy; HPV DNA testing is preferred.
- Endometrial sampling should be performed routinely for the finding of atypical endometrial cells.
- Endometrial sampling should be performed in women 35 years and older and in those with risk factors for endometrial cancer.
- Follow-up for AGC-NOS after negative findings is repeat cytology/HPV DNA testing at 6 months if they are initially HPV DNA-positive and 12 months if negative.
- Follow-up for AGC-favor neoplasia after a negative evaluation is a diagnostic excisional procedure, preferably cold-knife cone.
- AIS is managed by a diagnostic excisional procedure, preferably cold-knife cone.

Special Populations
- Pregnant women should be managed in an identical fashion to the general population with the exception that endometrial and endocervical biopsies are unacceptable.
- Benign-appearing endometrial cells on a Pap smear in a women older than 40 should be evaluated with endometrial biopsy.

LSIL

- LSIL carries the same risk of high-grade dysplasia as ASCUS + HPV and is therefore managed identically (colposcopy).
- Endocervical curettage is preferred in those with an unsatisfactory or negative colposcopic examination.
- A finding of less than CIN 2/3 can be followed by cytology at 6 and 12 months or HPV DNA testing at 12 months.

Special Populations
- Adolescents with LSIL should be followed by repeat cytology at 12 months and 24 months. A finding of HSIL or greater at 12 months or ASC-US or greater at 24 months merits colposcopy. Only immunosuppressed adolescents are now screened.

- Postmenopausal women can be managed by reflex HPV DNA testing, colposcopy, or repeat cytology at 6 and 12 months.
- Pregnant women with LSIL should have a colposcopic examination. Postpartum follow-up is also acceptable.

HSIL

- Due to the high risk of significant cervical disease, one approach is to "see and treat" with immediate LEEP.
- Colposcopy with endocervical curettage is also acceptable. An unsatisfactory colposcopy should be managed by a diagnostic excisional procedure.
- A satisfactory colposcopy that results in a diagnosis of less than CIN 2/3 can be followed by colposcopy/cytology at 6 and 12 months, excisional diagnostic procedure or review of the original pathologic material to verify the diagnosis.

Special Populations

- Adolescents with HSIL cytology should be referred to colposcopy. "See and treat" is unacceptable in this population due to the high rate of lesion regression and negative ramifications on future fertility.
  - A satisfactory colposcopy less than CIN 2/3 should be followed by colposcopy/cytology every 6 months for up to 2 years.
  - Persistent HSIL for 24 months should be evaluated with an excisional diagnostic procedure.
  - A high-grade colposcopic lesion or persistence of HSIL for 1 year should be evaluated by biopsy.
  - Two consecutive negative Pap smears and no high-grade lesions on colposcopy allow for resumption of normal screening schedule.
- Pregnant women with HSIL should be evaluated by colposcopy. Lesions suspicious for CIN 2/3 or cancer should be biopsied; it is unacceptable to biopsy other lesions.
  - Evaluation no sooner than 6 weeks postpartum should be performed for women with a diagnosis of less than CIN 2/3.

DIAGNOSTIC CATEGORIES: HISTOLOGY

- Colposcopy is used for the evaluation of abnormal cervical cytology.
- A colposcope is used to examine the cervix after the application of 3% acetic acid. The dilute acid preferentially dehydrates abnormal epithelial cells, yielding acetowhite changes.
- Colposcopy is considered satisfactory if the whole squamocolumnar junction is seen circumferentially and all lesions are completely visualized.
- See Table 42-1 for the natural history of untreated CIN 1, CIN 2, and CIN 3.

CIN 1

- CIN 1 is the histologic diagnosis applied to low-grade lesions; it is not equivalent to LSIL.
- It is estimated that 1 million women are diagnosed with CIN 1 annually in the United States and that the annual incidence of CIN 1 is 1.2 per 1,000 women.
- CIN 1 uncommonly progresses to CIN 2/3.

CIN 2/3

- CIN 2/3 is the histologic diagnosis applied to high-grade lesions, and it is not equivalent to HSIL.

TABLE 42-1	Natural History of Untreated CIN			
	Regression to Normal (%)	Persistent Dysplasia (%)	Progression to CIN 2/CIN 3 (%)	Progression to CIS (%)
CIN 1	57	30	11	0.3
CIN 2	43	35	—	14–22
CIN 3	32	48–56	—	12

CIN, cervical intraepithelial neoplasia; CIS, carcinoma in situ. Adapted from Mitchell MF, Tortolero-Luna G, Wright T, et al. Cervical human papillomavirus infection and intraepithelial neoplasia: a review. *J Natl Cancer Inst Monogr* 1996;(21):17–25.

- It is estimated that 500,000 women are diagnosed with CIN 2/3 annually in the United States and that the annual incidence of CIN 2/3 is 1.5 per 1,000 women.

AIS

- Unlike squamous lesions, AIS lesions are often multifocal. Therefore, negative margins do not reliably predict excision of all disease.

MANAGEMENT STRATEGIES: HISTOLOGIC ABNORMALITIES

CIN 1

- The management of CIN 1 depends on the cytology, as the risk of an occult high-grade lesion is greater when the referral cytology is HSIL or AGC (Fig. 42-2).
- CIN 1 preceded by ASC-US, ASC-H, or LSIL
  - Follow-up with repeat cytology at 6 and 12 months or HPV DNA testing at 12 months. A positive HPV DNA or cytology equal to or greater than ASC-US necessitates repeat colposcopy.
  - Two negative Pap smears or a single negative HPV DNA allows for resumption of standard screening.

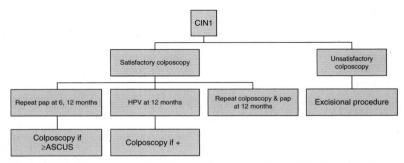

Figure 42-2. Triage strategy for CIN 1. (Adapted from Wright TC, Massad LS, Dunton CJ, et al. for the 2006 American Society for Colposcopy and Cervical Pathology-sponsored Consensus Conference. 2006 Consensus Guidelines for the Management of Women with Cervical Intraepithelial Neoplasia or Adenocarcinoma In Situ. *J Low Genit Tract Dis* 2007;11(4):223–239.)

- Persistent (≥2 years) CIN 1 can be followed as above or treated. Ablative and excisional procedures are acceptable given a satisfactory colposcopy. Ablation is unacceptable after unsatisfactory colposcopy.
- CIN 1 preceded by HSIL or AGC-NOS
  - Diagnostic excisional procedure or colposcopy/cytology at 6-month intervals is acceptable. Endocervical curettage should be performed if colposcopy is selected.
  - Unsatisfactory colposcopy or persistence of HSIL or AGC-NOS cytology requires a diagnostic excisional procedure.
  - Negative cytology/colposcopy for 1 year allows for resumption of routine screening.

Special Populations
- Adolescents with CIN 1 should be followed with yearly cytology. HSIL or greater at 1 year should be evaluated with colposcopy, as should ASC-US or greater after 24 months.
- Pregnant women with CIN 1 should be followed without treatment.

CIN 2 and CIN 3

- CIN 2/3 requires excision or ablation after a satisfactory colposcopy.
- Recurrent CIN 2/3 should be excised and ablation is unacceptable for CIN 2/3 and an unsatisfactory colposcopy.
- Hysterectomy is not acceptable management for CIN 2/3.
- After treatment, CIN 2/3 can be followed by HPV DNA testing at 6 to 12 months, cytology every 6 months, or cytology/colposcopy at 6 month intervals.
- Either HPV DNA positivity or ASC-US or greater on cytology require colposcopy with endocervical sampling.
- If testing is negative after posttreatment evaluation for 1 year, routine screening should be employed for at least 20 years.
- Hysterectomy is acceptable for persistent or recurrent CIN 2/3.
- Positive margins can be followed with either Pap smear, colposcopy, and ECC every 4 to 6 months or a further excisional procedure can be performed.

Special Populations
- Adolescents with CIN 2/3 can be followed by cytology/colposcopy at 6-month intervals for 2 years. Persistence of CIN 2/3 for 24 months should be excised while two consecutive normal colposcopic examinations and cytology permit return to routine screening.
- Pregnant women can be followed every 12 weeks with cytology/colposcopy. Repeat biopsy is only indicated if the appearance of the lesion worsens.

AIS

- Hysterectomy is the treatment of choice for AIS.
- Diagnostic excisional procedure can be considered for women who want to maintain fertility. An endocervical curettage needs to be performed at the time of the resection.

SUGGESTED READINGS

American Society for Colposcopy and Cervical Pathology website readings and resources. http://www.asccp.org/edu/practice.shtml.

Cervical Cytology Screening. ACOG Practice Bulletin Number 109. American College of Obstetricians and Gynecologists. *Obstet Gynecol* 2009;114:1409–1420.

Cervical cancer in adolescents: screening, evaluation, and management. Committee Opinion Number 463. American College of Obstetricians and Gynecologists. *Obstet Gynecol* 2010; 116:469–472.

Cervical Cancer

Michelle Khan and Teresa P. Díaz-Montes

Cervical cancer is the most common gynecologic malignancy in the world, and the second most frequently diagnosed cancer in women worldwide after breast cancer. The majority of cases occur in developing countries. In the United States, cervical cancer is the third most common gynecologic malignancy and the second most common cause of gynecologic cancer death. Mortality and incidence rates for cervical cancer have declined in most developed countries due to the introduction of routine Papanicolaou smear (Pap test) and, more recently, human papillomavirus (HPV) screening.

EPIDEMIOLOGY OF CERVICAL CANCER

Approximately 60% of women diagnosed with cervical cancer in developed countries have either never been screened or have not been screened in the preceding 5 years. The mean age for cervical cancer is 52.2 years, and the distribution of cases is bimodal, with peaks at 35 to 39 years and 60 to 64 years.

Risk Factors for Cervical Cancer

- The main **risk factors** for cervical cancer include exposure to HPV, smoking, parity, and immunosuppression; other factors that have been linked with cervical cancer are race/socioeconomic status and sexually transmitted infections.
  - **HPV infection** is present in 99.7% of all cervical cancers. Thus, traditional risk factors for cervical cancer include early age at first coitus, multiple sexual partners, multiparity, lack of barrier contraception, and history of sexually transmitted infections.
    - High-risk HPV types 16, 18, 31, 33, 35, 45, 52, and 58 are associated with 95% of squamous cell carcinomas of the cervix. HPV 16 is most commonly linked with squamous cell cervical cancer. HPV 18 is most commonly present in adenocarcinoma.
    - Most HPV infections are transient, resulting in either no change in the cervical epithelium or low-grade intraepithelial lesions that are often spontaneously cleared. The progression from high-grade lesion to invasive cancer takes approximately 8 to 12 years, yielding a long preinvasive state with multiple opportunities for detection.
  - **Cigarette smoking** is an independent risk factor in the development of cervical disease. Smokers have a 4.5-fold increased risk of carcinoma in situ (CIS) compared with matched controls. Additionally, an increased risk of cervical cancer has been noted in women exposed passively to tobacco smoke. The potential effect of smoking appears to be limited to squamous cell carcinoma of the cervix.
  - **Immunosuppression** may increase the risk of developing cervical cancer, with more rapid progression from preinvasive to invasive lesions. Patients with human immunodeficiency virus (HIV) infection present earlier and with more advanced

disease than noninfected patients. The Centers for Disease Control has described cervical cancer as an AIDS defining illness.

- **Race and socioeconomic status**
  - ○ The incidence per 100,000 women per year of cervical cancer in the United States varies by ethnicity/race.
    - – Blacks 11, Whites 8, Native Americans 12, Hispanics 6, Asians 7
  - ○ These differences are partially accounted for by the increased risk of cervical cancer among women of low socioeconomic status. When access to care is made equal, the excess risk of cervical cancer precursor lesions among African American women decreases.
  - ○ Racial differences are also apparent in survival; 58% of all African Americans with cervical cancer survive 5 years, compared with 72% of all whites.

SCREENING, PRESENTATION, AND DIAGNOSIS

Cervical neoplasia is presumed to be a continuum from dysplasia to CIS to invasive carcinoma. **Screening** for cervical cancer with the use of an exfoliative cytologic study (i.e., Pap smear) has significant effects on the incidence, morbidity, and mortality of invasive disease by facilitating the discovery and early treatment of precursor lesions. See Chapter 42.

Clinical Presentation

- **Early symptoms**
  - Abnormal vaginal bleeding may take the form of postcoital bleeding, intermenstrual, or postmenopausal bleeding.
  - Serosanguineous or yellowish vaginal discharge, at times foul smelling, may occur.
- **Late symptoms**
  - Hematometra due to occlusion of the endocervical canal by a cancer.
  - Symptomatic anemia
  - Pelvic pain. Sciatic and back pain can be related to sidewall extension, hydronephrosis, or metastasis.
  - Bladder or rectal invasion by advanced-stage disease may produce urinary or rectal symptoms (e.g., vaginal passage of stool or urine, hematuria, urinary frequency, hematochezia).
  - Lower extremity swelling from occlusion of pelvic lymphatics or thrombosis of the external iliac vein.

Diagnosis of Cervical Cancer

- Most women with cervical cancer have a visible cervical lesion.
  - On **speculum examination**, cervical cancer may appear as an exophytic cervical mass (Fig. 43-1) that characteristically bleeds on contact. Endophytic tumors develop entirely within the endocervical canal, and the external cervix may appear normal. In these cases, bimanual examination may reveal a firm, indurated, and often barrel-shaped cervix. The vagina should be inspected for extension of disease. Rectal exam provides information regarding the nodularity of the uterosacral ligaments and helps determine extension of disease into the parametrium.
  - On **general physical examination**, advanced cervical cancer may present with pleural effusions, ascites, and/or lower extremity edema. Unilateral lower extremity

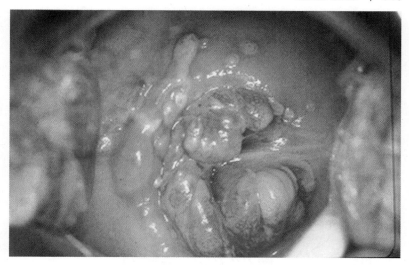

Figure 43-1. Photograph of the cervix demonstrating an exophytic cervical carcinoma. (Courtesy of Dr. Robert Giuntoli, The Johns Hopkins Hospital, Department of Gynecology and Obstetrics, Division of Gynecologic Oncology.)

edema may indicate involvement of the pelvic sidewall. Groin and supraclavicular lymph nodes may be indurated or enlarged, indicating spread of disease.

- With obvious exophytic lesions, cervical biopsy is usually all that is needed for histologic confirmation.
- In patients with a grossly normal cervix and abnormal cytology on Pap smear, colposcopic examination with directed biopsies and endocervical curettage (ECC) is necessary. See Chapter 42.
- If a definite diagnosis of cervical cancer cannot be made on the basis of office biopsies, diagnostic cervical conization may be necessary.

DISEASE PROGRESSION, STAGING, AND PROGNOSIS

Routes of Cervical Cancer Spread

- Cervical cancer usually spreads by **direct extension.**
  - **Parametrial extension.** The lateral spread of cervical cancer occurs through the cardinal ligament lymphatics and vessels, and significant involvement of the medial portion of this ligament may result in ureteral obstruction.
  - **Vaginal extension.** The upper vagina is frequently involved (50% of cases) when the primary tumor has extended beyond the confines of the cervix.
  - **Bladder and rectal involvement.** Anterior and posterior spread of cervical cancer to the bladder and rectum is uncommon in the absence of lateral parametrial disease.
- Cervical cancer may also progress via **lymphatic spread** (Fig. 43-2). The cervix is drained by preureteral, postureteral, and uterosacral lymphatic channels.
  - The following are considered first station nodes: obturator, external iliac, hypogastric, parametrial, presacral, and common iliac.

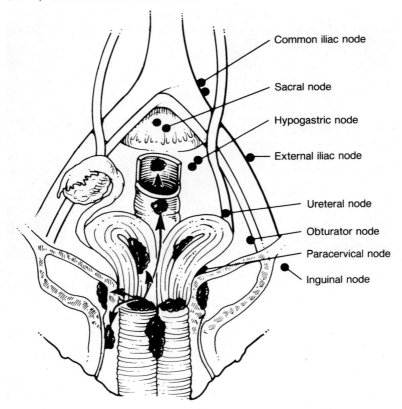

Common iliac node

Sacral node

Hypogastric node

External iliac node

Ureteral node

Obturator node

Paracervical node

Inguinal node

Figure 43-2. Possible sites of direct extension of cervical cancer to adjoining organs or metastases to regional lymph nodes. The uterus, cervix, and vagina are depicted bisected and opened to reveal the possible sites of tumor implantation. (From Scott JR, DiSaia PJ, Hammond CB, et al. *Danforth's Obstetrics and Gynecology,* 7th Ed. Philadelphia: Lippincott-Raven Publishers, 1997:909, with permission.)

- Paraaortic nodes are second station, are rarely involved in the absence of primary nodal disease, and are considered metastases.
- The percentage of involved lymph nodes increases directly with primary tumor volume and stage of disease.
- **Blood-borne metastases** from cervical carcinomas occur but are less frequent and are usually seen late in the course of the disease.

Staging of Cervical Cancer
- **Staging of cervical cancer** is based on clinical, rather than surgical, evaluation (Tables 43-1 and 43-2).
  - Routine laboratory studies should include a complete blood count (CBC), complete metabolic profile, and urinalysis. No tumor marker has achieved widespread acceptance.

- Inspection and palpation should begin with the cervix, vagina, and pelvis and continue with examination of extrapelvic areas, including the abdomen and supraclavicular lymph nodes.
- Lymphangiograms, arteriograms, computer tomography (CT), magnetic resonance imaging (MRI), positron emission tomography (PET), laparoscopy, or laparotomy findings are not used for clinical staging, but their results may be valuable for planning treatment. Imaging studies beyond the chest x-ray should be obtained only when the findings will have an impact on treatment.
- Cervical cancer is staged according to the **International Federation of Gynecology and Obstetrics (FIGO) system** (Table 43-1; Fig. 43-3). Lymph-vascular involvement does not alter the classification.
  - When doubt exists concerning the stage to which a tumor should be assigned, the earlier stage is chosen. Once a clinical stage has been determined and treatment has begun, subsequent findings do not alter the assigned stage. Overstaging and understaging of the parametria are problematic and may affect therapeutic decisions. FIGO stage correlates with prognosis, and strict adherence to the rules of clinical staging is necessary for comparison of results between institutions.
  - The distribution of patients by clinical stage is as follows: 38% stage I, 32% stage II, 25% stage III, 4% stage IV. Clinical stage of disease at the time of presentation is the most important determinant of survival regardless of treatment modality.
  - Five-year survival declines as FIGO stage at diagnosis increases from stage IA (95%) to stage IV (14%).
  - Only the subclassifications of stage I (IA1, IA2) require pathologic assessment.
- Vast discrepancies can exist between clinical staging and surgicopathologic findings, such that clinical staging fails to identify extension of disease to the para-aortic nodes in 7% of patients with stage IB disease, 18% with stage IIB, and 28% with stage III. Thus, some clinicians emphasize surgical staging in women with locally advanced cervical carcinoma to identify occult tumor spread and allow treatment of metastatic disease beyond the traditional pelvic radiation field.

Prognostic Factors for Cervical Cancer

- **Prognosis** is directly related to tumor characteristics including histologic subtype, histologic grade, FIGO stage, lymph node status, tumor volume, depth of invasion, and lymph-vascular space involvement (Table 43-3). Other prognostic variables include age, race, socioeconomic status, and immune status.

Histologic Subtype

- Conflicting data exist on the influence of histologic subtype on tumor behavior, prognosis, and survival.
  - **Invasive squamous cell carcinoma** is the most common histologic type of cervical cancer, comprising about 80% of cases. Squamous cell carcinomas are also subclassified according to cell type: **large cell keratinizing, large cell nonkeratinizing,** and **small cell** types. Rarer types include **verrucous carcinoma** and **papillary squamous cell carcinoma**
  - **Adenocarcinomas** comprise 15% of invasive cervical carcinomas. Grossly, cervical adenocarcinoma may appear as a polypoid or papillary exophytic mass. However, in nearly 15% of adenocarcinomas, the lesion is located entirely within the endocervical canal and escapes visual inspection.
    - **Mucinous adenocarcinoma** is the most common type and is well differentiated with plentiful mucin production.

TABLE 43-1 FIGO Staging System for Carcinoma of the Cervix (2009)

Stage	Description	Comments
I	**The carcinoma is strictly confined to the cervix (extension to the corpus would be disregarded)**	The diagnosis of both stage IA1 and IA2 cases should be based on microscopic examination of removed tissue, preferably a cone, which must include the entire lesion. The depth of invasion should not be more than 5 mm taken from the base of the epithelium, either surface or glandular, from which it originates. The depth of invasion should always be reported in mm, even in those cases with "early (minimal) stromal invasion" ~1 mm. The second dimension, the horizontal spread, must not exceed 7 mm. Vascular space involvement, either venous or lymphatic, should not alter the staging but should be specifically recorded because it may affect treatment decisions.
IA	Invasive carcinoma, which can be diagnosed only by microscopy, with deepest invasion ≤5 mm and largest extension ≤7 mm	
IA1	Measured stromal invasion of ≤3 mm in depth and extension of ≤7 mm.	
IA2	Measured stromal invasion of >3 mm and not >5 mm in depth with an extension of not >7 mm.	
IB	Clinically visible lesions limited to the cervix uteri or preclinical cancers greater than stage IA. All gross lesions, even with superficial invasion, are stage IB cancers.	As a rule, estimating clinically whether a cancer of the cervix has extended to the corpus or not in preclinical lesions higher than stage IA is impossible. Extension to the corpus should therefore be disregarded.
IB1	Clinically visible lesion ≤4 cm in greatest dimension.	
IB2	Clinically visible lesion >4 cm in greatest dimension.	

II	**Cervical carcinoma extends beyond the uterus but not to the pelvic wall or to the lower third of the vagina.**
IIA	Without parametrial invasion.
IIA1	Clinically visible lesion ≤4.0 cm in greatest dimension.
IIA2	Clinically visible lesion >4.0 cm in greatest dimension.
IIB	With obvious parametrial invasion.
III	**The tumor extends to the pelvic wall and/or involves the lower one third of the vagina and/or causes hydronephrosis or nonfunctioning kidney.**	On rectal examination, no cancer-free space is found between the tumor and the pelvic wall. Hydronephrosis or nonfunctioning kidney due to stenosis of the ureter by cancer and no other known cause permits a case to be allotted to stage III even if, according to the other findings, the case should be assigned to stage I or stage II.
IIIA	Tumor involves lower third of vagina, with no extension to the pelvic wall.
IIIB	Extension to the pelvic wall and/or hydronephrosis or nonfunctioning kidney.
IV	**The carcinoma has extended beyond the true pelvis or has involved (biopsy proven) the mucosa of the bladder or rectum**	The presence of bullous edema, as such, should not permit a case to be assigned to stage IV. Ridges and furrows in the bladder wall should be interpreted as signs of submucous involvement of the bladder if they remain fixed to the growth during palpation (i.e., examination from the vagina or the rectum during cystoscopy). A finding of malignant cells in cytologic washings from the urinary bladder requires further examination and biopsy of the wall of the bladder
IVA	Spread of the growth to adjacent organs.
IVB	Spread to distant organs.

Adapted from FIGO Committee on Gynecologic Oncology: Revised FIGO staging for carcinoma of the vulva, cervix, and endometrium. *Int J Gynecol Obstet* 2009;105:103–104.

TABLE 43-2	Staging Procedures for Cervical Cancer
Physical examination[a]	Palpation of lymph nodes Examination of vagina Bimanual rectovaginal examination (under anesthesia recommended)
Radiologic studies[a]	Intravenous pyelogram (IVP) Barium enema Chest radiograph Skeletal radiograph
Procedures[a]	Biopsy Conization Hysteroscopy Colposcopy Endocervical curettage Cystoscopy Proctoscopy
Optional studies[b]	*CT scan Lymphangiography Ultrasonography Magnetic Resonance Imaging (MRI) Radionuclide scanning Laparoscopy*

[a]Allowed for cervical cancer staging by International Federation of Gynecology and Obstetrics (FIGO).
[b]Information that is not allowed by FIGO to change the clinical stage but may be useful for treatment and planning. Adapted from Berek JS, Hacker NF, eds. *Practical Gynecologic Oncology*, 4th Ed. Baltimore: Williams & Wilkins, 2004.

- ○ **Endometrioid carcinoma**, 30% of cervical adenocarcinomas, resembles those typical of the uterine corpus.
- ○ **Clear cell carcinomas**, approximately 4% of adenocarcinomas, are nodular, reddish lesions with punctate ulcers and cells with abundant, clear cytoplasm. Diethylstilbestrol exposure is a risk factor.
- ○ **Minimal deviation adenocarcinoma**, or adenoma malignum, is reported to represent 1% of cervical adenocarcinomas.
- • Primary cervical carcinoma with both malignant-appearing glandular and squamous elements is referred to as **adenosquamous carcinoma**. The clinical behavior of these tumors is controversial, with some studies suggesting lower survival rates and others higher survival rates than with the more common squamous tumors.
- • **Small cell carcinomas** of the uterine cervix are similar to small cell neuroendocrine tumors of the lung and other anatomic locations. These tumors are clinically aggressive, with a marked propensity to metastasize. At diagnosis, disease is often disseminated, with bone, brain, and liver being the most common sites. Because of high metastatic potential, local therapy alone (surgery, radiation, or both) rarely results in long-term survival. Multiagent chemotherapy, in combination with external-beam and intracavitary radiation therapy, is the standard therapeutic approach.

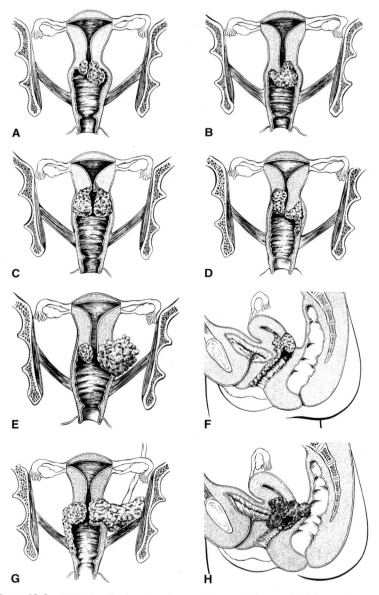

Figure 43-3. FIGO classification of carcinoma of the cervix. In stage I (**A,B**), only the cervix is involved. In stage II (**C,D,E**), the parametrium or upper two thirds of the vagina is involved. In stage III (**F,G**), the tumor involves the lower one third of the vagina or extends to the pelvic sidewall. In stage IV (**H**), areas beyond the true pelvis are involved or the bladder or rectal mucosa. (Adapted from Chi DS, Abu-Rustum NR, Hoskins WJ. Cancer of the cervix. In Rock JA, Jones HW III, eds. *TeLinde's Operative Gynecology,* 9th Ed. Philadelphia: Lippincott Williams & Wilkins, 2003:1378–1379, with permission.)

TABLE 43-3	Cervical Cancer Survival by FIGO Stage[a]
Stage	**5-Year Survival (%)**
IA	97.0
IB	78.9
IIA	54.9
IIB	51.6
IIIA	40.5
IIIB	27.0
IV	12.4

[a]Based on 1994 FIGO staging of carcinoma of the cervix uteri. From Kosary CL. FIGO stage, histology, histologic grade, age and race as prognostic factors in determining survival for cancers of the female gynecological system: an analysis of 1973–87 SEER cases of cancers of the endometrium, cervix, ovary, vulva, and vagina. *Semin Surg Oncol* 1994;10:31–46.

Histologic Grade
- Histologic differentiation of cervical carcinomas includes three grades.
  - Grade 1 tumors are **well differentiated** with mature squamous cells, often forming keratinized pearls of epithelial cells. Mitotic activity is low.
  - Grade 2 tumors are **moderately well-differentiated** carcinomas have higher mitotic activity and less cellular maturation accompanied by more nuclear pleomorphism.
  - Grade 3 tumors are composed of **poorly differentiated** smaller cells with less cytoplasm and often bizarre nuclei. Mitotic activity is high. Poorly differentiated tumors have lower 5-year survival rates.

Other Prognostic Factors
- The most important factor in the prognosis for cervical cancer is **clinical stage**.
- **Node status.** Among surgically treated patients, survival is related to the number and location of involved lymph nodes.
  - When pelvic nodes alone are involved, the 5-year survival rate is about 65%. Five-year survival drops to 25% when common iliac lymph nodes are positive, and involvement of para-aortic nodes further lowers survival. Bilateral pelvic lymph node involvement has a worse prognosis than unilateral disease.
- **Tumor volume.** Lesion size is an important predictor of survival, independent of other factors. Five-year survival rates for lesions <2 cm, 2 to 4 cm and >4 cm are approximately 90%, 60%, and 40%, respectively.
- **Depth of invasion.** Survival rates are inversely correlated with depth of stromal invasion.
- **Lymph-vascular space invasion.** No clear relationship exists between lymph-vascular space involvement and survival.

MANAGEMENT OF CERVICAL CANCER

Surgery and radiation therapy are the two modalities most commonly used to treat invasive cervical carcinoma.

Surgical Management
- In general, **primary surgical management** is limited to disease of stages I through IIA.

- Advantages of surgical therapy:
  - Allows for thorough pelvic and abdominal exploration, which can identify patients with a disparity between the clinical and surgicopathologic stages. These patients can be offered an individualized treatment plan based on their disease status.
  - Permits conservation of the ovaries with their transposition out of radiation treatment fields.
  - Avoids the use of radiation therapy and its complications.
- Disadvantages to surgical therapy:
  - Risks of surgery including bleeding, infection, damage to organs, vessels, and nerves.
  - Radical hysterectomy results in vaginal shortening; however, with sexual activity, gradual lengthening may occur.
  - Fistula formation (urinary or bowel) and incisional complications related to surgical treatment. These tend to occur early in the postoperative period and are usually amenable to surgical repair.
- Other indications for the selection of radical surgery over radiation:
  - Concomitant inflammatory bowel disease
  - Previous radiation for other disease
  - Presence of a simultaneous adnexal neoplasm
- The abdomen is opened through either a low transverse incision using the Maylard or Cherney method, or through a vertical midline incision. Once inside the peritoneal cavity, a thorough abdominal exploration should be performed to evaluate for visual or palpable metastases. Particular attention should be paid to the vesicouterine peritoneum for signs of tumor extension or implantation and palpation of the cardinal ligaments and the cervix. The para-aortic nodes should be palpated transperitoneally.
- Five distinct **classes of hysterectomy** are used in the treatment of cervical cancer (Table 43-4 and Fig. 43-4 for a brief comparison).
  - **Class I** hysterectomy refers to the standard **extrafascial total abdominal hysterectomy**. This procedure ensures complete removal of the cervix with minimal disruption to surrounding structures (e.g., bladder, ureters). This procedure may be performed in patients with stage IA1 cervical cancer.
  - **Class II** hysterectomy is also referred to as a **modified radical hysterectomy** or **Wertheim's hysterectomy** and is well suited for patients with stage IA2 and small lesions that do not distort the anatomy.
  - **Class III** hysterectomy, also known as **radical abdominal** or **Meigs' hysterectomy**, is recommended for stages IB and IIA.
  - **Class IV** or **extended radical hysterectomy** includes removal of the superior vesical artery, periureteral tissue, and up to three fourths of the vagina.
  - In a **class V** or **partial exenteration** operation, the distal ureters and a portion of the bladder are resected. Class IV and class V procedures are rarely performed today, because patients with disease extensive enough to require these operations can be more adequately treated using primary radiation therapy.
- In the past 15 years, surgeons have begun to investigate **minimally invasive methods** of treating early cervical cancers. These include laparoscopic procedures and, more recently, robotic laparoscopic procedures. Several small studies have compared laparoscopic and robotic radical hysterectomy with the open laparotomy approach. Findings include no significant differences in postoperative complications among the three groups, with longer mean operating times, shorter length of hospital

| TABLE 43-4 | Types of Abdominal Hysterectomy |

| | Type of Surgery | | | |
	Intrafascial	Extrafascial Class I	Modified Radical Class II	Radical Class III
Cervical fascia	Partially removed	Completely removed	Completely removed	Completely removed
Vaginal cuff	None removed	Small rim removed	Proximal 1–2 cm removed	Upper one-third to one-half removed
Bladder	Partially mobilized	Partially mobilized	Mobilized	Mobilized
Rectum	Not mobilized	Rectovaginal septum partially mobilized	Mobilized	Mobilized
Ureters	Not mobilized	Not mobilized	Unroofed in ureteral tunnel	Completely dissected to bladder entry
Cardinal ligaments	Resected medial to ureters	Resected medial to ureters	Resected at level of ureter	Resected at pelvic side wall
Uterosacral ligaments	Resected at level of cervix	Resected at level of cervix	Partially resected	Resected at postpelvic insertion
Uterus	Removed	Removed	Removed	Removed
Cervix	Partially removed	Completely removed	Completely removed	Completely removed

From Perez CA. Uterine cervix. In Perez CA, Brady LW, eds. *Principles and Practice of Radiation Oncology*, 2nd Ed. Philadelphia, PA: JB Lippincott, 1992, with permission.

stay, and smaller estimated blood loss for laparoscopic procedures compared with laparotomy.

Fertility-Preserving Surgical Options
- Fertility-preserving surgeries are used for younger women who have not completed childbearing and require treatment for early stage cervical cancer. These methods include **cervical conization** and **radical trachelectomy** (i.e., Dargent's operation) and appear to have similar recurrence rates to radical hysterectomy if candidates are selected appropriately.
  - Cervical conization is generally reserved for stage IA cervical cancers but has also been performed with lymphadenectomy for IB1 cancers. Of the few published studies, no recurrences were noted with a minimum of 14 months follow-up.
  - Radical trachelectomy can be performed for up to stage IB1 cancer with negative nodes, in patients with tumors <2 cm in diameter. The obstetric consequences for radical trachelectomy appear to be similar to those for loop electrosurgical excision

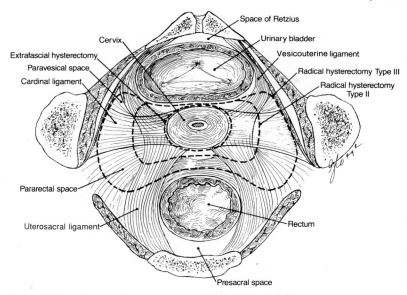

Figure 43-4. Diagram of pelvic anatomy and types of hysterectomy. (From Berek JS, Hacker NF. *Practical Gynecologic Oncology,* 4th Ed. Philadelphia: Lippincott Williams & Wilkins, 2005:356, with permission.)

procedure (LEEP) and conization, which include preterm delivery and low birth weight.

Primary Radiation Therapy

- **Radiation therapy** can be used for all stages of disease and for most patients, regardless of age, body habitus, or coexistent medical conditions. Radiation therapy should *not* be used in patients with diverticulosis, tubo-ovarian abscess, or pelvic kidney. Radiation therapy has evolved to include concurrent chemotherapy as a radiosensitizer, which results in improved disease-free progression and overall survival compared with radiation therapy alone.
- Preservation of sexual function is significantly related to the mode of primary therapy. Pelvic radiation produces persistent vaginal fibrosis and atrophy, with loss of both vaginal length and caliber. In addition, ovarian function is lost in virtually all patients who undergo tolerance-dose radiation therapy to the pelvis. Fistulous complications associated with radiation therapy tend to occur late and are more difficult to repair because of radiation fibrosis, vasculitis, and poorly vascularized tissues.
- The two main methods for delivering radiation therapy are external photon beam radiation and brachytherapy.
  - **External photon beam radiation** is usually delivered from a linear accelerator. Microscopic or occult tumor deposits from epithelial cancers require 4,000 to 5,000 cGy for local control. A clinically obvious tumor requires in excess of 6,000 cGy.
  - Once external therapy has been completed, **brachytherapy** can be delivered using various intracavitary techniques, including intrauterine tandem and vaginal

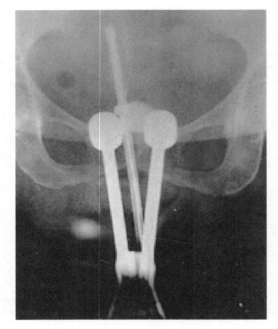

Figure 43-5. Brachytherapy: pelvic radiograph showing tandems and ovoids. (Image courtesy of Dr. Robert Giuntoli, The Johns Hopkins Hospital, Department of Gynecology and Obstetrics, Division of Gynecologic Oncology.)

colpostats, vaginal cylinders, or interstitial needle implants. The tandem is placed through the cervix into the uterus, and the ovoids are placed in the lateral vaginal fornices (Fig. 43-5). Brachytherapy can be delivered as low dose rates (LDR) or high-dose treatments. LDR treatments are inpatient over 3 to 4 days and receive 40 to 70 cGy/hr. High dose rate treatments may be delivered on an outpatient basis over five visits.

- ○ Two **reference points** are commonly used to describe the dose prescription for cervical cancer:
  - **Point A** is 2 cm lateral and 2 cm superior to the external cervical os and theoretically represents the area where the uterine artery crosses the ureter; and
  - **Point B** is 3 cm lateral to point A and corresponds to the pelvic sidewall and to the location of the obturator lymph nodes.
- ○ The cumulative dose to point A, regardless of method, adequate for central control is usually between 7,500 and 8,500 cGy. The prescribed dose to point B is 4,500 to 6,500 cGy, depending on the bulk of parametrial and sidewall disease.

Chemotherapy

- **Single agent chemotherapy** is used to treat patients with extrapelvic metastases as well as those with recurrent tumor who have been previously treated with surgery or radiation and are not candidates for exenteration procedures. The best candidates for chemotherapy are those with an excellent performance status and disease that is both outside of the field of radiation and not amenable to surgical resection. Cisplatin has been the most extensively studied agent and has demonstrated the most consistent clinical response rates (20% to 25%).

- The most active **combination chemotherapy** regimens for cervical cancer contain cisplatin. The agents most commonly used in combination with cisplatin are bleomycin, 5-fluorouracil, mitomycin C, methotrexate, cyclophosphamide, and doxorubicin. A limited number of randomized trials comparing dual agent regimens with either triple agent regimens or single agent regimens have demonstrated that combination therapy leads to a slightly higher response rate and a longer progression-free survival; however, no difference was found among the regimens in terms of overall survival.

Combined Modalities

- **Postoperative adjuvant radiation** therapy has been advocated for patients with microscopic parametrial invasion, pelvic lymph node metastases, deep cervical invasion, and positive or close surgical margins. Postoperative radiation therapy reduces the rate of pelvic recurrence after radical hysterectomy in high-risk patients.
- **Neoadjuvant chemotherapy.** Trials testing the efficacy of preoperative chemotherapy suggest improved outcomes, but results have been heterogeneous.
- **Chemoradiation** confers significant survival benefit over radiation alone in the treatment of cervical cancer. When combined with radiation, weekly cisplatin administration reduces the risk of progression for stage IIB through stage IVA cervical cancer. Cisplatin acts as a radiosensitizer, yielding a large reduction in the rate of local recurrence and a more modest reduction in the rate of distant metastases.

Management by Stage of Disease

- **Stage IA1.** Stage IA1 without lymph-vascular invasion is managed with conservative surgery, such as excisional conization or extrafascial hysterectomy. Conization may be used selectively if preservation of fertility is desired, provided that the surgical margins are free of disease. Patients treated with conization should be followed closely with Pap smear, colposcopy, and ECC every 3 months for the first year. For medically inoperable patients, stage IA carcinoma can be effectively treated with chemoradiation.
- **Stage IA2.** This is associated with positive pelvic lymph nodes in 5% of cases. The preferred treatment of these lesions is modified radical (class II) hysterectomy with pelvic lymphadenectomy. In patients who desire preservation of fertility, radical trachelectomy with laparoscopic or extraperitoneal lymphadenectomy may be performed.
  - In a **radical trachelectomy**, cervical and vaginal branches of the uterine artery are ligated, while the main trunk of the uterine artery is preserved. Once the blood supply has been controlled, the cervix is amputated at a point approximately 5 mm caudal to the uterine isthmus. The uterus is then suspended from the lateral stumps of the transected paracervical ligaments. Once the uterus has been suspended, isthmic cerclage is performed, using a technique similar to that used as prophylaxis against miscarriage. Subsequently, the vaginal and isthmic mucosa are reapproximated.
- **Stages IB1, IB2, IIA.** Radical hysterectomy (class III hysterectomy) and radiation are equally effective in treating stages IB and IIA carcinoma of the cervix (studies based on 1994 FIGO staging).
  - Management of patients with bulky stage I disease (IB2) is controversial. The two options are a class III hysterectomy or radiation. Often surgery is first performed

with postoperative radiation. Alternatively, a Gynecologic Oncology Group study showed that weekly cisplatin 40 mg/m^2 (six doses) with external radiation and a single implant to give 55 Gy at point B, followed by extrafascial hysterectomy, gave the best outcome.

- **Stages IIB, III, IVA, IVB.** Radiation therapy is the treatment of choice for patients with stage IIB and more advanced disease. Long-term survival rates with radiation therapy alone are approximately 70% for stage I disease, 60% for stage II disease, 45% for stage III disease, and 18% for stage IV disease. With the routine use of chemoradiation, long-term survival and disease-free progression are expected to increase for all stages of disease. Patients with stage IVB disease are usually treated with chemotherapy alone or chemotherapy in combination with local radiation. These patients have a uniformly poor prognosis regardless of treatment modality.

Treatment-Related Complications

- Modern surgical techniques and anesthesia have reduced the operative mortality rate. Febrile morbidity is common after radical hysterectomy due to typical postoperative reasons. Major causes of morbidity include lower extremity venous thrombosis, vesicovaginal fistulas (<1%), ureteral fistulas, permanent ureteral stenosis, voiding dysfunction, and pelvic lymphocyst formation.
- Acute complications of radiation therapy that occur during or immediately after therapy include uterine perforation, proctosigmoiditis, and acute hemorrhagic cystitis.
- Chronic complications that occur months to years after completing therapy include vaginal stenosis, rectovaginal and vesicovaginal fistulas, small bowel obstruction, and radiation-induced second cancers.

Posttreatment Surveillance

- Abdominal exam, leg and groin exam, speculum exam, bimanual rectovaginal examination, and evaluation of lymph nodes should be performed every 3 months for 3 years following treatment for cervical cancer. After the first 3 years, examinations should be done every 6 months for an additional 2 years, and every 6 months to 1 year thereafter. More frequent examinations are warranted if abnormal signs or symptoms develop. Pap smears should be obtained at every visit, with consideration for annual chest x-ray and IVP or abdominal pelvic CT.
- Cervical cancer detected within the first 6 months after therapy is termed **persistent cancer**. Disease diagnosed >6 months later is referred to as **recurrent disease**. Treatment of recurrent cervical cancer is dictated by the site of recurrence and by the mode of initial therapy. Only patients with central recurrence and no evidence of disease outside the pelvis are candidates for pelvic exenteration.

Special Management Issues

Cervical Cancer in Pregnancy
- Cervical cancer is the most common malignancy in pregnancy, ranging from 1 in 1,200 to 1 in 2,200 pregnancies. Cervical cancer coincident with pregnancy requires complex diagnostic and therapeutic decisions that may jeopardize both mother and fetus.
- The symptoms of cervical cancer are the same in pregnant patients and nonpregnant patients. Pregnant women are at risk of delay of diagnosis of cervical cancer. Directed cervical punch biopsies can be performed safely during pregnancy when high-grade intraepithelial lesions or microinvasion is suspected. ECC should be avoided due to the risk of rupturing the amniotic membranes. Cervical conization

should be performed only if it is strictly indicated and between 12 and 20 weeks' gestation.

- Pregnant women with cervical cancer should undergo the same evaluation as non-pregnant women. Because the bimanual examination may be difficult in pregnancy, MRI may be useful to identify extracervical disease.

- In patients with intraepithelial lesions or microinvasive disease stages IA1 and IA2, there appears to be no harm in delaying definitive therapy until after fetal lung maturity has been attained. Patients with less than 3 mm of invasion and no lymph-vascular space involvement may be followed to term and delivered vaginally. The major risk during delivery is hemorrhage due to tearing of the tumor. Recurrences of cervical cancer have been reported at the episiotomy site in women who deliver vaginally.

- Following vaginal delivery, these women should be reevaluated and treated at 6 weeks postpartum. If delivery is by cesarean section, extrafascial hysterectomy can be performed at the time of delivery or after a delay of 4 to 6 weeks if further childbearing is not desired. Patients with 3 to 5 mm of invasion or lymph-vascular invasion can also be safely followed until fetal lung maturity has been achieved. In these cases, however, surgical treatment should include a modified radical hysterectomy with pelvic lymph node dissection, performed either at the time of cesarean delivery or at 4 to 6 weeks postpartum. Radiation therapy is associated with survival rates comparable to those after surgical treatment.

- In patients with stages IB1, IB2, and IIA (studies based on 1994 FIGO staging), a delay in therapy in excess of 6 weeks may impact survival. If the diagnosis is made after 20 weeks' gestation, consideration may be given to postponing therapy until fetal viability because neonatal intensive care allows survival of greater than 90% for infants born after 28 weeks.

  - Standard treatment consists of classical cesarean delivery followed by radical hysterectomy and pelvic and para-aortic lymph node dissection; however, this procedure is associated with longer operative time and greater blood loss than in non-pregnant patients. Lower segment transverse cesarean section is not recommended because of the increased risk of cervical extension with this procedure that may increase intraoperative bleeding. Radiation therapy results in equivalent survival rates and may be preferable for patients who are poor surgical candidates.

Cervical Hemorrhage

- Profuse vaginal bleeding from cervical malignancies is a challenging therapeutic situation. Generally, conservative measures to control cervical hemorrhage are preferable to emergency laparotomy and vascular (i.e., hypogastric artery) ligation. Attention must first be directed toward the stabilization of the patient with appropriate intravenous fluid and blood product replacement.

- Immediate control of cervical hemorrhage can usually be accomplished with a vaginal pack soaked in Monsel's solution (ferric subsulfate). Topical acetone (dimethyl ketone) applied with a vaginal pack placed firmly against the bleeding tumor bed has also been used successfully to control vaginal hemorrhage from cervical malignancy.

- Definitive control of cervical hemorrhage can be accomplished with external radiation therapy of 180 to 200 cGy/day if the patient has not previously received tolerance doses of pelvic irradiation. Alternatively, arteriography can be used to identify the bleeding vessel(s), and Gelfoam or steel coil embolization can then be performed. Vascular embolization has the disadvantage of producing a hypoxic local tumor environment and potentially compromising the efficacy of subsequent radiation therapy.

SUGGESTED READINGS

Amant F, Van Calsteren K, Halaska MJ, et al. Gynecologic cancers in pregnancy: guidelines of an international consensus meeting. *Int J Gynecol Cancer* 2009;19(suppl 1): S1–12.

Green JA, Kirwan JM, Tierney JF, et al. Survival and recurrence after concomitant chemotherapy and radiotherapy for cancer of the uterine cervix: a systematic review and meta-analysis. *Lancet* 2001;358:781.

Hacker NF, Friedlander ML. Cervical cancer. In Berek JS, Hacker NF, eds. *Practical Gynecologic Oncology*, 4th Ed. Baltimore: Williams & Wilkins, 2005.

Schiffman M, Castle PE, Jeronimo J, et al. Human papillomavirus and cervical cancer. *Lancet* 2007;370:890–907.

44 Cancer of the Uterine Corpus

Alok C. Pant and Robert E. Bristow

Endometrial cancer is the fourth most common cancer in women and the most common gynecologic malignancy, accounting for 6% of all female cancers.

EPIDEMIOLOGY OF UTERINE CANCER

The American Cancer Society estimated 43,470 new cases and 7,950 deaths from endometrial cancer in 2010. The incidence has increased 0.8% each year since 1998. Seventy-two percent of cases will be localized at the time of diagnosis because endometrial cancer often presents with postmenopausal or irregular bleeding.

Risk Factors for Uterine Cancer

- A woman's risk of endometrial cancer increases with **age**. The median age at diagnosis is 61, and the peak incidence occurs from ages 55 to 70. Women over 50 account for 90% of the diagnoses of endometrial cancer and 5% develop disease before age 40.
- Other risk factors are based on **increased estrogen exposure**.
  - **Estrogen replacement** without concomitant progesterone carries a relative risk of 4.5 to 8.0 and persists for 10 years after treatment is stopped (Table 44-1).
  - **Chronic anovulation** states, such as seen in polycystic ovarian syndrome (PCOS), lead to constant estrogen stimulation of the endometrium and increase the risk of cancer due to the lack of a corpus luteum to produce progesterone.
  - **Obesity** increases endogenous estrogen by peripheral conversion of androstenedione to estrogen by aromatase in adipose tissues. Nearly 70% of early-stage endometrial cancer patients are obese. The relative risk of death increases with increasing body mass index (BMI), and a BMI >30 kg/m² will triple the risk of endometrial cancer.
  - **Nulliparity** (related to infertility) and **diabetes mellitus** are independent risk factors and have a relative risk of 2 to 3 for endometrial cancer while the association of **hypertension** seems related to obesity.
- A woman taking **tamoxifen** has an annual risk of 2 in 1,000 of developing endometrial cancer and 40% of women will develop cancer more than 12 months after stopping therapy.
- Women with **hereditary nonpolyposis colon cancer (HNPCC)** syndrome have a 39% risk of developing endometrial cancer by age 70.
- Some factors can decrease the risk of endometrial cancer.
  - Factors that decrease circulating estrogen, such as cigarette smoking and OCP use, may be protective.
  - OCPs decrease endometrial cancer risk by 40%, even up to 15 years after discontinuation, and this protection increases with length of use. Four years of use

TABLE 44-1	Risk Factors for Endometrial Cancer
Risk Factor	**Relative Risk**
Nulliparity	2.0
Estrogen replacement without progesterone	4–8
Obesity	
30–49 pounds	3.0
>50 pounds	10.0
Type 2 diabetes mellitus	2.8
Tamoxifen	2.2

From Barakat RR, Markman M, Randall ME, et al. Corpus: Epithelial tumors. In Hoskins WJ, Perez CA, Young RC, eds. *Principles and Practice of Gynecologic Oncology*, 2nd Ed. Philadelphia: Lippincott-Raven Publishers, 1997.

reduces risk by 56%, 8 years decreases risk by 67%, and 12 years of use decreases risk by 72%.

- **Hyperplasia** appears to be the precursor lesion for most endometrial cancer. A study that followed women for 10 years after a diagnosis of hyperplasia showed that the risk of progression to cancer increased from simple hyperplasia to complex, and the presence of atypia further increased the risk.
- A recent study revealed that 43% of hysterectomies performed in community hospitals for complex atypical hyperplasia will have endometrial cancer on final pathology.

PRESENTATION, EVALUATION, AND DIAGNOSIS

Clinical Presentation

- Endometrial cancer often presents as **postmenopausal bleeding**. In one study of women with postmenopausal bleeding, 7% had cancer, 56% had atrophy, and 15% had endometrial hyperplasia.
  - The likelihood that postmenopausal bleeding is due to cancer significantly increases with a woman's age. One study showed that 9% of women in their 50s with postmenopausal bleeding had endometrial cancer, whereas the rate was 16% for women in their 60s, 28% for women in their 70s, and 60% for women in their 80s.
- Although endometrial cancer is mostly a disease of postmenopausal women, 20% of cases are diagnosed before menopause. **Perimenopausal menometrorrhagia**, especially in women at high risk for endometrial cancer, should be investigated with endometrial biopsy.
- Likewise, **endometrial cells on a Pap smear** (obtained at a time remote from recent or impending menstrual period) in women over age 40 can signal endometrial cancer and should trigger a workup.
- The rate of endometrial adenocarcinoma in a woman over the age of 35 with a Pap smear result of **atypical glandular cells of undetermined significance** is 23%.
- Routine Pap smear will only detect 50% of cases of endometrial cancer and is not a screening test.

Tamoxifen

- Women who are on **tamoxifen** have an increased risk of developing endometrial cancer.
- Routine screening with ultrasound or endometrial biopsies has not been proven effective in providing earlier diagnosis and is therefore not recommended in this setting.
  - Use of ultrasound for screening is of limited use because tamoxifen causes subepithelial stromal hypertrophy and therefore increases the thickness of the endometrial stripe and may result in unnecessary surgical procedures.
- Women on tamoxifen should be followed with yearly pelvic exams and should report any vaginal bleeding. Any episode of vaginal bleeding should trigger an evaluation.
- After discontinuing tamoxifen, patients should be closely followed for symptoms of abnormal vaginal bleeding as the median time from cessation of therapy to developing endometrial cancer is 33 months.

HNPCC

- Women with HNPCC have such a high risk of endometrial cancer (as high as 50% lifetime) that prophylactic hysterectomy should be considered. Only six prophylactic hysterectomies need to be performed to prevent one case of endometrial cancer.

Evaluation and Diagnosis of Postmenopausal Bleeding

- The appropriate evaluation for postmenopausal bleeding is much debated. Ultrasound and endometrial biopsy are the two main tools available.

Ultrasound

- **Pelvic ultrasound** measurement of the endometrial stripe can be used with a minimum cutoff of 5 mm in thickness.
- The Postmenopausal Estrogen/Progestins Interventions (PEPI) trial showed that with a 5 mm stripe cutoff, pelvic ultrasound has a positive predictive value of 9%, a negative predictive value of 99%, a sensitivity of 90%, and a specificity of 48% for endometrial cancer.
- Meta-analysis shows that the posttest probability of cancer following a pelvic ultrasound with a stripe <5 mm is 2.5%. If the stripe is >5 mm, the posttest probability of cancer is 32%.
- If ultrasound is used as the first step, 50% of women will require further evaluation.

Biopsy

- **Endometrial biopsy** provides a cancer detection rate of 99.6% in premenopausal women and 91% in postmenopausal women. Specificity is 98%, and sensitivity is 99%. The false-negative rate is between 5% and 15%.
- The posttest probability of endometrial cancer is 82% if the biopsy is positive and 0.9% if it is negative. However, a biopsy read as "insufficient sample" should trigger further evaluation because 20% of these women will be found to have pathology on further investigation, and 3% will have cancer.

Further workup

- No matter which method is used for initial evaluation, if bleeding persists or clinical suspicion is high, further evaluation with a **dilation and curettage (D&C)** should be pursued. The false-negative rate of a D&C is 2% to 6%.
- **Hysteroscopy** with D&C has a positive predictive value of 96%, a negative predictive value of 98%, a sensitivity of 98%, and a specificity of 95%. If hysteroscopy is performed, consideration should be given to using CO_2 as the distention medium

rather than fluid, so as to minimize the risk of iatrogenically introducing malignant cells into the peritoneal cavity via transtubal migration.

- A recent Gynecology Oncology Group (GOG) prospective study demonstrated the difficulty in diagnosing complex atypical hyperplasia (CAH). One third of cases of CAH were deemed to be "less than" CAH by study pathologists, 1/3 were deemed to be "greater than" CAH (i.e., endometrial cancer), and 1/3 of the diagnoses were consistent with the original diagnosis of CAH.

STAGING AND PROGNOSIS

Surgical Staging Procedures

- Staging for endometrial cancer is done surgically, and because many patients have early-stage disease at the time of diagnosis, this is often the only intervention necessary. **Surgical staging** includes exploratory laparotomy, peritoneal cytologic washings, total hysterectomy and bilateral salpingo-oophorectomy, cytoreduction of all visible disease, and pelvic and periaortic lymph node dissection.
- The lymphatics of the uterine fundus drain to the aortic nodes; the lower uterine segment drains to the internal and external iliac lymph nodes; and the round ligaments can drain to the superficial inguinal lymph nodes. **Pelvic and para-aortic lymph node dissection** is required for surgical staging of endometrial cancer. Morbid obesity may make a lymph node dissection more challenging, but it is still a required component of the procedure if indicated based on histologic and pathologic risk factors (see below).
  - The decision as to whether or not to proceed to lymph node dissection is often made in the operating room based on frozen section evaluation of the uterus for histologic cell type, tumor differentiation (grade), and depth of myometrial invasion.
  - Lymph node dissection, if deemed surgically possible, should be pursued in the following instances: the presence of invasion to the outer one third of the myometrium (any grade), high-grade differentiation with any myometrial invasion, clear cell histology, papillary serous histology, tumor size >2 cm in maximal diameter, lymph-vascular space invasion, cervical or lower uterine segment invasion, adnexal involvement, clinically bulky lymph nodes, or disease outside of the uterus.
- Women without any of these risk factors have <5% risk of positive lymph nodes and >90% 5-year survival rate with a TAH-BSO. However, with the presence of any of these risk factors, the risk of positive lymph nodes increases to >10% and 5-year survival rate decreases to 70% to 85% without further treatment (Table 44-2).
- The presence of lymph-vascular space invasion (LVSI) is also predictive of positive lymph nodes. LVSI portends a 27% risk of positive pelvic nodes, and a 19% chance of positive para-aortic lymph nodes.
- Recent data have shown a >50% incidence of any myometrial invasion in patients with a preoperative diagnosis of complex atypical hyperplasia.
- Routine computed tomography scan rarely alters management and is a poor predictor of nodal disease, and magnetic resonance imaging has not been shown to have sufficient accuracy to predict myometrial invasion. Neither modality should be used to determine which patient should undergo lymphadenectomy.
- Approximately 50% of positive lymph nodes will be <1 cm. Palpation and visual evaluation of retroperitoneal lymph nodes should not be considered diagnostic. Additionally, gross examination of myometrial invasion should not be utilized to

TABLE 44-2	Lymph Node Metastasis by Grade and Depth of Invasion of Endometrial Cancer		
	Pelvic Lymph Nodes (%)		
Grade	**No Invasion**	**Inner 1/3**	**Mid 1/3**	**Outer 1/3**
1	0	3	0	11
2	3	5	9	19
3	0	9	4	34
	Para-aortic Lymph Nodes (%)		
1	0	1	5	6
2	3	4	0	14
3	0	4	0	23

From Creasman W, et al. Surgical pathologic spread patterns of endometrial cancer. A Gynecologic Oncology Group Study. *Cancer* 1987;60:2035–2041.

determine who should undergo lymphadenectomy, as this is less accurate than frozen section evaluation.
- Multiple recent series from different institutions have shown the feasibility and accuracy of **laparoscopic and robotic staging** for endometrial cancer. Minimally invasive surgical staging is generally well tolerated and results in equivalent overall survival and recurrence rates. A survey of the members of the Society of Gynecologic Oncology showed that >50% of its members utilize some form of laparoscopic-assisted staging.
  - A recent meta-analysis including 331 patients demonstrated fewer postoperative complications, less blood loss, longer operating time, shorter hospital stay, and no significant difference between overall survival and recurrence when minimally invasive surgical techniques were utilized versus open surgery for endometrial cancer.
  - The GOG conducted a prospective trial following 2,213 women, of whom 76% were successfully staged laparoscopically. Laparotomy was required in 23% of cases. No difference was noted in peritoneal cytology, lymph node metastases or stage.

Staging of Endometrial Cancer
- Staging is based on surgical findings, as described in the FIGO 2009 staging criteria. In this new staging system, positive cytology no longer changes the stage, but is still reported.
  - Stage **IA**: cancer confined to the uterus and anything <50% of the myometrium.
  - Stage **IB**: myometrial invasion that is equal to or >50% of the myometrium but still confined to the uterus.
  - Stage **II**: tumor invades cervical stroma but does not extend beyond the uterus.
    ○ Endocervical glandular involvement is considered Stage I.
  - Stage **IIIA**: tumor invades the serosa of the corpus uteri and/or adnexae. Positive cytology has to be reported separately without changing the stage.
  - Stage **IIIB**: vaginal and/or parametrial involvement.
  - Stage **IIIC**: metastases to pelvic and/or para-aortic lymph nodes.
    ○ **IIIC1**: positive pelvic nodes.

○ **IIIC2**: positive para-aortic lymph nodes with or without positive pelvic lymph nodes.
- Stage **IVA**: tumor invasion of bladder and/or bowel mucosa
- Stage **IVB**: distant metastases, including intra-abdominal metastases and or inguinal lymph nodes

Histopathologic Factors for Endometrial Cancer

- **Type I** endometrial cancers are estrogen dependent, arise in a background of hyperplasia, and are of endometrioid histology.
- **Type II** tumors are not estrogen dependent, arise in a background of endometrial atrophy, are poorly differentiated, and are often of a serous or clear cell histology.
- Endometrioid cancers make up 75% to 80% of endometrial cancers. Clear cell cancers are 5% of endometrial cancers. Uterine papillary serous (UPSC) make up 5% to 10% of endometrial cancers. These cancers histologically resemble papillary serous ovarian cancers. Some recent reports link BRCA1 or BRCA2 mutations with UPSC.
- The PTEN tumor suppressor gene, K-ras oncogene, and microsatellite instability resulting from mutations in DNA mismatch repair proteins (e.g., MLH1, MSH2, or MSH6) are associated with endometrioid cancer pathogenesis and complex atypical hyperplasia.
- UPSC tends to metastasize early (72% have extrauterine spread at the time of diagnosis) and metastasize more like an ovarian cancer by spreading throughout the peritoneal cavity. Therefore, omentectomy along with upper abdominal and peritoneal biopsies should be performed as part of surgical staging for a known UPSC.
- Sarcomas (including mixed müllerian mesodermal tumors [MMMTs], leiomyosarcomas [LMSs], and endometrial stromal sarcomas [ESSs]) make up the remaining 2% to 5% of uterine cancers.
- **Tumor grade** affects the risk of spread and recurrence and is therefore important in determining the need for adjuvant therapy.
  - **Grade 1** tumors have <5% solid, nonsquamous, or morular component.
  - **Grade 2** tumors are 6% to 50% composed of these features.
  - **Grade 3** tumors have these features in >50% of the tumor.

Prognostic Factors for Endometrial Cancer

- The most significant prognostic factors for recurrence and survival are stage, grade, and depth of myometrial invasion. Age, histologic type, LVSI, and progesterone receptor activity also have prognostic significance. LVSI is associated with a 35% rate of recurrence.
- Positive peritoneal cytology is controversial as a prognostic factor. Multiple large studies show conflicting results. While positive peritoneal cytology is associated with adverse features such as extrauterine disease, therapy for this finding as an isolated result does not improve survival.
- Prognosis for the more aggressive histologic types is less favorable. Even without myometrial invasion, 36% of UPSC cancers will have positive lymph nodes.
  - Five-year survival for disease stages I to II is 36% and is unusual for more advanced disease
  - Clear cell cancer portends a 72% 5-year survival for stage I disease and a 60% 5-year survival for stage II disease.
  - Overall 5-year survival for the aggressive histologic subtypes is 40%
- Relapses tend to occur distally, often in the lungs, liver, or bones.

MANAGEMENT OF ENDOMETRIAL CANCER

Appropriate treatment is determined by stage, grade, histologic type, and the patient's ability to tolerate therapies (Table 44-3).

- Patients with **low-risk endometrial cancer** of endometrioid type require no further therapy beyond surgery. Stage IA Grade 1 and 2 and Stage IA Grade 3 without any LVSI are considered low risk. The risk of recurrence for these low-risk patients is 3.2% over 10 years. These data may need to be updated in light of the new staging system.

Management of High Risk Endometrial Cancer

- Treatment for women with higher risk disease is more controversial. Multiple studies have sought to define the appropriate role for adjuvant therapy.

Radiation Therapy
- The Post Operative Radiation Therapy in Endometrial Carcinoma (PORTEC) study randomized women with stage IC Grade 1, stage IB and stage IC Grade 2, or stage IA Grade 3 (under 1988 FIGO Staging). All women were treated with TAH-BSO without a lymph node dissection. These women were then randomized to receive or not receive **pelvic radiation** with 4,600 cGy.
  - Local recurrence occurred in 4.2% of radiated women versus 13.7% of those not radiated. However, the rate of death from cancer was not statistically different between the two groups (9.2% vs 6.0%, respectively).
  - Additionally, radiation therapy for vaginal recurrence in the nonradiated group was successful in inducing a complete response in 89%, and 5-year survival of this salvage radiation group was 65%. Therefore, postoperative radiation can significantly increase local control but does not appear to impact survival. The authors concluded that postoperative radiation should be limited to women with two out of three risk factors: greater than age 60, stage IC, or grade 3.
  - One problem with the PORTEC data was the lack of full surgical staging. The GOG addressed this in a phase III trial of 392 intermediate-risk patients who underwent TAH/BSO and lymph node surgery followed by observation (12% recurrence and 86% 4 year survival) versus radiation therapy (3% recurrence and 92% 4 year survival) and found similar results to the PORTEC data.
- A multicenter retrospective trial demonstrated an 81% response rate to salvage radiation for isolated vaginal recurrences in surgical Stage I patients who did not initially receive adjuvant radiation.

Cytoreductive Surgery
- Stage II uterine cancer significantly increases the risk for vaginal recurrence. If cervical involvement is known preoperatively, a **radical hysterectomy** should be considered, which has been shown to result in a 75% 5-year survival rate. A combination of extrafascial hysterectomy followed by radiation is associated with a 5-year survival rate of 70%. If the diagnosis is made postoperatively, vaginal brachytherapy should be offered.
- These data may need to be updated in light of the new staging system.
- For stages III and IV cancers, **optimal cytoreductive surgery** has been shown to improve survival. Adjuvant therapy after cytoreduction is advised; however, the optimal mode of adjuvant therapy is unclear.

TABLE 44-3   Management Recommendations For Uterine Cancer by Stage and Grade

Stage[a]	Grade 1	Grade 2	Grade 3
IA	Observe	Observe	Observe or vaginal brachytherapy or pelvic radiation with or without vaginal brachytherapy
IB	Observe	Observe or vaginal brachytherapy or pelvic radiation with or without vaginal brachytherapy	Vaginal brachytherapy or pelvic radiation with or without vaginal vaginal brachytherapy
IC	Observe or vaginal brachytherapy or pelvic radiation with or without vaginal brachytherapy	Pelvic radiation with or without vaginal brachytherapy	Pelvic radiation with or without vaginal brachytherapy
IIA myometrial invasion (<50%)	Observe or vaginal brachytherapy	Vaginal brachytherapy	Pelvic radiation and vaginal brachytherapy
IIA myometrial invasion (>50%)	Pelvic radiation and vaginal Brachytherapy	Pelvic radiation and vaginal brachytherapy	Pelvic radiation and vaginal brachytherapy
IIB	Pelvic radiation and vaginal brachytherapy	Pelvic radiation and vaginal brachytherapy	Pelvic radiation and vaginal brachytherapy
IIA Positive cytology only, tumor confined to fundus, noninvasive	Observe	Observe	Observe or vaginal brachytherapy or pelvic radiation with or without vaginal brachytherapy.
IIIA all others	Pelvic radiation or whole abdomino-pelvic radiation with or without vaginal brachytherapy or chemotherapy on protocol only	Pelvic radiation or whole abdomino- pelvic radiation with or without vaginal brachytherapy or chemotherapy on protocol only	Pelvic radiation or whole abdomino- pelvic radiation with or without vaginal brachytherapy or chemotherapy on protocol only

[a]Recommendations are based on 1988 FIGO staging criteria. From Benedet JL, Bender H, Jones H 3rd, et al. FIGO staging classifications and clinical practice guidelines in the management of gynecologic cancers. FIGO Committee on Gynecologic Oncology. *Int J Gynaecol Obstet* 2000 Aug;70(2):209–262.

- Complete **salvage cytoreduction** for recurrent disease has been associated with a prolonged postrecurrence survival (39 months) versus patients with gross residual disease (13.5 months).

Chemotherapy
- Chemotherapy can also be used; however, the optimal chemotherapy regimen for endometrial cancer is unknown. Single-agent response rates are low. Multiple trials have been conducted with various regimens.
- Cisplatin and doxorubicin together have a 43% response rate. The addition of paclitaxel to the cisplatin and doxorubicin regimen in a randomized trial conducted by the GOG resulted in an increase in response rate and survival. There was a significantly higher rate of peripheral neuropathy in the group treated with paclitaxel.
- Neither Megace combined with cyclophosphamide, doxorubicin, and fluorouracil nor Megace combined with fluorouracil and melphalan has proven to be superior to single-agent regimens.
- Patients who fail first-line chemotherapy generally have a very poor prognosis with a response rate to second- and third-line agents of <10% and overall survival of <9 months.

Posttreatment Surveillance

- After treatment, surveillance for recurrence should include an examination every 3 to 6 months for 2 years and then annually. Vaginal cytology should be performed every 6 months for 2 years and then each year. If serum CA125 was elevated at the time of diagnosis, it can be followed at each visit. Most recurrences are diagnosed by symptoms.

Special Problems

Clear Cell and UPSC Endometrial Cancer
- These are often treated with adjuvant therapy regardless of stage. Adjuvant chemotherapy and pelvic radiation are appropriate. Despite therapy, these tumors are often very aggressive.
- The overall 5-year disease-free survival for clear cell endometrial cancers is only 40%. Relapses are often distant and tend to occur in the lungs, liver, and bone.
- As opposed to Type I endometrial cancers, the precursor lesion to UPSC is endometrial intraepithelial carcinoma not endometrial hyperplasia. UPSC usually shows evidence of LVSI, and 36% of women with no myometrial invasion will have positive lymph nodes. Five-year survival is only 30% to 50% for stage I disease.
- As in ovarian cancer, chemotherapy regimens with carboplatinum and taxol have been the most successful.
- Multiple recent reports have suggested that Stage IA patients, after undergoing complete surgical staging, may not require adjuvant therapy. Three year overall survival rates range from 95% to 100%. These data may need to be updated in light of the new staging system.

Fertility Preservation
- Women with very early endometrial cancer who wish to preserve their fertility have been treated with progesterone rather than surgery. A review of 81 patients with stage IA1 endometrial cancer treated with progesterone revealed the following:
  - Seventy-six percent responded with median time to response of 12 weeks, and median duration of treatment was 24 weeks. Of those who responded, 24% recurred, and median time to recurrence was 19 months.

- Forty-seven percent of the women who recurred were retreated, and seventy-two percent had a second complete response.
- A multicenter prospective study examined 28 women with endometrial carcinoma and 17 women with atypical hyperplasia who were treated with progesterone.
  - Complete response was noted in 55% of the patients with carcinoma and 82% of those with atypical hyperplasia. The patients were followed for 3 years during which there were 12 pregnancies and a 47% recurrence rate.
- A recent prospective trial followed 105 women with endometrial hyperplasia treated with a levonorgestrel-releasing intrauterine device and showed a 90% regression rate after 2 years.
- Women who wish to retain their fertility should be counseled that risks are associated with such an approach, and a TAH-BSO is recommended after childbearing is completed.
- D&C should be done to confirm pathology. An MRI is recommended to assess for myometrial invasion. D&C should be repeated every 3 months to assess response.

Incomplete Surgical Staging
- Treatment depends on risk factors.
- Grade 1 or 2 tumors with <50% myometrial invasion have a <10% risk of having positive lymph nodes and >90% 5-year survival without any further treatment.
- However, any grade 3 cancer or grade 1 and 2 cancers with more than 50% invasion pose a >10% risk of positive pelvic lymph nodes, and 5-year survival is decreased to 70% to 85% without further treatment. Therefore, restaging or use of adjuvant radiation is appropriate. Laparoscopic node dissection can be used for patients who were incompletely staged at their initial surgery. Additionally, FDG-PET scanning may hold promise for evaluating lymphadenopathy but further study is needed.

Medical Contraindications to Surgery
- Women who are medically unable to undergo surgery can be treated with pelvic radiation alone. However, 5-year survival for clinical stage I disease is decreased to 69% with this approach versus 87% for surgery alone.
- It has been shown that for stage I disease with a preoperative CA-125 of <20 U/mL, the risk of extrauterine spread was only 3%. In these cases, vaginal hysterectomy is a therapeutic option for those women unable to undergo a more extensive operation.
- In a small series of patients with a well-differentiated endometrial adenocarcinoma, a progestin-secreting intrauterine device has been shown to be effective therapy.

UTERINE SARCOMA

Sarcomas represent 5% of uterine cancers. They usually present with postmenopausal bleeding, and often on exam the woman will be found to have a fungating mass protruding from her cervix. They are divided based on their sarcomatous elements.

Staging of Uterine Sarcoma
- In 2009, a **staging system for uterine sarcomas** was defined:
  - Stage **IA**: tumor limited to the uterus and <5 cm.
  - Stage **IB**: tumor ≥5 cm.
  - Stage **IIA**: adnexal involvement.
  - Stage **IIB**: tumor extends to extrauterine pelvic tissue.
  - Stage **IIIA**: tumor invades into one site of abdominal tissue.

- Stage **IIIB**: tumor invades into more than one site of abdominal tissue.
- Stage **IIIC**: metastasis to pelvic and/or para-aortic lymph nodes.
- Stage **IVA**: tumor invades bladder and/or rectum.
- Stage **IVB**: distant metastasis.

Mixed Müllerian Mesodermal Tumors

- **Mixed müllerian mesodermal tumors** are carcinosarcomas and the most aggressive of the sarcomas. They are often large and necrotic. Carcinosarcoma is an independent predictor of survival with a hazard ratio of 3.2 for recurrence compared to the other histologies. Thus, carcinosarcoma should be studied separately from high-risk endometrial cancers given the difference in behavior. Previous pelvic radiation is associated with the development of carcinosarcoma.
- The 5-year survival rate is 50% for stage I tumors and 20% for stage IV.
- Lymph node dissection has not been shown to be therapeutic for these tumors. Stage and mitotic grade are the most predictive of disease course.
- Chemotherapy regimens, including cisplatin, doxorubicin, ifosfamide, and paclitaxel, have been used for MMMT.

Leiomyosarcoma

- **Leiomyosarcomas** are the next most aggressive uterine sarcoma. They usually arise in the myometrium and rarely in fibroids. Vaginal bleeding is the most common presenting symptom. Ten percent of patients will have lung metastases at the time of diagnosis. The typical picture is a postmenopausal woman with a rapidly enlarging fibroid.
- In a series of 1,432 patients who underwent a hysterectomy for a fibroid uterus, only 0.49% were found to have LMS. Another series of 1,332 patients who underwent hysterectomy for fibroids had a subset of patients with "rapidly growing fibroids" and only 0.2% were found to have LMS.
- These tumors appear like leiomyomas but have >10 mitoses per 10 high power fields and diffuse nuclear atypia. Additionally, the presence of coagulative necrosis is suggestive of LMS.
- No benefit of adjuvant radiation has been noted.

Endometrial Stromal Sarcoma

- **Endometrial stromal sarcomas (ESS)** arise from the endometrium and can be separated into low and high grade. They represent 10% of sarcomas. They are the least aggressive uterine sarcomas. However, even in low-grade ESS, 36% will relapse and 10% will die from the disease.
- Low-grade ESS often responds to progestins and aromatase inhibitors. Higher grade ESS should be treated with surgery and pelvic radiation. Chemotherapy has not been shown to be beneficial; however, with metastatic disease, doxorubicin and ifosfamide have been used.

Prognosis for Uterine Sarcoma

- A retrospective study including women with all forms of sarcoma showed a 3-year survival rate of 82%, 60%, and 20% for sarcomas with low-, medium-, and high-grade histology, respectively.
- Three-year survival was 56%, 45%, 33%, and 5% for stages I, II, III, and IV sarcomas. These data may need to be updated in light of the revised staging criteria.

- Survival rates of 77%, 60%, and 30% were seen for sarcomas treated with surgery and then pelvic radiation with vaginal brachytherapy, surgery with just pelvic radiation, and no adjuvant therapy, respectively.

SUGGESTED READINGS

Ben-Shachar I, Pavelka J, Cohn DE, et al. Surgical staging for patients presenting with grade 1 endometrial carcinoma. *Obstet Gynecol* 2005;105:487–493.

Bristow RE, et al. Salvage cytoreductive surgery for recurrent endometrial cancer. *Gynecol Oncol* 2006;103:281–287.

Chan JK, Cheung MK, Huh WK, et al. Therapeutic role of lymph node resection in endometrioid corpus cancer: a study of 12,333 patients. *Cancer* 2006;107:1823–1830.

Chung HH, Kang SB, Cho JY, et al. Accuracy of MR imaging for the prediction of myometrial invasion of endometrial carcinoma. *Gynecol Oncol* 2007;104:654–659.

Lin F, Zhang QJ, Zheng FY, et al. Laparoscopically assisted versus open surgery for endometrial cancer—a meta analysis of randomized controlled trials. *Int J Gynecol Cancer* 2008;18(135):1315–1325.

Management of endometrial cancer. ACOG Practice Bulletin Number 65. American College of Obstetricians and Gynecologists. *Obstet Gynecol* 2005;65:413.

Mutch DG. The new FIGO staging system for cancers of the vulva, cervix, endometrium and sarcomas. *Gynecol Oncol* 2009;115:325–328.

Thomas MB, Mariani A, Cliby WA, et al. Role of systematic lymphadenectomy and adjuvant therapy in stage I uterine papillary serous carcinoma. *Gynecol Oncol* 2007;107:186–189.

Trimble CL, Kauderer J, Zaino R, et al. Concurrent endometrial carcinoma in women with a biopsy diagnosis of atypical endometrial hyperplasia: a Gynecologic Oncology Group study. *Cancer* 2006;106:812–819.

von Gruenigen VE, Tian C, Frasure H, et al. Treatment effects, disease recurrence, and survival in obese women with early endometrial carcinoma: a Gynecologic Oncology Group study. *Cancer* 2006;107:2786–2791.

Zaino RJ, Kauderer J, Trimble CL, et al. Reproducibility of the diagnosis of atypical endometrial hyperplasia: a Gynecologic Oncology Group study. *Cancer* 2006;106:804–811.

Ovarian Cancer

Joyce N. Barlin and Robert L. Giuntoli, II

Ovarian cancer accounts for 3% of cancers in women and is the fifth leading cause of cancer-related death in American women, after lung, breast, colorectal, and pancreatic cancers. Ovarian cancer is the second most common gynecologic cancer, following cancer of the uterine corpus.

EPIDEMIOLOGY OF OVARIAN CANCER

For women in the United States, lifetime risk of developing the disease is estimated to be 1 in 70 (1.4%). This likelihood increases with age, with a median age at diagnosis of 63 years.

- The risk of malignancy in an adnexal mass is 7% in a premenopausal woman and rises to 30% in a postmenopausal woman. Each year an estimated 21,650 women will be diagnosed, and 15,520 will die from their ovarian cancer. Ovarian cancer has the highest mortality of all female reproductive system malignancies.
- Ovarian neoplasms, 80% of which are benign, are divided into three major groups: epithelial, germ cell, and sex cord–stromal tumors (Table 45-1). The ovary can also be a site of metastatic cancer, particularly from the breast or the gastrointestinal tract (e.g., Krukenberg's tumors).

EPITHELIAL OVARIAN TUMORS

Tumors derived from the coelomic epithelium are the most common ovarian neoplasms, accounting for 65% of ovarian neoplasms and 90% of ovarian cancers. Types include serous, mucinous, endometrioid, clear cell, and transitional (Brenner's).

Risk Factors

- Age over 40 years, white race, nulliparity, infertility, history of endometrial or breast cancer, and family history of ovarian cancer consistently have been found to increase the risk of invasive epithelial cancer. Higher parity, use of oral contraceptive pills (OCPs), history of breast-feeding, tubal ligation, and hysterectomy have been associated with a decreased risk of ovarian cancer.
- Patients with a **family history** of ovarian, breast, endometrial, or colon cancer are at increased risk of developing ovarian carcinoma.
  - Hereditary familial ovarian cancer accounts for approximately 10% of all newly diagnosed cases. Women with one first-degree relative with ovarian cancer have a 5% lifetime risk of developing the disease and those with two first-degree relatives with ovarian cancer have a 7% risk.
  - There are three distinct autosomal dominant syndromes that have been termed familial ovarian cancer: site-specific ovary, breast-ovary, and hereditary nonpolyposis colorectal cancer (HNPCC, or Lynch syndrome).

TABLE 45-1	Classification of Ovarian Neoplasms

Epithelial Tumors
Serous (histology resembles the lining of the fallopian tube)
Mucinous (histology resembles endocervical epithelium)
Endometrioid (histology resembles endometrial lining)
Clear cell (histology resembles vaginal mucosa)
Transitional cell (Brenner's; histology resembles bladder)

Germ Cell Tumors
Dysgerminoma
Endodermal sinus tumor
Embryonal carcinoma
Polyembryoma
Choriocarcinoma
Teratoma:
• Immature
• Mature

Sex Cord–Stromal Tumors
Granulosa-stromal cell
• Granulosa cell
• Thecoma-fibromas
Sertoli-Leydig cell
Sex cord tumor
Sex cord tumor with annular tubules
Gynandroblastoma

Unclassified and Metastatic

- **HNPCC** is an autosomal dominant cancer susceptibility syndrome. Lynch syndrome II describes a familial predisposition to other cancers (endometrial, ovarian, genitourinary tract) in addition to HNPCC.
  - Women with HNPCC have a 40% to 60% lifetime risk for endometrial cancer and 12% lifetime risk for ovarian cancer. Mutations in three DNA mismatch repair genes, MLH1, MSH2, and MSH6, account for over 95% of mutations found with Lynch syndrome.
- **BRCA.** Two breast and ovarian cancer susceptibility genes (BRCA1, located on chromosome 17q, and BRCA2, located on chromosome 13q) have been identified. These genes, involved in DNA repair, have been linked to familial breast cancer, breast-ovary, and site-specific ovarian cancer syndromes.
  - Women with BRCA gene mutations have a lifetime risk of breast cancer of 82% and lifetime risk of ovarian cancer of 25% to 60% for BRCA1 carriers and 15% to 25% for BRCA2 carriers. These women also develop the disease at an earlier age than women without the mutations. Screening tests for these genes are available.
- **Environmental factors** may play a role in ovarian cancer. A recent meta-analysis does not support a causal relationship between talc exposure and ovarian cancer.
- Reproductive factors play an important role in ovarian cancer risk. Increasing **parity** is associated with decreased relative risk of developing ovarian cancer, whereas **nulliparity** is associated with increased risk.

- The use of **OCPs** also has been associated with a decreased relative risk.
- Women with a history of **breast-feeding** have a lower risk of ovarian cancer than nulliparous women and parous women who have not breast-fed.
- Women with **infertility** have an elevated risk of ovarian cancer, independent of nulliparity. Although fertility drugs have been implicated in the development of ovarian cancer, their association has not been clearly separated from the risk that nulliparity and infertility confer.
- **Tubal ligation** and **hysterectomy** with ovarian preservation both appear to lower the risk of ovarian cancer, although the mechanisms are unclear.

Screening and Prevention

- Early ovarian cancer is often asymptomatic. No available screening test has sufficient positive predictive value for early-stage ovarian cancer.
- **Routine yearly pelvic examination** is currently recommended for the general population as a screening tool, but it has poor sensitivity for detecting early disease.
- **Cancer antigen 125 (CA-125)**, first described in the 1980s, is a biomarker for ovarian cancer. A level >35 U/mL is usually considered abnormal. Approximately 50% of ovarian cancer cases confined to the ovary and >85% of advanced ovarian cancer cases have elevated CA-125 levels. However, this biomarker alone is neither sufficiently sensitive nor specific enough to be diagnostic for ovarian cancer.
  - CA-125 levels may be elevated in several benign conditions, including pelvic inflammatory disease, endometriosis, fibroids, pregnancy, hemorrhagic ovarian cysts, liver disease, and any other lesion that can promote peritoneal irritation, as well as other malignant conditions, including breast, lung, pancreatic, gastric, and colon cancer. In addition, CA-125 is normal in approximately half of women with stage I ovarian cancer. The most important use is following serial CA-125 levels in monitoring response to treatment and detecting recurrence in women with known ovarian cancer.
- **Other biomarkers.** CA 19-9, CA 15-3, CA 72-4, lipid-associated sialic acid, lysophosphatidic acid, OVX1, and osteopontin are being investigated.
- **Transvaginal ultrasonography** also has been considered as a screening tool. Characteristics suggestive of malignancy include complex ovarian cysts with solid components, the presence of septations, papillary projections into the cyst, thick cyst walls, surface excrescences, ascites, and neovascularization. However, transvaginal ultrasonography has a poor positive predictive value when used to screen the general population. When limited to postmenopausal women with pelvic masses, a sensitivity of 84% and a specificity of 78% have been reported.
- **Multimodal screening** using CA-125 measurement with transvaginal sonography yields a higher specificity and positive predictive value than either modality alone. In postmenopausal women, the combination of transvaginal ultrasound and a CA-125 >65 U/mL increased sensitivity to 92% and specificity to 96%. Prospective trials are underway to determine the appropriateness of multimodal screening for ovarian cancer.
- **Current recommendations for screening.** According to the US Preventive Services Task Force, no existing evidence suggests that any screening test, including CA-125, ultrasound, or pelvic examination, reduces mortality from ovarian cancer; therefore, routine screening is not recommended. The American College of Obstetricians and Gynecologists (ACOG) agrees that routine screening tests are not beneficial for low-risk, asymptomatic women. ACOG advises the obstetrician-gynecologist to remain vigilant for the early signs and symptoms of ovarian cancer and then evaluate with

a pelvic examination. The American Cancer Society does not recommend routine screening but states that women at high risk of ovarian cancer should be offered a combination of a thorough pelvic exam, transvaginal ultrasound, and CA-125.

- **Prophylactic bilateral salpingo-oophorectomy.** Women over age 45 who are undergoing any pelvic surgery may consider prophylactic removal of the ovaries. A bilateral salpingo-oophorectomy will essentially eliminate her risk for developing ovarian cancer. The potential for surgical menopause must be weighed against the potential benefit of averting ovarian malignancy. Women at high risk of ovarian cancer (e.g., Lynch syndrome, BRCA mutations) should consider prophylactic bilateral salpingo-oophorectomy when childbearing is complete.

- **OCP prophylaxis.** The overall estimate of protection with OCPs is approximately 40%. Increased duration of OCP use appears to be associated with decreased risk, and the protective effect persists for ten or more years after discontinuation. The OCP is the only documented method of chemoprevention for ovarian cancer, and the effect is substantial.

Presentation and Diagnosis

- **Presentation.** Only 19% of ovarian cancer cases are diagnosed while the cancer is localized (stage I), and approximately 68% of patients with epithelial ovarian cancer have advanced (stage III or greater) disease at time of diagnosis. Although some women with early disease experience symptoms, the majority are asymptomatic.
  - When symptoms develop, they are nonspecific and can include abdominal bloating, early satiety, weight loss, constipation, anorexia, urinary frequency, dyspareunia, fatigue, and irregular menstrual bleeding.
  - On physical examination, a pelvic mass is an important sign of disease. In more advanced stages of disease, abdominal distention may develop, and chest examination may reveal evidence of pleural effusion.

- **Workup.** Evaluation of a pelvic mass varies depending on the patient's age, significant medical and family history, and the sonographic characteristics of the mass. Women with pelvic masses that are suspicious for malignancy should be referred to a gynecologic oncologist (Table 45-2). In premenopausal women, an adnexal mass

TABLE 45-2	Pelvic Mass Evaluation: Criteria for Gynecologic Oncology Referral
Premenopausal Women	**Postmenopausal Women**
Very elevated CA-125 (>200 U/mL)	Elevated CA-125
Ascites	Ascites
Evidence of abdominal or distant metastasis	Evidence of abdominal or distant metastasis
Family history of one or more first-degree relatives with ovarian or breast cancer	Family history of one or more first-degree relatives with ovarian or breast cancer
	Nodular or fixed pelvic mass

From American College of Obstetricians and Gynecologists. ACOG Committee Opinion No. 280. The role of the generalist obstetrician-gynecologist in the early detection of ovarian cancer. *Obstet Gynecol* 2002;100:1413–1416, with permission.

<8 to 10 cm with no other concerning features is typically monitored with serial sonograms. After the decision is made to proceed to surgical evaluation, the preoperative evaluation should include a full history and physical examination, including a pelvic examination and a pap smear.

- Additional tests should be performed on the basis of a patient's risk factors and underlying medical status. Consideration should be given to performing a CT scan of the chest, abdomen, and pelvis to evaluate for metastatic disease. All patients who undergo surgery must have available a surgeon capable of performing an adequate staging procedure, preferably a gynecologic oncologist, to optimize outcome.

TABLE 45-3	FIGO Staging System for Carcinoma of the Ovary (1988)
Stage	**Tumor characteristics**
I	**Growth limited to the ovaries**
IA	Growth limited to one ovary; no ascites; no tumor on the external surface; capsule intact
IB	Growth limited to both ovaries; no ascites; no tumor on the external surfaces; capsule intact
IC	Tumor either stage IA or IB but with tumor on surface of one or both ovaries; or with capsule ruptured; or with ascites present containing malignant cells; or with positive peritoneal washings
II	**Growth involving one or both ovaries with pelvic extension**
IIA	Extension or metastases to the uterus or tubes
IIB	Extension to other pelvic tissues
IIC	Tumor either stage IIA or IIB but with tumor on surface of one or both ovaries; or with capsule ruptured; or with ascites present containing malignant cells; or with positive peritoneal washings
III	**Tumor involving one or both ovaries with peritoneal implants outside the pelvis and/or positive retroperitoneal or inguinal nodes. Superficial liver metastasis equals stage III. Tumor is limited to the true pelvis but with histologically proven malignant extension to small bowel or omentum**
IIIA	Tumor grossly limited to the true pelvis with negative nodes but with histologically confirmed microscopic seeding of abdominal peritoneal surfaces
IIIB	Tumor of one or both ovaries with histologically confirmed implants of abdominal peritoneal surfaces, none exceeding 2 cm in diameter; nodes are negative
IIIC	Abdominal implants >2 cm in diameter or positive retroperitoneal or inguinal nodes
IV	**Growth involving one or both ovaries, with distant metastases. If pleural effusion is present, cytologic findings must be positive to allot a case to stage IV. Parenchymal liver metastasis equals stage IV**

From Current FIGO staging for cancer of the vagina, fallopian tube, ovary, and gestational trophoblastic neoplasia. FIGO Committee on Gynecologic Oncology. *Int J Gynecol Obstet* 2009;105:3–4.

Staging and Prognosis

- Ovarian cancer is **surgically staged** (Table 45-3). The importance of complete surgical staging in developing a proper treatment plan and prognosis cannot be overemphasized. The standard surgical approach involves a vertical midline incision to allow for adequate exposure, although more recent advances in laparoscopic surgery have made minimally invasive options available (Table 45-4).
- Epithelial ovarian tumors are classified by cell type and behavior as benign, atypically proliferating, or malignant. Atypically proliferating tumors are also referred to as tumors of low malignant potentials (LMPs) or "borderline" tumors.
- Ovarian cancer can spread by direct extension, by exfoliation of cells into the peritoneal cavity (transcoelomic spread), via the bloodstream, or via the lymphatic system. The most common pathway of spread is transcoelomic. Cells from the tumor are shed into the peritoneal cavity and circulate, following the clockwise path of the peritoneal fluid. All peritoneal surfaces are at risk. Lymphatic spread to the pelvic and para-aortic lymph nodes can occur. Hematogenous spread to the liver or lungs can occur in advanced disease.

Prognostic Factors

- Most important are stage, grade, histology of the tumor, the amount of residual disease remaining after initial debulking surgery, and the age of the patient.
- The 5-year survival rate of patients with epithelial ovarian cancer correlates directly with **tumor stage** (Table 45-5).
- Within each **histologic category**, a spectrum of subgroups is present, including benign, LMP, and malignant.
  - **Serous.** The serous histologic subtype resembles cells of the fallopian tube and is the most common, accounting for over 50% of all malignant ovarian tumors. Approximately one third are malignant, one sixth are LMP, and half are benign. The mean age of patients at diagnosis is 57 years. Psammoma bodies are present in 25%.

TABLE 45-4	Surgical Staging Procedures for Ovarian Cancer

Obtain ascites for cytologic evaluation
Washings from the pelvis, gutters, and diaphragm
Systematic exploration of all organs and surfaces
Hysterectomy[a]
Bilateral salpingo-oophorectomy[a]
Infracolic omentectomy
Sampling pelvic and para-aortic lymph nodes
Multiple biopsy specimens from peritoneal sites
    Pelvic side walls
    Surfaces of the rectum and bladder
    Cul-de-sac
    Lateral abdominal gutters
    Diaphragm

---

[a]May be preserved in select patients, particularly if future fertility is desired. From Young RC, Decker DG, Wharton JT, et al. Staging laparotomy in early ovarian cancer. *JAMA* 1983;250(22):3072–3076; and Trimbos JB, Schueler JA, van Lent M, et al. Reasons for incomplete surgical staging in early ovarian carcinoma. *Gynecol Oncol* 1990;37:374–377.

TABLE 45-5	Five-Year Survival for Epithelial Ovarian Cancer, by Stage (2010)		
Stage	**5-Year Survival (%)**	**Stage**	**5-Year Survival (%)**
IA	94	**IIC**	57
IB	91	**IIIA**	45
IC	80	**IIIB**	39
IIA	76	**IIIC**	35
IIB	67	**IV**	18

From American Cancer Society SEER data, last updated July 07, 2010. Available at www.cancer.org/Cancer/OvarianCancer/OverviewGuide/ovarian-cancer-overview-survival-rates. Accessed 09/20/2010.

- **Mucinous** tumors are lined by cells that resemble the cells of the endocervical glands. Primary ovarian mucinous tumors account for 3% to 4% of epithelial tumors. Sixty percent of mucinous tumors are stage I, and most are unilateral. They are typically large, often filling the abdominal cavity, cystic, and multiloculated. The mean age of patients diagnosed with malignant mucinous tumors is 54 years. CA-125 levels may not be markedly elevated.
  ○ Pseudomyxoma peritonei is a condition associated with mucinous neoplasms, usually of gastrointestinal origin, and is characterized by gelatinous mucus or ascites in the abdomen.
- **Endometrioid** tumors resemble the histology of the endometrium and account for 6% of epithelial tumors. Most are malignant; 20% may be LMP. The mean age of patients diagnosed with malignant tumors is 56 years. About 14% of women will also have endometrial cancer, and 15% to 20% or more will also have endometriosis. Endometrioid tumors appear to have a better prognosis than serous tumors, most likely because of their early stage at diagnosis.
- **Clear cell** carcinomas account for 3% of epithelial ovarian cancers. These tumors are the most chemoresistant type of ovarian cancer and are most commonly associated with paraneoplastic syndromes. Endometriotic implants are commonly present (30% to 35% cases). About 50% of patients present in stage I. Tumors are large, with a mean diameter of 15 cm. Histologically, hobnail-shaped cells are characteristic of the clear cell carcinomas. The mean age at diagnosis is 57 years.
- **Transitional cell** tumors histologically resemble the bladder. The two types of malignant transitional cell tumors are Brenner's tumors and transitional cell carcinomas. Approximately 10% to 20% of advanced stage ovarian carcinomas contain a transitional cell carcinoma component. The mean age for malignant Brenner's tumors is 63 years.
- **Grade** is an important independent prognostic factor, particularly in patients with early-stage disease.
  - Grade 1 is well differentiated, grade 2 is moderately differentiated, and grade 3 is poorly differentiated.
- Debulking, also called **cytoreduction**, is defined as removal of as much tumor as possible during surgical exploration. Optimal cytoreduction implies that tumor nodules no larger than 1 cm in diameter are left behind and survival improves as the amount of residual disease decreases.

- **Tumor ploidy** has been demonstrated to be an independent prognostic variable. Diploid tumors are often stage IA, whereas aneuploid tumors are often seen in more advanced cancer.

Management of Epithelial Ovarian Cancer

- Treatment of epithelial ovarian cancer depends on the stage and grade of the disease, type of disease (i.e., primary or recurrent), previous treatment, and the patient's performance status.

Tumors of LMP

- These tumors show a different pattern of behavior than malignant ovarian disease. Approximately 15% of all epithelial ovarian malignancies are LMPs and are often found in younger patients. These tumors are most commonly of serous histology (85%), followed by mucinous.
- Serous LMPs with invasive implants tend to behave as low-grade carcinomas with a mortality rate of 34%.
- Mucinous LMPs confined to the ovary have a survival rate approaching 100%, whereas those with advanced-stage disease have a survival rate of 40% to 50%. Mucinous LMPs may be associated with a concurrent appendiceal primary tumor, and affected patients should also undergo appendectomy. Mucinous LMPs that display aggressive behavior are associated with pseudomyxoma peritonei, which is of appendiceal origin.
- Surgical staging of LMPs is advocated because of the possibility of identifying an invasive cancer on final pathology. Because of the indolent growth of LMPs, adjuvant therapy is not recommended even in patients with advanced disease. If disease recurs, it recurs an average of ten years after initial diagnosis, and resection can be performed again at the time of recurrence. Most patients die *with* the disease rather than *from* the disease.
- In addition, early-stage disease in women who want to maintain fertility may be treated with unilateral salpingo-oophorectomy, or even with unilateral cystectomy, with good results.

Early Invasive Disease (Stage I or II)

- **Initial surgical resection** is necessary for establishing a histologic diagnosis and appropriate staging. Options exist for young patients who wish to preserve fertility. If intraoperative findings are consistent with stage I disease and the contralateral ovary is normal in appearance, unilateral salpingo-oophorectomy with thorough surgical staging may be performed. The uterus and normal-appearing contralateral ovary may remain in situ. The patient needs to understand the potential for a second primary in the preserved ovary, and a total abdominal hysterectomy and removal of the remaining tube and ovary should be considered after childbearing is completed.
- **Chemotherapy.** For patients with stage IA, grade 1 or 2 disease, chemotherapy is not required. For patients with early-stage disease with prognostic factors placing them at higher risk for recurrence, postoperative chemotherapy is recommended. The appropriate chemotherapy regimen for patients with early-stage disease is still being evaluated in clinical trials.
- **Radiation.** Radiation therapy is very infrequently used today as effective chemotherapy is available.

Advanced Invasive Disease

- **Advanced disease** requires surgical staging, debulking, and a course of platinum-based chemotherapy.

- Primary **cytoreductive surgery**, or debulking, is central in the treatment of advanced disease because maximal cytoreduction is one of the most powerful predictors of survival in patients with advanced cancer.
  - The determination of residual disease upon closure of the procedure does not include the total volume of tumor cells left behind but rather the diameter of the largest single residual nodule. For example, a patient with one unresected nodule measuring 2.5 cm has not undergone optimal debulking, whereas debulking is considered to be optimal in a patient with residual miliary studding of the entire peritoneal cavity.
- **Neoadjuvant therapy** has been associated with a lower overall survival compared to initial surgery. However, it may be an appropriate alternative for patients whose performance status prohibits initial surgery. In addition, for patients in whom suboptimal debulking is likely, neoadjuvant chemotherapy has been used as an alternate strategy before surgery in an attempt to increase the likelihood of optimal tumor debulking.
- **Combination chemotherapy** is most often used as postoperative (adjuvant) treatment for advanced epithelial ovarian cancer. Combination chemotherapy with six cycles of carboplatin plus paclitaxel is the treatment of choice for patients with advanced disease. A cycle is given every 3 weeks, with monitoring of tumor status by physical examination, CA-125 levels, and CT imaging.
- **Intraperitoneal chemotherapy.** Recent data have shown a substantial improvement in overall survival and progression-free survival in patients with newly diagnosed, optimally debulked stage III ovarian cancer by the administration of cisplatin and paclitaxel via an intraperitoneal (IP) port rather than the conventional intravenous (IV) administration. The median survival was 65.6 months in the IP group compared to 49.7 months in the IV group. However, an increase in toxic events and catheter-related complications is a disadvantage of this therapeutic approach and can prevent completion of all six cycles.
- **Alternative therapies**, including biologic therapy using autologous tumor-infiltrating lymphocytes and monoclonal antibodies, are under investigation.
- **Consolidation treatment.** Eighty percent of patients who complete optimal tumor debulking followed by six cycles of carboplatin and paclitaxel will achieve a clinical remission. Consolidation treatment strategies to lengthen time to recurrence are currently being investigated. Administration of tamoxifen or aromatase inhibitors to patients with estrogen positive primary tumors can be considered.

Posttreatment surveillance

Asymptomatic Patients
- Appropriate follow-up for asymptomatic patients after primary surgery and chemotherapy should include a physical examination with rectovaginal examination, CA-125 testing, and CT scan. Patients should be seen every 3 months for the first 2 years.
  - In patients whose CA-125 level was elevated preoperatively, CA-125 is a reliable marker of disease recurrence. The combination of thorough physical examination and CA-125 testing has been shown to detect recurrent disease in 90% of patients. Combined positron emission tomography imaging and CT may have clinical use in detecting disease recurrence in select patients.
- **Second-look surgery** by laparotomy or laparoscopy can be performed on patients with advanced epithelial ovarian cancer who have undergone primary debulking followed by chemotherapy and who have no clinical evidence of disease. The use of second-look surgery remains controversial and should be performed only in the

setting of a clinical trial or on an individualized basis, as no data exist to prove that it prolongs survival. Patients need to be counseled that the procedure is not therapeutic but may provide prognostic information.

Recurrent or Persistent Disease

- **Secondary debulking.** Patients with recurrent or persistent disease may be candidates for further surgical therapy, or secondary cytoreduction. Surgery should be reserved for patients in whom therapy has a good chance of prolonging life or palliating symptoms. Those with longer disease-free intervals (at least 6 to 12 months) and fewer sites of recurrence are the best candidates for secondary cytoreduction.
- **Second-line chemotherapy.** Response rates for second-line chemotherapy are in the range of 20% to 40%. A host of chemotherapy options are available for recurrent ovarian cancer.
- **Hormone therapy** has been used as salvage treatment. Both megestrol acetate (Megace) and tamoxifen have been used to treat recurrent disease. Response rates are low.
- **Experimental studies.** Many investigators are currently studying the underlying molecular biology of epithelial ovarian cancer. Microarray analysis and proteomics provide insight into the differential expression of mRNA and proteins, respectively. Translational studies to further characterize these molecular changes, as they relate to the clinical disease state, provide an opportunity to develop novel therapeutic agents. Clinical trials are also currently investigating antiangiogenic drugs.

Complications of Advanced Ovarian Cancer

- **Intestinal obstruction.** Many women with ovarian cancer develop intestinal obstruction, either at initial diagnosis or with recurrent disease. Obstruction may be related to mechanical blockage or carcinomatous ileus. Correction of intestinal obstruction at initial treatment is usually possible; obstruction associated with recurrent disease, however, is a more complex problem. Some of these obstructions may be treated conservatively with IV hydration, total parenteral nutrition, and gastric decompression. The decision to proceed with palliative surgery must be based on the physical condition of the patient and her expected survival. If patients are unable to undergo surgery or are judged to be poor operative candidates, placement of a percutaneous gastric tube may offer some relief.
- **Ascites.** Initial ascites on presentation with ovarian cancer is almost always improved by debulking surgery and several courses of chemotherapy. Persistent ascites is difficult to manage and is a very poor prognostic sign. Ascites is best managed by repeated paracenteses and chemotherapy.

Survival

- **Age.** Overall survival rate 5 years after diagnosis in women younger than age 65 is nearly twice that of women over age 65 (57% and 28%, respectively).
- **Stage.** Patients with stage I disease have up to a 94% 5-year survival rate. In contrast, overall survival for women with distant disease on presentation is 29% (Table 45-5).
- **Performance status.** The Karnofsky Performance Scale Index (Table 45-6) classifies patients according to their functional impairment and can be used to assess prognosis in individual patients. Lower scores are associated with worse survival for most serious illnesses.

Peritoneal Carcinoma

- The primary malignant transformation of the peritoneum is termed **primary peritoneal carcinoma**, which clinically and pathologically resembles serous epithelial ovarian cancer. Primary peritoneal carcinoma can therefore appear with a clinical

TABLE 45-6	The Karnofsky Performance Scale

Description	%
Normal; no complaints; no evidence of disease	100
Able to carry on normal activity; minor signs, and symptoms of disease	90
Normal activity with effort; some signs and symptoms of disease	80
Cares for self; unable to carry on normal activity or do work	70
Requires occasional assistance but is able to care for most personal needs	60
Requires considerable assistance and frequent medical care	50
Disabled; requires special care and assistance	40
Severely disabled; hospitalization indicated although death not imminent	30
Very sick; hospitalization necessary; requires active support treatment	20
Moribund; fatal processes progressing rapidly	10
Dead	0

Originally published by Karnofsky DA, Burchenal JH. The clinical evaluation of chemotherapeutic agents in cancer, in Macleod CM, ed. *Evaluation of Chemotherapeutic Agents.* New York: Columbia University, 1949:199–205.

presentation similar to ovarian cancer in patients with a history of oophorectomy or with pathologically normal-appearing or minimally involved ovaries. Extensive upper abdominal disease is common, and clinical course, management, and prognosis are similar to those for epithelial ovarian cancer.

FALLOPIAN TUBE CANCER

- **Epidemiology.** Carcinoma of the fallopian tube is very rare, accounting for <1% of cases of gynecologic cancer in women. Carcinoma of the fallopian tube is seen most often in the fifth and sixth decades of life.
- **Histology.** To confirm a histologic diagnosis of fallopian tube cancer, most of the tumor must be present in the fallopian tube, the mucosa of the tube must be involved, and a demonstrable transition from benign to malignant tubal epithelium must exist. Over 90% of tumors are papillary serous adenocarcinoma, resembling ovarian serous carcinoma.
- **Clinical presentation and diagnosis.** The triad of symptoms of fallopian tube carcinoma is watery vaginal discharge (hydrops tubae profluens), a pelvic mass, and pelvic pain. However, only 15% of patients present with this triad. Vaginal discharge or bleeding is the most common presenting symptom (50% to 60%), followed by abdominal pain and an abdominal mass. As in ovarian cancer, presentation may be nonspecific. Ascites may be present if the disease is advanced. Unlike ovarian cancer, fallopian tube carcinoma more often presents at an early stage. A preoperative diagnosis of fallopian tube cancer is made in only a minority of patients; the usual clinical diagnosis is ovarian tumor or pelvic inflammatory disease. The majority of patients will have elevated CA-125 levels.
- **Natural history and patterns of spread.** Tubal cancers spread in a similar fashion to ovarian cancers.

- **Staging.** The ovarian cancer staging system has been adapted for the fallopian tube.
- **Treatment** is similar to that of ovarian cancer, with surgical debulking as the mainstay of treatment, followed by combination platinum-based chemotherapy. Chemotherapy for early-stage disease is the subject of controversy.
- **Prognosis and survival** are related to the stage of disease. Data on 5-year survival rates are as follows from stage I to IV: 95%, 75%, 69%, and 45%.

GERM CELL OVARIAN TUMORS

Epidemiology

- Approximately 20% of all ovarian tumors are of germ cell origin, with only 2% to 3% of these being malignant. Types include the following: dysgerminoma, endodermal sinus tumor, embryonal, polyembryoma, choriocarcinoma, and teratoma.
- Roughly 70% to 80% of all germ cell tumors occur before age 20, and approximately one third of these are malignant. The median age of women diagnosed with a malignant germ cell tumor is 16 to 20 years. About 50% to 75% of patients with malignant germ cell tumors present with stage I disease. Overall survival rates, including those with advanced disease, are 60% to 80%.
- The most common germ cell tumor is the dermoid (benign cystic teratoma), and the most common malignant tumor is the dysgerminoma.

Pathology

- Germ cell tumors are derived from the primordial germ cells of the ovary; however, they are a heterogeneous group of tumors. They gradually differentiate to mimic tissues of embryonic origin (ectoderm, mesoderm, endoderm) and extraembryonic origin (trophoblast, yolk sac). They are aggressive tumors, frequently unilateral, and usually curable if treated early.

Diagnosis

- Clinically, germ cell malignancies grow quickly and are often characterized by acute pelvic pain. The pain can be caused by distention of the ovarian capsule, hemorrhage, necrosis, or torsion. A palpable pelvic mass is a common finding on presentation. Abdominal distention and abnormal vaginal bleeding may also be the presenting complaint. The tumors are often large at presentation, with a median diameter of 16 cm.
- Ovarian masses that are 2 cm or larger in premenarchal girls or 8 to 10 cm or larger in premenopausal patients are concerning and generally require exploratory surgery. See Chapter 31.
- **Preoperative workup.** Measurement of serum tumor markers may assist in the diagnosis of germ cell malignancies (Table 45-7). Workup should include measurement of serum hCG, alpha-fetoprotein (AFP) titers, lactate dehydrogenase (LDH) levels, a CBC, and liver function tests. A chest radiographic study is important to rule out pulmonary metastases. A preoperative CT scan should be considered to assess for the presence or absence of liver metastases and retroperitoneal lymphadenopathy.

Germ Cell Tumor Types

- **Dysgerminomas** are the most common malignant germ cell tumor, comprising up to 50%. All dysgerminomas are malignant; however, not all are aggressive. Seventy-five percent of dysgerminomas occur in the second and third decades of life. They

| TABLE 45-7 | Serum Markers for Germ Cell and Sex Cord Stromal Ovarian Tumors | | | | | | | |

Tumor	LDH	AFP	hCG	E_2	Inhibin	Testosterone	Androgen	DHEA
Dysgerminoma	±	−	±	−	−	−	−	−
Embryonal	−	±	+	−	−	−	−	−
Endodermal sinus tumor	−	+	−	−	−	−	−	−
Polyembryoma	−	±	+	−	−	−	−	−
Choriocarcinoma	−	−	+	−	−	−	−	−
Immature teratoma	−	±	−	±	−	−	−	±
Granulosa cell	−	−	−	±	+	−	−	−
Thecoma-fibroma	−	−	−	−	−	−	−	−
Sertoli-Leydig	−	−	−	−	±	+	+	−
Gonadoblastoma	−	−	−	±	±	±	±	±

LDH, lactate dehydrogenase; AFP, alpha-fetoprotein; hCG, human chorionic gonadotropin; E2, estradiol; DHEA, dehydroepiandrosterone.

are the only germ cell tumor that tends to be bilateral (10% to 15% of cases). The 5-year survival rate for stage IA disease is 95% and for all stages is 85%.

- **Endodermal sinus tumors** (yolk sac tumors) are derived from cells of the primitive yolk sac and are the second most common malignant germ cell tumor, accounting for 20%. Pathologically, they are characterized by Schiller-Duval bodies. These tumors tend to grow rapidly and aggressively. They secrete AFP. The disease-free survival rate for all stages is >80%.
- **Embryonal carcinoma.** These tumors are extremely rare and occur in children and young adults. They may secrete both hCG and AFP. Patients may present with sexual precocity and vaginal bleeding.
- **Polyembryoma.** These tumors are exceedingly rare and highly malignant. They resemble early embryos and may secrete AFP or hCG.
- **Choriocarcinoma.** Pure, nongestational choriocarcinoma is very rare and is histologically similar to gestational choriocarcinoma. Almost all patients are premenarchal. The tumor often produces high levels of hCG. Precocious puberty is seen occasionally, and patients may present with vaginal bleeding. This tumor has historically had a poor prognosis but does respond to combination chemotherapy.
- **Immature malignant teratomas** contain tissues resembling those in an embryo. They account for 20% of malignant germ cell tumors and 1% of ovarian malignancies. Half of immature teratomas occur in patients between ages 10 and 20. These tumors may secrete AFP. The most important prognostic factor is the grade of the tumor. The 5-year survival rate is 95% for stage I disease and 75% for advanced disease.
- **Mixed germ cell tumors** account for 10% of malignant germ cell tumors and contain elements of two or more of the germ cell tumors discussed previously.

Management of Germ Cell Tumors

- **Surgical.** Primary treatment for all germ cell tumors is surgical and should include proper surgical staging to rule out the presence of extraovarian microscopic disease. Because most of the patients are of reproductive age, preservation of fertility is important.

- Unilateral oophorectomy is performed along with unilateral pelvic and para-aortic lymphadenectomy. A frozen section should be performed. Bilateral involvement is rare in germ cell tumors, with the exception of dysgerminomas (10% to 15% bilaterality). The contralateral ovary should be inspected, and a biopsy may be performed if there is suspicion of involvement, but the ovary should be removed in a young patient only if disease is present. The remaining pelvic organs may be left in situ to preserve fertility.
- For patients who have completed childbearing, a total abdominal hysterectomy with bilateral salpingo-oophorectomy is reasonable. When the disease is metastatic on initial surgery, cytoreductive surgery is recommended, although data are limited.
- Surgical therapy alone is recommended for stage IA dysgerminomas and stage IA, grade I immature teratomas. These patients have a 5-year survival of >90%. Approximately 15% to 25% will recur but can be treated successfully at the time of presentation. For endodermal sinus tumors, staging is not always recommended because chemotherapy should be given regardless.
- **Adjuvant therapy.** The decision to administer adjuvant therapy depends on the histologic type of germ cell tumor. All patients, except those with stage IA, grade I immature teratoma and stage IA dysgerminoma, require postoperative chemotherapy. Dysgerminomas are very sensitive to radiation therapy; however, fertility is lost as a consequence of irradiation. Therefore, chemotherapy is the first-line treatment. Combination therapy with three agents (bleomycin, etoposide, and cisplatin, or BEP) is recommended. Prognosis has significantly improved with platinum-based chemotherapy.
- Ninety percent of patients with germ cell tumors who experience a **recurrence** will do so in the first 2 years after therapy. If initially treated with surgery alone, BEP chemotherapy can be used. Patients who initially received chemotherapy can be treated with a platinum-based agent.

SEX CORD-STROMAL OVARIAN TUMORS

Sex cord–stromal tumors are derived from the sex cords and mesenchyme of the embryonic gonad and account for 5% to 8% of all ovarian neoplasms. Most of these tumors are hormonally active (Table 45-7). Types include the following: granulosa-stromal cell, Sertoli-Leydig, sex cord tumor, and gynandroblastoma.

Granulosa Cell Tumor

- **Incidence.** The granulosa cell tumor is the most common malignant sex cord–stromal tumor, accounting for 70%. Adult granulosa cell tumors occur primarily in the perimenopausal years, with a mean age of 52 at presentation. Two forms exist: an adult form (95%) and a much rarer juvenile form (5%). The tumor is bilateral in <10% of cases.
- **Diagnosis and presentation.** In the majority of cases, the tumor secretes estrogen and inhibin. Histologically, Call-Exner bodies are seen. Patients may present with abnormal vaginal bleeding, abdominal distention, pain, or a mass, most >10 cm in diameter. Granulosa cell tumors are characteristically hemorrhagic and can present with a hemoperitoneum.
  - The incidence of concurrent endometrial hyperplasia is over 50%, and the incidence of concurrent endometrial adenocarcinoma ranges from 3% to 27%. The majority (90%) of affected patients present with stage I disease, mainly because the hormonal effects of the tumor cause symptoms early in the disease. In juvenile

type, patients present with pseudo precocious puberty and have elevated serum estradiol.

- **Treatment.** Surgery alone is usually sufficient treatment only for disease of stage IA or IB. For all other stages, chemotherapy is recommended. Similar regimens utilized for germ cell tumors such as BEP are often employed. Radiation, chemotherapy, or both are used for recurrent disease. If the patient desires to maintain fertility, a unilateral salpingo-oophorectomy is adequate for treating stage IA tumors, and a staging operation should also be performed. If the patient has completed her childbearing, a total abdominal hysterectomy and bilateral salpingo-oophorectomy should be performed. If the uterus is left in situ, dilation and curettage should be performed to rule out endometrial hyperplasia or adenocarcinoma. Chemotherapy after surgery does not prevent recurrence of the disease.
- **Prognosis and survival.** Granulosa cell tumors have a propensity for late recurrence, with recurrence reported as many as 30 years after treatment for primary tumor. The 10-year and 20-year survival rates are 90% and 75%, respectively.

Sertoli-Leydig Cell Tumor

- **Incidence.** Sertoli-Leydig cell tumors account for only 0.2% of cases of ovarian neoplasms. The average age at diagnosis is 25. The tumors are most frequently low-grade malignancies, and nearly all patients (97%) present at stage I.
- **Diagnosis and presentation.** Sertoli-Leydig cell tumors often produce androgens. Patients present with virilization (30% to 50%), menstrual disorders, and other symptoms related to an abdominal mass. Average size of mass is about 16 cm. These tumors may produce testosterone, androstenedione, or AFP.
- **Treatment.** In young patients, unilateral salpingo-oophorectomy with staging may be performed to preserve fertility. In older patients, a total abdominal hysterectomy and bilateral salpingo-oophorectomy should be performed as well. Treatment in those with higher stage and/or grade typically includes chemotherapy.
- **Prognosis and survival.** Prognosis is related to stage and histologic grade. The 5-year survival rate is 70% to 90%.

SPECIAL CONSIDERATIONS IN OVARIAN CANCER

- **Metastatic tumors** account for 5% to 20% of ovarian malignancies and are often, but not always, bilateral.
- **Gastrointestinal tract tumors** are the most likely to metastasize to the ovary. Krukenberg tumors are usually bilateral and account for 30% to 40% of metastatic tumors to the ovary. The tumor is characterized histologically by signet-ring cells, in which the nucleus is flattened against the cell wall by the accumulation of cytoplasmic mucin. In postmenopausal women who undergo evaluation for an adnexal mass, metastatic colon cancer should be ruled out, if possible, using colonoscopy.
- **Breast cancer** is the second most likely cancer to metastasize to the ovary.
- **Lymphomas** can also metastasize to the ovary. Burkitt's lymphoma may affect children or young adults. Rarely, ovarian lesions are the primary manifestation of disease in lymphoma patients.
- **Metastatic gynecologic tumors** may involve the ovaries. Fallopian tube cancer is the most common malignancy to metastasize to the ovaries and occurs by direct extension. Cervical cancer very rarely spreads to the ovaries. Endometrial cancer may metastasize to the ovaries; however, synchronous endometrioid adenocarcinoma, primary to both the ovary and the endometrium, can also occur.

- **Malignant mixed-mesodermal tumors** of the ovary are extremely rare. These lesions are very aggressive, and treatment consists of surgical resection followed by combination chemotherapy.
- **Ovarian tumors during pregnancy** are very rare. The incidence of an adnexal mass during pregnancy is approximately 1 in 800. The majority of adnexal masses discovered during the first trimester resolve by the second trimester. However, approximately 1% to 6% of these masses are malignant.
  - Germ cell tumors (primarily dysgerminoma) account for approximately 45% of ovarian malignancies diagnosed in pregnancy.
  - The masses are usually diagnosed during routine ultrasonography or at the time of cesarean section. The majority of patients (74%) are diagnosed with stage I disease.
  - Early-stage disease can be treated with conservative surgery in the second trimester of pregnancy, usually with good maternal and fetal results. Late-stage and high-grade disease should be treated aggressively after appropriate counseling of the patient.

SUGGESTED READINGS

Armstrong DK, Bundy B, Wenzel L, et al. Gynecologic Oncology Group. Intraperitoneal cisplatin and paclitaxel in ovarian cancer. *N Engl J Med* 2006;354:34–43.

Bristow RE, Chi DS. Platinum-based neoadjuvant chemotherapy and interval surgical cytoreduction for advanced ovarian cancer: a meta-analysis. *Gynecol Oncol* 2006;103(3): 1070–1076.

Hoskins WJ, Perez CA, Young RC, eds. *Principles and Practice of Gynecologic Oncology,* 4th Ed. Philadelphia: Lippincott Williams & Wilkins, 2005.

Kauff ND, Domchek SM, Friebel TM, et al. Risk-reducing salpingo-oophorectomy for the prevention of BRCA1- and BRCA2-associated breast and gynecologic cancer: a multicenter, prospective study. *J Clin Oncol* 2008;26(8):1331–1337.

46 Gestational Trophoblastic Disease

Alaina Johnson and Stefanie Ueda

Gestational trophoblastic disease (GTD) is a heterogeneous group of interrelated but distinct neoplasms derived from the placenta. Lesions range from the premalignant complete and partial hydatidiform moles to the malignant invasive mole, choriocarcinoma, placental site trophoblastic tumor (PSTT), and epithelioid trophoblastic tumor (ETT). Most women with GTD can be cured with their fertility preserved.

EPIDEMIOLOGY OF GTD AND TYPES OF TROPHOBLASTIC CELLS

Incidence of GTD varies widely throughout the world, with the highest rates reported in Asia, Africa, and Latin America.
- In the United States, hydatidiform moles are observed in 1 in 600 therapeutic abortions and 1 in 1,000 to 1,200 pregnancies. Approximately 20% of patients require treatment for malignant sequelae after evacuation of hydatidiform mole.
- Gestational choriocarcinoma, by comparison, occurs in about 1 in 20,000 to 40,000 pregnancies.
- Although much less common than hydatidiform mole or choriocarcinoma, PSTT and ETT can develop after any type of pregnancy.

Risk Factors for GTD
- Risks for GTD include:
  - **Extremes of reproductive age.** Women over age 40 have a 5.2-fold increased risk, whereas women less than age 20 have a 1.5-fold increased risk. Persistent GTD occurs more frequently in older patients.
  - Obstetric **history of spontaneous abortions**.
  - **History of previous hydatidiform mole.** The risk of a subsequent hydatidiform mole rises by 10- to 20-fold. With two previous molar pregnancies, the risk multiplies by 40-fold. Conversely, term pregnancies and live births produce a protective effect.
  - **Race.** Asians demonstrate a higher risk of being diagnosed with GTD, while African-Americans have lower risk.
  - **Low socioeconomic status** and **dietary factors**.

Types of Cells and Hormone Secretion
- Three types of trophoblastic cells have been identified: syncytiotrophoblast, cytotrophoblast, and intermediate trophoblast.
  - **Syncytiotrophoblasts** are well-differentiated cells that interface with the maternal circulation and produce most of the placental hormones. No mitotic activity

is evident. Syncytiotrophoblasts demonstrate **human chorionic gonadotropin (hCG)** production at 12 days of gestation. Secretion rapidly increases and peaks by 8 to 10 weeks, with a decline thereafter. By 40 weeks, hCG is present only focally in syncytiotrophoblasts. At 12 days, **human placental lactogen (hPL)** is also present in syncytiotrophoblasts. Production continues to rise throughout pregnancy.

- **Cytotrophoblasts** are primitive trophoblastic cells that are polygonal to oval in shape. They exhibit a single nucleus and clearly defined borders. Mitotic activity is evident. Cytotrophoblasts do not produce either hCG or hPL.
- **Intermediate trophoblasts** show infiltrative growth into decidua, myometrium, and blood vessels. Intermediate trophoblasts characteristically invade the wall of large vascular channels until the wall is completely replaced. Intermediate trophoblasts are the predominant cell of PSTT and exaggerated placental sites. As early as 12 days after conception, **hCG** and **hPL** are present focally in intermediate trophoblasts. However, at 6 weeks, hCG production disappears, while secretion of hPL peaks at 11 to 15 weeks' gestation.

CLASSIFICATION OF GTD

Gestational trophoblastic neoplasms are unique among human neoplastic disorders because they are genetically related to fetal tissues. The molecular pathogenesis of these tumors is an area of active research interest.

Hydatidiform Mole

- In both partial and complete hydatidiform moles, the placental villi become edematous, forming small grape-like structures. Despite the cytogenetic, pathologic, and clinical differences in these disease processes (Table 46-1), the management of patients is similar.
- Ultrasound establishes the diagnosis, identifying a mixed echogenic pattern as villi and blood clots replace normal placental tissue. Medical complications occur in approximately 25% of patients, being more prominent in those with uterine enlargement >14 to 16 weeks' gestational size.

TABLE 46-1	Comparison of Complete Versus Partial Hydatidiform Mole	
	Complete	**Partial**
Karyotype	Most commonly 46,XX or 46,XY	Most commonly 69,XXX or 69,XXY
Uterine size		
Large for gestational age	33%	10%
Small for gestational age	33%	65%
Diagnosis by ultrasonography	Common	Rare
Theca lutein cysts	25–35%	Rare
β-hCG (mIU/mL)	>50,000	<50,000
Malignant potential	15–25%	<5%
Metastatic disease	<5%	<1%

Adapted from Soper JT. Gestational trophoblastic disease. *Obstet Gynecol* 2006;108(1):176–187.

Complete Mole
- **Clinical findings.**
  - Presentation is between 11 and 25 weeks' gestation, with an average gestational age of 16 weeks.
  - Vaginal bleeding is the most common presenting symptom, occurring in 97% of cases. Uterine size is often greater than expected for gestational age.
  - Severe hyperemesis and pregnancy-induced hypertension can develop in up to 25% of women, with hyperthyroidism in 7% of cases.
  - In approximately 1/3 of patients, the uterus is small for gestational dates. Ovarian enlargement caused by theca lutein cysts occurs in 25% to 35% of cases.
  - Levels of β-hCG are generally above 50,000 mIU/mL.
  - Ultrasonography often, but not always, shows a classic "snowstorm" appearance
- **Pathologic features.**
  - Gross findings include massively enlarged, edematous villi that give the classic grape-like appearance to the placenta and lack embryonic tissue.
  - Microscopic examination shows hydropic swelling in the majority of villi, accompanied by a variable degree of trophoblastic proliferation. Complete moles have widespread, diffuse immunostaining for hCG; moderately diffuse staining for hPL; and focal staining for placental alkaline phosphatase (PLAP).
- **Chromosomal abnormalities.**
  - Most complete moles are diploid, with a 46,XX karyotype; rare examples of triploid or tetraploid moles have been reported.
  - In most cases, all of the chromosomal complements are paternally derived. The XX genotype typically results from duplication of a haploid sperm pronucleus in an empty ovum. Three to thirteen percent of complete moles have a 46,XY chromosome complement, presumably as a result of dispermy, in which an empty ovum is fertilized by two sperm pronuclei.

Incomplete Mole
- **Clinical findings.**
  - Commonly, patients present between 9 and 34 weeks' gestation.
  - These tumors are consistently associated with embryonic/fetal tissue.
  - Patients report abnormal uterine bleeding in about 75% of cases. A clinical diagnosis of a missed or spontaneous abortion is made in 91% of women with incomplete molar pregnancy.
  - Uterine size is generally small for gestational dates; excessive uterine size is observed in less than 10% of patients.
  - Serum hCG level is in the normal or low range for gestational age.
  - Pre-eclampsia occurs with lower incidence (2.5%) and presents much later with a partial mole than with complete moles but can be equally severe.
- **Pathologic features.**
  - Gross findings reveal fetal tissue in nearly all instances, although its discovery may require careful examination, because early fetal death normally takes place (i.e., 8 to 9 weeks' gestational age).
  - Microscopic examination finds two populations of chorionic villi: one of normal size and the other grossly hydropic. Partial moles show focal to moderate immunostaining for hCG and diffuse staining for hPL and PLAP.
- **Chromosomal abnormalities.**
  - Karyotype of partial moles most frequently shows triploidy (i.e., 69 chromosomes), with two paternal and one maternal chromosome complement.

- The chromosomal complement is XXY in 70% of cases, XXX in 27% of cases, and XYY in 3% of cases. The abnormal conceptus in these cases arises from the fertilization of an egg with a haploid set of chromosomes either by two sperm, each with a set of haploid chromosomes, or by a single sperm with a diploid 46,XY complement.

Invasive Mole

- **Invasive mole** is an important complication of hydatidiform mole, representing 50% of cases of persistent GTD. Other common names include chorioadenoma destruens, penetrating mole, malignant mole, or molar destruens.
- **Pathologic features.**
  - Histologically, hydropic chorionic villi migrate into the myometrium, vascular spaces, or outside of the pelvis in 20% of cases to the vagina, perineum, or lungs.
  - Grossly, invasive moles present as erosive, hemorrhagic lesions extending from the uterine cavity into the myometrium. Metastasis can range from superficial penetration to extension through the uterine wall, with subsequent perforation and life-threatening hemorrhage. Molar vesicles are often apparent.
  - Microscopically, the diagnostic feature of invasive mole is the presence of molar villi and trophoblast within the myometrium or at an extrauterine site. Lesions at distant sites are usually composed of molar villi confined within blood vessels, without invasion into adjacent tissue.

Choriocarcinoma

- **Gestational choriocarcinoma** is a highly malignant epithelial tumor that can be associated with any type of gestational event, most often a complete hydatidiform mole. In the United States, choriocarcinoma occurs in 1 in 20,000 to 40,000 pregnancies. Approximately 25% of gestational choriocarcinomas develop after term pregnancies, 50% after molar gestations, and 25% after abortion or ectopic pregnancies. Early systemic hematogenous metastasis often takes place.
- **Clinical findings.**
  - Eighty percent of patients with extrauterine disease show pulmonary metastases, while approximately 30% demonstrate extension to the vagina. Ten percent of women also exhibit liver and CNS involvement.
- **Pathologic features.**
  - On gross examination, these tumors appear as dark red, hemorrhagic masses with shaggy, irregular surfaces. Metastatic lesions outside the uterus are well circumscribed. On microscopic examination, sheets of syncytiotrophoblasts and cytotrophoblasts are seen *without chorionic villi* invading surrounding tissue or permeating vascular spaces.

Placental Site and Epithelioid Trophoblastic Tumor (PSTT and ETT)

- **PSTT** and **ETT** are rare gestational trophoblastic neoplasms, accounting for 1% of persistent GTD. Both can develop long after prior gestational events. Most cases of PSTT and ETT are benign, especially those tumors that are confined to the uterus, but about 15% to 25% of cases are malignant and present with local invasion and distant metastasis.
- **Clinical features.**
  - PSTTs and ETTs usually remain confined to the uterus and metastasize late. In some cases, recurrent or metastatic PSTT/ETTs can occur in patients long after initial treatment.
  - These tumors produce only small amounts of β-hCG, and hCG levels are typically low despite a large tumor burden. Serum hPL produced by the intermediate

trophoblasts that predominate serves as a better marker for disease progression or recurrence.

- Approximately 15% of lesions metastasize to extrauterine sites (e.g., lungs, liver, abdominal cavity, and brain). In contrast to other trophoblastic tumors, these tumors are relatively insensitive to chemotherapy, and surgical excision is usually the best treatment modality.
- **Pathologic features.**
  - By contrast to the normal implantation site where invasion of the extravillous intermediate trophoblast is tightly regulated and confined to the inner third of the myometrium, tumor cells of PSTT and ETT are invasive and infiltrate deeply into the myometrium.
  - Although PSTT and ETT share similar clinical features, careful examination of tumor histology and gene-expression patterns shows that PSTT and ETT are composed of different extravillous trophoblastic cells.
  - Gross lesions may be barely visible or may result in diffuse nodular enlargement of the myometrium. Most tumors are well circumscribed. Microscopically, invasion may extend to the uterine serosa and, in rare instances, extends to adnexal structures.

DIAGNOSIS AND MANAGEMENT OF MOLAR PREGNANCY

- The **pathologic diagnosis** of hydatidiform mole is typically made following dilation and curettage (D&C) performed for an incomplete abortion or because of suspicion of hydatidiform mole based on clinical findings.
  - The following tests should be performed preoperatively:
    - Quantitative serum β-hCG level
    - Complete blood count (CBC)
    - Prothrombin time, partial thromboplastin time
    - Comprehensive metabolic panel with renal and liver function tests
    - Blood type and screen
      - Rh-negative patients must be given $Rh_O(D)$ immune globulin (RhoGAM)
    - Chest radiograph
- The **primary treatment** for hydatidiform mole is suction D&C.
  - The following steps should be taken before suction D&C:
    - Stabilization of medical complications
    - Full operating room support in a hospital setting
    - Large-bore intravenous (IV) access with possible central line monitoring
    - Induction of regional or general anesthesia
    - Initiation of oxytocin drip (during D&C)
  - Uterine evacuation is accomplished with the largest cannula that can be safely introduced through the cervix. IV oxytocin is begun after the cervix is dilated and suction is initiated, and it is continued postoperatively for several hours.
- Post evacuation **follow-up** should include:
  - β-hCG level 48 hr after evacuation
  - Weekly β-hCG level until three consecutive negative results, then monthly until results are negative for 6 consecutive months (Fig. 46-1).
  - Regular pelvic examinations to monitor involution of pelvic organs and for detection of metastasis.
  - Repeat chest radiograph if the β-hCG titer plateaus or rises.
  - Effective contraception for the entire interval of β-hCG follow-up testing. Preventing pregnancy is crucial as a rising β-hCG titer due to a normal pregnancy cannot be distinguished from persistent GTD.

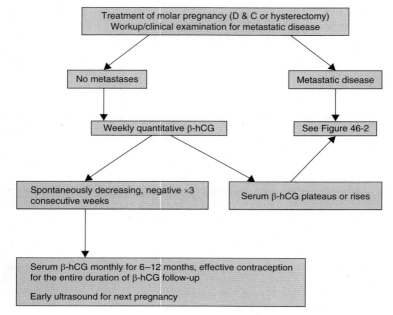

Figure 46-1. Follow-up of molar pregnancy. (Adapted from Diagnosis and treatment of gestational trophoblastic disease. ACOG Practice Bulletin Number 53. American College of Obstetricians and Gynecologists. *Obstet Gynecol* 2004;103:1365–1377.)

- Because of increased risk (1% to 2%) of a second mole in subsequent pregnancies, all future pregnancies should be evaluated by ultrasonography early in their course.
- **Complications** include anemia, infection, hyperthyroidism, pregnancy-induced hypertension or pre-eclampsia, and theca lutein cysts.

DIAGNOSIS AND MANAGEMENT OF PERSISTENT GTD

Persistent GTD includes invasive mole, choriocarcinoma, and PSTT. Persistent disease occurs in approximately 20% of cases of complete mole; approximately 15% develop invasive GTD and <5% develop metastatic GTD.
- Over 95% of malignant sequelae occur within 6 months after surgical evacuation. If β-hCG plateau or rise, immediate workup is required, and treatment for persistent GTD may be indicated.
- **Risk factors** for persistent GTD include large-for-dates uterus, ovarian enlargement due to theca lutein cysts, recurrent molar pregnancy, uterine subinvolution, advanced maternal age, significantly elevated β-hCG level, and acute pulmonary compromise. The risk of persistent GTD is considerably lower for partial moles than for complete moles.

Diagnosis of Persistent GTD

- A plateau or rise in β-hCG titers is typically the first indication of persistent GTD. Patients may also present with recurrent vaginal bleeding after D&C.
- Other presenting signs and symptoms are related to the anatomic sites involved with metastatic disease: chest pain, hemoptysis, or persistent cough with pulmonary

involvement; bleeding from vaginal extensions; and focal neurologic deficits from cerebral hemorrhage.

- Rarely, the diagnosis of persistent GTD is made via histologic evidence of choriocarcinoma. Given the risk of hemorrhage associated with biopsy, pathologic specimens are usually not obtained.
- **Criteria** for persistent GTD include
  - hCG level plateau of four measurements ±10% recorded over a 3-week duration (days 1, 7, 14, and 21)
  - hCG level increase of >10% for three measurements over a 2-week duration (days 1, 7, and 14)
  - Detectable hCG for >6 months after molar evacuation
  - Histological diagnosis of choriocarcinoma
- The diagnosis of persistent GTD is based on the quantitative pattern of serum β-hCG level, D&C findings, presence of metastatic disease, and histology. Both invasive mole and choriocarcinoma are typically detected by a plateau or elevation in the β-hCG titer. It may not be possible to distinguish clinically between these lesions.
  - Obtaining a tissue diagnosis is not necessary (because the treatment for both is the same) and may be associated with significant hemorrhage. PSTTs and ETTs typically demonstrate low β-hCG levels; however, serum hPL level is often elevated and may be a more useful serologic marker.
- All patients suspected of having persistent GTD should undergo the following workup to evaluate the extent of disease (Fig. 46-2):
  - Complete history and physical examination
  - Serum β-hCG level, possibly serum hPL level
  - Liver, thyroid, and renal function tests
  - CBC
  - Pelvic ultrasonography to evaluate for intrauterine pregnancy

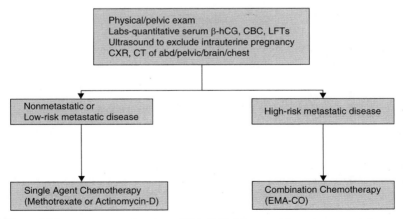

Figure 46-2. Management of persistent GTD. EMA-CO, etoposide, methotrexate, actinomycin D, cyclophosphamide (Cytoxan), and vincristine sulphate; LFT, liver function test; CXR, chest radiograph. (Adapted from Diagnosis and treatment of gestational trophoblastic disease. ACOG Practice Bulletin Number 53. American College of Obstetricians and Gynecologists. *Obstet Gynecol* 2004;103:1365–1377.)

- Chest radiograph
- CT of pelvis, abdomen, and brain
- Stool guaiac test

Treatment of Persistent GTD

- **Treatment** depends on the stage of disease (Table 46-2) and risk assessment based on the World Health Organization (WHO) prognostic scoring system (Table 46-3).

TABLE 46-2	FIGO Staging System for Gestational Trophoblastic Neoplasia
Stage	**Description**
I	Strictly confined to uterus
II	Extension outside uterus but limited to pelvic structures
III	Extension to lungs
IV	All other metastatic sites

Each stage is divided into high or low risk using the WHO Prognostic Scoring Index. From Current FIGO staging for cancer of the vagina, fallopian tube, ovary, and gestational trophoblastic neoplasia. *Int J Gynecol Obstet* 2009;105:3–4.

TABLE 46-3	FIGO/WHO Prognostic Scoring Index for Gestational Trophoblastic Neoplasia			
Score	**0**	**1**	**2**	**4**
Age	<40 yr	≥40 yr		
Antecedent pregnancy	Mole	Abortion	Term	
Time since pregnancy	<4 mo	4–6 mo	7–12 mo	>12 mo
Initial hCG levels (mIU/mL)	<1,000	1,000–9,999	10,000–99,999	≥100,000
Largest tumor size (in cm, including uterus)	<3	3–4	5 or more	
Site of metastases	Lung, vagina	Spleen, kidney	Gastrointestinal tract	Brain, liver
Number of metastases	0	1–4	5–8	>8
Prior failed chemotherapy	None		Single drug	≥2 drugs

The total score is obtained by adding the scores for individual prognostic factors. Scores from 0 to 6 are categorized as low risk, while a score of 7 or higher is high risk. Adapted from Kohorn EI. The new FIGO 2000 staging and risk factor scoring system for gestational trophoblastic disease: description and clinical assessment. *Int J Gynecol Cancer* 2001;11:73–77.

Nonmetastatic Disease and Low-Risk Metastatic Disease
- Disease falls into the category of low risk based on a WHO prognostic score ≤6 (Table 46-3).
- **Treatment** is with single-agent chemotherapy with either methotrexate (MTX) or actinomycin D is the recommended primary therapy.
  - MTX is alternated with folinic acid in most institutions and given with a fixed window of 7 to 14 days between courses. Some evidence suggests that dactinomycin may provide slightly higher remission rates than MTX but is associated with more toxicity. Pulsed dactinomycin generally is used more frequently than the 5-day regimen.
  - Systemic treatments are administered until hCG levels normalize for two or more consecutive assessments. An additional one to three cycles of consolidation chemotherapy can be given after a negative serum hCG is obtained.
  - If hCG titers plateau or rise after two courses, the patient is considered resistant to that particular chemotherapeutic agent, and the alternative single-agent chemotherapy is promptly instituted. If no response is seen after both single agents, then combination chemotherapy is required.
- For patients who have completed childbearing, hysterectomy should be considered for refractory disease confined to the uterus.
- Patients with nonmetastatic disease are less likely to require second-line therapy than patients with low-risk metastatic disease. Overall, 85% to 95% of patients can be cured with single-agent chemotherapy without hysterectomy. The cure rate for patients with low-risk disease approaches 100% with recurrence rates <5%.

High-risk Metastatic Disease
- Disease may be deemed high risk based on a WHO prognostic score ≥7 (Table 46-3).
- For patients with high-risk metastatic disease, the recommended **treatment** is combination chemotherapy with etoposide, MTX, actinomycin D, cyclophosphamide (Cytoxan), and vincristine sulfate (EMA-CO). Recurrent or refractory disease, particularly in cases of chemoresistant PSTT and ETT, may respond better to platinum-etoposide combinations such as EMA-EP.
  - Chemotherapy is given until negative hCG levels are achieved in 3 consecutive weeks or until intolerable side effects occur. After the normalization of hCG levels, an additional two courses should be given as consolidation therapy.
- For patients with **complications** of metastatic disease specific to the organ involved, the following interventions can be instituted:
  - **Vaginal involvement.** These lesions can bleed profusely. Bleeding can be controlled with packing for 24 hr. Prompt radiation to the affected region may provide further hemostasis. Although infrequently used, embolization of the pelvic vessels may also be implemented in women with life-threatening or recurrent hemorrhage.
  - **Pulmonary metastases.** These lesions usually respond to chemotherapy. Occasionally, thoracotomy is required to remove a persistent viable tumor nodule. Not all chest lesions clear radiographically due to scarring and fibrosis from the injury and healing process.
  - **Hepatic lesions.** If these lesions fail to respond to systemic chemotherapy, other options include hepatic arterial infusion of chemotherapy or partial hepatic resection to remove resistant tumor.

- **Cerebral metastases.** Whole-brain irradiation (approximately 3,000 cGy) is initiated as soon as the extent of disease is confirmed. Radiation and chemotherapy reduce the risk of spontaneous cerebral hemorrhage.
- **Extensive uterine disease.** Hysterectomy is indicated in cases with large intrauterine tumor burden, infection, or hemorrhage.
- Following EMA-CO, the overall remission rate is 80% to 90%. Approximately 25% of high-risk patients demonstrate incomplete responses to first-line therapy and relapse. When brain metastases are present, the overall remission rate drops to 50% to 60%. Higher failure rates are also seen with stage IV disease, greater than eight metastatic lesions, and a history of previous chemotherapy.
- For patients with refractory or recurrent disease after EMA-CO treatment, salvage therapies often consist of platinum etoposide combinations. Bleomycin and ifosfamide (VIP, ICE) have also been utilized with limited success. Experimental protocols may be investigated in these patients.

SUGGESTED READINGS

Berkowitz RS, Goldstein DP. Gestational trophoblastic disease in Berek JS, ed. *Berek & Novak's Gynecology*. 14th Ed. Philadelphia, PA: Lippincott Williams & Wilkins, 2007.

Schorge JO, Schaffer JI, Halvorson LM, eds. Gestational trophoblastic disease. In: *Williams Gynecology*. New York: McGraw-Hill, 2008.

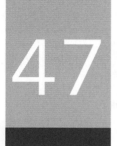

47 Chemotherapy and Radiation Therapy

Kimberly Levinson and Edward Trimble

Treatment of gynecologic cancer may involve one or more modalities of treatment, including surgery, **chemotherapy**, and **radiation therapy**. When more than one modality is used in a treatment regimen, they may be delivered sequentially or at the same time, as with chemoradiation or intra-operative radiation therapy.

- The sequence of treatment is delineated by adjectives such as "**primary**," referring to initial treatment; "**adjuvant**," referring to secondary treatment given to treat micrometastatic disease after primary therapy; "**neoadjuvant**," referring to induction chemotherapy, radiation therapy, or both given before definitive therapy; and "**salvage**," referring to treatment at time of recurrence. Recently, patient advocates have objected to use of the term "salvage," which they believe suggests that patients are objects that must be salvaged.

- All modalities used to treat gynecologic cancer can cause damage to normal tissue. The goal of cancer treatment is the removal or destruction of all viable cancer cells while limiting damage to normal tissues, as well as preserving health-related quality of life and normal function to the greatest extent possible. The governing principle of both chemotherapy and radiation therapy is to attain maximal therapeutic cytotoxic effects upon cancer cells without extreme toxicity to normal tissues. Unfortunately, it is not always possible to obtain a therapeutic effect without temporarily or, in some instances, permanently altering the functions of other healthy cells, tissues, organs, or systems.

- The term **therapeutic index** is the ratio of the toxic dose to the dose that is curative. The optimal treatment goal is to utilize chemotherapy agents and radiation prescriptions that have a high therapeutic index.

CELL CYCLE

The kinetic behavior of individual tumor cells has been well described, and a classic cell cycle model has been developed (Fig. 47-1). There are both **cell cycle–specific chemotherapeutic agents** and **cell cycle–nonspecific chemotherapeutic agents**.

- Cell cycle–specific agents depend on the proliferative capacity of the cell and on the phase of the cell cycle for their action. They are effective against tumors with relatively long S phases, and rapid proliferation rates.

- Cell cycle–nonspecific drugs kill cells in all phases of the cell cycle, and their effectiveness is not dependent on a tumor's proliferative capacity. Radiation therapy is not cell cycle dependent.

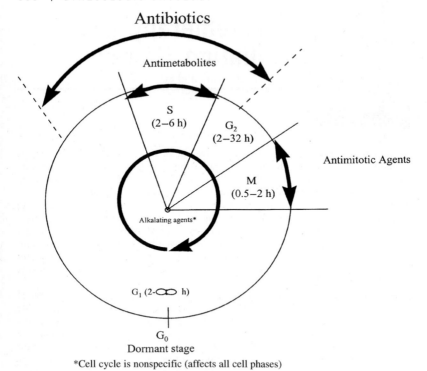

Figure 47-1. Phases of the cell cycle, relative time intervals, and sites of action of the various classes of antineoplastic agents. (From Trimble EL, Trimble CL. *Cancer Obstetrics and Gynecology*. Philadelphia: Lippincott Williams & Wilkins, 1999:60, with permission.)

CHEMOTHERAPY

Types of Chemotherapy

- Chemotherapeutic agents commonly used for the treatment of gynecologic cancer may be grouped into the following categories (Table 47-1):
  - **Alkylating agents** are cell cycle nonspecific. They contain an alkyl group that forms a covalent bond with the DNA helix, preventing DNA duplication. They also function by attaching to free guanine bases of DNA, thus preventing their action as templates for new DNA formation.
  - **Antimetabolites** are similar in chemical structure to compounds required by normal and tumor cells for cell division. These antimetabolites may be incorporated into new nuclear material or combined with enzymes to inhibit cell division.
  - **Plant alkaloids** are derived from various plants and trees, including the periwinkle plant (*Vinca rosea*), the may apple (*Podophylum peltatum*), and the Pacific yew

TABLE 47-1	**Chemotherapeutic Agents Frequently Used in Gynecologic Cancer and their Most Common Toxicities**

Chemotherapeutic Agent	Toxicity
Alkylating Agents	
Cyclophosphamide (Cytoxan)	Myelosuppression (WBCs > platelets), hemorrhagic cystitis, bladder fibrosis, alopecia, hepatitis, amenorrhea
Ifosfamide	Myelosuppression, hemorrhagic cystitis, CNS dysfunction, renal toxicity
	Myelosuppression (platelets > WBCs), nausea and vomiting, secondary malignancies (leukemia)
Alkylating-like Agents	
Cis-dichloro-diamino-platinum (Cisplatin)	Nephrotoxicity, nausea and vomiting, tinnitus and hearing loss, myelosuppression, peripheral neuropathy characterized by paresthesia of the extremities
	• Renal insufficiency is the major dose-limiting toxic effect causing elevations in BUN, serum creatinine, and serum uric acid levels within 2 wk of treatment. Irreversible renal damage can occur. Prevention with IV hydration and diuretics is important during treatment. 24-hr creatinine clearance is measured to establish baseline renal function before treatment
	• Tinnitus or high-frequency hearing loss may be observed and may be cumulative and possibly irreversible. Audiograms may be obtained before and during treatment to assess hearing loss.
Carboplatin	Less neuropathy, ototoxicity, and nephrotoxicity but more myelosuppression than cisplatin
Antitumor Antibiotics	
Actinomycin D (Dactinomycin)	Nausea and vomiting, skin necrosis, mucosal ulceration, myelosuppression
Bleomycin sulfate	Pulmonary toxicity, fever, anaphylactic reactions, dermatologic reactions
	• May cause significant *pulmonary fibrosis*, and careful attention should be given to the lung examination. Generally, this side effect is both dose and age related, but it can be idiopathic. Pulmonary function tests are performed to assess baseline pulmonary capacity

(Continued)

| TABLE 47-1 | Chemotherapeutic Agents Frequently Used in Gynecologic Cancer and their Most Common Toxicities (Continued) |

Chemotherapeutic Agent	Toxicity
Bleomycin sulfate (*continued*)	before the first dose is administered and are repeated as needed. • Can cause anaphylaxis, skin reactions, fever, and chills. Because of the high incidence of allergic reactions, patients are given a test dose of 2–4 U intramuscularly before the first dose of drug.
Doxorubicin hydrochloride (Adriamycin)	Myelosuppression, cardiac toxicity, alopecia, mucosal ulcerations, nausea and vomiting Irreversible cardiomyopathies that involve progressive congestive heart failure, pleural effusions, heart dilation, and venous congestion. These are generally cumulative; therefore, dosages are kept under the maximum. Multiple-gated acquisition (MUGA) scans are commonly obtained before treatment to obtain a baseline ejection fraction and may be repeated as necessary.
Liposomal doxorubicin (Doxil)	Myelosuppression, skin and mucosal toxicity, hand-foot syndrome
Antimetabolites	
5-FU	Myelosuppression, nausea and vomiting, anorexia, alopecia
Methotrexate sodium (MTX)	Myelosuppression, mucosal ulceration (stomatitis and mucositis), hepatotoxicity, acute pulmonary infiltrates that respond to steroid therapy
Gemcitabine hydrochloride (Gemzar)	Mild myelosuppression, flu-like syndrome
Plant Alkyloids	
Vincristine sulfate (Oncovin)	Neurotoxicity (peripheral, central, and visceral neuropathies that are cumulative), alopecia, myelosuppression, cranial nerve palsies
Epipodophyllotoxin (etoposide, VP-16)	Myelosuppression, alopecia, hypotension, allergic reaction
Paclitaxel (Taxol)	Myelosuppression, alopecia, allergic reactions, cardiac arrhythmias, neuropathies • Asymptomatic and transient bradycardia (40–60 beats a minute), ventricular tachycardia, and atypical chest pain during infusion. These symptoms resolve with slowing of infusion.

(Continued)

TABLE 47-1	Chemotherapeutic Agents Frequently Used in Gynecologic Cancer and their Most Common Toxicities (Continued)
Chemotherapeutic Agent	**Toxicity**
	• Hypersensitivity reactions with characteristic bradycardia, diaphoresis, hypotension, cutaneous flushing, and abdominal pain. Premedications of diphenhydramine hydrochloride, dexamethasone, and ranitidine are given prophylactically.
Docetaxel (Taxotere)	Myelosuppression, hypersensitivity; cutaneous reactions, alopecia
Miscellaneous	
Topotecan hydrochloride (Hycamptin; topoisomerase 1 inhibitor)	Myelosuppression

(*Taxus brevifolia*). They bind to tubules, which block microtubule formation and interfere with spindle formation. This leads to the arrest of metaphase and inhibits mitosis.

- **Antitumor antibiotics** have many different modes of action, including increasing cell membrane permeability, inhibiting DNA and RNA syntheses, and blocking DNA replication.
- **Miscellaneous agents** have different modes of action than those previously mentioned.

Common Side Effects of Chemotherapy

- **Myelosuppression** can be the most dangerous and life-threatening side effect of chemotherapy and varies in severity according to the drug administered. A nadir in white cell, red cell, or platelet count is usually observed 7 to 14 days after drug administration. Most agents are readministered every 3 to 4 weeks if the patient has recovered from myelosuppression. Pancytopenia is the major dose-limiting toxicity associated with chemotherapy treatment.
- **Neutropenia** causes susceptibility to bacterial infection. Recombinant human granulocyte colony–stimulating factor (**G-CSF**) (filgrastim, **Neupogen**) may be started after the onset of a febrile neutropenic episode and is often given prophylactically when the absolute neutrophil count (ANC) is <500/µL. In addition, G-CSF may be given prophylactically between chemotherapy cycles for patients at significant risk of severe neutropenia. Use of G-CSF is contraindicated during the actual administration of chemotherapy. Another G-CSF, pegylated filgrastim (**Neulasta**), can be administered within 24 to 72 hr after chemotherapy and may be re-dosed if the ANC remains below 10,000/µL.
- **Anemia** can be treated with **erythropoietin** (epoetin α [Epogen, Procrit]), which is administered SC. After 8 weeks of therapy, the dose may be increased if a rise in hemoglobin level of more than 1 g/dL has not been achieved. The target is a hemoglobin level of 12 g/dL or hematocrit of 36% to 40%.

- **Thrombocytopenia** is treated with platelet transfusion when the platelet count drops below 15 K to 20 K/µL, or if clinical signs of spontaneous bleeding are evident. **Thrombopoietin** (oprelvekin, Neumega) may also be given.
- **Infections** caused by organisms associated with granulocytopenic defects are more common in individuals receiving chemotherapy and may be more severe. Common causes of infection include enteric Gram-negative bacteria, Gram-positive bacteria (*Staphylococcus epidermidis*, *S. aureus*, and diphtheroids), viruses (herpes simplex and herpes zoster), and fungi (*Candida* and *Aspergillus* species). Infections are generally related to the severity and duration of the patient's neutropenia and to alterations in the integrity of the mucous membranes and skin. Fever in a neutropenic patient is sufficient evidence of occult infection to warrant initiation of empiric antibiotic therapy after blood and urine culture specimens have been obtained. The administration of broad-spectrum antibiotics is recommended.
- **Nausea and vomiting** are two of the most common and distressing side effects of chemotherapy. The severity and incidence of these symptoms vary greatly, but the inability to effectively control them can result in patient refusal to carry out potentially curative treatment. Nausea and vomiting can be
  - *acute*—occurring during or immediately after chemotherapy administration
  - *delayed*—occurring several days after chemotherapy administration
  - *anticipatory*—occurring before the administration of chemotherapy

  The incidence and severity are related to the emetogenic potential of the drug, the dose, the route and time of day of administration, patient characteristics, and the combination of drugs used. Emetogenic potential of commonly used chemotherapeutic agents is listed in Table 47-2. Gastrointestinal (GI) obstruction must be considered if abdominal distention or obstipation is present.
  - **Ondansetron hydrochloride** and **granisetron hydrochloride**, both serotonin 5-HT$_3$ receptor-blocking agents, have been shown to be particularly effective in reducing acute emesis from highly emetogenic drugs. For delayed emesis, prevention is critical; patients should therefore be encouraged to take antiemetics as prescribed for 3 to 4 days after receiving chemotherapy.
- **Diarrhea** may occur in association with chemotherapy and is most likely not infectious in origin.

TABLE 47-2	Emetogenic Potential of Commonly Used Chemotherapeutic Agents		
Very High (>90%)	**High (60%–90%)**	**Moderate (30%–60%)**	**Low (<30%)**
Cisplatin	Carboplatin	Etoposide	Bleomycin
Cyclophosphamide	Cyclophosphamide	Ifosfamide	sulfate
(high dose)	Dactinomycin	Topotecan	5-Fluorouracil
		hydrochloride	Methotrexate
			sodium
			Paclitaxel
			Vincristine
			sulfate

Percentage of patients experiencing nausea/vomiting without anti-emetics. Adapted from Hawks RG. Nausea. In Carroll WL, Finlay JL, eds. *Cancer in Children and Adolescents.* Sudbury, MA: Jones and Bartlett Publishers, 2010:533.

- **Dehydration** may occur following chemotherapeutic treatment. Patients are encouraged to increase their fluid intake to prevent postchemotherapy dehydration, with its risk of secondary side effects, such as nephrotoxicity or electrolyte disturbances.
- **Acute allergic reactions** may occur with the use of chemotherapeutic agents. For agents that may cause **anaphylaxis**, such as bleomycin, a test dose should be given prior to administration. For agents that cause **hypersensitivity**, such as paclitaxel, premedications of diphenhydramine hydrochloride, dexamethasone, and ranitidine are given prophylactically.
- **Hepatic side effects** including transient elevations in transaminase and alkaline phosphatase levels may occur with chemotherapy. Cholangitis, hepatic necrosis, and hepatic veno-occlusive disease, although rare, must be considered.
- **Stomatitis and mucositis** occur most commonly following therapy with antimetabolites. Treatment is with either **Larry's solution** (three equal parts diphenhydramine hydrochloride elixir [Benadryl], magnesia and alumina oral suspension [Maalox], and viscous lidocaine) or **nystatin**, swish and swallow. Severe cases may require hospitalization for enteral or parenteral nutrition, intravenous (IV) hydration, and pain management.
- **Neurologic side effects** of chemotherapy include damage to peripheral nerves as well as subtle changes in cognitive function, also known as "chemobrain." Peripheral nerve damage may range from transient paresthesias, such as "pins-and-needles" sensation, to chronic loss of sensitivity and fine motor control. Changes in cognitive function are generally perceived as difficulties with concentration and short-term memory. To date, there are no interventions proven to prevent or ameliorate this neurologic damage.
- **Fatigue** is commonly reported by patients undergoing chemotherapy. The mechanisms causing fatigue are not well understood; however, correction of anemia, good sleep hygiene, and regular exercise can all help reduce symptoms of fatigue.
- **Local and dermal side effects** include **alopecia** (which is reversible after treatment stops) and **photosensitivity**. In addition, administration of IV chemotherapy can cause **phlebitis**, and local infiltration or extravasation can lead to tissue necrosis. Extravasation may be treated with topical steroids, local injection of hyaluronidase, or sodium thiosulfate, depending on the specific drug involved.
- **Hemorrhagic cystitis** can occur with ifosfamide and cyclophosphamide treatment. Preventive measures include hydration and administration of diuretics. Treatment includes dosage reduction or discontinuation of the drug. **Mesna**, a uroprotector, is always administered simultaneously with ifosfamide to protect against bladder toxicity. Mesna acts to detoxify *acrolein*, the common metabolite of both cyclophosphamide and ifosfamide.

RADIATION THERAPY

Destruction of tumor and normal cells by x-rays or gamma rays relies on the conversion in tissues of photon energy into kinetic energy of electrons and the subsequent chemical changes within molecules. Permanent cell damage occurs with the creation of oxygen-free radicals and a multitude of other reactions resulting in DNA injury.

- The absorption of energy by tissue is measured in rads. One gray (Gy) = 100 rad and 1 centigray (cGy) = 1 rad. The **inverse square law** states that the dose of radiation at a given point is inversely proportional to the square of the distance from the source of radiation.

Clinical Radiation Sources

- **Teletherapy** is external-beam radiation. During external-beam radiation, the patient may be in either the prone or the supine position. The usual total dose to the pelvis ranges from 4,000 to 5,000 cGy, given in daily fractions of 180 to 200 cGy over 5 weeks.
- **Brachytherapy** involves placement of a radiation device either within or close to the target tumor volume (i.e., interstitial and intracavitary irradiation); the radiation dose to the tissue is determined largely by the inverse square law.
- The radiation applicators are called **intrauterine tandems** and **ovoids/colpostats**. Intrauterine tandems are placed in the uterine cavity while the patient is under anesthesia, and their position is confirmed with radiographic studies. Vaginal ovoids or colpostats are designed for placement in the vaginal vault and support the position of the tandem but they may also be loaded with radioactive sources themselves. Commonly, radiation doses for brachytherapy are reported as the total dose delivered to **point A** (defined as 2 cm above the lateral vaginal fornix and 2 cm lateral to the endocervical canal) and **point B** (3 cm lateral to point A).
- Vaginal, endometrial, and cervical cancers may be treated by either high- or low-dose-rate intracavitary implants. Replacing low-dose-rate (usually **cesium**) with high-dose-rate intracavitary brachytherapy treatments (usually **iridium-192**) is becoming increasingly common in the United States and Europe. Among the advantages of high-dose-rate applications are that placement does not require anesthesia or operating room time, and radiation exposure is 10 to 20 minutes for each outpatient visit (usually four to six visits are required), whereas use of low-dose-rate cesium implants requires hospitalization for 48 to 72 hr.
- **Interstitial implants** are another form of brachytherapy configured as radioactive wires or seeds and placed directly within tissues. Hollow guide needles are inserted in a geometric pattern to deliver a relatively uniform dose of radiation to a target tumor volume. After the position of the guide needles is confirmed radiologically, they can be threaded with the radioactive sources (loaded) and the hollow guides removed. Interstitial implants are sometimes used in the treatment of locally advanced cervical cancer, or for women with pelvic recurrences of endometrial or cervical cancer.

Common Side Effects of Radiation Therapy

- **Skin reaction** severity depends upon the total dose of radiation, dose fraction, treatment volume, and radiation energy. An acute skin reaction commonly becomes evident during the third week of therapy. The reaction is characterized by erythema, desquamation, and pruritus and should resolve completely within 3 weeks of the end of treatment. Topical corticosteroids or moisturizing creams may be applied several times a day for symptomatic palliation and to promote healing. If the skin reaction worsens, it may be necessary to stop treatment and apply zinc oxide or silver sulfadiazine to the affected area until it improves enough to continue treatment. The perineum is at greater risk for skin breakdown because of its increased warmth, moisture, and lack of ventilation. The patient should be taught to keep the perineal area clean and dry in an effort to prevent skin breakdown. In addition, late subcutaneous fibrosis can develop, especially with doses higher than 6,500 cGy.
- **Myelosuppression** is dependent upon the volume of marrow irradiated and the total radiation dose. In adults, 40% of active marrow is in the pelvis, 25% is in the vertebral column, and 20% is in the ribs and skull. Extensive radiation to these sites may result in the need for blood transfusions or administration of erythropoietin to support the patient's hematologic function during therapy.

- **GI effects** may be either acute or chronic. Nausea, vomiting, and diarrhea commonly occur 2 to 6 hr after abdominal or pelvic irradiation. The severity of the effect increases with the fraction size and treatment volume. Supportive therapy with hydration and administration of antiemetics and antidiarrheals such as Loperamide hydrochloride (Imodium) are generally used for first-line therapy. This may be followed by diphenoxylate hydrochloride (Lomotil) if necessary. If the patient is having severe diarrhea, opiates such as opium tincture, paregoric elixir, or codeine may be used to decrease peristalsis. Occasionally, a reduction in fraction size or a break in treatment is necessary to control the acute GI effects. Finally, octreotide acetate (Sandostatin) may be given to reduce the volume of persistent high-output diarrhea. Chronic diarrhea, obstruction caused by bowel adhesions, and fistula formation are serious complications of irradiation that occur in fewer than 1% of cases. Small bowel and rectovaginal fistulas can be caused by radiation effects or by recurrent disease. Fistulas are often associated with a foul odor, and good hygiene, charcoal-impregnated dressings, skin cleansers, and air deodorizers help to eliminate the odor. After recurrent disease is ruled out as a cause of the fistula, the patient may require a temporary or permanent colostomy to allow healing of the affected bowel.
- **Cystitis** is characterized by inflammation of the bladder, with associated symptoms of pain, urgency, hematuria, and urinary frequency. The bladder is relatively tolerant of radiation, but doses higher than 6,000 to 7,000 cGy over a 6- to 7-week period can result in cystitis. A diagnosis of radiation cystitis may be made after a normal urine culture result has been obtained. Hydration, frequent sitz baths, and, possibly, the use of antibiotics and antispasmodic agents may be necessary for treatment. **Hemorrhagic cystitis** may lead to symptomatic anemia that requires blood transfusions and hospitalization. Clot evacuation of the bladder with continuous bladder irrigation is often necessary. Bladder irrigation with 1% alum or 1% silver nitrate can alleviate bleeding. Persistent bleeding on continuous bladder irrigation or significant gross hematuria in the unstable patient requires immediate cystoscopic evaluation to localize and control the bleeding.
- **Vesicovaginal fistulas and ureteral strictures** are possible long-term complications of radiation therapy. Placement of nephrostomies, insertion of ureteral stents, and, less commonly, surgical intervention may be necessary.
- **Vulvovaginitis** occurs secondary to erythema, inflammation, mucosal atrophy, inelasticity, and ulceration of the vaginal tissue. Adhesions and stenosis of the vagina are common and can result in pain on pelvic examination and/or intercourse. Treatment involves vaginal dilation, either by frequent sexual intercourse or by the use of a vaginal dilator. Vaginal dilation should be performed at least two to three times per week for up to 2 years. In addition, the use of estrogen creams is useful in promoting epithelial regeneration. Infections, including candidiasis, trichomoniasis, and bacterial vaginosis, may be associated with radiation-induced vaginitis.
- **Fatigue** is often reported by women undergoing radiation therapy and may continue for several months after completion of therapy. As with chemotherapy-induced fatigue, correction of anemia, good sleep hygiene, and regular exercise can help decrease fatigue.
- **Constipation** is usually encountered with radiation in patients who have neurogenic GI atony resulting from chemotherapy with vinca alkaloids. In severe cases, ileus may ensue. Treatment includes hydration and administration of stool softeners (docusate sodium), laxatives (milk of magnesia), enemas, cathartics, and/or bulking agents.

OTHER ANTICANCER AGENTS

- **Monoclonal antibodies** are monospecific antibodies that bind to one biological substance. **Bevacizumab**, which is directed against vascular-endothelial growth factor, has demonstrated single-agent activity in ovarian cancer. It is currently undergoing phase III evaluation as part of primary therapy for epithelial ovarian cancer (EOC). Potential complications of monoclonal antibody therapy include allergic reactions, anaphylactic shock, generalized pain, hyponatremia, fever, rigors and chills, rash, paresthesias, weakness, chronic refractory postural hypotension, serum sickness, cytokine release syndrome, and tumor lysis syndrome.
- **Hormonal agents**, which have been studied extensively in gynecologic cancer, include **tamoxifen** (which has both antiestrogenic effects in breast tissue as well as estrogen-stimulatory effect in endometrial and myometrial tissues), **medroxyprogesterone acetate** (Provera), and progesterone-releasing intrauterine devices. These agents take advantage of the fact that both normal and well-differentiated neoplastic gynecologic tissues generally have both estrogen and progesterone receptors. These receptors are commonly lost as tumors become less well differentiated.

PRIMARY TREATMENT MODALITIES ACCORDING TO CANCER SITE

Epithelial Ovarian Cancer (EOC)

- Women with EOC need comprehensive surgical staging to confirm the diagnosis and guide treatment planning. Stage III and IV EOC requires effective surgical cytoreduction, preferably to no residual disease, either at time of initial surgery or after three to four cycles of neoadjuvant chemotherapy. Carcinoma of the fallopian tube and primary peritoneal carcinoma should be managed in the same way as epithelial ovarian carcinoma.
- Patients with stage IA and IB, grades 1 to 2 disease do not benefit from adjuvant chemotherapy. Patients with stage IC, all grades, and those with stage IA-B, grade 3, disease should receive three to six cycles of IV **platinum-based adjuvant chemotherapy**, which has been shown to improve both recurrence-free and overall survival.
- Patients with stages III to IV EOC should be treated with at least six cycles of platinum-taxane based chemotherapy. As mentioned above, neoadjuvant chemotherapy may also be considered for patients unfit for surgery at the time of presentation. Women with stage III EOC who have minimal or no residual disease after primary surgery should be considered for combined IV and intraperitoneal (IP) chemotherapy. In the most recent phase III trial, the combined IV/IP arm included both IV and IP paclitaxel, as well as IP cisplatin. The combined IV/IP regimens are associated with greater neurologic, metabolic, and hematologic toxicity than IV regimens. Nonetheless, the combined regimen is associated with a significant improvement in both progression-free survival and overall survival.
- EOCs, which persist or progress despite surgery and primary platinum-based chemotherapy are termed "platinum refractory." EOCs, which recur within 6 months of the last platinum-based treatment are termed "platinum resistant," while neoplasms that recur more than 6 months later than the last platinum-based treatment are considered "platinum sensitive." Drugs commonly used for the treatment of women with platinum-refractory or platinum-resistant disease include topotecan, liposomal doxorubicin, docetaxel, gemcitabine, weekly paclitaxel, and bevacizumab. Patients with platinum-sensitive disease are generally treated with a combination of platinum and another active agent.

Ovarian Germ Cell Cancers

- As with EOC, comprehensive surgical staging is critical for patients with ovarian germ-cell cancers. Young patients with stage I pure dysgerminoma and low-grade (grade 1) immature teratoma who wish to preserve fertility are adequately treated with unilateral salpingo-oophorectomy alone. All other patients with stage I to IV disease should undergo adjuvant chemotherapy with three courses of **bleomycin, etoposide, and cisplatin** after primary surgery. Postoperative radiation is an option for patients with dysgerminoma.

Cervical Cancer

- Surgery, chemotherapy, and radiation therapy may all play a role in the management of women with cervical cancer limited to the pelvis (stages IA to IVA). Treatment options for a woman with stage IA cervical cancer may include cervical conization, total hysterectomy, radical hysterectomy, or intracavitary radiation therapy. Treatment options for women with stage IB to IIA disease include radiation therapy, platinum-based chemoradiation, radical hysterectomy and bilateral pelvic lymphadenectomy, and neoadjuvant chemotherapy followed by radical hysterectomy. Treatment options for women with stage IIB to IVA disease include radiation, platinum-based chemoradiation, and neoadjuvant chemotherapy followed by radical hysterectomy.
- In general, the addition of concomitant platinum improves both progression-free and overall survival for women with cervical cancer who require radiation as part of their treatment. For women who cannot tolerate platinum, other chemosensitizing agents, such as 5-fluorouracil (5-FU), should be considered. It is important to note, however, that patients who undergo both surgery and radiation (or chemoradiation) for the treatment of their cervical cancer will experience more short- and long-term toxicity than those who are treated with one modality alone.
- Treatment for women with stage IVB disease should focus on symptom control as these patients are not cureable with currently available treatment options. Radiation may be used for palliation of central disease and/or distant metastases. Drugs with known activity include cisplatin, ifosfamide, paclitaxel, irinotecan, and the two-drug combinations of cisplatin with ifosfamide, paclitaxel, or gemcitabine. Women who experience a pelvic recurrence after primary surgery for cervical cancer should be considered for chemoradiation or pelvic exenteration, both of which have cure rates <50%. The same chemotherapeutic agents listed for women with stage IVB disease also may be considered for women with distant recurrent disease.

Vulvar Cancer

- The goals for treatment of vulvar cancer should include efforts to decrease the extent of surgery and preserve normal urinary, rectal, and sexual functions in addition to providing curative therapy. Early vulvar cancer may be treated with radical local excision, with bilateral inguinal and femoral node dissection as indicated. Locally advanced disease may be treated with either neoadjuvant chemoradiation followed by surgery or primary surgery followed by chemoradiation. The most active agents used in chemoradiation are **cisplatin** and **5-fluroruracil**. There is no effective chemotherapy yet identified for patients with distant metastatic vulvar cancer.

Vaginal Cancer

- Early vaginal cancer may be treated with either surgery or radiation (intracavitary with or without interstitial radiation). More advanced disease is generally treated with radiation alone or a combination of surgery and radiation. Platinum-based chemoradiation is also commonly used, in light of the data supporting the use of chemoradiation in cervical, vulvar, and rectal cancers.

Endometrioid Endometrial Carcinoma

- Endometrioid endometrial carcinomas are thought to arise in the hormonal milieu of estrogen excess relative to progesterone. Prolonged progesterone therapy has been shown to induce histologic regression of cancer in about 50% of women with well-differentiated endometrioid endometrial carcinoma confined to the endometrium. Hormonal therapy, therefore, may be a treatment option among young women who wish to preserve fertility, as well as among patients with multiple comorbidities for whom the operative risks of hysterectomy are considered too great.
- Hysterectomy and bilateral salpingo-oophorectomy are the standard of care for women with stage I disease and radical hysterectomy and bilateral salpingo-oophorectomy for women with stage II disease. Pelvic and para-aortic lymphadenectomy are also advocated to complete surgical staging. Pelvic radiation, whether vaginal cuff brachytherapy or external beam radiation, has been shown to improve local control but not to increase overall survival. Patients found to have metastatic disease at time of hysterectomy (stages III to IV) will benefit from radiation directed at sites of disease as well as systemic chemotherapy. The most active combination includes cisplatin, doxorubicin, and paclitaxel, with G-CSF support. The two-drug combination of carboplatin and paclitaxel is less toxic, although its equivalence in efficacy to the three-drug combination has not yet been established.
- Patients found to have endometrial cancer recurring in the pelvis may benefit from surgical resection and radiation. Patients with distant metastatic disease should receive the same combination chemotherapy as those with stage III to IV disease. The small subset of women with recurrent grade 1 disease may benefit from hormonal therapy.

Uterine Carcinosarcomas

- The primary treatment for uterine carcinosarcomas is total abdominal hysterectomy and bilateral salpingo-oophorectomy. Adjuvant pelvic radiation will reduce the risk of local recurrence but not improve overall survival. The benefit of adjuvant chemotherapy has not yet been established. Active single agents for patients with recurrent disease include ifosfamide, doxorubicin, paclitaxel, and cisplatin. The two-drug combination of ifosfamide and paclitaxel has been shown to be more effective than ifosfamide alone.

Uterine Leiomyosarcomas

- The primary treatment for leiomyosarcomas remains total abdominal hysterectomy and bilateral salpingo-oophorectomy. Adjuvant pelvic radiation will reduce the risk of local recurrence but not improve overall survival. The benefit of adjuvant chemotherapy has not yet been established. The most active agents for women with recurrent or metastatic disease include ifosfamide and doxorubicin.

Gestational Trophoblastic Tumors

- Hydatidiform mole is generally treated with cervical dilatation and uterine curettage, with chemotherapy reserved for those with persistent disease, as evidenced by serum HCG levels, which rise or plateau. Women with persistent disease are generally treated with a combination of methotrexate with leucovorin or single-agent dactinomycin. Women with recurrent gestational trophoblastic tumors (GTT) after primary chemotherapy are treated with a five-drug combination of etoposide, methotrexate, actinomycin-D, cyclophophamide, and vincristine (Oncovin). This combination is commonly abbreviated as **EMA-CO**. A more dose-intense regimen, EMA-CE, substitutes etoposide and cisplatin for vincristine and cyclophosphamide. Hysterectomy may be indicated for patients with disease that persists after multi-drug therapy. Surgical resection of persistent disease in metastatic sites may also be required. Women with recurrent GT metastatic to the brain should be treated with both whole brain radiation therapy and chemotherapy with ifosfmaide, carboplatin, and etoposide. Placental site trophoblastic tumors are not sensitive to chemotherapy; they should be treated with primary hysterectomy.

SUGGESTED READINGS

Baekelandt MM, Castiglione M. ESMO Guidelines Working Group. Endometrial carcinoma: ESMO recommendations for diagnosis, treatment and follow-up. *Ann Oncol* 2008;19(Suppl 2):ii19–ii20.

Byrd LM, Swindell R, Webber-Rookes D, et al. Endometrial adenocarcinoma: an analysis of treatment and outcome. *Oncol Rep* 2008;20:1221–1228.

Chemotherapy for Cervical Cancer Meta-Analysis Collaboration. Reducing uncertainties about the effects of chemoradiotherapy for cervical cancer: a systematic review and meta-analysis of individual patient data from 18 randomized trials. *J Clin Oncol* 2008;26:5802–5812.

Clinical management guidelines for obstetricians-gynecologists. Management of endometrial cancer. ACOG Practice Bulletin, Number 65. American College of Obstetricians and Gynecologists. *Obstet Gynecol* 2005;106(2):413–425.

Fiorelli JL, Herzog TJ, Wright JD. Current treatment strategies for endometrial cancer. *Expert Rev Anticancer Ther* 2008;8:1149–1157.

Gershenson DM. Management of ovarian germ cell tumors. *J Clin Oncol* 2007;25: 2938–2943.

Greer BE, Koh WJ, Abu-Rustum N, et al. Cervical cancer. *J Natl Compr Canc Netw* 2008;6(1):14–36.

Haie-Meder C, Morice P, Castiglione M, ESMO Guidelines Working Group. Cervical carcinoma: ESMO recommendations for diagnosis, treatment and follow-up. *Ann Oncol* 2008;19(Suppl 2):ii17–ii18.

Kyrgiou M, Salanti G, Pavlidis N, et al. Survival benefits with diverse chemotherapy regimens for ovarian cancer: meta-analysis of multiple treatments. *J Natl Cancer Inst* 2006;98: 1655–1663.

Morgan RJ Jr, Alvarez RD, Armstrong DK, et al. Ovarian cancer: clinical practice guidelines in oncology. *J Natl Compr Canc Netw* 2008;6:766–794.

Pectasides D, Kamposioras K, Papaxoinis G, et al. Chemotherapy for recurrent cervical cancer. *Cancer Treat Rev* 2008;34(7):603–613.

Reed NS. The management of uterine sarcomas. *Clin Oncol (R Coll Radiol)* 2008;20: 470–478.

Temkin SM, Fleming G. Current treatment of metastatic endometrial cancer. *Cancer Control* 2009;16:38–45.

Palliative Care

Kimberly Levinson, K. Joseph Hurt, and Sydney Dy

This chapter presents medical issues commonly encountered in **palliative care** and suggests management options for alleviating symptoms and supporting the patient and her family.

DEFINITION OF PALLIATIVE CARE

- **Definition and characteristics** of palliative care:
  - Care of patients with advanced disease that aims to alleviate symptoms and prevent suffering;
  - Focus is on quality of life;
  - Holistic in nature, addressing physical, social, and psychological aspects of care.
- Palliative care has a role in all medical treatments and should not be withheld during other treatments.
- Definition of **hospice**:
  - Both a mindset and an organization, focused on providing palliative care to patients;
  - Focuses on providing symptom control, psychosocial care, nursing support, bereavement support, and respite care at the end of life;
  - Depending on insurance coverage, the individual hospice organization, and patient needs and preferences, hospice can sometimes be provided together with chemotherapy, radiation, or other disease-modifying therapy;
  - Hospice provides support and care for both patients and families;
  - Often patients are enrolled very near death but can also benefit from earlier admission.
- Qualifications for hospice:
  - Projected life expectancy of 6 months or less
  - To receive Medicare hospice, the patient must select hospice over regular Medicare part A care.
    - Physician Medicare benefits are maintained, and patients can sign back on to Medicare whenever they wish.
    - The physician must certify that a patient has <6-month life expectancy assuming that the disease progresses as expected; there are no penalties for outliving the 6-month limit.
- In general, comfort and quality of life are the primary goals. A "do not resuscitate" (DNR) order is not necessary.

ETHICAL CONSIDERATIONS

Do Not Resuscitate/Do Not Intubate (DNR/DNI)

- DNR/DNI is often a difficult discussion that patients expect their doctors to initiate.
  - In general, the conversation should address the goals of treatment and the patient's priorities, including how much emphasis to place on prolongation of life versus

quality of life, specific issues such as DNR status, preferences for life-sustaining therapies, and goals for pain management.

- A patient can decide to be DNR/DNI but still pursue aggressive treatment; likewise, a patient can decide to pursue palliative treatment and still desire full resuscitation.
- Data show that resuscitation and intubation efforts in oncology patients are rarely successful.
- DNR/DNI discussion is urgently indicated if:
  - Death is imminent or the patient is otherwise at high risk for intubation or resuscitation (e.g., compromised pulmonary function);
  - The patient expresses a desire to die;
  - The patient or her family want to discuss hospice options;
  - The patient has been recently hospitalized for progressing illness;
  - Or the patient has significant suffering coupled with a poor prognosis.
- DNR/DNI preferences should be considered when addressing:
  - Prognosis;
  - Treatment options that have a low probability of success;
  - The patient's hopes and fears;
  - Any time the doctor anticipates that the patient is likely to die within 6 to 12 months.

Legal Considerations

- The patient's decision may not always be the same as that of her physician or family.
- The principle of autonomy is an important consideration in American medicine.
  - Living wills and DNR orders can ensure that patients' wishes are carried out.
  - Situations in which patients' surrogate decision makers may disagree with previously formulated advance directives are common.
    - Legally and ethically, a surrogate decision maker must clearly follow the advance directive formulated by a competent patient.
- Patients have the right to refuse or to withdraw care.
- Permitting death by not intervening is distinct from the action of killing.
- Physician-assisted suicide (i.e., a doctor provides a patient with the means to commit suicide with knowledge of the patient's intent) is legal only in Oregon and Washington states.
- Voluntary euthanasia (i.e., an intervention to end a patient's life with her consent) is illegal in all states.
- Difficulties can arise when patients and their families request treatments considered futile or inappropriate by their physicians.
  - No legal or societal consensus exists for situations in which patients and families disagree with physicians' recommendations to stop treatment.
  - Consultation with an ethics committee or palliative care can be helpful.
  - Excellent communication regarding educational, spiritual, and psychosocial needs can often resolve these conflicts.

PAIN MANAGEMENT

- One of the most common and frightening symptoms for patients with terminal illness.
- Pain should be addressed aggressively with multimodal therapy.
  - The World Health Organization (WHO) pain ladder provides guidelines for pain control escalation (Fig. 48-1).

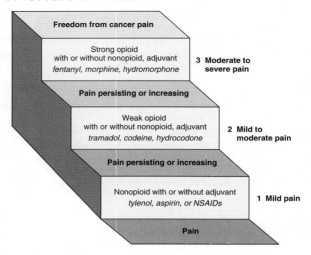

Figure 48-1. The WHO three-tier analgesia ladder depicts a rationale for escalating combination pain treatments as necessary to achieve pain control goals. Pain medications should be administered in order (nonopioids, then mild opioids like codeine, then strong opioids like morphine) until pain relief is achieved. Analgesics should be scheduled rather than given as needed. (Adapted from World Health Organization. *Cancer Pain Relief and Palliative Care: Report of a WHO Expert Committee.* Geneva: World Health Organization, 1990:7–21.)

- Adjuvants include medicines, interventions, and alternative/complementary approaches designed to reduce fear or relieve anxiety.
- Pain can be visceral, somatic, or neuropathic; many patients have multifactorial pain.

Pain Management

Nonsteroidal Anti-Inflammatory Drugs (NSAIDs)
- First step in the WHO pain treatment ladder.
- Can act synergistically with opioids.
- Should be given around the clock if pain is constant—twice daily options can aid in compliance.
- No NSAID has greater efficacy than another.
- Side effects include platelet inhibition (some nonsteroidals, such as trilisate, do not inhibit platelets), GI effects, and nephrotoxicity. These can be especially pronounced in older, frail patients.
- Often contraindicated in clinical trials or while receiving chemotherapy. GI prophylaxis usually indicated for long-term palliative use.
- Acetaminophen is often just as effective and may be safer in some situations

Opiates
- Second and third steps in the WHO ladder.
- Opioids can be considered first-line for terminal patients, especially those with severe pain.

TABLE 48-1	Opioid Analgesics: Equivalent Dosing for Various Narcotic Formulations			
Analgesic	Parenteral IM/IV Dose (mg)	Oral Dose (mg)	Half-life[a] (h)	Peak Effect[a] (hr)
Morphine	10	30	2–3	0.5–1
Hydromorphone	1.5	7.5	2–3	0.5–1
Meperidine	75	300	2–3	0.5–1
Fentanyl	0.1	Variable	3–12	0.1–0.25
Levorphanol	2	4	12–15	0.5–1
Oxycodone	NA	20	2–3	1
Codeine	130	200	2–3	1.5–2
Hydrocodone	NA	30	4–6	0.5–1
Methadone	10	20	12–190	0.5–1.5

Use rows to convert dosing route and columns to convert between medications. [a]Parenteral dosing except for oral only medications. NA, not available (oral only). Adapted from Barakat RR, Markman M, Randall ME. *Principles and Practice of Gynecologic Oncology*. Philadelphia, PA: Lippincott Williams & Wilkins, 2009:993.

- When pain is constant, escalate to round-the-clock dosing or longer acting narcotics with rescue doses as needed.
- There are various formulations and routes of administration:
  - Long acting options include morphine, oxycodone, and the fentanyl patch.
  - For patients unable to tolerate oral intake, intravenous medications and highly concentrated (20 mg:1 mL) sublingual morphine, oxycodone, fentanyl lollipop, lozenges, or patch may be helpful.
  - Meperidine (Demerol) should be avoided, especially in renal failure, because its metabolite can accumulate and cause seizures.
  - Partial agonist/antagonists (nalbuphine or buprenorphine) should be avoided because they can precipitate withdrawal.
  - Refer to dosing guidelines (see equianalgesic table, Table 48-1), as intravenous (IV) opioids are three times more potent than oral doses. Hydromorphone and fentanyl are much more potent than other opiates.

Severe Pain Crisis
- Treat with a rapid taper of a fast-acting IV narcotic, or with IV patient-controlled analgesia (PCA).
- Once acute pain is controlled, calculate the dose and convert to a long-acting form.

Side Effects
- To alleviate side effects: decrease the dose, change to a different narcotic, change the route, or simply treat the symptoms.
  - See below for treatment of nausea and vomiting.
  - Constipation is frequently a problem for patients on around-the-clock opioid. A bowel regimen should be prescribed; senna is often the first choice.
  - Sedation is common, although tolerance often develops.
  - Treat pruritus with Benadryl or low-dose nalbuphine or naloxone.

Adjuvant Treatment
- Used to supplement or synergize with other pain medications.
- Can be used to reduce narcotic dose and side effects.
- **Tricyclic antidepressants** are especially good for neuropathic pain.
  - Side effects are related to their anticholinergic properties: sedation, urinary retention, dry mouth, constipation, dysphoria, and blurred vision
  - Can cause cardiac conduction abnormalities and decrease seizure threshold.
- Other types of antidepressants (SSRIs) also have some evidence for efficacy. They are particularly helpful in patients with both depression and neuropathic pain.
- **Anticonvulsants** can be used for neuropathic pain.
  - **Carbamazepine** can be started at 100 mg po bid and titrated up rapidly.
    - Side effects include sedation, vertigo, hyponatremia, bone marrow suppression, and hepatotoxicity.
    - CBC and liver function tests should be followed.
  - **Phenytoin** can be loaded as 20 mg/kg or 1,000 mg (whichever is less) IV and then 100 mg tid.
    - Side effects include anemia, anorexia, nausea/vomiting, hepatotoxicity, ataxia, bone marrow suppression, hypersensitivity (fever, rash, hepatitis).
  - **Gabapentin/pregabelin** shows good efficacy in some randomized controlled trials for cancer; must be started at low dose and titrated slowly; sedation principal side effect.
- All adjuvants for neuropathic pain generally take weeks for efficacy. Acute pain should be treated with acetaminophen, NSAIDs, and/or opioids.
- Topical **lidocaine**—for sores or mucositis; lidocaine patch for herpes zoster.
- **Capsaicin** can be effective for neuropathic pain (especially Zoster) but may burn when applied. Mechanism of action is depletion of substance P.
- **Bisphosphonates** are useful to treat bone metastasis, breast pain, and possibly other cancers. They also prevent skeletal complications.
- Visceral crampy abdominal pain may be relieved by treating coexisting constipation or with anticholinergics such as **hyoscyamine**.

Nonmedical and Invasive Treatments
- About 30% of cancer patients will have inadequate pain control despite large doses of opiates or will have intolerable side effects at opiate doses that do control pain.
- **Radiation** may be useful for bone metastasis and bulk effects.
- **Chemotherapy** may be useful for tumor effects, such as bowel obstruction.
- **Anesthesia/neurosurgical procedures**
  - Myofascial injections may work for pain from localized muscle contractions.
    - Relief lasts from days to weeks.
  - Neurostimulation (implanted device) has an unclear mechanism of action.
    - Stimulation can be given to the spinal cord or thalamic nuclei.
    - Spinal cord stimulators—electrodes placed in the epidural space.
      - Very expensive and require patient involvement—not ideal for end of life.
  - Epidural or spinal PCA can decrease narcotic doses and reduce side effects.
  - Somatic nerve block works for pain localized to a single nerve, plexus, or dermatome.
    - A temporary injection is used to test for effectiveness.
    - A neurolytic block can then be used for longer relief.
    - The block can disrupt motor, sensory, or autonomic pathways.

- Sympathetic blocks can relieve visceral pain.
  - Do not cause somatosensory or motor dysfunction
  - A celiac plexus block can treat pain from the upper abdomen.
    - Performed under fluoroscopic or CT guidance.
    - Almost all patients have transient hypotension, diarrhea, back pain.
    - Other complications include unilateral paresis and retroperitoneal bleeding.
  - Superior hypogastric plexus blocks relieve pain from the pelvic viscera.
    - Seventy-nine percent of patients achieve pain relief with a low complication rate.
- **Surgery**
  - May be necessary for the most severe and persistent pain.
  - Vertebral body collapse and long bone fractures are treated best with prompt surgical intervention.
- **Psychotherapy support groups, cancer counseling, spiritual support**
  - Help patients deal with their diagnosis, decrease cognitive dissonance, and assist with coping skills.
  - Cognitive behavior techniques (progressive muscle relaxation, focused breathing, and meditation) require an alert patient but can be very helpful.
- Topical warm and cold treatments—few side effects.
  - Can provide relief for muscle pain
- Transcutaneous electrical nerve stimulation and acupuncture.
  - No proven effect in randomized trials but virtually no side effects.

END OF LIFE CARE: SYMPTOM MANAGEMENT

Respiratory Symptoms

Dyspnea
- **Dyspnea** is the sensation of uncomfortable breathing or shortness of breath.
- Differential diagnosis includes: pulmonary embolus, pleural effusion, anemia, lung metastasis, pneumonia, anxiety, and fatigue/weakness.
- Treatment of the underlying cause (e.g., with antibiotics, anticoagulation, blood transfusion, thoracentesis) can provide relief.
- Oxygen and opiates can also relieve the sensation and reduce fear and anxiety.
- Increase opiates about 25% above baseline, just as for escalating pain treatment, for comfort.
- Benzodiazepines, corticosteroids, and bronchodilators may be useful.

Gastrointestinal Symptoms

Anorexia/Cachexia
- Usually a symptom of, not the cause of, functional decline. May be a symptom of the dying process.
- **Anorexia** refers to decreased appetite.
- **Cachexia** implies wasting; seen in cancer patients at the end of life.
  - The pathophysiology of cachexia is not completely understood, but it appears to be related to decreased intake and increased cytokine levels.
  - Cachexia does not respond well to nutritional supplements.
- Force feeding often produces no weight gain and can increase patient discomfort and nausea.
- Treatment
  - Appetite stimulants can restore appetite briefly, but have multiple side effects and are not associated with improved survival.

- ○ Use when appetite is a significant quality of life issue and potential benefits outweigh side effects.
- Only two classes of drugs are well supported by multiple randomized trials:
  - ○ Dexamethasone 4 mg daily; side effects are those associated with chronic steroid use.
  - ○ Megace 400 to 800 mg daily; liquid and long-lasting forms are available. Also significant side effects.
- Artificial nutrition is indicated only for patients who are unable to eat (e.g., bowel obstruction) and have relatively good prognosis (3 months or greater). Also has substantial adverse effects.

Nausea/Vomiting
- May result from chemotherapy, opiates, or disease progression.
- The type of nausea may determine treatment strategy:
  - ○ *acute* (within 24 hr of a treatment or procedure)
  - ○ *delayed* (after 24 hr)
  - ○ *anticipatory* (a conditioned response after severe nausea and vomiting in the past).
- Treatment: Around-the-clock dosing with rescue and escalation regimens using drugs from different categories is often successful. Multiple receptor-signaling pathways in the area postrema have been suggested to mediate nausea and vomiting:
- **Anticholinergic** drugs act mainly on muscarinic receptors.
  - ○ Scopolamine 1.5 mg transdermally q72h.
  - ○ Side effects include dry mouth, drowsiness, and visual changes.
- **Antihistamines** have sedation as their greatest side effect.
  - ○ Diphenhydramine (Benadryl) 25 to 50 mg po q6h or 10 to 50 IV.
  - ○ Dimenhydrinate (Dramamine) 50 mg po q4h.
  - ○ Cyclizine (Marezine) 50 mg po/IM q4 or 100 PR q4h.
  - ○ Meclizine (Antivert) 25 to 50 mg po qd.
  - ○ Promethazine (Phenergan) 12.5 to 25 mg po/IM q4h or PR q12h.
- **Dopamine receptor antagonists**
  - ○ Phenothiazines may lead to extrapyramidal reactions which can be treated with diphenhydramine.
  - ○ Prochlorperazine (Compazine) 5 to 10 mg po q6h or 2.5 to 10 IM/IV q3h or 25 mg PR q12h.
  - ○ Chlorpromazine (Thorazine).
  - ○ Haloperidol (Haldol).
  - ○ Side effects include akathisia, dystonia, and tardive dyskinesia.
  - ○ Metoclopramide (5 to 10 mg po/IV/IM q6h) is a modest antiemetic and increases gastric emptying.
- **Serotonin antagonists** are highly efficacious but very expensive. Side effects are mild, including headache and constipation. Granisetron, dolasetron, and palonosetron are in this category and have equivalent efficacy.
- **Neurokinin receptor antagonists** are a newer option.
  - ○ Aprepitant is approved for short-term use only, with highly emetogenic chemotherapy.
- Other antiemetics have unclear mechanisms of action.
  - ○ Corticosteroids are especially effective for chemotherapy-induced nausea.
  - ○ Cannabinoids have modest antiemetic effects.
    - – Dronabinol 5 to 10 mg po q6h is the legal prescribable form.

○ Benzodiazepines are weak antiemetics but are very good at treating anxiety, which can contribute to nausea.

○ Small studies have shown that acupuncture has some antiemetic effects.

• Prophylaxis
  • The appropriate method depends on the emetogenic property of the chemotherapy.
  • If severe nausea has occurred with a particular regimen, treatment should be escalated.
  • Agents with very low emetogenic risk usually require no prophylaxis.
  • Low-risk regimens: dexamethasone 20 mg IV or prochlorperazine 10 mg po once before chemotherapy.
  • Moderate- to high-risk regimens: serotonin antagonist, such as ondansetron (oral dosing equivalent to IV) plus dexamethasone 8 mg IV prior to chemo, followed by dexamethasone 4 to 8 mg po bid × 2 more days to prevent delayed nausea.
  • Extremely high-risk chemotherapy (especially cisplatin): serotonin antagonist plus dexamethasone 8 mg IV plus aprepitant 125 mg po prior to chemo, followed by dexamethasone 8 mg po qd × 3 days and aprepitant 80 mg po qd × 2 days.
  • Anticipatory nausea can be treated with alprazolam 0.5 to 2 mg prn.

Ascites
• A frequent problem in late-stage ovarian cancer.
• Not many treatment options are available.
  • High-dose spironolactone has shown some benefit in small trials.
  • Therapeutic large volume paracentesis can be performed for acute relief:
    ○ Mean duration of relief is only 10 days.
    ○ Large volume drainage leads to hypovolemia.
    ○ Repetitive taps increase the risk of infection.
    ○ If more than 5 L are drained, albumin can be given.
  • Permanent catheters (PleurX) are available and may reduce infection risk; patients can drain ascites at home.

Bowel Obstruction
• Bowel obstruction is frequent in ovarian cancer patients.
• **Small bowel obstruction (SBO)**
  • Usually managed conservatively with bowel rest and decompression (i.e., nasogastric tube) unless bowel ischemia or strangulation is present.
  • Further intervention depends upon the clinical situation.
    ○ Surgery should not occur routinely in patients with very poor prognosis (e.g., massive ascites, multiple sites of obstruction, diffuse carcinomatosis, or poor performance status).
    ○ Obstruction can be relieved by surgery, but perioperative morbidity and mortality are high. Reobstruction is common.
  • A percutaneous gastrostomy tube can be placed for venting.
  • Hyoscyamine or octreotide (0.3 to 0.6 mg SQ) decreases gastric secretion and slows intestinal motility, thereby decreasing the nausea/vomiting associated with (SBO). This is supported by several randomized trials.
• **Colonic obstruction**
  • Less frequent than SBO.
  • Surgical correction is indicated.
  • Endoscopic stents may work for palliative treatment.

- **Acute colonic pseudo-obstruction**
  - Mimics anatomic obstruction which must be ruled out by imaging.
  - Follow with serial abdominal exams and daily x-rays.
  - Supportive care with bowel rest is often enough to reverse the pseudo-obstruction.
  - Low magnesium, calcium, and potassium should be replaced.
  - Neostigmine 2 mg IV × 1 can be used; however, some patients experience bradycardia and should be monitored in an intensive care setting, with atropine available.
  - Endoscopic decompression with placement of a rectal tube may be attempted if neostigmine fails, if evidence of decompensation exists, or if the bowel diameter is >13 cm.
  - Surgery should be attempted if the above measures fail.

Constipation

- **Constipation** is common for patients on opiates. Both prophylaxis and treatment are indicated.
- Treatment regimens should incorporate multiple mechanisms of action.
  - Fiber and bulk-forming laxatives are usually contraindicated for palliative care.
  - Hyperosmolar laxatives draw water into the stool (polyethylene glycol 240 to 720 mL a day; lactulose 15 to 30 mL bid; sorbitol 120 mL of 25% solution daily; and glycerine 3 g PR daily or 5 to 15 mL enemas).
  - Saline laxatives are also hyperosmolar (magnesium sulfate 15 g daily, magnesium citrate 200 mL daily).
  - Stool softeners are usually ineffective when used alone (docusate sodium 100 mg po bid, mineral oil 15 to 45 mL a day).
  - Stimulants increase bowel motility (bisacodyl 30 mg po qd or 10 mg PR qd and senna 1 to 4 tsp qd).
- Fecal impaction should be treated aggressively.
  - Can be extremely painful and even lead to mental status changes.
  - Mechanical disimpaction is required, followed by enemas. Colonic cleanout with polyethylene glycol is important, and aggressive bowel therapy should be started to prevent a recurrence.

Constitutional Symptoms

Fatigue

- The pathophysiology of **fatigue** from cancer is unclear.
- Can significantly decrease quality of life.
- Differential diagnosis includes anemia, chronic stress reaction, inflammation/immune reaction, disrupted circadian rhythm or sleep disturbance, hormonal changes, depression, and direct CNS toxicity.
  - Evaluation of reversible causes should be initiated.
- Workup includes evaluation of disease progression, medication effects and interactions, hematocrit, electrolytes, pain assessment, depression risk, and medical comorbidities.
- At the end of life, reassurance for the family may be the most appropriate step.
- Treatments:
  - Severe anemia may be treated with red cell transfusion, erythropoietin injection, iron, folic acid, and vitamin B_{12} supplementation.
  - Moderate exercise may reduce fatigue and improve functional status in healthier patients. Energy conservation (including limiting/scheduling activities) is more appropriate in patients with more advanced illness.

- Sleep hygiene and cognitive-behavioral therapy can increase the effectiveness of sleep.
- Psychostimulant use is not well supported (methylphenidate 5 mg po every morning and noon to start; modafinil, a nonamphetamine activating agent, 100 to 200 mg every morning and at noon can be used in some situations).
- Antidepressants may decrease fatigue associated with depression. Nortriptyline has sedative properties but can be useful for insomnia and poor sleep hygiene contributing to fatigue; alternatively, bupropion is more activating.

Neurologic Symptoms

Insomnia
- Often alleviated by treating underlying pain, anxiety, depression, or by addressing psychosocial/spiritual issues. Consider delirium in the diagnosis.
- When initial treatment is ineffective, a hypnotic agent can be used short term.
- In patients already on hypnotics, reduced dosing may restore normal sleep patterns.
- Sleep hygiene is often helpful.

Delirium/Agitation
- Mental status changes can be very distressing for families and can complicate home care.
- Workup depends on the patient's status and preferences.
- The mnemonic delirium can be helpful:
D: drugs (e.g., anticholinergics, ranitidine, lorazepam, opiates)
E: electrolytes, emotions (e.g., hyponatremia, hypophosphatemia, hyperammonemia)
L: low O_2, lack of drugs (e.g., pneumonia, pulmonary embolus, withdrawal)
I: ictal (e.g., stroke, brain metastases, seizure disorder)
R: retention (e.g., of CO_2, urine, or stool)
I: ischemia, infection (e.g., TIA, stroke, meningitis, urosepsis, pneumonia)
U: uremia (e.g., renal failure)
M: myocardial (e.g., infarction, arrhythmia, heart failure)
- Rapid sedation with haloperidol 0.5 to 1 mg IV/po/sq, repeated as needed and coupled with lorazepam 0.5 to 1 mg po/IV q1 to 2h may be helpful.

Symptoms from Distant Metastases

Bone Metastases
- Can be very painful and lead to pathologic fractures.
- Localized radiation provides pain relief in 35% to 100% of patients but has toxicity including mucositis, enteritis, dermatitis, and bone marrow suppression.
- Can often be relieved with single treatment (well supported by randomized trials) but may take several weeks for full efficacy.
- Hemibody radiation can be used for diffuse metastasis but has complications including radiation pneumonitis.
- Surgical fixation is appropriate for fractures and some impending fractures.
- Bisphosphonates decrease the rate of skeletal complications in breast cancer, but their role in the treatment of bone pain and in other cancers is less clear.
- Consider NSAIDs and steroids.
- Calcitonin has not been shown to relieve bone pain from metastasis.

Brain Metastases
- Initial presentation may be seizures, nausea/vomiting, persistent headache, neurologic symptoms, or cognitive/personality changes.
- MRI is usually necessary for diagnosis.
- Symptomatic patients receive dexamethasone 10 mg then 4 mg po every 6 hr.
  - Response is usually within 24 to 72 hr.
  - Patients are at risk for opportunistic infections. Start Bactrim prophylaxis for PCP.
  - Protein pump inhibitor prophylaxis is appropriate.
- Wean steroids to lowest effective dose.
- Prophylactic seizure medication is not required, but treatment is necessary if seizure persist.
- Radiation can reduce symptoms and improve survival, depending on patient prognosis.

Spinal Metastases
- Cause bone pain, cord compression, fractures, leptomeningeal metastasis, malignant plexopathy.
- Epidural spinal cord compression requires rapid diagnosis and treatment to avoid permanent paralysis.
  - Presentation is pain progressing to weakness and hyperreflexia, followed by bowel and bladder dysfunction and paralysis.
  - An MRI should be obtained on all cancer patients with new or worsening back pain.
- Treatment:
  - Steroids relieve pain and decrease the rate of neurologic complications.
    - Low-dose regimen: 10 mg load then 16 mg a day tapered over 2 weeks.
    - High-dose regimen: 100 mg IV load then 24 mg tid for 3 days, tapered over 10 days. There are significant side effects with this dosing regimen.
- Spinal cord compression requires urgent radiation treatment or surgical decompression.
  - Radiation treats pain and stabilizes neurologic function.
  - Eighty to one hundred percent of patients who are walking at the time of radiation will retain function; patients who have lost function are unlikely to regain it.

Other Considerations

Hydration
- The decision to begin or continue hydration can be difficult at the end of life; treatment should be formulated in consultation with the patient and her family.
- There is no evidence that hydration improves patient comfort.
- Dry mouth is best treated with mouth swabs.
- May prolong death process, increase secretions and edema. IV access may be difficult.
- May decrease electrolyte-induced delirium.

Palliative Sedation
- Rarely used except for extreme symptom control.
- Use of benzodiazepines or phenobarbital at end of life should be discussed.
- Palliative care consultation may be helpful before initiating heavy sedation.

Death Rattle
- The course rasps at the end of life are sometimes described as a "death rattle."
- A scopolamine patch can help decrease these distressing sounds.

Depression
- Adjustment reaction to a terminal diagnosis is expected; however, depression should be formally evaluated and treated when diagnosed.
- Counseling and cognitive-behavioral therapy are useful adjuncts.
- All antidepressants have side effects, which should be considered in the choice of treatment.
  - Tricyclic antidepressants are sedating and have anticholinergic effects (e.g., dry mouth, constipation, urinary retention)
  - Selective serotonin reuptake inhibitors (SSRIs) are less sedating and less anticholinergic than tricyclics.
  - Bupropion can lower seizure threshold.

Anxiety
- Benzodiazepines are the mainstay of acute treatment.
  - Short acting: Alprazolam 0.25 to 1 mg po tid or qid; lorazepam 0.5 to 2 mg po/IV/IM q3 to 6h.
  - Longer acting: Clonazepam 1 to 2 mg po bid; diazepam 2.5 to 10 mg po/IV/IM q3 to 6h.
- Many antidepressants, especially SSRIs, also have anxiolytic effects.
- Neuroleptics may be used if benzodiazepines are ineffective: thioridazine 10 to 25 mg po tid; haloperidol 0.5 to 5 po/IV/sq q2 to 12h.
- Other options include methotrimeprazine 10 to 20 mg IM/IV/sq q4 to 8h and chlorpromazine 12.5 to 50 mg po/IM/IV q4 to 12h. These are more sedating but are also analgesic.
- Atypical antipsychotics:
  - Olanzapine 2.5 to 10 po qd and risperidone 0.5 to 4 po qd may be useful in frail, older patients.
  - Buspirone 10 po tid may be used for chronic anxiety; takes 5 to 10 days to see any effect.

Spiritual/Existential Issues
- Concerns about maintaining personal dignity, lack of closure in relationships, inability to discern meaning in life, and spiritual crisis are often very distressing to patients.
- Counseling and early involvement of a spiritual counselor can often give comfort.

SUGGESTED READINGS

Chase DM, Monk BJ, Wenzel LB, et al. Supportive Care for women with gynecologic cancers. *Expert Rev Anticancer Ther* 2008;8(2):227–241.

Doyle D, Woodruff R. *The IAHPC Manual of Palliative Care*. 2nd Ed. Houston: The International Association for Hospice and Palliative Care: Promoting Hospice and Palliative Care Worldwide, IAHPC Press.

Grant M, Elk R, Ferrell B, et al. Current status of palliative care clinical implementation, education, and research. *Cancer J Clin* 2009;59:327–335.

Sepulveda C, Marlin A, Yoshida T, et al. Palliative care: The World Health Organization's Global Perspective. *J Pain and Symptom Manage* 2002;24(2):91–96.

Index

Page numbers followed by f indicate a figure; page numbers followed by t indicate a table

E